W0043459

European Archives of

Oto-Rhino-Laryngology

Official Journal of the European Federation
of Oto-Rhino-Laryngological Societies (EUFOS)

Affiliated with the German Society for
Oto-Rhino-Laryngology – Head and Neck Surgery

Supplement

**Proceedings of the
VIIth International Symposium
on the Facial Nerve
Cologne, June 9–14, 1992**

Editor:
E. R. Stennert

Co-Editors:
G. W. Kreutzberg
O. Michel
M. Jungehülsing

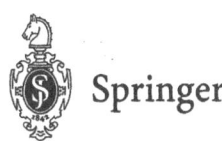

Springer

E. R. Stennert (Editor)

G. W. Kreutzberg · O. Michel
M. Jungehülsing (Co-Editors)

The Facial Nerve

An Update on Clinical
and Basic Neuroscience Research

Springer-Verlag

Berlin Heidelberg New York
London Paris Tokyo
Hong Kong Barcelona Budapest

E. R. Stennert

Universität zu Köln
Klinik und Poliklinik
für Hals-, Nasen- und Ohrenheilkunde
Joseph-Stelzmann-Str. 9
D-50924 Köln, Germany

G. W. Kreutzberg

Max-Planck-Institut
für Psychiatrie und Neuromorphologie
Am Klopferspitz 18 a
D-82152 Martinsried, Germany

O. Michel

Ltd. Oberarzt
Klinik und Poliklinik
für Hals-, Nasen- und Ohrenheilkunde
Joseph-Stelzmannstr. 9
D-50924 Köln, Germany

M. Jungehülsing

Wiss. Mitarbeiter
Klinik und Poliklinik
für Hals-, Nasen- und Ohrenheilkunde
Joseph-Stelzmann-Str. 9
D-50924 Köln, Germany

ISBN-13:978-3-540-57686-0   e-ISBN-13:978-3-642-85090-5
DOI: 10.1007/978-3-642-85090-5

Production: PRODUserv Springer Produktions-Gesellschaft, Berlin
Typesetting: Fotosatz-Service Köhler OHG, Würzburg

SPIN 10426711   25/3020-5 4 3 2 1 0-Printed on acid-free paper.

Honor Lecture for Professor John J. Conley

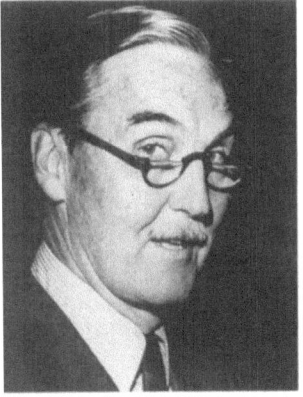

Distinguished guests, dear friends, I am glad that you have come here to join me in welcoming Dr. and Mrs. Conley to our meeting. We are here to honor Dr. Conley. What are the reasons for people to honor somebody? What is their motivation? First, they feel that the person who will be honored has qualifications superior to others. The high professional qualifications of our guest of honor do not need any documentation. Nevertheless, it is stimulating to focus our attention on his curriculum vitae. These are no more than highlights, just a collection of some fascinating items, forming a brilliant mosaic upon which we can reflect.

John Conley was borne June, 1, 1912, in Carnegie, Pennsylvania, and thus celebrated his 80th birthday just a few days ago. He received his undergraduate and graduate degrees at the University of Pittsburg. He became resident in Internal Medicine, and in Otolaryngology and Endoscopy at Kings County Hospital in Brooklyn, New York. During his military service from 1941 to 1945 at Tilton General Hospital he not only rose to Chief of the Sections of Ear Nose and Throat, Endoscopy, General Plastic Surgery and Maxillo-Facial Surgery, but also to Chief of the Neurosurgical Section, Ward Officer in General Surgery, and as an early signal for one of his later passions, painting, Chief of the Photographics Laboratories. This early phase of his career ended with an honorable discharge from the military with the rank of major at the end of the Second World War.

During that time, he was already in the process of creating a meritorious professional and academic career. He bacame Professor of Otolaryngology at Columbia University in New York, Attending Otolaryngologist at Columbia Presbyterian Medical Center, Chief of the Head and Neck Service at St. Vincent's Medical Center, Director of the Head and Neck Department of the Pack Medical Foundation and Consultant at the Manhattan Eye, Ear and Throat Hospital. He has been member of 12 professional societies. He was elected President of the American Academy of Ophthalmology and Otolaryngology, the American Society of Head and Neck Surgery and the American Academy of Facial Plastic and Reconstructive Surgery. He has been invited to give honorary lectures more than 20 times during his academic life. He has been distinguished by nine awards, including the "Distinguished Philantropist Award" of the American College of Surgeons. Last but not least, in 1980 he received an Honorary Doctorate from the University of Göttingen.

Ladys and Gentlemen, as you see, John Conley's professional qualifications are self-evident. These are good reasons to honor him.

However, I want amplify my introductory questions: What is *our motivation* for honoring him this evening? Dr. Conley, your contributions to our profession are our motivation for honoring you! Yesterday evening, you told me that you consider your major contribution to have been the introduction of new operative techniques – arising from the evolution of plastic surgery in the course of treating the wounds of our cancer patients.

John Conley's research comprises the development of new operative techniques for the rehabilitation of the larynx, the improvement of speech after laryngology, mandibular reconstruction, the development of regional and myocutaneous flaps for rehabilitation in the head and neck, the treatment of many forms of cancers of the head and neck area, especially melanomas and adenoid cystic carcinomas. His work also includes the development of new techniques of facial nerve grafting and the application of hypoglossal-facial nerve anastomoses with or without masseter muscle transfer. This immensely innovative work is contained in more than 280 original papers, in 11 published monographs and in 16 chapters in books. Dr. Conley's first publication concerning new techniques of facial nerve grafting in the treatment of parotid gland tumors was published in 1955. From that moment, and that means throughout all our Facial Nerve Symposia, John Conley has been one of the leading protagonists of this International Symposium and a model for other scientists: powerful, creative and stimulating. We all have to thank him for his impetus.

From the very beginning, Dr. Conley has been very stimulating especially with respect to surgical problems of the VII cranial nerve. Dr. Conley has that undefinable "something" which is not easy to describe. It is part of his character and it is a determining factor of his personality: His statements and comments are always balanced, obvious, fair and serious. He has never needed to criticize others to prove his own value and has never used arrogance or presumtion in proving a point. This part of his character, in combination with his qualification as a surgeon and clinical scientist, have made him a true authority.

Dear Dr. Conley, I remember the exact moment when we first met. It was in 1976 during the Third International Facial Nerve Symposium in Zurich. Somebody had presented a paper and you commented on it. I was immediately impressed by what I would term "your charisma". So I asked my neighbor: "Who is this man?" and he answered: "It's the famous John Conley, ...*Sir* John." In my opinion this is another reason why we must thank you. You demonstrated to us the quiet use of culture with authority in scientific discussion. I am sorry that I can only honor, but not ennoble you as "Sir John Conley".

Before I come to a last reason for being grateful to you, I feel that it would be necessary to modify once more the initial question: What is *my personal motivation* for honoring you?

In 1958 you invited my teacher Professor Miehlke to visit you in New York. In your very frank, open and generous manner you instructed him in all aspects and skills you had gained in the field of facial nerve surgery. Again you were the one who became the inspirator for the establishment of the "Miehlke-School" of facial nerve surgery, which disseminated your knowledge not only in Germany but in the whole of Europe. It was your personal influence that encouraged your friend and pupil Professor Miehlke, which had three main consequences. First, the early visible result of your influence on the academic life in the ENT Department of the University in Göttingen was the publication of Miehlke's book "Facial Nerve Surgery". Second, at the time when the final preparation for the second edition of this monograph was being prepared, I started my training in this department. My new boss Professor Miehlke directed me to help with the manuscript. So, your heritage has personally influenced my academic life from the very beginning. In other words, your are the spiritureal mentor of the "Miehlke School" and I feel like one of your grandsons. Third, this grandson has meanwhile been elected chairmen of the ENT Department of the University of Cologne. As a consequence, it is also your impact and influence that has brought us all together to carry out the *VII International Symposium on the Facial Nerve* here in Cologne.

Before I come to the end of my speech, I would like to add a few other remarkable pieces to the mosaic of John Conley's attributes. Eleven years ago, in June, 1981, I had the privilege of visiting him in New York and accompanying him during his daily work for 5 weeks. I was deeply impressed by the fascinating facility and the elegance of his surgery. I often thought that he could bring to a perfect end the most difficult operation even if there were an electrical failure in the operation theater were. I was equally impressed by his most sensitive way of handling patients, who seemed to lose every fear, even if they suffered from a life-threatening cancer. I was, moreover, impressed by his permanent search for new experiences, free from any from of prejudice. For example, he once called me to see a lady who needed resection tumor huge. He had already prepared different skin flaps for the reconstruction of her face, and of course there was no better expert in the world to solve this difficult task. Nevertheless, he asked me, an unknown youngster, about my ideas concerning the reconstructive strategy. This behavior was the result of his permanent and everlasting curiousity to learn from someone else if there might be a new idea or approach, not yet known to him. On another occasion he told me: "It is not our job to criticize others, it is our task to listen and to learn".

Yes, Dr. Conley, you are right: Although we have alreaedy learned so much from you, we would all like to gon on listening to you! Distinguished guests, dear friends, to complete the exceptional mosaic of Professor Conley, I finally have to mention that he is not only a brilliant surgeon, wonderful doctor, and a most effective clinical researcher and scientist, but also an extremely creative and successful painter and poet.

E. R. Stennert

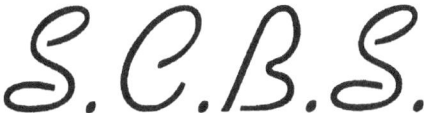

The Sir Charles Bell Society

The Sir Charles Bell Society (S.C.B.S) was founded in 1992 during the VIIth International Symposium on the Facial Nerve (President: Professor E. Stennert) in Cologne. This unique international multidisciplinary organization is dedicated to the collection, dissemination and exchange of ideas relating to the facial nerve and its diseases. The Society maintains a database with addresses of the researchers and research projects to aid in planning future meetings and symposia. A newsletter will be published regularly. There are no fees for memberships.

If you are interested, please send a fax to or call

> Prof. Kedar Karim Adour, Co-Coordinator for the SCBS
> 1000 Green Street #1203, San Fransisco, CA 94133, USA
> Telephone 001-415-474 4046
> Fax 001-415-474-3541

In Germany interested persons should contact

> Priv.-Doz. Dr. O. Michel, University-HNO-Klinik
> Joseph-Stelzmann-Str. 9, D-50924 Cologne, Germany
> Telephone: +49-221-478-4750
> Fax: +49-221-478-4793.

Preface

The intention of the VIIth International Symposium on the Facial Nerve was to create a platform for an extensive exchange of knowledge and scientific information between clinicians and basic research workers. This aim could only be realized on the basis of a common interest in the facial nerve, which unites the interdisciplinary scientific efforts of otologists, neurosurgeons, facial plastic surgeons, neurologists, neurophysiologists, and neuroanatomists. Therefore, a meeting of this kind remains in its aim to exchange ideas over scientific disciplines which do not come unique together normal conditions.

The symposium has been held every four years since 1966. The VIIth symposium was preceded by symposia in Stockholm (1966), Osaka (1970), Zürich (1976), Los Angeles (1980), Bordeaux (1984) and Rio de Janeiro (1988), and marked an important milestone in the continuously developing knowledge about the facial nerve, its physiology, disorders, diagnostics and treatment. In contrast to the previous meetings this symposium extended in vitations to both clinicians and basic research workers.

More than 350 scientists from 25 different nations met in Cologne, Germany, in June 1992 and their high-level presentations contributed to the overwhelming success of this international meeting. The symposium took place in the vicinity of the old cathedral of Cologne, itself a vivid symbol of never-ending efforts to create something perfect and lasting.

May I present my special thanks, not only to all speakers, but also to the team in Cologne who worked for over two years to make this meeting a successful one. We have made every effort to include in this volume all the texts that were submitted, thus preserving the content of the symposium both for current use and as a guideline for future improvements in our field of facial nerve research.

E.R. Stennert

Contents

Anatomy

Eur Arch Otorhinolaryngology (1994) [Suppl]: S3–S5

G. Székely and C. Matesz

Comparative Anatomy of the Central Representation of the Facial Nerve

The branchiomotor (ventrolateral) column of cranial nerve nuclei is one of the brain structures which is often described in a rather ambiguous and contradictory manner even in the present literature. The reason for these problems is twofold. First, the nomenclature of these structures was created by early comparative neuroanatomists. With the techniques at their disposal, they could not make a distinction between structures acquired early or late in phylogenesis and this caused confusion in terminology. Second, the facial nerve innervates the derivatives of the second visceral arch, and a number of these structures merge with the derivatives of the first visceral arch. Therefore, the relations of the fifth and seventh nerves and their periphery must be also considered in the study of their central representation. Some years ago, we developed a technique to stain the dendritic geometry of selected neurons. With a neuromorphological approach to these problems, we were able to classify different neuron types in the cranial nerve motor nuclei and establish their relative appearance in phylogenesis on a comparative neurohistological basis; with the aid of the new data we were able to correct some of the ambiguities still present in modern descriptions.

The technique utilizes the advantageous property of Co^{3+} ions, which, by some unexplained mechanism, is transported by the axoplasma both in the cellulipetal and cellulifugal directions. To achieve transport into the cranial nerve nuclei the proximal stumps of the cut nerves were incubated in a solution of cobalt for varying periods of time. After killing the animal, corresponding parts of the brain stem were dissected and immersed in a buffer solution saturated with H_2S. This treatment transformed the Co^{3+} ions into insoluble CoS compound. Following regular histological processing, serial sections were made from the tissue block, and the specimens were intensified with a physical developer, which, by virtue of its silver content,

enlarged and made visible the otherwise invisible CoS precipitate. This labeling procedure showed the dendritic arbor and the trajectory of the axon to their full extent in most of the cases (for details see [4, 8]). For comparative reasons the morphology of motoneurons of cranial nerves was studied in frogs, lizards, and rats. As indicated, we concentrate on the trigeminal (nV) and the facial (nVII) motor nuclei in this presentation.

In the frog, the nV and nVII constitute two separate neuron groups [6]. The nV is bigger and consists of three morphologically distinct neuron types. The first type can be characterized by relatively large (approximately 40 µm) polygonal perikarya from which a dorsomedial and a ventrolateral dendritic array emerges. The first array expands in a fan-like manner, whereas the ventrolateral dendrites form a compact broom-like bundle. After an initial dorsal course, the axon bends ventrally. This type of neuron occupies the rostral part of the nucleus and innervates the closer muscles of the jaw. The second type of neuron is found in the caudal part of the nucleus. The ovoid or spindle-shaped perikaryon is smaller (approximately 32 µm), the dorsomedial dendritic array is less extensive, and the ventrolateral broom-like dendrite bundle is well developed. The axon has a similar trajectory as in the first type. These neurons innervate the muscles of the floor of the mouth (C. Matesz and Z. Hevessy, unpublished). The third type innervates an orbital muscle, which cannot be found in higher vertebrates: the muscle and its motoneuron pool disappear in phylogenesis. The nVII is composed of the morphological counterpart of the second type of neuron, contributes to the innervation of the floor of the mouth, and supplies the jaw opener muscle.

In the lizard, the organizaton of the nV and nVII is very similar to in the frog [10]. The first type of neuron has a larger range of size (11–45 µm) than in the frog, but the arborization pattern of the dendrites is very similar. A characteristic and stable feature is the dorsal origin of the axon, which runs medially, turns back at the lateral aspect of the medial longitudinal fasciculus (mlf), and cruises laterally to the root exit. In view of their rostral position

G. Székely (✉) and C. Matesz
Department of Anatomy, University Medicine School,
4012 Debrecen, Hungary

within the nV, these neurons innervate the closer muscles of the jaw. Another type of neuron which is found in the caudal part of the nV is the counterpart of the second type of neuron in the frog nV. These neurons innervate the muscles of the floor of the mouth. The third type of neuron and the orbital muscle are missing in the lizard. The nVII consists of a lateral subgroup, which contains small, probably preganglionic neurons, and a medial subgroup, which is composed of the counterpart of the second type of trigeminal neurons. These neurons contribute to the innervation of the floor of the mouth and supply the jaw opener muscle.

In conclusion, it may be stated that the organization of the nV and nVII nuclear complex is very similar in the frog and the lizard. Neurons innervating the jaw closer muscles can be clearly distinguished from neurons which innervate the floor of the mouth and the jaw opener muscles. While the "closer" neurons are more differentiated as far as the dendritic arborization is concorned, the morphology of the "opener" neurons is more conservative in the two animal species.

Profound changes occur in the orofacial region during evolution of mammalian species [2]. The primary mandibular joint, which is found in submammalian tetrapodes, is a two-armed lever, and due to structural restrictions it permits only an opening and closing of the mouth. These animals can grasp and swallow the food but they cannot chew and grind it. Muscles that act on this joint can be classified into a closer and an opener group. This simple joint is replaced by the secondary mandibular joint with very complex articular facets in mammals. The closer muscles give place to the masticatory muscles which act upon the joint along a variety of lines of force. Due to the structural changes of the joint, its opening is performed by the suprahyoid muscle group. The secondary palate develops, which separates the oral and nasal cavities. Gomphotic teeth replace the cemented teeth in the upper and the lower jaws. A new muscle group appears in the facial nerve region: the muscles of facial expression. These changes render the animal capable of chewing. In fact, *all* these changes are indispensable for, and contribute to, the complex action of mastication; the facial muscle group performs, in addition, a variety of other functions involved mainly in orientation and communication.

In the rat brain stem, we find similarly profound changes [9]. If the trigeminal nerve is labeled with cobalt in the rat, we find three morphologically distinct types of neurons. The first type provides the bulk of the neurons in the trigeminal motor nucleus. They have polygonal somata from which the dendrites radiate out in all directions. The axons emerge from the ventral aspect of the neurons, run along a straight course toward the root exit, and innervate masticatory muscles. This type of neuron is not found in the submammalian nV. The second type of neuron presents an ovoid or spindle-shaped body from which a dorsal and a ventral dendritic array originates. The axons emerge from the dorsal aspect of the neurons, make a dorsal loop

or a hair-pin turn at the lateral aspect of the mlf, and join the trigeminal motor root. One cannot fail to recognize the second neuron type (opener) of the submammalian nV. These neurons form a separate group which is known as the accessory trigeminal nucleus (nVa) and innervate the anterior suprahyoid muscles (mylohyoid, anterior digastricus). The third type of neuron is outside the classically defined nV and is half the size of the former types. These neurons innervate the tensor tympani muscle [3].

Labeling of the facial nerve reveals four morphologically different neuron types. The first type is very similar to the "masticatory" neurons in the nV and forms the classically defined nVII. The axons turn dorsally, form a complex whirl-like structure at the lateral aspect of the abducens nucleus, and then turn ventrally toward the root exit. They innervate the mucles of facial expression. This type of neuron is not found in the submammalian nVII, and the facial genu is conspicuously different from the dorsal loops, or hair-pin turns, of facial axons in submammalian species. The second type is the counterpart of neurons which form the nVa. These neurons form an elongated group dorsal to the rostral pole of the nVII, called the accessory facial nucleus (nVIIa). It is the caudal extension of the nVa. The innervation of the posterior suprahyoid muscles (stylohyoid, posterior digastricus) originates in the nVIIa. The third type is found largely between the rostral pole of the nVII and the superior olive. These neurons are half the size of the facial neurons and innervate the stapedius muscle [7]. The fourth type is represented by the parasympathetic preganglionic neurons. They are found in the small-celled part of the reticular formation scattered between the nVII and the internal genu. A number of these neurons form ill-defined aggregates in this area, and the most dorsal neurons constitute the rostral pole of the classically defined dorsal motor nucleus of the vagus. These neurons supply the sphenopalatine and submandibular ganglia [1].

As a conclusion concerning the organization of the mammalian facial nucleus, we may state the following:

1. The main nucleus which innervates the facial muscles can be found only in mammals. Although it is a new acquisition in evolution, the musculotopic organization is remarkably conservative in all mammalian species investigated. The individual muscles are represented in longitudinal columns of neurons. Neurons supplying nasolabial muscles are located in the lateral column, posterior auricular and scalp muscles in the medial column, platysma and neck muscles in the intermediate column, lower lip muscles in the ventral part, and ocular muscles in the dorsal part of the intermediate column. Depending on the variety of the function of facial muscles, these representation areas vary greatly in size in different species [5, 11].

2. The posterior suprahyoid muscles are innervated by the "ancient" facial nucleus. These neurons occupy a different location and probably receive central connections

which are different from the main nucleus. Functionally speaking, the nVIIa relates more to the trigeminal than to the facial nuclear complex.

3. Neurons innervating the stapedius muscle are located outside the classically defined nVII. They form a common column with neurons of the tensor tympani muscle in the ventral part of the pontine tegmentum. Regarding their function and position, they form an independent nucleus which does not belong either to the facial or the trigeminal nuclear complex.

References

1. Contreras RJ, Gomez MM, Norgren R (1980) Central origins of cranial nerve parasympathetic neurons in the rat. J Comp Neurol 190:373–394
2. Crompton AW (1989) The evolution of mammalian mastication. In: Wake DB, Roth G (eds) Complex organismal functions: integration and evolution in vertebrates. Wiley, Chichester, pp 23–40
3. Friauf E, Baker R (1985) An intracellular HRP-study of cat tensor tympani motoneurons. Exp Brain Res 57:499–511
4. Görcs T, Antal M, Oláh E, Székely G (1979) An improved cobalt labelling technique with complex compounds. Acta Biol Acad Sci Hung 30:79–86
5. Hinrichsen CFL, Watson CD (1984) The facial nucleus of the rat. Representatio of facial muscles revealed by retrograde transport of horseradish peroxidase. Anat Rec 209:407–415
6. Matesz C, Székely G (1978) The motor column and sensory projections of the branchial cranial nerves in the frog. J Comp Neurol 178:157–176
7. Shaw MD, Baker R (1983) The loalizations of stapedius and tensor tympani motoneurons in the cat. J Comp Neurol 216:10–19
8. Székely G, Gallyas F (1975) Intensification of cobaltous sulphide precipitate in frog nervous tissue. Acta Biol Acad Sci Hung 26:175–188
9. Székely G, Matesz C (1982) The accessory motor nuclei of the trigeminal, facial and abducens nerves in the rat. J Comp Neurol 210:258–264
10. Székely G, Matesz C (1988) Topography and organization of cranial nerve nuclei in the sand lizard, Lacerta agilis. J Comp Neurol 267:525–544
11. Welt C, Abbs JH (1990) Musculotopic organization of the facial motor nucleus in Macaca fascicularis: a morphometric and retrograde tracing study with cholera toxin B-HRP. J Comp Neurol 291:621–636

Eur Arch Otorhinolaryngology (1994) [Suppl]: S6–S9

H. Schröder

The Facial Nerve – Peripheral and Central Connections of Proprioception

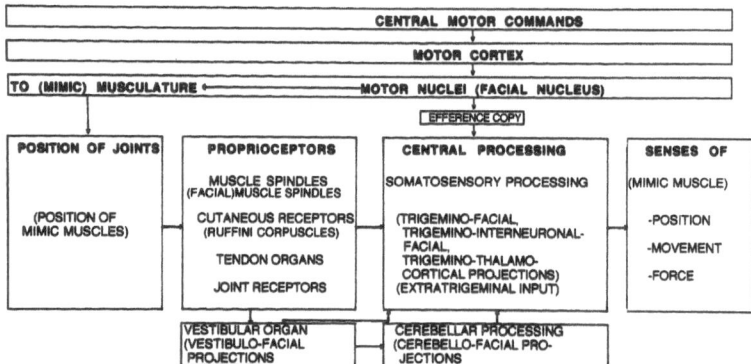

Fig. 1 Synoptic survey of the general organization of proprioception. Facial-specific components are given in brackets. (Modified according to [21])

Introduction

Proprioception is the awareness of the position and movements of body parts. Proprioceptor-linked sensory afferents convey kinesthetic signals to the appropriate motor nuclei (Fig. 1). Facial proprioceptors monitor movement and position of mimic muscles, ensuring adequate motor performance. The switch-over of facial nucleus (FN) activation and proprioception to the hypoglossal nucleus (HN) is a crucial issue in hypoglossal-facial anastomosis [23]. The functional anatomy of the best-studied model of FN connectivity, the cat, will be discussed, including human data wherever possible.

H. Schröder
Institute II for Anatomy, University of Cologne,
Joseph-Stelzmann-Strasse 9
50931 Cologne, Germany

Facial Proprioceptors and Afferent Sensory Nerves

Mimic muscles insert into and act on the skin, which is equipped with mechanoreceptors. Among these – fast-adapting type I (FA I) Meissner, (FA II) Pacininian corpuscles, slow-adapting (SA I) Merkel cell complexes, SA II Ruffini corpuscles (RC) – only the latter, subcutaneous pressure receptors composed of encapsulated nerve fibers, exist in human skalp skin [9]. Muscle spindles (MSp), encapsulated small myocytes with efferent and afferent endings, convey muscle tension-related data to the central nervous system (CNS). In cats, no facial MSp, but sensory afferent-like myelinated fibers [19], and in man only few facial MSp were observed [14]. Stretching of the skin or contraction of facial muscles elicits distinct on-off responses in human infraorbital nerve during the dynamic phases of stimulation [17]. Static discharge is less pronounced. Spontaneously active stretch-sensitive SA II units with large receptive fields most likely correspond to RC. Some

Table 1 Survey of functionally important input into the cat facial nucleus

Functional system	Area/Nucleus	Ipsi-lateral	Contra-lateral	Projection to HN
1. Somatosensory proprioceptive afferents (trigeminal nerve)	Spinal trigeminal nucleus	+	(+)	+
2. Reticular formation interneurons	Lateral RF	(+)	+	+
3. Pyramidal motor system	Motor cortex[a]	(+)	+	+
4. Extrapyramidal motor system	Globus pallidus[b]	(?)	+	
	Interstitial nucleus	+[d]	+[d]	+(Opossum)
	Red Nucleus	−	+[e]	
	Nucleus of Darkshevitsch	+[d]	+[d]	
5. Visual system	Colliculus superior	+	+[f]	
6. Hypothalamus	Lateral hypothalamus	(?)	+	
7. Vestibular system	Vestibular nucleus	+	(+)	
8. Cerebellum	Interposital/dentate nucleus[c]	(?)	+	

Data compiled from [4–7, 10–13, 18, 20, 22, 24, 26, 28].
RF, reticular formation; HN, hypoglossal nucleus.

[a] Also via the nucleus reticularis parvocellularis of the medulla and the spinal trigeminal nucleus.
[b] Via the interstitial nucleus of Cajal.
[c] Via the interstitial nucleus of Cajal, the nucleus of Darkshevitsch, and the red nucleus.
[d] Via tegmental pathways.
[e] Via rubrospinal pathway.
[f] Via tectobulbar tracts, paralemniscal region, pontine RF, and via tectospinal pathway.

stretch-sensitive units may also have MSp in perioral muscles. Since there is no evidence for proprioceptive afferents in the human facial nerve, most likely the trigeminal nerve (n. V) contains the afferents of intramuscular and cutaneous receptors [17]. The latter are probably the main proprioceptors for mimic movements.

Trigeminofacial Connections and the Role of Interneurons

The blink reflex is a model for integration of proprioceptive n.V afferents and FN motor responses. As shown electrophysiologically in cats, the early reflex response is conveyed via a three-neuronal disynaptic pathway [27]. Stimulation of the supraorbital nerve elicits a response in the spinal trigeminal nucleus (STN) that projects in turn to the FN. Efferent motor fibers activate the orbicularis oculi muscle, resulting in closure of the eye. Morphologically, different n.V branches have been shown to converge on STN neurons from where mostly ipsilateral projections reach the FN, which also receives collateral input from STN efferents to abducens and trigeminal motor nuclei [4, 5, 24, 26]. In addition, a second, interneuron-mediated pathway has been shown electrophysiologically [27]. In man, Stennert and Limberg [23], based on electrophysiological studies, postulated the involvement of an interneuron in facial proprioceptive movement control. Morphologically, STN connections with the bulbar reticular formation (RF) [24] and RF interneurons projecting to the FN [11, 25] have been shown. Bilateral RF projections to the FN may subserve the late bilateral response of

the blink reflex. Most interestingly, RF interneurons projecting to the FN and those connected with the HN are located roughly in the same area [11]. Furthermore, direct ipsilateral projections from the STN to the HN have been shown in cat [24] and rat [2]. Thus, after hypoglossal-facial anastomosis preexisting trigeminohypoglossal connections as in the cat CNS may subserve the transposition of tasks from the FN to the HN (see Table 1).

Proprioception-related extratrigeminal projections to the FN are described below (Table 1).

Metencephalon – Vestibular Nuclei

Tract tracing and electrophysiology have revealed vestibular monosynaptic bilateral projections to the FN [22] coordinating facial, eye, and head movements for an integrated orientation response.

Nucleus Reticularis Parvocellularis of the Medulla

The nucleus reticularis parvocellularis of the medulla (NRP) is a relay nucleus transmitting corticofugal influences to the FN. NRP stimulation evokes an excitatory FN response probably mediated by a monosynaptic connection [7].

Mesencephalon – Pretectal Area

The pretectal area (PTE), mediating the pupillary reflex and the generation of compensatory eye movements, projects to the FN [13], probably evoking monosynaptic excitatory responses [7].

Colliculus Superior

The colliculus superior (CS) provides rapid orientation of sensory organs towards new relevant objects in space. Bilateral pathways to the FN via the paralemniscal area are suggested by electrophysiological and anatomical studies [8, 10, 28].

Nucleus of Darkshevitsch (ND), Interstitial Nucleus of Cajal (INC)

The nucleus of Darkshevitsch (ND), the interstitial nucleus of Cajal (INC), and red nucleus (RN; vide infra) belong to the extrapyramidal motor system. ND and INC receive afferents from the globus pallidus and from vestibular nuclei. The INC is probably involved in the maintenance of vertical eye position [3]. Bilateral projections from ND and INC to the FN have been shown by means of tract tracing [12] and electrophysiology, revealing a probably monosynaptic connection [7]. In the opossum, a projection from the INC to the HN has been shown [18].

Red Nucleus

The RN mediates corticofugal influences to the FN, as shown electrophysiologically [7]. Tracing techniques have revealed a contralateral pathway from RN to the FN [12].

Cerebellum

Cerebellum input from the interposital and dentate nuclei into the FN may be mediated via the INC, ND, and RN (see [7]).

Telencephalon – Cerebral Cortex

Man and cat have direct bilateral, contralaterally predominant motor cortex projections to the FN [15, 20]. In cats, indirect pathways via the STN are also known to exist [11, 16]. Cortex stimulation elicits excitatory and inhibitory FN responses [6].

Conclusions

Trigeminofacial connections subserving proprioceptive movement control as well as trigeminohypoglossal projections have been shown in the cat. Sensitive histochemical techniques [1] enable tract-tracing experiments in autopsied brains. Such techniques will be a valuable tool for the evaluation of trigeminofacial projections and the involvement of interneurons in the human CNS. Postmortem investigations of patients with hypoglossal facial anastomosis will reveal possible anatomical changes underlying functional transposition.

References

1. Beach TG, McGeer EG (1987) Tract-tracing with horseradish peroxidase in the postmortem human brain. Neurosci Lett 76:37–41
2. Borke R, Nau EM (1987) The ultrastructural morphology and distribution of trigemino-hypoglossal connections labeled with horseradish peroxidase. Brain Res 422:235–241
3. Büttner-Ennever JA, Büttner K (1988) The reticular formation. In: Büttner-Ennever JA (ed) Neuroanatomy of the oculomotor system. Elsevier, Amsterdam, pp 119–176
4. Carpenter MB, Hanna GR (1961) Fiber projection from the spinal trigeminal nucleus in the cat. J Comp Neurol 117:117–125
5. Durand J, Gigan P, Guéritaud JP, Horcholle-Bossavit G, Tyc-Dumont S (1983) Morphological and electrophysiological properties of trigeminal neurones projecting to the accessory abducens nucleus of the cat. Exp Brain Res 53:118–128
6. Fanardjian VV, Manvelyan LR (1987a) Mechanisms regulating the activity of facial nucleus motoneurons. III. Synaptic influences from the cerebral cortex and subcortical structures. Neuroscience 20:835–843
7. Fanardjian VV, Manvelyan LR (1987b) Mechanisms regulating the activity of facial nucleus motoneurons. IV. Influences from the brainstem structures. Neuroscience 20:845–853
8. Grantyn R (1988) Gaze control through superior colliculus: structure and function: In: Büttner-Ennever JA (ed) Neuroanatomy of the oculomotor system. Elsevier, Amsterdam, pp 273–333
9. Halata Z, Munger BL (1981) Identification of the Ruffini corpuscles in human hairy skin. Cell Tissue Res 219:437–440
10. Henkel CK, Edwards SB (1978) The superior colliculus control of pinna movements in the cat: possible anatomical connections. J Comp Neurol 182:763–776
11. Holstege G, Kuypers HGJM, Dekker JJ (1977) The organization of the bulbar fibre connections to the trigeminal, facial and hypoglossal motor nuclei. II. An autoradiographic tracing study. Brain 100:265–286
12. Holstege G, Tan J, Van Ham J, Boss A (1984) Mesencephalic projections to the facial nucleus in the cat. An autoradiographical tracing study. Brain Res 311:7–22
13. Itoh K, Takada M, Yasiu Y, Mizuno N (1983) A pretectofacial projection in the cat: a possible link in the visually triggered blink reflex pathways. Brain Res 275:332–335
14. Kadanoff D (1956) Die sensiblen Nervenendigungen in der mimischen Muskulatur des Menschen. Z Mikrosk Anat Forsch 62:1–15
15. Kuypers HGJM (1958a) Corticobulbar connections to the pons and lower brain stem in man. Brain 81:364–388
16. Kuypers HGJM (1958b) An anatomical analysis of corticobulbar connections to the pons and lower brain stem in the cat. J Anat 92:198–218
17. Nordin M, Hagbarth K-E (1989) Mechanoreceptive units in the human infra-orbital nerve. Acta Physiol Scand 135:149–161
18. Panneton WM, Martin GF (1979) Midbrain projections to the trigeminal facial and hypoglossal nuclei in the opossum. A study using axonal transport techniques. Brain Res 168:493–511

19. Radpour S, Gacek RR (1985) Anatomic organization of the cat facial nerve. Otolaryngol Head Neck Surg 93:591–596

20. Schmitt J, Gacek RR (1986) Anatomical investigation of the corticonuclear projections of the facial nerve nucleus in the cat. Laryngoscope 96:129–134

21. Schmitt RF, Thews G (eds) (1989) Human physiology. 2nd edn. Springer, Berlin Heidelberg New York

22. Shaw MD, Baker R (1983) Direct projections from the vestibular nuclei to the facial nucleus in cats. J Neurophysiol 50: 1265–1280

23. Stennert E, Limberg CH (1982) Central connections between fifth, seventh and twelfth cranial nerves and their clinical significance. In: Graham MD, House WF (eds) Disorders of the facial nerve. Raven, New York, pp 57–65

24. Stewart WA, King RB (1963) Fiber projections from the nucleus caudalis of the spinal trigeminal nucleus. J Comp Neurol 121: 271–286

25. Takada M, Itoh K, Yasui Y, Mitani A, Nomura S, Mizuno N (1984) Distribution of premotor neurons for orbicularis oculi motoneurons in the cat with particular reference to possible pathways for blink reflex. Neurosci Lett 50:251–255

26. Takeuchi Y, Nakano K, Uemura M, Matsura K, Matsushima R, Mizuno N (1979) Mesencephalic and pontine afferent fiber system to the facial nucleus in the cat: a study using horseradish peroxidase and silver impregnation techniques. Exp Neurol 66:330–342

27. Tamai Y, Iwamoto M, Tsujimoto T (1986) Pathway of the blink reflex in the brainstem of the cat: interneurons between the trigeminal and the facial nucleus. Brain Res 380:19–25

28. Vidal P-P, May PJ, Baker R (1988) Synaptic organization of the tectal-facial pathways in the cat. I. Synaptic potentials following collicular stimulation. J Neurophysiol 60:769–797

Eur Arch Otorhinolaryngology (1994) [Suppl]: S 10 – S 15

S. Radpour and R. R. Gacek

Facial Nerve Fiber Orientation, Linkage Between Central Nervous Organization and Muscular Function

Introduction

Conflicting descriptions [1 – 9] of the anatomical organization of the facial nerve motor neurons have bee reconciled recently, through the use of neuroanatomical tracers [10 – 12] in combination with anterograde tracer and axonal degeneration techniques [13]. These observations have provided an anatomical basis for explaining some of the clinical phenomenon related to the facial nerve.

The separate localization of the motor neuron pools to the various individual regional muscle groups of the face and the multifascicular arrangement of the facial nerve at the root entry zone and tympanic portion of the temporal bone suggested that a discrete compartmentalization of the axons from each of these motor neuron pools was maintained throughout the peripheral course of the facial nerve.

However, recent studies [10 – 11] using retrograde transport of horseradish peroxidase (HRP) within the motor axons [12] and axonal degeneration studies using Marchi and Osmium stain [13] following total and partial lesions of the facial nerve at the level of the internal auditory canal clearly demonstrated that no compartmentalization of the regional motor axon group exists in facial nerve (Figs. 1 – 6). Instead, the fibers to all peripheral branches are distributed throughout the nerve at all levels before peripheral branching occurs. The axonal degeneration studies have the advantage that only the motor axons are affected, while sensory neurons within the facial nerve are preserved intact.

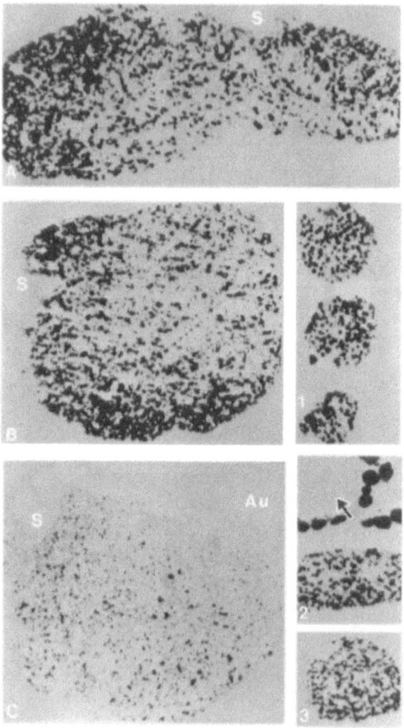

Fig. 1A–C Composite of cross-sections taken through tympanic (**A**), upper vertical (**B**), and lower vertical (**C**) segments of facial nerve trunk 6 days after complete transection at internal auditory meatus. Numbers **1, 2,** and **3** are sections through zygomatico-orbital (1), superior buccolabial (buccal) (2), and inferior buccolabial (mandibular) (3) branches of facial nerve. Fragments of degenerating myelinated fibers are stained *black* with Marchi solution, while nondegenerated sensory fibers are *unstained. Arrow* in (2) points to sensory fascicle in buccal branch. *S,* nervus intermedius; *AU,* auricular branch of vagus nerve

S. Radpour (✉)
Richard L. Roudebush Veterans Affairs Medical Center,
Indiana University Medical School,
Clinical Professor Otolaryngology-H&NS, 1481 W. 10th Street,
Indianapolis, IN 46202, USA

R. R. Gacek
Department Otolaryngology-H&NS, Upstate Medical Center,
750 E. Adams Street,
Syracuse, NY 13210, USA

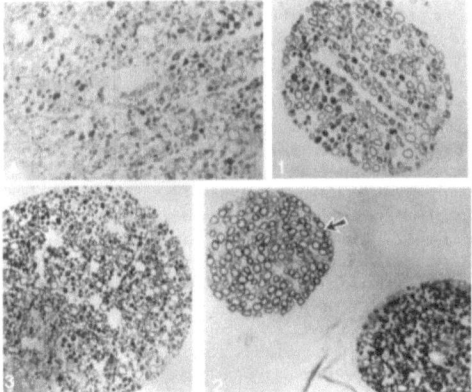

Fig. 2 Postfixed osmium technique 6 days after total transection of facial nerve at internal auditory meatus. Degenerating motor axons appear as darkened, shrunken configurations, while intact sensory fibers are represented by intact myelin sheaths. **A** High-power section through lower vertical segment of facial nerve trunk. **1** Zygomatico-orbital branch. **2** Superior buccolabial (buccal) branch. **3** Inferior buccolabial (mandibular) branch. Arrow in **2** points to intact sensory fasicle that regularly accompanied buccal branch. *Bar* in **2**, 29 µm

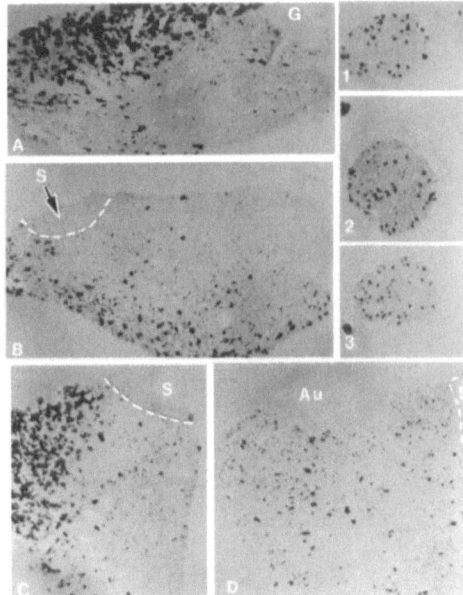

Fig. 4A–D Composite of comparable levels of the facial nerve and branches shown in Fig. 3, 5 days after transection of caudal fascicle of facial nerve in internal auditory meatus. Degenerated fibers travel together dorsal and medial to geniculate ganglion (**G**) in labyrinthine segment (**A**). They spread out along medial aspect of tympanic segment (**B**), but come together in posteromedial aspect of upper vertical segment (**C**). However, these degenerated fibers become scattered throughout lower vertical segment (**D**) and supply the three peripheral branches evenly (**1–3**). *Arrow* points to sensory fascicle in buccal branch (**2**). **S**, nervus intermedius; **Au**, auricular branch (sensory) of vagus nerve. (From [13])

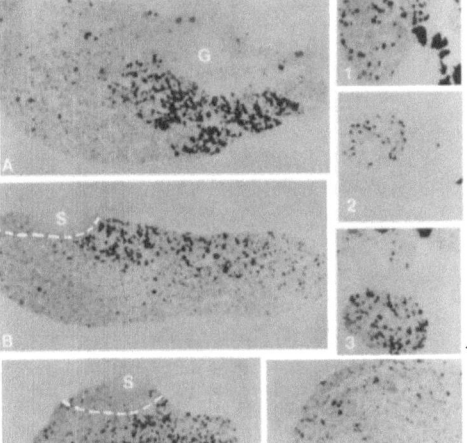

◀**Fig. 3A–D** Composite of representative sections through labyrinthine (**A**), tympanic (**B**), and upper vertical (**C**) segments of facial nerve trunk and branches stained by Marchi method 6 days after transection of rostral fascicle of nerve in internal auditory meatus. **A–C** show localized group of degenerated fibers traveling ventral to geniculate ganglion (**G**) and sensory nervus intermedius (**S**) on lateral (toward middle ear) aspect of nerve trunk. These degenerated fibers are widely dispersed in lower vertical segment of nerve (**D**) and are distributed to peripheral branches (**1**, **2**, and **3**) in almost equal numbers. *Arrows* point to sensory fascicles in buccal branch (**2**). (From [13])

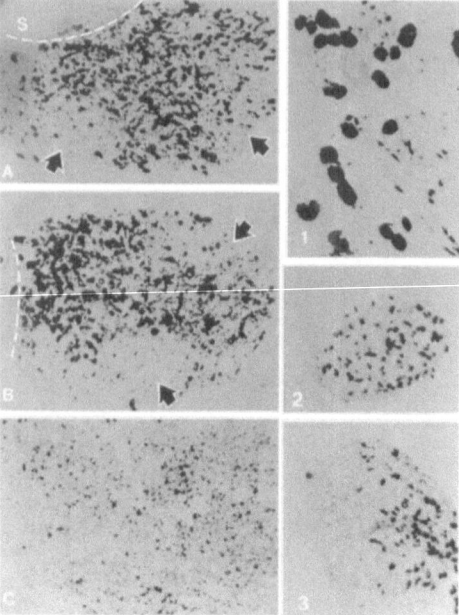

mately equal numbers (Figs. 3–6). This demonstrated that the motor axons to the peripheral facial nerve branches are distributed throughout the cross-section of the facial nerve trunk. These degeneration studies also demonstrated that there are two sensory neuronal components to the facial nerve: (1) the nervus intermedius carrying preganglionic autonomic axons as well as the gustatory sensory neurons located in a compact, small fiber group which is consistently localized at the lateral and posterior margin of the facial nerve trunk intratemporally and (2) the sensory component, comprising at least 15%–20% of the nerve, wich is scattered throughout the cross-section of the nerve trunk. Some of these fibers are large (greater than 10 μm) in size while others are small (2–3 μm). The location of the cell bodies for the general sensory component is not clear, but may be found in the geniculate ganglion or may represent afferent axons which are derived from the trigeminal nerve.

Fig. 5 A–C Composite of sections through tympanc (**A**), upper vertical (**B**), and lower vertical segments (**C**) of facial nerve 6 days after transection of central portion of nerve at internal auditory meatus. Zone of degenerated fibers remained limited to central part of nerve until lower vertical segment (**C**) was reached. Note that zones which contain fibers from rostral and caudal fascicles of nerve are now relatively free of degenerated fibers (*arrows*). Degenerated fibers were found in all three peripheral branches (**1–3**)

The result of a corticonuclear projection study showed a small, but bilateral projection to the facial nucleus from motor neurons located in the frontal lobe with contralateral predominance [14].

Materials and Methods

The details of the technique and preparation of these experimental studies are described elsewhere [13–14]. The Marachi method selectively stains degenerated myelinated fibers (Figs. 1–5) and the postfixed osmium stain demonstrates both degenerated and normal myelinated fibers (Figs. 2, 6). The retrograde HRP studies [12] fills both motor and sensory fibers.

Following the placement of discrete partial transections of various portions of the facial nerve at the level of the internal auditory canal, degenerated motor axons were found in all peripheral facial nerve branches in approxi-

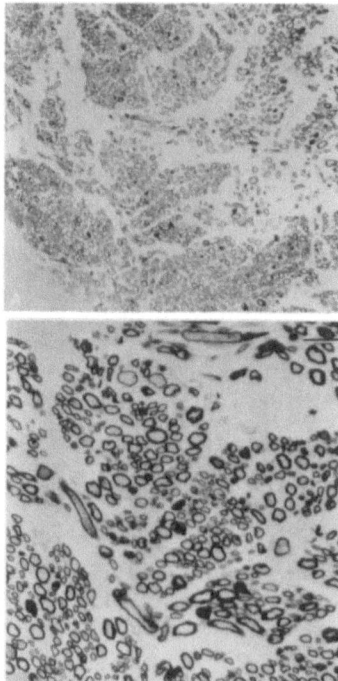

Fig. 6 A, B Low-power (**A**) and high-power (**B**) photomicrographs of lower vertical segment of facial nerve postfixed-stained with osmium 6 days after transection of rostral fascicle of nerve. Degenerated motor axons are represented by *solidly dark fibers* scattered among intact normal fibers. *Bar* in **B**, 29 μm

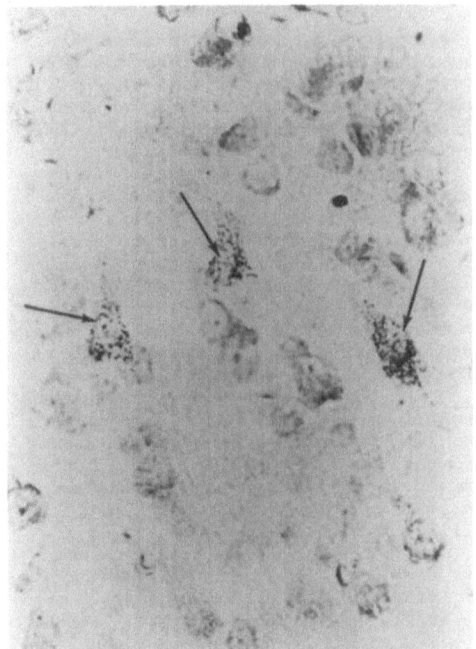

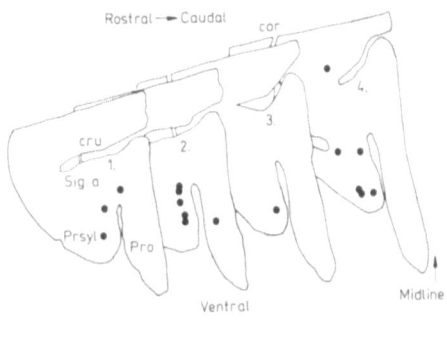

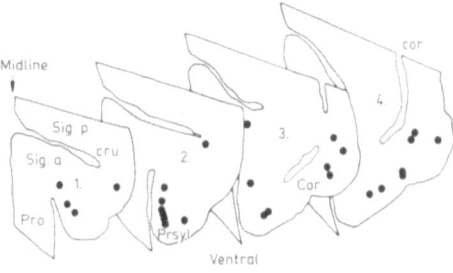

Fig. 7 Three labeled pyramidal-shaped neurons (*arrow*) in layer V of frontal lobe cortex. (Original magnification, ×374)

Fig. 9 Computer reconstruction of coronal sections through right (*top*) and left (*bottom*) frontal lobe cortex in at no. 14. The sections were trimmed dorsally for clarity. Location of labeled neurons is marked by *black dots*. *cru*, Cruciate sulcus; *cor*, coronal sulcus; *Prsyl*, presylvian gyrus; *Sig. a*, anterior sigmoid gyrus; *Sig. p*, posterior sigmoid gyrus. (Original magnification, ×5)

Fig. 8 Transverse section of brain stem in cat no. 14 demonstrating localized horseradish peroxidase (HRP) reaction product in the right facial nucleus (*arrow*). **FN**, contralateral facial nucleus; **C**, cochlear nucleus; **P**, pyramidal tracts; **V**, spinal trigeminal tract; **RB**, restiform body

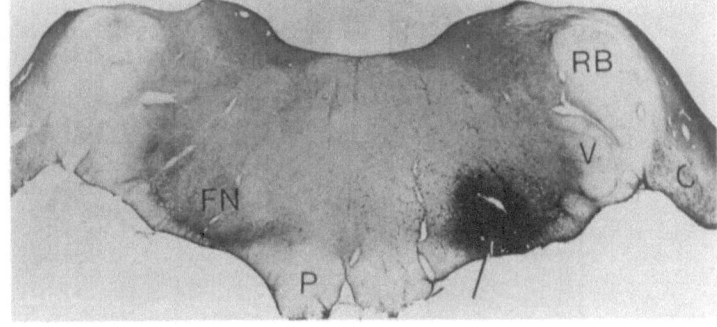

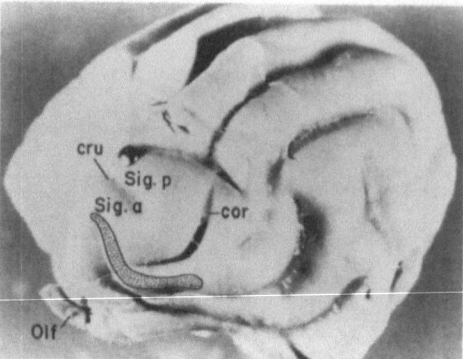

Fig. 10 Left cerebral hemisphere in the cat. The *stippled* area represents the facial motor cortex as indicated by the retrograde transport of horseradish peroxidose (HRP). *Olf,* olfactory tract; *cru,* cruciate sulcus; *cor,* coronal sulcus; *Sig. a,* anterior sigmoid gyrus; *Sig. p,* posterior sigmoid gyrus

A demonstration of corticonuclear projections to the facial nucleus was accomplished by injection of HRP through a dorsal or ventral approach to the facial nerve nucleus (posterior fossa and skull base). Labeled pyramidal-shaped neurons were found bilaterally in layer V of the anterior sigmoid, presylvian, and coronal gyri of the frontal cerebral cortex [14] (Figs. 7–10). This area has also been shown physiologically to contain neurons which excite the facial nerve [15]. This pathway is better developed in primate species. The increase in the magnitude of these projections with ascending species is related to the need and ability to perform voluntary and sophisticated facial muscle contractions in the higher species.

Discussion

Although it has been shown that the motor neurons supplying each peripheral facial muscle group are located in discrete portions of the facial nerve nucleus [10], it does not follow that the fibers which comprise individual branches exist throughout the facial trunk as a compact group of fibers. Examination of the central course of the facial nerve revealed that the multifascicular pattern exists back only to the point lateral to its central genu.

The axonal degeneration study [13] showed that the motor nerve fibers, although they travel in a straightforward course throughout the labyrinthine, tympanic, and upper vertical portions of the facial nerve, become dispersed as the lower vertical portion is reached. The fibers in a discret portion of the facial nerve, including the internal auditory canal, contain contributions to all peripheral branches.

Two groups of non-motor sensory fibers have been demonstrated in the axonal degeneration studies. The nervus intermedius portion of the facial nerve travels in a compact bundle on the lateral surface of the facial nerve throughout its temporal course, forming the chorda tympani (small diameter, 1–2 µm myelinated fibers).

A second group of myelinated afferent fibers were scattered throughout the facial nerve and its branches with a wide diameter spectrum of 1–12 µm. This group of sensory fibers were present as nondegenerated fibers in the facial nerve. They therefore represent fibers either arising from cell bodies in the geniculate ganglion or·other afferents which may enter the facial nerve branches from an extraneous source such as the trigeminal nerve. It is well known that the trigeminal nerve forms anastomotic connections with the facial nerve branches [16].

Although large myelinated fibers (up to 10–12 µm) have been reported as innervating muscle spindles, these structures have not been observed in the facial muscles. Nevertheless, these sensory fibers, which travel in the facial nerve and its branches, may partly explain the sensory changes often noted by patients who experience Bell's palsy or other forms of peripheral facial nerve paralysis.

It is well known that lesions of the temporal and internal auditory canal portions of the facial nerve produce weakness in all divisions of the face rather than selective regions. Our study and description of the fibers offers a logical explanation for this observation. The mixed arrangement of motor fibers in the facial nerve trunk also accounts for the regular occurrence of a disorganized and misdirected regeneration of fibers after severe facial trauma. Therefore, repair of the facial nerve by primary anastomosis or by free nerve grafting cannot result in organized reinnervation of the facial muscles, no matter how precisely the repair of the nerve segment is carried out.

The diffuse arrangement of facial nerve motor axons furthermore demonstrates why slow compressive lesions of the nerve at the internal auditory canal, such as acoustic neurinoma, rarely produce any noticeable facial weakness, even when the facial nerve is significantly smaller. The reduction in size of the facial nerve associated with such benign tumors reflects the decreased number of functioning motor axon units which are present without clinical manifestations or paralysis.

Finally, the mixed arrangement of motor axons in the facial nerve favors the otologic surgeon when operating on the nerve. The diffuse arrangement of motor fibers may partly account for the fact that routine uncovering of the facial nerve at surgery rarely results in any noticeable facial weakness, even though a certain degree of trauma may be associated by this procedure. An additional margin of safety in facial nerve surgery is provided by the lateral location of the nervus intermedius in the nerve trunk throughout its tympanic and mastoid segments.

The bilaterality of the projection with a contralateral predominance supports the notion that certain muscles supplied by the facial nucleus may be bilaterally innervated [10–11]. We have demonstrated that the orbicularis oculi and oris muscles (major muscles of facial expression) are located in the lateral division of the facial nerve nucleus, while the platysma, digastric, and auricular muscles are represented in the medial division of the facial nerve nucleus (all minor muscles of the facial expression). Only frontalis muscle motor neurons are located in both lateral and medial divisions of the facial nucleus [10–11]. This may provide an explanation for the clinical phenomenon where an upper motor neuron lesion will produce a unilateral facial paralysis of all muscle groups except for the frontalis muscle.

It is possible that the medial portion of the facial nerve nucleus is more favorably located to receive bilateral cortical nuclear innervation, while the lateral portion of the nucleus may receive only a contralateral cortical nuclear projection [14].

References

1. Kempke LF (1989) Topical organization of the distal portion of the facial nerve. J Neurosurg 52:671–673
2. Crumley R (1980) Spatial anatomy of facial nerve fibers – a preliminary report. Laryngoscope 90:274–276
3. May M (1973) Anatomy of the facial nerve (spatial orientation of fibers in the temporal bone). Laryngoscope 83:1311–1329
4. Miehlke A (1958) Über die Topographie des Faserverlaufes in Facialisstamm. Arch Ohren Nas Kehlk 171:340–347
5. Miehlke A (1964) Normal and anomalous anatomy of the facial nerve. Trans Am Acad Opthalmol 68:1030–1044
6. Sunderland S, Cossar DF (1953) The structure of the facial nerve. Anat Rec 116:147–166
7. Harris WD (1968) Topography of the facial nerve. Arch Otolaryngol 88:264–267
8. Scoville WD (1955) Partial section of proximal VIIth nerve trunk for facial spasm. Surg Gynecol Obstet 101:495–497
9. Sade J (1975) Facial nerve reconstruction and its prognosis. Ann Otol Rhinol Laryngol 84:695–703
10. Radpour S (1977) Organization of the facial nerve nucleus in the cat. Laryngoscope 87:557–574
11. Radpour S, Gacek R (1980) Facial nerve nucleus in the cat, further study. Laryngoscope 90:685–692
12. Thomander D, Aldeskogius H, Grant G (1981) Motor fiber organizatin in the nerve studies with the horseradish peroxidase technique. Acta Universtatis Upsaliensis 40 (iii):1–24
13. Gacek R, Radpour S (1982) Fiber orientation of the facial nerve. Laryngoscope 92:547–556
14. Gacek R, Schmitt J (1986) Anatomical investigation of the corticonuclear projection to the facial nerve nucleus of the cat. Laryngoscope 96:129–134
15. Nieoullon A, Rispal-Padel L (1976) Somatotopic localization in cat morot cortex. Brain Res 105:405–422
16. Baumel JJ (1974) Trigeminal facial communications. Their function in facial muscle innervation and re-innervation. Arch Otolaryngol 99:34–44

Eur Arch Otorhinolaryngology (1994) [Suppl]: S 16–S 17

J. M. Schröder

Changing Ratio Between Myelin Thickness and Axon Caliber in Developing Human Facial Nerves

"The facial nerve is generally regarded as being one of the most complex of the cranial nerves" [9]. For evaluating pathological changes in any given nerve we need to know details about the number and the quality of its nerve fibers. In addition, reactive changes of axons, myelin sheaths, Schwann cells, and connective tissue elements, including endoneurial, perineurial, and epineurial components, blood vessels, and occasionally also lymph vessels have to be considered.

The number of nerve fibers is given per area (usually per 1 mm ^{2}) or per whole nerve cross-sectional area (total number of nerve fibers). In the facial nerve, we studied the number of myelinated nerve fibers on both sides of its extracranial portion in 11 autopsy cases [8]. There was an average of 7097 (range: 5048–10543) on the right and 6800 (range: 5077–7323) on the left side, which is in good agreement with previous counts [4, 9]. The zygomatic branch comprised most of the fibers (30%), whereas the frontal branch contained only 18%, the buccal branch 29%, and the cervical branch 21% of the fibers.

In addition, the quality of nerve fibers is important. In particular, we need to know details concerning the normal development of axons and myelin sheaths in order to recognize developmental disturbances, such as total lack of myelin (amyelination) or hypomyelination, and progressive demyelinating, or axonal and neuronal disorders. The facial nerve shows similar changes in the axon to myelin ratio during development and a similar asynchronous development of axon calibers and myelin sheath thickness as noted in sural, femoral, ulnar, and trochlear nerves [6, 7].

For the present study, six facial nerves were obtained at autopsy immediately distal to their exit at the base of the skull from individuals without clinical evidence of peripheral neuropathy. The nerves were evaluated morpho-

metrically by light and electron microscopy at the age of 4.4, 13.7, 48.5, 62.3, 191.6, and 203.4 months. The mean caliber of the 20 largest nerve fibers, evaluated by ocular micrometer measurements, was approximately 2 μm smaller than of the axons in the femoral nerve. The difference in the myelin sheaths in these nerve fibers, however, was minor. The values for the ulnar, trochlear, and sural nerves were between those for the facial and the femoral nerve. When axons had already reached their maximal diameter at 5 years, maximal myelin sheath thickness was not attained before 16–17 years of age, i.e., more than 10 years later. The slope of the regression lines for the ratio between axon diameter and myelin sheath thickness was significantly steeper in older than in younger individuals. It also differed if small and large fibers with more or less than 50 myelin lamellae were evaluated separately.

The developmental changes at the node of Ranvier are more complicated, since the myelin lamellae are attached by transverse bands to the paranodal axon and to each other by desmosomes and tight junctions. Despite its importance for maintenance of structure and function of peripheral nerve fibers in general, normal, fine structural, developmental changes at the paranodal axon-myelin sheath complex (during axonal expansion and myelin lamellar growth) have only recently been studied in man [2] although some developmental data on normal feline nerves are already available [1]. The ratio between internodal and paranodal axon diameters remains remarkably constant during development. It ranges between 1.8 and 2.0, i.e., the axonal diameter at the paranode is only about half as thick as at the internode, with all the consequences to conduction velocity and axonal transport.

The myelin lamellae transiently lose their special devices for attachment to the underlying axolemma and to each other during developmental expansion. Some of the myelin loops pile up within the paranodal myelin segment to form the so-called bracelets of Nageotte. This mechanism, as well as the narrowing of the paranodal myelin lamellae, assures that the paranodal myelin attachment zone of the axolemma does not increase in proportion to

J. M. Schröder

Institut für Neuropathologie der Medizinischen Fakultät der RWTH Aachen, Pauwelsstrasse 30, 52057 Aachen, Germany

the development of the myelin sheath thickness, but is kept within a rather narrow range. Teleologically speaking, this limitation of the paranodal narrowing of axons may be of advantage concerning axonal conduction velocity and axonal flow. These normal developmental changes have to be taken into account if pathological changes are to be identified.

Although we have not been able to study facial nerves in Guillain Barré syndrome (GBS), we were able to see evidence of demyelination, remyelination, and axonal degeneration and regeneration in a sural nerve biopsy from a 47-year-old man with severe GBS and bilateral facial nerve paralysis. There was good recovery from peripheral motor and sensory symptoms, but facial paresis persisted at last for more than 2 months after onset of symptoms.

In a biopsy of the frontal branch of the facial nerve after trauma and cross-facial anastomosis that we happened to see because of failure of the autograft, we found very few myelinated nerve fibers; however, most bands of Büngner had remained noninnervated despite persistence of the whole nerve structure at approximately 6 months after surgery.

These two examples illustrate that motor nerves alone and especially the facial nerve are usually not the subject of pathomorphological studies. Examination of the facial nerve, because of ethical and other reasons, is often avoided even at autopsy. Thus, very few neuropathological data on this particular nerve are available [5], but it is assumed that it reacts as other human nerves do, at least in its extracranial portion. The intracanalicular portion is different, and it would be of major interest to study it at the fine structural level and with modern immunohistochemical techniques.

References

1. Berthold H-C (1978) Morphology of normal peripheral axons. In: Waxman SG (ed) Physiology and pathology of axons. Raven, New York, pp 3–63
2. Bertram M, Schröder JM (1992) Developmental changes at the node and paranode in human sural nerves: morphometric and fine structural evaluation. Brain Res (submitted)
3. Beuche W, Friede RL (1985) A new approach toward analyzing peripheral nerve fiber populations. II. Foreshortening of regenerated internodes corresponds to reduced sheath thickness. J Neuropathol Exp Neuropathol Exp Neurol 44:73–84
4. Kullman GL, Dyck PJ, Cody DTR (1971) Anatomy of the mastoid portion of the facial nerve. Arch Ololaryngol 93:29–33
5. Podvinec M, Ulrich J (1980) Neuropathologische Befunde bei der peripheren Fazialislähmung. Akt Probl Otolaryng 3:32–38
6. Schröder JM, Bohl J, Brodda K (1978) Changes of the ratio between myelin thickness and axon diameter in the human developing sural nerve. Acta Neuropathol (Berl) 43:169–178
7. Schröder JM, Bohl J, von Bardeleben U (1988) Changes of the ratio between myelin thickness and axon diameter in human developing sural, femoral, ulnar, facial, and trochlear nerves. Acta Neuropathol (Berl) 76:471–483
8. Sogard I, Samii M, Schröder JM (1981) Distribution of nerve fibers in the extratemporal branches of the facial nerve. In: Samii M, Jannetta PJ (eds) The craial nerves. Springer, Berlin Heidelberg New York, pp 403–404
9. Van Buskirk C (1945) The seventh nerve complex. J Comp Neurol 82:303–333

The Denervated Muscle

Eur Arch Otorhinolaryngology (1994) [Suppl]: S 21 – S 23

T. Gordon

To What Extent Can Poor Functional Recovery of Denervated Muscles Be Attributed to Incomplete as Opposed to Inappropriate Reinnervation After Surgical Repair of Severed Nerves?

Introduction

The motor unit, i. e. the nerve and the muscle fibers that it supplies, is the functional unit of movement, being the smallest unit of force which is controlled by synaptic drive in the central nervous system. Normally, any movement involves the progressive recruitment of motor units in the appropriate muscles with the force of each muscle unit being controlled by modulating the firing rate of the unit [16, 17, 26].

When the motor unit is disrupted by peripheral nerve injuries, the size of the axotomized nerve and paralyzed denervated muscle fibers declines dramatically [3, 7, 9, 10, 15, 21]. This atrophy may be reversed if nerve regeneration leads to reformation of functional nerve-muscle connections [11]. Atrophy mean literally without food, so that atrophic changes after axotomy and denervation show that trophic interaction between nerve and muscle is essential for the normal structural and functional integrity of the mature motor unit [15, 26]. Changes in gene expression in axotomized neurons appear to revert the neuron back to a more immature growth mode for regeneration [7], and, in the denervated muscles, altered gene expression is associated with an expression of a more immature state which is permissive for reinnervation [26]. Reformation of functional nerve-muscle connections reverses these states back to the mature phenotype.

Recovery of denervated musculature depends on how many nerves regenerate and their capacity to supply all available denervated muscle fibers. This recovery is independent of the source of innervation, because directing a foreign nerve to reinnervate the denervated muscle will result in formation of functional connections and reversal

T. Gordon
Division of Neuroscience, University of Alberta,
525 Heritage Medical Research Center, Edmonton, Alberta,
T6G 2S3 Canada

of axotomy and denervation changes [6, 11, 12, 13]. Recovery of motor control, however, is more complicated and requires that nerves regenerate to their former target muscles to allow for activation of the appropriate muscle. In addition, normal control of force depends on the wide range of force, contractile speed, and endurance of motor units in each muscle which normally allows for smooth gradation of muscle contraction during movement [16, 17].

Misdirection of Regenerating Nerves and Synkinesis

Recovery of function is generally more complete after compression injuries, in which nerve fibers regenerate back to their former targets, presumably because the perineurial sheaths remain intact [18, 21]. In contrast, recovery of function is often disappointing after injuries which disrupt the continuity of Schwann cell tubes, despite considerable surgical skills and development of microsurgical repair techniques. Synkinesis, the phenomenon of inappropriate cocontraction of muscles, is a well-recognized clinical problem which has been well described in the laryngeal muscles after injuries to the recurrent laryngeal nerve [1, 8], in the facial muscles after facial nerve injuries [2], and in the hand muscles after ulnar nerve injuries [22]. Synkinesis has been attributed, at least in part, to misdirection of regenerating nerves to inappropriate target muscles [1, 2, 4, 8, 19, 22]. Under some circumstances, synkinesis may be so severe that reinnervation of muscles is counterproductive and reinnervated muscles may be functionally ineffective. An example is when antagonistic muscles of the larynx cocontract, the stronger adductor muscles counteract abduction, and the vocal folds are immobilized despite muscle innervation and activation. In our study of reinnervated hand muscles [22], we used needle and surface electromyographic (EMG) recording to record from the adductor digiti minimi (ADM) or first dorsal interosseus muscles and identified the source of reinnervation of the muscle by asking the patient to voluntarily activate each of the ulnar innervated muscles, including the lumbrical and adductor pollicis muscles. For example, the integrated EMG was recorded when subjects moved their little finger consistent with the motoneuron innervating the appropriate muscle. However, the surface EMG showed that several motoneurons which formerly innervated other ulnar innervated muscles also reinnervated the ADM. Unitary EMG signals were also recorded with the bipolar needle electrode in the ADM, for example when the patient voluntarily activated a muscle on the opposite side of the hand. The collation of data from several patients showed that reinnervation appeared to be random [22]. The considerable misdirection of regenerating nerves could explain why fine movements of the fingers were almost impossible for the patients.

Reversal of Denervation Atrophy Depends on Number of Reinnervated Motor Units

The number of regenerating nerves which make functional connections will depend on the type of injury and the success of the surgical repair. Often, regenerating fibers will fail to cross the suture line and only a fraction of the nerves will reinnervate muscles. In studies in cat and rat hindlimb muscles, we experimentally reduced the number of motor units to determine whether reduced numbers of motor nerves can reinnervate all the available muscle fibers to reverse denervation atrophy and to establish the minimal motor unit complement for muscle recovery. One of three contributing lumbar spinal nerves was cut unilaterally under aseptic conditions and the animals divided into two groups. In the first group (corresponding to a partial denervation), the nerve to the muscle of interest, the medial gastrocnemius in the cat and the tibialis anterior of the rat, was left intact. In a second group (corresponding to complete muscle denervation), the muscle nerve was cut and resutured. At least 4 months later, motor unit size was determined indirectly by measuring motor unit isometric force and directly by counting the number of muscle fibers in an isolated and glycogen-depleted motor unit.

In partially denervated muscles, enlargement of the remaining motor units by sprouting was sufficient to rescue all denervated muscle fibers unless the root section reduced the number of units to less than 15% [20]. In more extensively denervated muscles, denervated muscle fibers continued to atrophy with the result that muscle weight and force did not recover to normal levels. We found that regenerated nerves were as able to enlarge their motor units. Regenerated nerves reinnervated all the denervated muscle fibers only if regeneration restored at least 30% of the normal complement of motor units in the denervated muscle [14]. Otherwise, muscles were smaller and weaker, containing less muscle fibers than normal.

Size and Properties of Motor Units in Reinnervated Muscle

Under conditions in which the majority of axotomized nerves regenerate and reinnervate denervated muscles, the size and properties of the reinnervated motor units are similar to normal [11–14, 23–25]. Reinnervation restores the same skewed distribution of unit force that is seen normally with more small motor units than large, and contractile force and speed are well correlated with motor nerve size [11–13, 23–24]. Furthermore, motor units and muscle fibers may be classified using the same criteria, although there is a poorer correlation between muscle force and susceptibility to fatigue than is seen normally [6, 13, 25].

Muscle fibers in the reinnervated motor unit are more heterogeneous than normal with respect to their myosin heavy chain and metabolic enzyme content [5]. Nevertheless, all fibers are homogeneous, as in normal motor units in their histochemical type [18, 24, 25]. With a few exceptions, the muscle fiber type corresponds well with the physiological unit type [25]. This matching of motoneuron size and properties with size and properties of the muscle unit cannot be accounted for simply by regenerating nerves reinnervating their former muscle fibers, which they do not, except after crush injuries. Muscle fibers in reinnervated motor units have a different distribution to normal, with many fibers adjacent to one another [18, 24]. The regenerating nerve supplies muscle fibers which belonged to several different motor units and converts the muscle fibers to the same histochemical type, although the fibers still appear to differ from each other in size [24, 25]. This conversion accounts for the recovery of motor unit contractile speed and fatigue properties. However, differences in muscle fiber cross-section area, which accounted in part for the range of motor unit force in normal muscles, were not seen after reinnervation. Rather, the normal range of motor unit force was reestablished in reinnervated muscles by the differences in the number of muscle fibers supplied by the motoneurons [24]. Because the unit force correlates well with motor nerve size in reinnervated muscles, it follows that the number of muscle fibers per motoneuron increases in the same order as force. In turn, the correlation between unit force and motor nerve size indicates that reestablishment of the normal range of motor unit force in the reinnervated muscles can be attributed to a size-dependent branching of the regenerating nerve [11–13, 24].

Under conditions where the number of motor units was experimentally reduced, we observed that all motor units enlarged by the same factor and the normal relationships between motor unit force, innervation ratio, and motor nerve size could be demonstrated [14, 20]. In other words, even where motor unit number may be substantially lower than normal after partial or complete nerve injuries, where regeneration success is low and motor units enlarge, branching of the motoneurons maintains the normal range of unit size. As a result, muscle contraction may still be adequately controlled by recruitment of progressively larger motor units. The same range of contractile speed in reinnervated muscles permits the normal rate coding to modulate muscle contraction within motor units.

Conclusions

Our experiments show that the scope of recovery of denervated muscles may be considerable, even when relatively few nerves get back. Under conditions in which at least 30% of the normal complement of motor units is restored by reinnervation of denervated muscles after nerve injury, successful nerve regeneration may completely reverse denervation atrophy and restore a normal range of motor unit force and contractile properties. However, even where reinnervation is complete, recovery of movement is not guaranteed, particularly after nerve injuries which disrupt large nerve branches. Regenerating nerves which fail to reinnervate their former target muscle can lead to inappropriate activation of antagonistic muscles, particularly when motor nerves which, formerly supplied one muscle reinnervate more than one muscle. Thus progressive recruitment of motor units may not simply grade muscle force in the appropriate muscle, but lead to unwanted contractions in other muscles, which may actually oppose the required movement, leading to so-called synkinesis. This problem remains a major challenge to surgeons who repair injured peripheral nerves and therapists who train patients to use their muscles in the most appropriate way possible.

Acknowledgements The collaboration of my colleagues, including Dr. Thomas, Dr. Stein, Dr. Gillespie, Dr. Totosy de Zepetnek, and Dr. Murphy, my technicians, Mrs. Serap Erdebil and Neil Tyreman, and graduate students, Victor Rafuse and Susan Fu, is gratefully acknowledged. My thanks also to the Medical Research Council and Muscular Dystrophy Association of Canada for their financial support for this work and the Alberta Foundation for Medical Research for my personal support as a Heritage Scientist.

References

1. Crumley RL (1989) Laryngeal synkinesis: its significance to the laryngologist. Ann Otol Rhinol Laryngol 98:87–92
2. Crumley RL (1979) Mechanisms of synkinesis. Laryngoscope 89:1847–1854
3. Davis LA, Gordon T, Hoffer J, Jhamandas J, Stein RB (1978) Compound action potentials recorded from mammalian peripheral nerves following ligation and resuturing. J Physiol (Lond) 285:543–559
4. Flint PW, Downs DH, Coltrera MD (1991) Laryngeal synkinesis following reinnervaton in the rat. Neuroanatomic and physiologic study using retrograde fluorescent tracers and electromyography. Ann Otol Rhinol Laryngol 100:797–806
5. Fu S, Gordon T, Parry DJ, Tyreman N (1992) Immunohistochemical analysis of fiber types within physiologically typed motor units of rat tibialis anterior muscle after long-term cross-reinnervation. Soc Neurosci 18:1557
6. Gillespie MJ, Gordon T, Murphy PA (1987) Motor units and histochemistry in the rat lateral gastrocnemius and soleus muscles: evidence for dissociation of physiologial and histochemical properties after reinnervation. J Neurophysiol 57:921–937
7. Gordon T (1983) The dependence of peripheral nerves on their target organs. In: Burnstock G, Vrbova G, O'Brien R (eds) Somatic and autonomic nerve-muscle interactions. Elsevier, New York, pp 289–325
8. Gordon T (1992) Mechanisms for functional recovery of the larynx after surgical repair of injured nerves. J Voice 8:70–78
9. Gordon T, Davis LA (1986) Electrical activity in injured peripheral nerves. In: Nix WA, Vrbova G (eds) Electrical stimulation and neuromuscular diseases. Springer, Berlin Heidelberg New York, pp 64–74
10. Gordon T, Gillespie J, Orozco R, Davis L (1991) Axotomy-induced changes in rabbit hindlimb nerves and the effects of chronic electrical stimulation. J Neurosci 11:2157–2169
11. Gordon T, Stein RB (1982) Time course and extent of recovery in reinnervated motor units of cat triceps surae muscles. J Physiol (Lond) 323:307–323
12. Gordon T, Stein RB (1982) Reorganization of motor-unit properties in reinnervated muscles of the cat. J Neurophysiol 48:1175–1190
13. Gordon T, Stein RB, Thomas C (1986) Motor unit organization in extensor muscles cross-reinnervated by flexor motoneurones. J Physiol (Lond) 374:443–456
14. Gordon T, Totosy de Zepetnek JE, Rafuse V, Erdebil S (1991) Motoneuronal branching and motor unit size after complete and partial nerve injuries. In: Wernig A (ed) Motoneuronal plasticity. Springer, Berlin Heidelberg New York, pp 207–216
15. Gutmann E (1976) Neutrotrophic relations. Annu Rev Physiol 38:177–216
16. Henneman E, Mendell LM (1981) Functional organization of the motoneuron pool and its inputs. In: Brooks VB (ed) Handbook of physiology, sect 1, vol II. Williams and Wilkins, Baltimore, pp 423–508
17. Kernell D (1992) Organized variability in the neuromuscular system: a survey of task-related adaptations. Arch Ital Biol 130:19–66
18. Kugelberg E, Edstrom L, Abbruzzese M (1970) Mapping of motor units in experimentally reinnervated rat muscle. J Neurol Neurosurg Psychiatry 33:319–329
19. Nahm I, Shin T, Shiba T (1990) Regeneration of the recurrent laryngeal nerve in the guinea pig. Reorganization of motoneurons after freezing injury. Am J Otolaryngol 19:33–37
20. Rafuse VF, Gordon T, Orozco R (1992) Proportional sprouting in partially denervated triceps surae muscles in the cat. J Neurophysiol (in press)
21. Sunderland S (1978) Nerve and nerve injuries. Churchill Livingstone, London
22. Thomas CK, Stein RB, Gordon T, Lee R, Elleker G (1987) Patterns of reinnervation and motor unit recruitment in human hand muscles after complete ulnar and median nerve section and resuture. J Neurol Neurosurg Psychiatry 50:259–268
23. Totosy de Zepetnek J, Gordon T, Stein RB, Zung HV (1991) Comparison of force and EMG measures in normal and reinnervated tibialis anterior muscles of the rat. Can J Physiol Pharmacol 69:1774–1783
24. Totosy de Zepetnek J, Zung HV, Erdebil S, Gordon T (1992) Innervation ratio is an important determinant of force in normal and reinnervated rat tibialis anterior muscles. J Neurophysiol 67:1385–1403
25. Totosy de Zepetnek J, Zung HV, Erdebil S, Gordon T (1992) Motor units categorization on the basis of contractile and histochemical properties: a glyogen depletion analysis of normal and reinnervated rat Tibialis Anterior muscle. J Neurophysiol 67:1404–1415
26. Vrbova G, Gordon T, Jones R (1978) Nerve-muscle interaction. Chapman and Hall, London

Eur Arch Otorhinolaryngology (1994) [Suppl] : S24–S27

INVITED LECTURES

H. H. Goebel, I. Schneider, D. S. Tews, A. Gunkel, E. Stennert, and W. F. Neiss

Morphologic Studies on Human and Rodent Facial Muscles

Introduction

Denervation of skeletal muscle fibers results in their atrophy. Early morphologic consequences of acutely denervated human muscle fibers are largely unknown. Conversely, morphologic features of human denervated and neurogenically atrophic muscle fibers have been amply established in chronic disorders such as spinal muscular atrophies and neuropathies. The dynamics of these denervating disorders, which include precise onset, velocity of evolution, and completion of denervation and thereby the nerve-supplied metabolic and electrophysiological inputs from the nerve to the corresponding muscle fibre, are morphologically unexplored.

Two additional aspects further complicate interpretation of spontaneous neurogenic processes in human skeletal muscles: reinnervation due to sprouting of axons and a lack of innervation in infantile spinal muscular atrophy and in malformations of the spinal cord. Furthermore, in man our knowledge of denervation is largely based on findings from limb muscles.

Facial muscles are largely exempt from spontaneously occurring spinal muscular atrophies and neuropathies. Denervation of human facial muscles is almost exclusively of the acute type, e. g., by trauma, in the wake of the removal of a tumor, or as Bell's palsy. Myopathology of post-traumatic and spontaneous denervation of facial muscles may be the same, but little is known about it, especially when using modern techniques [9]. Morphologic features of normal human muscle fibers, based on modern enzyme histochemical and morphometric techniques, have also been scantily reported (8); some only in abstracts [4, 5, 7].

H. H. Goebel (✉), I. Schneider, D. S. Tews, A. Gunkel,
E. Stennert, and W. F. Neiss
Abteilung für Neuropathologie der Univ. Mainz,
Langenbeckstrasse 1,
55131 Mainz, Germany

Conventional Morphologic Aspects of Denervation in Human Skeletal Muscle

For decades, groups of atrophic muscle fibers have been considered as evidence of denervation. These muscle fibers comprise both type I and type II fibers using the standard ATPase preparation. At the electron microscopic level, denervated muscle fibers have lost sarcomeres and myofilaments, have decreased in volume, and often may show a separated, shrivelled basal lamina as evidence of shrinkage of the intrinsic myofibers. The arrangement of the sarcotubular network and proliferation of transverse tubules may present additional ultrastructural features of denervated muscle fibers.

Myofibers of angular shape often display increased activity of nonspecific esterase and loss of reciprocity associated with strong enzyme activity of the reduced nicotinamide adenine dinucleotide (NADH) tetrazolium reductase and the menadione-linked α-glycerophosphate dehydrogenase (MAG). When atrophy of reinnervated muscle fibers has completely subsided and normal fiber diameters have been reestablished, fiber type grouping may be the only evidence of a neurogenic process. Strong reactivity and loss of reciprocity in NADH and MAG preparations of angular atrophic denervated muscle fibers may also subside with reinnervation. It is the broad spectrum of ongoing denervation and of subsequent reinnervation of muscle fibers that renders interpretation of human skeletal muscle affected by a spontaneous neurogenic process difficult.

Because of this inability to identify denervation of individual muscle fibers with precision, it is not surprising that immunohistochemical techniques have been employed in analyzing neurogenic processes in muscle. Respective antibodies have been directed against various antigens. These include antibodies against fetal heavy chain myosin to identify possibly noninnervated small myofibers [3], against acetylcholine receptor proteins, against neural cell adhesion molecule (N-CAM), against desmin, the muscle

Fig. 1 A, B Scattered small myofibers are normal in human facial muscles (**A**, m. orbicularis oris), compared to fibers of uniform size in normal human limb muscle (**B**, m. biceps bracchii). ATPase preparation after acid (pH 4.5) preincubation, × 160

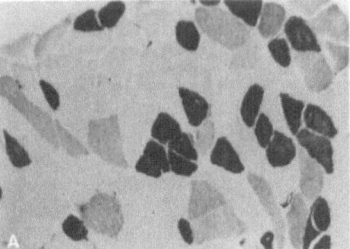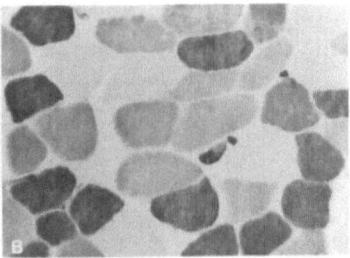

fiber-specific intermediate filament, and against tenascin, an extracellular glycoprotein. While experimental studies of denervated muscle might have brought forth reliable data as to the significance of these antigens with regard to denervation, myopathology of human neurogenic processes is fraught with two further complicating aspects. First, not all atrophic myofibers within neurogenic processes may be labeled, possibly due to the length of the denervation period, i.e., remoteness of the "moment" of complete denervation. Second, certain antigens not necessarily expressed in normal muscle fibers may reappear not only after denervation, but also during regeneration. As reinnervation of denervated atrophic muscle fibers is also associated with regeneration of muscle fibers contents, the state of denervation may be difficult to be distinguished from ongoing reinnervation.

Normal Human Facial Muscles

Based on enzyme histochemical and morphometric techniques, normal human facial muscle fibers show lower mean diameter values than normal human limb muscle fibers. They measure some 45 μm in the adult platysma [6], whereas our own earlier studies [8] revealed somewhat lower values for the platysma, i.e., 40 μm for type II fibers and 33 μm for type I fibers. Similarly, normal type I fibers were slightly smaller than normal type II fibers in the levator labii, zygomaticus major, and orbicularis oris muscles (Fig. 1). The same human facial muscles showed a higher number of type II fibers [8]. Both in our findings [8] and in the studies by Krarup [6], type IIB fibers were found most frequently in the normal human platysma. The distribution in the platysma of fibers types most closely resembled that in normal human limb muscles. The other four human facial muscles showed a predominance of type IIA fibers and a very low frequency of type IIB fibers [8]. Our studies also revealed normal variability coefficients of some 325 in normal facial muscles, above those of normal human limb muscles of 250. The content of neuromuscular junctions in randomly sampled normal human facial muscle is high (Fig. 2). Other structural features at the light and electron microscopic levels are identical in normal human facial and limb muscles [1, 2].

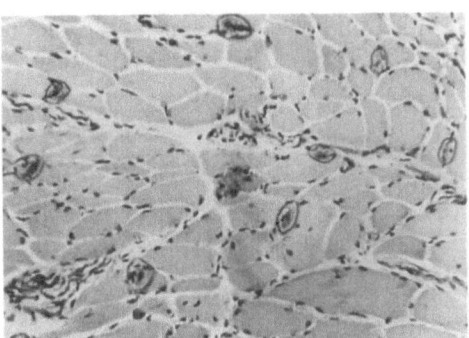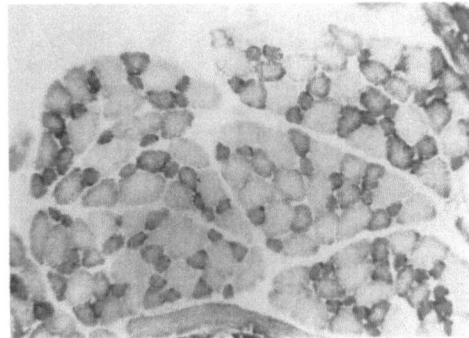

Fig. 2 Numerous motor end plates in a normal human m. orbicularis oris. Acetylcholine esterase preparation, × 168

Fig. 3 Numerous scattered small type I fibers (*dark*) in a normal m. levator labii of the rat. Reduced nicotinamide adenine dinucleotide (NADH) tetrazolium reductase, × 140

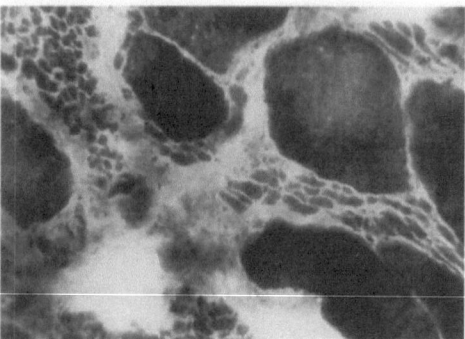

Fig. 4 Groups of highly atrophic fibers and a few scattered large myofibers, human m. orbicularis oris 13 years after denervation due to head trauma. Modified trichrome stain, ×160

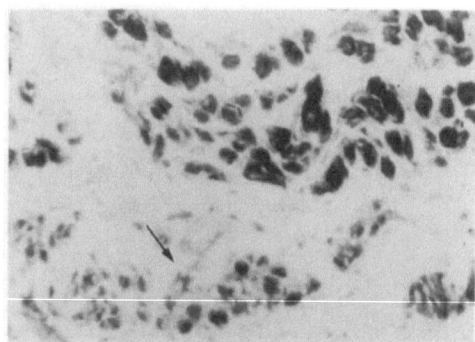

Fig. 5 Group of atrophic muscle fibers (*arrow*) without precise typability in the m. levator labii of the rat 20 weeks after denervation. Reduced nicotinamide adenine dinucleotide (NADH) tetrazolium reductase, ×212

Normal Rodent Facial Muscles

Our preliminary studies on the normal levator labii muscle in the rat also showed a population of small, disseminated type I fibers. Type II fibers were considerably larger in size than type I fibers. The respective frequency for the different fibers types was 33% for type I fibers, 25% for type IIA fibers, and 42% for type IIB fibers (Fig. 3).

Denervated Human Facial Muscles

In denervated human facial muscles [9], atrophy of muscle fibers persists for many years (Fig. 4). Typability of fibers is often lost, though acid ATPase preparations still distinguish type I and type II muscle fibers. A particular feature is fibrosis, the degree of which correlates with length of denervation. These studies were based on 17 samples of zygomatic, orbicularis oris, and levator labii muscles denervated for 1 month to 36 years due to either Bell's palsy or surgical trauma [9]. The wealth of neuromuscular junctions encountered in normal human facial muscles was also absent from denervated facial muscle tissue.

In the auricularis posterior muscle, atrophy of muscle fibers due to denervation appears no earlier than $2^1/_2$ weeks after denervation, with further reduction in fiber diameters over more than 1 year [2]. The ultrastructural features encountered in denervated human facial muscles [2] are similar to those seen in denervated human limb muscles, but a variety of peculiar inclusions such as nemaline, cytoplasmic, filamentous bodies, and tubular structures were encountered in denervated human facial muscles [1].

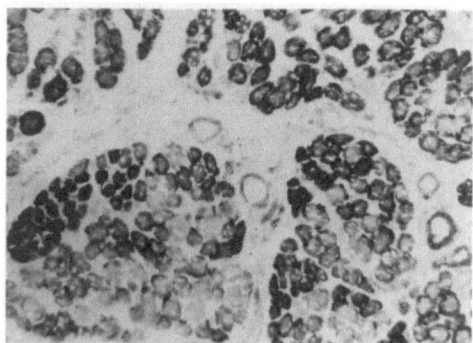

Fig. 6 Grouping of type I (*dark*) and type II (*light*) myofibers in the m. levator labii of the rat 20 weeks after experimental denervation and immediately followed by surgical reanastomosis. Reduced nicotinamide adenine dinucleotide (NADH) tetrazolium reductase, ×120

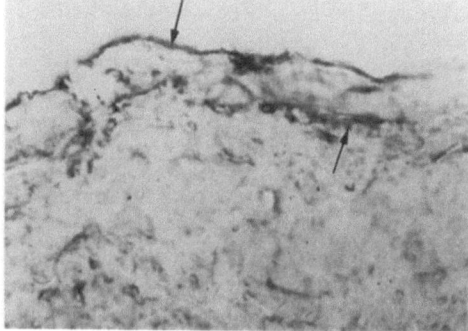

Fig. 7 Muscle fiber surrounded by neutral cell adhesion molecule (N-CAM; *arrows*), m. levator labii of the rat 20 weeks after denervation, ×550

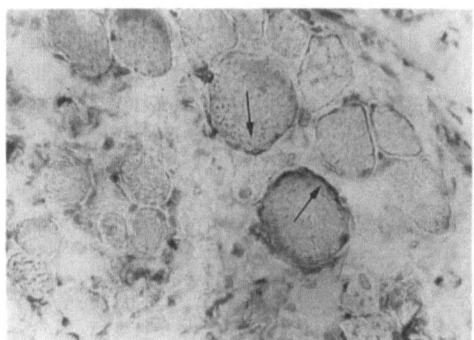

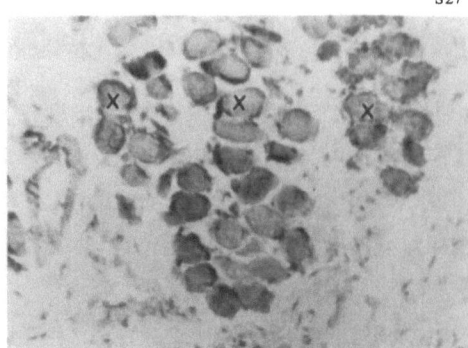

Fig. 8 Neutral cell adhesion molecule is still present around muscle fibers of the m. levator labii of the rat 20 weeks after experimental severance and immediately surgical reanastomosis, ×300

Fig. 9 Numerous myofibers of the m. levator labii of the rat display increased content of desmin 7 weeks after experimental severance of the facial nerve and immediate surgical reanastomosis as evidence of regeneration and reinnervation, ×240

Denervated Rodent Facial Muscles

We recently started an experimental series of denervation and reinnervation by immediate postoperative reanastomosis of the experimentally severed distal facial nerve with the proximal hypoglossal nerve. While denervation alone produced the expected atrophy of myofibers as well as loss of typability (Fig. 5), immediate reanastomosis resulted in fiber type grouping at the same postdenervation and post-reinnervation period (Fig. 6). N-CAM, the extracellular protein appearing after denervation, was also present around denervated muscle fibers (Fig. 7), but was occasionally also seen around muscle fibers after reanastomosis (Fig. 8). The effect of both denervation and reinnervation was also evident in desmin-positive muscle fibers (Fig. 9).

Comment

Samples of biopsied denervated human facial muscle provided data commensurate with those obtained from biopsied denervated limb muscles. It may be the exact timing of the denervation process affecting human facial muscles that enables testing of the usefulness of recent immunohistochemical techniques and the validity of particular denervation-related antigens. Moreover, experimental denervation and reinnervation by reanastomosis may provide additional information on reinnervation that may then aid in the interpretation of the corresponding human data.

Acknowledgements This study was financially supported by the Deutsche Forschungsgemeinschaft (Ne 412/1-1) and the Deutsche Gesellschaft zur Bekämpfung der Muskelkrankheiten e. V. Dr. Faisser kindly provided antibodies against tenascin and B. Schoser introduced its immunohistochemical demonstration into our laboratory. We are grateful to Andrea Schollmayer and Margarete Schlie for light microscopic preparations, to Walter Meffert for photography, to Amanda Bastian for linguistic assistance, and to Astrid Wöber for secretarial aid.

References

1. Bardosi G, Goebel HH, Stennert E (1987) The ultrastructure of normal and denervated human facial muscle. Plast Reconstr Surg 79:171–176
2. Belal A Jr (1982) Structure of human muscle in facial paralysis. J Laryngol Otol 96:325–334
3. Biral D, Scarpini E, Angelini C, Salvati G, Margreth A (1989) Myosin heavy chain composition of muscle fibers in spinal muscular atrophy. Muscle Nerve 12:43–51
4. Blaivas M, Nelson C (1990) Aging changes in human orbicularis oculi muscle (abstract). J Neuropathol Exp Neurol 49:298
5. Blaivas M, Nelson CC (1991) Ultrastructural characteristics of human orbicularis oculi muscle at various ages. J Neuropathol Exp Neurol 50:351 (abstr)
6. Krarup C (1977) Electrical and mechanical responses in the platysma and in the adductor pollicis muscle: in normal subjects. J Neurol Neurosurg Psychiatry 40:234–240
7. Nelson C, Blaivas M (1990) Histologic and histochemical characteristics of eye brow and eyelid muscles. J Neuropathol Exp Neurol 49:298 (abstr)
8. Schwarting S, Schröder M, Stennert E, Goebel HH (1982) Enzyme histochemical and histographic data on normal human facial muscles. ORL J Otorhinolaryngol Relat Spec 44:51–59
9. Schwarting S, Schröder M, Stennert E, Goebel HH (1984) Morphology of denervated human facial muscles. ORL J Otorhinolaryngol Relat Spec 46:248–256

Eur Arch Otorhinolaryngology (1994) [Suppl] : S28–S30

A. Irintchev and A. Wernig

Denervation and Reinnervation of Muscle: Physiological Effects

Introduction

The degree of motor function recovery after peripheral nerve injury is determined by different factors such as type of nerve trauma, duration of the denervation period, correct reestablishment of motor and sensory connections, degree of reinnervation, and status of the muscle. In this paper we consider muscle reinnervation after long-term denervation, changes in the denervated nerve stem, and functional effects of myoblast implantation into adult muscles.

Reinnervation after Long-Term Denervation

To study the impact of a long delay in muscle reinnervation in the mouse, we recently used repeated local freezing of the sciatic nerve to maintain muscles denervated over a long period of time (7 months) [7]. This procedure leads to a rapid and extensive muscle atrophy; maximum isometric muscle tension of denervated muscles is reduced to less than 10% of the contralateral muscles by the end of the second month and further declines thereafter.

The prolonged denervation and repeated nerve injury negatively affected axon regeneration. Regrowth and/or myelination of axons were largely delayed, since the number of myelinated axons in soleus nerves reached control values only after 3 months of reinnervation (compare, e.g., with 220% of control 1 month after three repeated nerve freezings, [12]). Axon numbers increased to 150% of control after 6 months reinnervation and declined thereafter (125% at 9–10 months). Production of supernumerary

axons usually occurs in regenerating nerves and is even enhanced after repeated injury [12, 13, 21]. The changes in axon numbers during the reinnervation period are accompanied by synaptic rearrangements, i.e., remodeling of motor units in the muscle, as can be seen from continual changes in muscle fiber type composition ([7], see [26] for a review). Strikingly though, nerve fiber diameters remained abnormally small; even after 10 months of reinnervation fiber diameters were unimodally distributed with a mean diameter of 3.3 µm, in contrast to the bimodal distribution in intact nerves (mean values, 3.9 and 9.0 µm, respectively; Fig. 1). Thus, despite the presence of supernumerary axons, total fiber cross-sectional area per nerve remained around 50% of contralateral nerves, at 10 months after reinnervation. Finally, the relative thickness of the myelin sheath (g ratio, i.e., axon to fiber diameter) did not return to normal until 9–10 months.

Soleus muscle force improved quite slowly during the reinnervation period. Maximal, though incomplete, recovery was achieved after 5 months, but peak tetanic tension

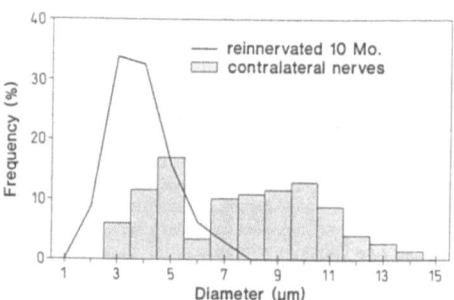

Fig. 1 Frequency distributions of myelinated nerve fiber diameters in regenerated (three nerves and 240 nerve fibers measured) and intact contralateral (two nerves and 148 nerve fibers measured) soleus nerves at 10 months of reinnervation

A. Irintchev, A. Wernig (✉)
Institute of Physiology/Neurophysiology
University of Bonn, Wilhelmstrasse 31,
53111 Bonn, Germany

did not reach on average more than 85% of age-matched intact muscles. Since total numbers of muscle fibers and specific muscle force (tension per unit muscle weight) were similar in reinnervated and control soleus muscles, the deficit in muscle force is solely due to the reduced muscle fiber diameters observed.

Denervated Nerve Stem

Growth of injured peripheral axons is largely dependent on the cellular and molecular environment in the distal nerve stem (see also W. Tetzlaff, this volume). Prolonged denervation has negative impacts on this environment, e.g., progressive reduction of the proliferative and myelinating capacity of the Schwann cells, loss of the growth substrate laminin, and endoneurial changes [15, 17, 18]. Special attention in this context should be paid to cell adhesion and extracellular matrix molecules, e.g., the neural cell adhesion molecule (N-CAM and tenascin/J1, which are upregulated in denervated or regenerating nerves and are known to be involved in cell-cell and cell-matrix interactions [11, 16]. Recent experiments in our laboratory [27] show delay in muscle reinnervation after application of antibodies to tenascin/J1 onto short-term denervated muscles, suggesting that such molecules play a functional role in early peripheral reinnervation.

Little is known about the consequences of prolonged denervation on the regenerative capacity of motoneurons. Observations of reduced motoneuron soma size [10] and reduced RNA levels [23] after prolonged denervation indicate a profound central impact. In the most dramatic case, when establishment of peripheral connections is impossible (leg amputations in humans), numerous motoneurons die within several years [9]. In this respect, trophic factors such as a recently discovered motoneuron survival factor (ciliary neurotrophic factor [20]) and synaptic phenomena such as synaptic stripping (post-traumatic deafferentation) of the motoneuron somata [2, 4] deserve special attention.

Implantation of Myogenic Cells

Muscle fiber loss after denervation lasting many months or years has been observed both in man and in animals [6, 22]. Recent investigations show continual degeneration and necrosis of muscle fibers in chronically denervated muscles, which, however, is accompanied by an increased myogenic activity of satellite cells serving to preserve muscle tissue [1, 3, 19]. Yet it is also clear that the proliferative capacity of the satellite cell pool is gradually exhausted with time and at some point (probably dependant on muscle type and species) muscle fiber death becomes dominant [1]. Therefore, a major factor on the part of the muscle which determines recovery after reinnerva-

tion appears to be the degree of preservation of the myogenic capacity of the muscle satellite cell pool.

Exhaustion of the satellite cell pool might cause or possibly also contribute to muscle weakness in other muscle diseases. We are therefore currently interested in whether implantation of isolated and in vitro expanded myogenic cells might contribute to the functional recovery of diseased muscles (for a review of myoblast transfer see [14]). Experiments with some permanent lines of mouse myoblasts showed positive effects of implantation in muscles reinnervated after long-term denervation, paralyzed with botulinum toxin A, or regenerating after cryodamage [25]. The implanted cells survived and gave progeny to extensive numbers of new muscle fibers, which in turn became functionally innervated and significantly improved muscle force. Largest effects were observed in cryodamaged muscles: increase in muscle tension by 57%, in muscle weight by 82%, and in the total number of muscle fibers by 400% as compared to spontaneously regenerated muscles at 8–18 weeks postimplantation.

On the other hand, the positive functional results of transplantation of permanent mouse myoblast lines were marred by late development of tumors in the injected limbs [25]. While this might prove to be particularly frequent in the case of permanent (i.e., transformed) cell lines, a general possibility for expanded primary cultures cannot at present be excluded. Furthermore, immune rejection of implanted myoblasts, even in case of host-donor histocompatibility, appears to be common (see, e.g., [8, 24] for human studies see [5]). In regenerating mouse muscles such rejection has serious consequences in that muscle force by maximal recovery remained only 50%–60% of control [24].

Acknowledgements The investigations reported here were supported by grants from the Deutsche Forschungsgemeinschaft (We 859) and the Hermann und Lilly Schilling Stiftung.

References

1. Anzil AP, Wernig A (1989) Muscle fibre loss and reinnervation after long-term denervation. J Neurocytol 18:833–845
2. Blinzinger K, Kreutzberg G (1968) Displacement of synaptic terminals from regenerating motoneurons by microglial cells. Z Zellforsch Mikrosk Anat 85:145–157
3. Carraro U, Morale D, Mussini I, Lucke S, Cantini M, Betto R, Catani C, Libera LD, Betto DD, Noventa D (1985) Chronic denervation of rat hemidiaphragm: maintenance of fibre heterogeneity with associated increasing uniformity of myosin isoforms. J Cell Biol 100:161–174
4. Graeber MB, Kreutzberg GW (1988) Delayed astrocyte reaction following facial nerve axotomy. J Neurocytol 17:209–220
5. Gussoni E, Pavlath GK, Lanctot AM, Sharma KR, Miller RG, Steinman L, Blau HM (1992) Normal dystrophin transcripts detected in Duchenne muscular dystrophy patients after myoblast transplantation. Nature 356:435–438
6. Gutmann E, Zelená J (1962) Morphological changes in the denervated muscle. In: Gutmann E (ed) The denervated muscle. Czechoslovak Academy of Sciences, Prague, pp 57–102

7. Irintchev A, Draguhn A, Wernig A (1990) Reinnervation and recovery of mouse soleus muscle after long-term denervation. Neuroscience 39:231–243

8. Irintchev A, Wernig A, Lange G (1992) Transient protection of incompatible myoblast grafts in the mouse by cyclosporin A. Eur J Neurosci Suppl 5:115

9. Kawamura Y, Dyck PJ (1989) Permanent axotomy by amputation results in loss of motor neurons in man. J Neuropathol Exp Neurol 40:658–666

10. Lieberman AR (1971) The axon reaction: a review of the principal features of perikaryal responses to axon injury. Int Rev Neurobiol 14:42–124

11. Martini R, Schachner M, Faissner A (1990) Enhanced expression of the extracellular matrix molecule J1/tenascin in the regenerating adult mouse sciatic nerve. J Neurocytol 19:601–616

12. Mira JC (1979) Quantitative studies of the regeneration of rat myelinated nerve fibres: variations in the number and size of regenerating fibres after repeated localized freezings. J Anat 129:77–93

13. Ohara S, Ikuta F (1988) Schwann cell responses during regeneration after one or more crush injuries to myelinated nerve fibers. Neuropathol Appl Neurobiol 14:229–245

14. Partridge TA (1991) Myoblast transfer: a possible therapy for inherited myopathies? Muscle Nerve 14:197–212

15. Pellegrino RG, Spencer PS (1985) Schwann cell mitosis in response to regenerating peripheral axons in vivo. Brain Res 341:16–25

16. Rieger F (1990) Localization and potential role of cell adhesion molecules and cytotactin in the developing, diseased, and regenerating neuromuscular system. In: Edelman GM, Cunningham BA, Thiery JP (eds) Morphoregulatory molecules. Wiley, New York, pp 421–441

17. Röyttä M, Salonen V (1988) Long-term endoneurial changes after nerve transection. Acta Neuropathol 76:35–45

18. Salonen V, Peltonen J, Röyttä M, Virtanen I (1987) Laminin in traumatized peripheral nerve: basement membrane changes during degeneration and regeneration. J Neurocytol 16:713–720

19. Schmalbruch H, Al-Amood WS, Lewis DM (1991) Morphology of long-term denervated rat soleus muscle and the effect of chronic electrical stimulation. J Physiol (Lond) 441:233–241

20. Sendtner M, Kreutzberg GW, Thoenen H (1990) Ciliary neurotrophic factor prevents the degeneration of motor neurons after axotomy. Nature 345:440–441

21. Toft PB, Fugleholm K, Schmalbruch H (1988) Axonal branching following crush lesions of peripheral nerves of rat. Muscle Nerve 11:880–889

22. Tower SS (1939) The reaction of muscle to denervation. Physiol Rev 19:1–48

23. Watson WE (1968) Observation on the nucleolar and total cell body nucleic acid of injured nerve cells. J Physiol (Lond) 196:655–676

24. Wernig A, Irintchev A (1992) Immune rejection of implanted myogenic cells in MHC-compatible hosts. Eur J Neurosci Suppl 5:115

25. Wernig A, Irintchev A, Härtling A, Zimmermann K, Starzinski-Powitz A (1991) Formation of new muscle fibres and tumours after injection of cultured myogenic cells. J Neurocytol 20:982–997

26. Wernig A, Salvini TF, Langenfeld-Oster B, Irintchev A, Dorlöchter M (1991) Endplate and motor unit remodelling in vertebrate muscles. In: Wernig A (ed) Plasticity of motoneuronal connections. Restorative neurology, vol 5. Elsevier, Amsterdam, pp 85–100

27. Wernig A, Langenfeld-Oster B, Faissner A (1992) Tenascin antibodies delay reinnervation of mammalian endplates. Eur J Neurosci Suppl 5:188

Eur Arch Otorhinolaryngology (1994) [Suppl]: S31–S36

INVITED LECTURES

A. Belal

Postdenervation Muscular Changes in Facial Paralysis

Introduction

Though facial paralysis is primarily manifested by weakness of the facial muscles, the study of denervation changes in these muscles has received little attention by researchers and clinicians working in this field. The present report reviews what happens in the facial muscles following facial paralysis of varying duration.

Review of Literature

Animal Experiments

M. Lyon and L. Malmgren (1982, personal communication) reported on the histochemical characteristics of the stapedius muscle of the cat. The major fiber type present was the fast oxidative glycolytic type (77%). Two other types of fibers were found. One had little staining with actinomysin ATPase, while the other stained densely for this enzyme. They concluded that the stapedius muscle is capable of fast repetitive contractions. The other two types of fibers may represent some specialized sensory structures, i. e., unencapsulated muscle spindles. Other morphological [6] and ultrastructural [7] studies on the stapedius muscle of the cat and rabbit were reported.

Iwano et al. [8] and Kanasaki et al. [9] reported the postdenervation changes in the facial muscles of the rat. Atrophic changes were evident 8 weeks following facial nerve transection. These were associated with histochemical changes in mycosin ATPase and actomyosin ARPase.

Abdel-Baki et al. [1] reported the postdenervation changes in the facial muscles of 15 rabbits 3–5 weeks following facial nerve transection. Atrophic changes were evident 3 weeks after denervation. They claimed that electrotherapy for 2 weeks delays the appearance of these changes.

Human Pathological Studies

Belal [2, 4] reported the normal light microscopic and ultrastructural characteristics of the human stapedius muscle and auricularis posterior. He also reported the effects of denervation of these muscles in 14 patients with total facial paralysis with varying duration ranging from 10 days to 6 years. He recommended muscle biopsy [2, 3] in long-standing facial paralysis and facial paralysis at birth. Similar recommendations were made by Crumley [5]. Stennert et al. [13] reported on the morphology of human mimetic musculature and the effect of facial paralysis from 1 month to 36 years on this musculature. They found that even after 36 years of facial paralysis, muscle fibers were still present, though highly atrophic.

Saito et al. [11] reported the temporal bone findings in a patient with Mobius syndrome. Though the facial nerve disappeared in the horizontal segment, the stapedius muscle was normally developed. This suggested that stapedius muscle may have a different brain stem nucleus separate from other facial mimetic muscles.

Normal Facial Muscles

Facial muscle fibers such as striated muscles of the body are grouped together in bundles or fascicles which are separated by perimysial connective tissue. Striated muscle fibers are multinucleated cylindrical cells with nuclei placed at the periphery under the sarcolemmic membrane.

Each muscle fiber is made up of filaments of contractile proteins which are arranged in bundles of hundreds to thousands of myofibrils. Each muscle fiber is surrounded by endomysial connective tissue and the fibers are grouped together into bundles or fascicles, which are in turn separated from each other by perimysial connective tissue. The sarcolemma consists of an inner plasma membrane dotted by invaginations and an outer basement membrane. The subsarcolemmic nuclei are elliptical in shape with well-

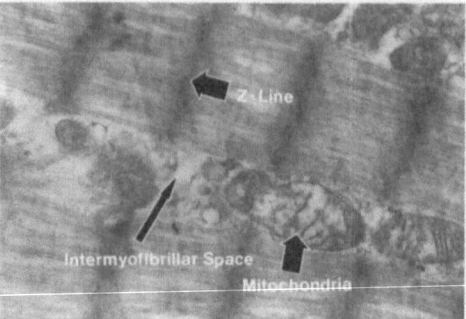

Fig. 1 Transmission electron microscopy (TEM) photograph of normal human auricularis posterior muscle. Muscle was biopsied during the course of tympanoplasty. The myofibrils show the cross-striated pattern and intact Z lines characteristic of normal fibers. Original, ×36 100

defined nucleoli and finely stippled nucleoplasm. The cross-striated pattern of the myofibrils is made by the repetition of light A bands alternating with dark I bands. Under the electron microscope (Fig. 1), the larger of the proteins, myosin, can be seen as a thick filament. These thick filaments are arranged in parallel fashion and each extends throughout the length of the A band. Interdigitating with the thick filaments are thin filaments made up of actin. These are also arranged in parallel fashion and are attached to the Z line, which is situated in the middle of the I band. One sarcomere is that part of the myofibril between two adjacent Z lines. Each myofibril is separated from its neighbor by the intermyofibrillar space. This space contains aqueous sarcoplasm, mitochondria, sarcoplasmic reticulum, the transverse tubular system (T system), glycogen particles, fat droplets, myoglobin, and enzymes. Mitochondria are small stuctures recognized by the complex cristae of their inner membrane and are most frequently located in the intermyofibrillar space on either side of the Z line. The tubules of the sarcoplasmic reticulum are arranged in a longitudinal way irregularly surrounding the myofibrils. The transverse tubular system (T system), on the other hand, extends transversely across the fiber from its connection to the sarcolemma. Glycogen granules are not limited to any one part of the muscle fiber, but tend to occur in greater numbers in the I band. Various other structures may be present in associaton with muscle fibers, including satellite cells, muscle spindles, blood vessels, and nerves.

Morphologic Characteristics

The normal adult human facial muscle fibers differ from human limb muscle fibers in that they are 50% smaller in

diameter. The average diameter of auricularis posterior muscle fibers is 14.8 μm [2]. There are as many or more type II fibers than there are type I fibers [13].

Muscle Characteristics

The stapedius muscle differs from the rest of the facial mimetic musculature in that it consists mainly of type II (red) fibers, which have thicker Z lines, more mitochondria, less glycogen, and more compactly arranged myofibrils (Fig. 2).

Species Characteristics

Human normal facial muscles differ from the rabbit's facial muscles in the following: The rabbit's facial muscle fibers have a smaller diameter and there is a higher proportion of type II fibers (ATPase reaction), reflecting a high speed of contraction. The type II fiber population, in these muscles can be further subdivided into A (light) and B and C (intermediate) groups. The stapedius muscle consists of type II B and C fibers, while the rest of the facial muscles have 50% type II B and C fibers. This may reflect the speed of contraction and fatigue index of these muscles.

Denervated Facial Muscles

Light Microscopy Changes

Very few of the histological changes, if any, are pathognomonic of denervation changes (see Table 1).

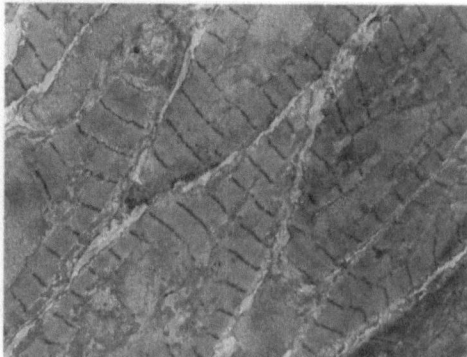

Fig. 2 Transmission electron microscopy (TEM) photograph of normal human stapedius muscle taken during the course of acoustic tumor removal. The muscle fibers are mostly type II fibers. Magnification, ×9000

Table 1 Postdenervation light microscopy changes in facial muscles

Structure	Pathological change
Subsarcolemmic nuclei	Prominent Central migration Noticeable increase in number Altered shape (small) Altered staining (pyknotic)
Myofibrils	Changes in fiber size Distinct population of small atrophic and large normal fibers, small or large group atrophy Degeneration
Cellular reactions	Endomysial fibrosis
Blood vessels	Congestion

Changes in Fiber Size

The earliest change in the size of myofibrils is noticed $2^{1}/_{2}$ weeks following denervation. The reduction in the size of the fibers is uniform. Distinct atrophy of a group of fibers is apparent $1^{1}/_{2}$ months following denervation. At 13 months many muscle fibers are atrophied.

Abnormalities in Fiber Distribution

It is characteristic of denervation atrophy that the pathological changes are not uniformly distributed throughout the muscle, but are more marked in some areas than in others. Atrophy of small groups of fibers surrounded by relatively normal-sized fibers is noted $1^{1}/_{2}$ months following facial paralysis, while large segments of atrophied muscle lying next to muscle fascicles which are relatively normal are noted 1 year following facial paralysis.

Changes in Subsarcolemmic Nuclei

The subsarcolemmic nuclei appear to be enlarged and vesicular and are present in increased numbers in the early stages of degeneraton, but later on the nuclei appear small and pyknotic and are clumped into groups.

Atrophy and Degeneration

While atrophy of the muscle fibers (reduction in the size of the filament while its form is conserved) is observed as early as $1^{1}/_{2}$ months after facial paralysis, these muscles seem resistant to degeneration. Degeneration (destruction of the muscle fiber to the point that it is unrecognizable) starts about 1 year following facial paralysis. Degenerated muscle fibers are seen in biopsy specimens in the form of a coarse granular material which has replaced the fiber structure.

Cellular Reactions

No evidence of cellular response is seen within the muscle fibers or in the supporting tissues. There is apparent proliferation of endomysial fibrous tissue in chronic cases.

Ultrastructural Changes

Changes in the fine structure of human skeletal muscle following denervation are summarized in Table 2.

Sarcolemma

The plasma and basement membranes are intact as a rule, even when myofibrils degenerate, and the latter often retain their normal relationship to the basement membrane. In some fibers, the basement membrane becomes dissociated from the plasma membrane and appears as a loose, scalloped layer. In other fibers the sarcolemma shows mitochondria-laden outpouchings.

Subsarcolemmic Nuclei

The subsarcolemmic nuclei often have deeply infolded, nucleolar membranes. A common finding is the migraton of one or more nuclei to a central location in a muscle cell. There is an apparent increase in the number of nuclei arranged in chains (Fig. 3) and the nuclei show peripheral chromatin aggregations.

Myofilaments

Loss of myofilaments and disruption of the normal banding patterns are the most striking changes noticed under the electron microscope. The extent of filament disruption is variable and focal disruption appears as early as $2^{1}/_{2}$ weeks following denervation. After 1 year some fibers show dissolution (Fig. 4), although such fibers have normal-appearing sarcolemmas surrounding closely packed gray amorphous material (fibrillary debris). Within this latter material are an occasional myofibril, mitochondria, glycogen particles, and variably shaped tubules. With the

Table 2 Postdenervation ultrastructural changes in facial muscles

Structure	Pathological change
Sarcolemma	Dissociation of plasma and basement membranes Mitochondria-laden outpouchings
Subsarcolemmic nuclei	Increased number Peripheral chromatin aggregations Dispersal of nucleolar substance Infoldings of nucleolar membrane Pinching off Central location
Myofilaments	Irregularity of Z Line Fragmentation of Z line Disruption of myofilament Dissolution of myofilament
Mitochondria	Subsarcolemmic aggregates Abnormally large Increased ribosomes
Otner organelles	Aggregates of tubular structures Lipofuscin granules Collagen fibers

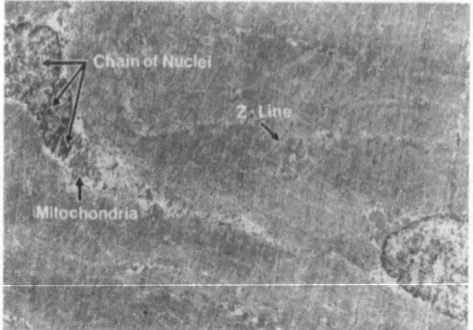

Fig. 3 Transmission electron microscopy (TEM) photograph of human auricularis posterior muscle 10 days after the onset of facial palsy associated with herpes zoster cephalicus. Muscle was biopsied during the course of facial nerve decompression. The subsarcolemmic nuclei are arranged like a chain and show peripheral chromatin aggregations. Original, ×6460

loss of myofilaments, the Z line shows focal irregularity and fragmentation. At a later stage, dissolution of the Z line occurs, as represented by the appearance of dense osmiophilic granules scattered throughout the sarcoplasm.

Mitochondria

Subsarcolemmic aggregation of mitochondria results in outpouchings of the sarcolemmic membrane. These organelles are of normal shape and density. Large mitochondria, oval in shape and with abnormally arranged cristae, are seen infrequently.

Other Subcellular Organelles

There is an increase in the number of ribosomes and in the amount of sarcoplasmic reticulum in the subsarcolemmic region. The ribosomes are abnormally large and the sarcoplasmic reticulum has abnormal aggregates of tubular structures. Densely osmiophilic particles thought to represent lipofuscin pigment accumulation are occasionally seen.

Natural History Of Denervation Changes

The first evidence of denervation muscular atrophy (see Table 3) is noticed 10 days following facial paralysis. The subsarcolemmic nuclei show deep infoldings of the nucleolar membrane; peripheral chromatin aggregations and nuclei are arranged in chains. Focal disruption and dissolution of myofilaments starts as early as $2\frac{1}{2}$ weeks following denervation. This is associated with fragmentation of Z lines and subsarcolemmic mitochondrial hyperplasia. Decrease in the size of the muscle fibers is noticed as early as $1\frac{1}{2}$ months following paralysis. Atrophy of small and large groups of muscle fibers can be seen $1\frac{1}{2}$ and 13 months after denervation, respectively. Decrease in the size of muscle fibers is associated with central migration of subsarcolemmic nuclei, scalloping and indentation of the sarcolemmic membrane, and the appearance of abnormal aggregates of subcellular organelles and particles. Degeneration of some myofibrils starts as early as 1 year after denervation, but progresses slowly in the facial muscles and may not be complete even 36 years after denervation [13].

Fig. 4 Transmission electron microscopy (TEM) photograph of human auricularis posterior muscle 13 months after facial paralysis following translabyrinthine removal of an acoustic tumor. Muscle was biopsied during the course of facial-hypoglossal nerve anastomosis. The degenerated muscle fiber has a normal-appearing sarcolemma surrounding closely packed fibrillary debris consisting of a few myofibrils, mitochondria, glycogen particles, and variably shaped tubules. Original, ×11400

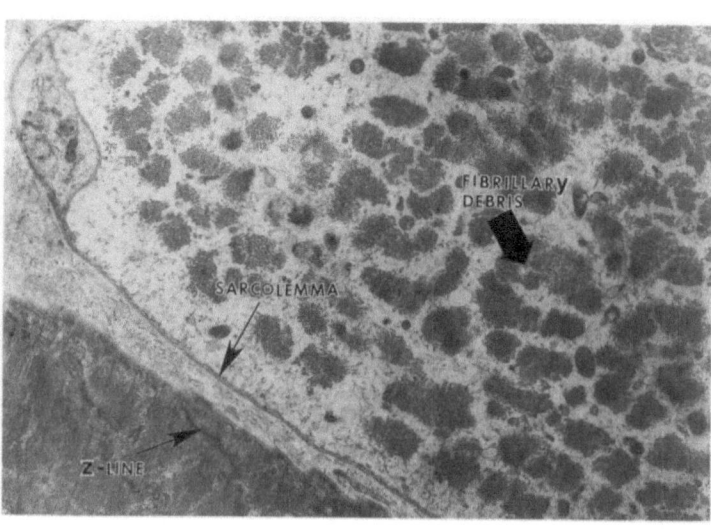

Table 3 Natural history of facial muscle atrophy following denervation

Time after onset of facial paralysis	Pathological change
10 days	Chains in subsarcolemmic nuclei Infoldings of nucleolar membrane No myofibrillar changes
2.5 weeks	Focal myofibrillar disruption Fragmentation of Z line Subsarcolemmic mitochondrial hyperplasia Indentations of sarcolemma
1.5 months	Small group atrophy of myofibrils Central migration of nuclei Disruption of some myofibrils
13 months	Large group atrophy of myofibrils Degenerated myofibrils
6 years	Large group atrophy of myofibrils Dissociation of plasma and basement membranes Increased collagen filaments

Facial Muscle Characteristics

Atrophy and degeneration affects both types of facial muscle fibers (I and II) equally and thus fiber grouping, usually encountered in human limb muscles, is absent [13].

Muscle Characteristics

The stapedius myofibrils are less liable to degneration than the rest of the facial mimetic muscles. This may be attributed to the fact that the stapedius muscle may have a different brain stem nucleus, thus possibly facial paralysis may be incomplete and regeneration is faster than in the rest of the facial muscles.

Species Characteristics

Denervation of facial muscles in experimental animals differs from humans in the following: degenerative changes and inflammatory reaction are evident as early as 4 weeks after nerve transection (Fig. 5). Eight weeks after denervation, almost all muscle fibers disappear and are replaced by fibrous tissue. These changes are similar to those occurring in very fast contracting oxidative muscles.

Clinical Applications

The applications of the knowledge we gained from studying the effect of denervation on the facial muscles seems to be concentrated on three clinical entities: facial paralysis at birth, long-standing facial paralysis, and difficult cases of facial paralysis.

Facial paralysis noticed at birth may be caused either by trauma, e.g., forceps delivery, or as a congenital anomaly. The differentiation of these two entities is important both from the medicolegal and the therapeutic point of view.

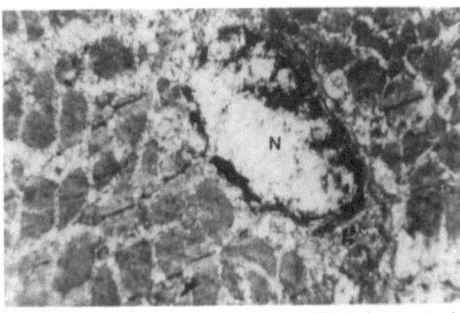

Fig. 5 Transmission electron microscopy (TEM) photograph of rabbit's buccinator 3 weeks following facial nerve transection (*N*, nucleus)

This differentiation is also important for the parents as far as future babies are concerned. Congenital facial palsy may occur alone or in association with other anomalies, e. g., Möbius syndrome. It may be uni- or bilateral, segmental or complete. The majority of cases are less than complete, and the lower lip is usually spared. The vertical part of the facial nerve is absent; this can be detected on CT scan. The stapedius nerve and chorda tympani are intact. Electrical testing of the facial nerve is of limited value up to 2 years of age, because the nerve myelin is immature and there is no cooperation from the baby.

Auditory brain-stem response (ABR) testing may show prolonged III and V waves. This may be associated with cranial nerve dificits, minor deformities of the external ear, and other developmental anomalies. Möbius syndrome is a specific clinical entity that entails unilateral or bilateral facial dysplasia, cranial nerve plasies, and extremity deformities.

Muscle biopsy of the facial muscles in congenital facial plasy reveals uniform distribution of hypoplastic muscle fibers. The muscles biopsied for this purpose should be the muscles of interest to the surgeon, e. g., levator labii superioris in the nasolabial fold for the buccal smile muscles and orbicularis oculi through a lateral brow incision for eye closure muscles.

Surgical decompression of the facial nerve is contraindicated in these cases. Should this be done, the vertical part of the facial nerve is usually represented by a fibrovascular tissue. Biopsy of this structure confirms the developmental nature of the case.

The primary concern in these cases is reanimation of eye closure muscles by using a lid spring. Muscle transfer or free neuromuscular vascular pedicles may be tried at a later age.

Traumatic facial paralysis noticed at birth, on the other hand, may be associated with a history of forceps delivery, ecchymosis over the mastoid process, and other signs of trauma to the face or limbs. CT scan may reveal fracture lines in the temporal bone, and electromyography may show fibrillation potentials. Muscle biopsy in these cases reveals a neurogenic pattern of two distinct populations of muscle fibers – small and large. Atrophic muscle fibers show pyknotic nuclear clumps, small angulated fibers, and other abnormalities of sarcolemma and mitochondria. Surgical decompression of the facial nerve in these cases is helpful if complete facial paralysis does not recover.

Cases of long-standing facial paralysis, i.e., 2–4 years or more, usually present a therapeutic dilemma to the otologist. The choice of reanimation technique in these cases is between reinnervating the facial muscles or using myofacial slings to replace the already degenerated fibrosed muscles. Obviously, the choice depends on two factors: the condition of the facial nerve and the status of the facial muscles.

Biopsy of the facial nerve in cases of long-standing paralysis [15] have shown that the nerve axons decrease in size and number by almost half in the first 3 months following paralysis. By the end of 4 years, the distal stump of the transected facial nerve is almost replaced by a fibrous cord.

Conclusion

The study of postdenervation changes in the facial muscles has shown that by the end of 1 year postparalysis there is atrophy of large groups of muscle fibers. Degeneration of myofibrils followed subsequently by their disappearance and replacement with fibrous tissue starts after 1 year of paralysis, but it may not be complete even after 36 years of paralysis [13].

There are individual variations as regards these degenerative changes in terms of when they start and the extent to

which they occur. To conclude, a case of long-standing facial paralysis can be handled by nerve biopsy of the distal stump of the facial nerve for nerve fibers, axon-myelin ratio, and fibrosis, as well as muscle biopsy for muscle fibers and fibrosis. The technique of facial reanimation depends on the results of these biopsies.

One in a while, a case of facial paralysis presents a diagnostic dilemma to the clinician. Such is the case with bilateral, alternating, recurrent facial paralysis or cases associated with generalized myopathic syndromes. Table 4 summarizes genetic and acquired myopathies associated with facial paralysis. Muscle biopsies in these cases show diffuse abnormality of all muscle fibers, in which fiber splitting and necrosis, internal nuclei, phagocytosis, basophilia, and fibrosis are observed. Sahashi et al. [14] reported involvement of the facial muscles in chronic progressive external ophthalmoplegia. This condition results from functional and biogenetic abnormalities of intracellular mitochondria.

Table 4 Facial myopathies

Genetic Myopathies
  Muscular dystrophies
    Facioscapulohumoral dystrophy
    Scapuloperoneal dystrophy
    Ocular and oculopharyngeal dystrophy
    Congenital muscular dystrophy
    Mobius syndrome
    Learns-Sayre syndrome
  Myotonic disorders
    Myotonic dystrophy
  Specific congenital myopathies
    Centronuclear myopathy

Acquired Myopathies
  Inflammatory myopathies
    Polymyositis complicating:
      Periarteritis nodosa
      Melkerson-Rosenthal syndrome
      Sjogren's syndrome
      Granulomateous myositis, e.g., sarcoidosis
  Endocrine myopathies
    Acromegaly
    Hyperthyroidism
    Hypothyroidism
  Toxic myopathies
    Alcohol
    Drugs

References

1. Abde-Baki F et al. (1987) The effect of denervation on facial muscles of rabbit and the role of electrotherapy: histological and electron microscopic study. Egypt J Otolaryngol 4:25–32
2. Belal A (1982) Auricularis posterior muscle biopsy. Am J Otol 3:216–220
3. Belal A (1984) Muscle biopsy in facial palsy. In: Portmann M (ed) Proceedings of the 5th international symposium of the facial nerve, pp 194–197
4. Belal A (1985) Structure of human muscle in facial paralysis: role of muscle biopsy. In: May M (ed) The facial nerve, pp 99–106
5. Crumley R (1982) Current status of muscle biopsy in facial paralysis. Facial paralysis study group. AAO, Dollars, Texas
6. Densert O, Wersall J (1974) The morphology of middle ear muscles in mammals. In: Keidel WD, Neff WD (eds) Handbook of sensory physiology, vol 5. Springer, Berlin Heidelberg New York
7. Hirayama M, Daly JF (1974) Ultrastructure of the middle ear muscles in the rabbit. I. Stapedius muscle. Acta Otolaryngol 77:13–18
8. Iwano F, Kituchi A, Koike Y (1984) Post-denervation changes in facial muscles in rats. Facial N Res Jpn 4:61–63
9. Kawasaki K et al. (1986) Changes in the facial muscles of rats after denervation – biochemical and histological observation of myosin ATPase. Facial N Res Jpn 6:54–56
10. Sahgal V, Hast MH (1986) Effect of denervation on primate laryngeal muscles: a morphologic and morphometric study. J Laryngol Otol 100:553–560
11. Saito H, Kishimoto S, Furuta M (1981) Temporal bone findings in a patient with Möbius syndrome. Ann Otol Rhinol Laryngol 90:80–84
12. Schwarting S et al. (1984) Morphology of denervated human facial muscles. ORL 46:248–256
13. Stennert H, Goebel H, Schwarting S, Schroder M (1984) Morphology of human mimic musculature. In: Portmann M (ed) Proceedings of the 5th international symposium of the facial nerve, pp 194–197
14. Sahashi M et al. (1990) Facial muscle involvement in chronic progressive external ophthalmoplegia. Facial N Res Jpn 10:92
15. Ylikoski JS, Hitselberger WE, House WF (1981) Degenerative changes in the distal stump of the severed human facial nerve. Acta Otolaryngol 92:239

Eur Arch Otorhinolaryngology (1994) [Suppl]: S37–S41

E. Stennert, C. Böschen, A. Gunkel, and H. H. Goebel

Effects of Electrostimulation Therapie: Enzyme-Histological and Myometric Changes in the Denervated Musculature

Introduction

Electrostimulation therapy is a widely accepted method applied to denervated skeletal muscles in order to prevent or retard muscular atrophy [1, 4, 13, 24, 25]. Following the proposal made by Duchenne in 1855, electrostimulation therapy has also been applied to mimic muscles in cases of facial palsy [6]. Animal experiments done on skeletal muscles have shown that an indispensable prerequisite for the success of electrostimulation therapy are isometric muscle contractions, which the skeletal muscles are able to perform due to bony insertions [1, 7, 11, 13, 16, 24]. Since mimic muscles do not, or only partially insert in bone and therefore cannot perform isometric contractions, it was concluded that electrostimulation of the paralyzed mimic musculature would be of no therapeutic value [16]. However, this statement has never been verified clinically or experimentally. The aim of the present investigation was to study whether electrostimulation therapy can prevent or retard muscular atrophy.

Materials and Methods

The right facial nerve of 48 Wistar rats on standard laboratory chow and tap water was severed at the stylomastoid foramen under light ether anaesthesia and after injection of 0.1 ml pentobarbital (Nembutal) intraperitoneally. The severed nerve stumps were folded back and secured with metal clips to avoid nerve sprouting. Postoperatively, animals showed an immobility of the right side of the whisker pad and right upper eyelid as well as hanging of the right

E. Stennert (✉), C. Böschen, A. Gunkel, and H. H. Goebel
Klinik und Poliklinik für Hals-, Nasen- und Ohrenheilkunde
der Universität Köln, Joseph-Stelzmann-Strasse 9,
50924 Köln, Germany

angle of the snout. Twenty-four of the animals underwent electrostimulation therapy of the right levator labii superior muscle with triangular impulses (4 Hz of 50 ms duration and 200 ms intervals for 30 days, twice per day, 8 min per session) (Neuroton 626, Siemens, Munich, Germany). Correct application of the electric current was controlled by surveying synchronous contractions and erections of the whisker pad.

The other 24 animals with facial palsy did not receive electrostimulation therapy, nor did the control left side of all 48 rats. On day 30 of the experiment, all animals were killed by an overdose of ether and the right and left levator labii superior muscles were removed. Visualization under the operation microscope checked during surgery that no reinnervation had taken place. The proximal ends of the muscles were embedded in Tissue Tec, shockfrozen at $-160.5\,°C$ and stored airtight at $-80.5\,°C$ [3].

The distal ends of the muscles were weighed, stored at $-80.5\,°C$ and used within 8 h for quantification of creatine kinase (CK) and lactate dehydrogenase (LDH) activity. For enzyme quantification, the frozen distal ends of the muscles were thawed slowly and cut into pieces. After addition of extraction buffer (sodium phosphate buffer pH 7.55, 50 mmol/l; potassium chloride 150 mmol/l; and mercaptoethanol 11 mmol/l) per gram muscle, the samples were homogenized three times for 30 min (Braun Homogenisator S, Frankfurt, Germany). After centrifugation for 30 min at 25000 rpm, the supernatant was removed and assayed for LDH and CK activity according to standard methods [8, 9]. Tissue blocks of the shock-frozen proximal muscles were cut on a cryostat (Kryostat Mikrotom, according to Pearse, Sloe, Mainz, Germany) into 10-μm sections and were stained with hematoxylin and eosin (HE) and Gomori Trichrome [10], and were stained histochemically for acetylcholinesterase (ACE), nicotinamide-adenine dinucleotide hydrogen (NADH), menadione-bound glycerophosphate dehydrogenase (MAG) and adenosinetriphosphate (ATP) [5, 12, 14, 21, 22, 23].

Muscle fiber diameters were measured on NADH-stained sections because this allowed differentiation into type I and type II fibers. We measured the diameter vertical to the largest diameter of 12 muscles of the denervated/stimulated muscle group and denervated/nonstimulated muscle group, as well as the control group [3, 12]. One whole section of each measured muscle was photographed at 500 × magnification and was computer analyzed using a computed video plan (Kontron-Messgeräte GmbH) for smallest diameter, mean fiber diameter and standard deviation. Histograms were made at 2 μm diameter differences of 50 type I and type II fibers.

Results

Quantitation of Enzyme Activities and Muscle Weight

The weight of the denervated/stimulated right levator labii superior muscle was reduced to 73% and CK and LDH activity were reduced to 33% and 37%, respectively, when compared with the control left side (Table 1). This decrease in muscle weight and CK and LDH activity was more pronounced in the denervated/nonstimulated muscles, with an average reduction to 50%, 24%, and 25%, respectively, in comparison with the control.

The absolute values as well as the mean values for muscle weight and CK activity of the denervated/stimulated muscles were highly significantly greater and for LDH activity they were significantly greater, than in the denervated/nonstimulated muscles, as tested by variance analysis.

Morphology

Light microscopy of the control side levator labii superior muscles (Fig. 1a) showed an uniform picture of polygonal muscle fibers, surrounded by a thin layer of connective tissue. The nuclei lay in the periphery of cross-sectioned fibers. Blood vessels were without infiltrate. The denervated/stimulated muscle fibers (Fig. 1b) were considerably smaller, and in some fibers the nuclei were central, the surrounding connective tissue had thickened and contained atrophic muscle fibrils and aggregated nuclei. These changes were much more pronounced in the denervated/nonstimulated muscles (Fig. 1c), in which only a few peripheral nuclei could be seen and the fibrils had rounded, losing their typical polygonal appearance.

In addition, sections stained with Gomori Trichrome allowed differentiation into type I and type II fibrils and estimation of mitochondrial activity. In the control muscles (Fig. 2a) type I fibrils contained more mitochondria than type II fibrils; in the denervated/stimulated muscles (Fig. 2b) the type I fibrils showed an increased content in mitochondria. When the muscles were not stimulated after denervation (Fig. 2c) the number of mitochondria increased in the type I as well as type II muscle fibrils.

Enzyme Histochemistry

In addition to the morphologic picture described above, staining for ACE revealed only a few motoric endplates in normal levator labii superior muscles and in muscles after denervation and electrostimulation, except for two denervated/stimulated muscles, which showed an increased content in motoric endplates.

Type I and type II fibrils were differentiated by the NADH tetrazolium diaphorase stain according to Brooke and Engel [3]. Type I fibrils took up more stain and were smaller than type II fibrils. In denervated/nonstimulated muscles, the distinction between type I and type II fibrils could not be made in all cases. Using the staining method for MAG, all muscles in all groups showed a reversed picture with type II fibrils staining darker than type I fibrils.

Table 1 Enzyme activity and muscle weight

Superior levator labii muscle (U/g)	Weight (mg)		CK activity (U/g)		LDH activity	
	Mean	SD	Mean	SD	Mean	SD
Group I						
Denervated/stimulated	257.5	52.4**	148.5	30.0**	53.1	14.1*
Control side (untreated)[a]	351.9	63.0	451.3	68.1	144.5	22.7
Group II						
Denervated/non-stimulated	179.9	44.1**	103.8	14.2**	37.2	3.8*
Control side (untreated)[a]	357	57.8	438.3	49.9	147.6	16.0

CK, creatinine kinase; LDH, lactate dehydrogenase.

* $\alpha = 5\%$, ** $\alpha = 1\%$ for differences between the two denervated muscle groups.
The difference between denervated muscles and controls were in all cases $\alpha = 1\%$; α was determined by the U-test by Mann and Whitney.
[a] Control side, the untreated contralateral side (left side) in both groups (denervated/stimulated; denervated/non-stimulated).

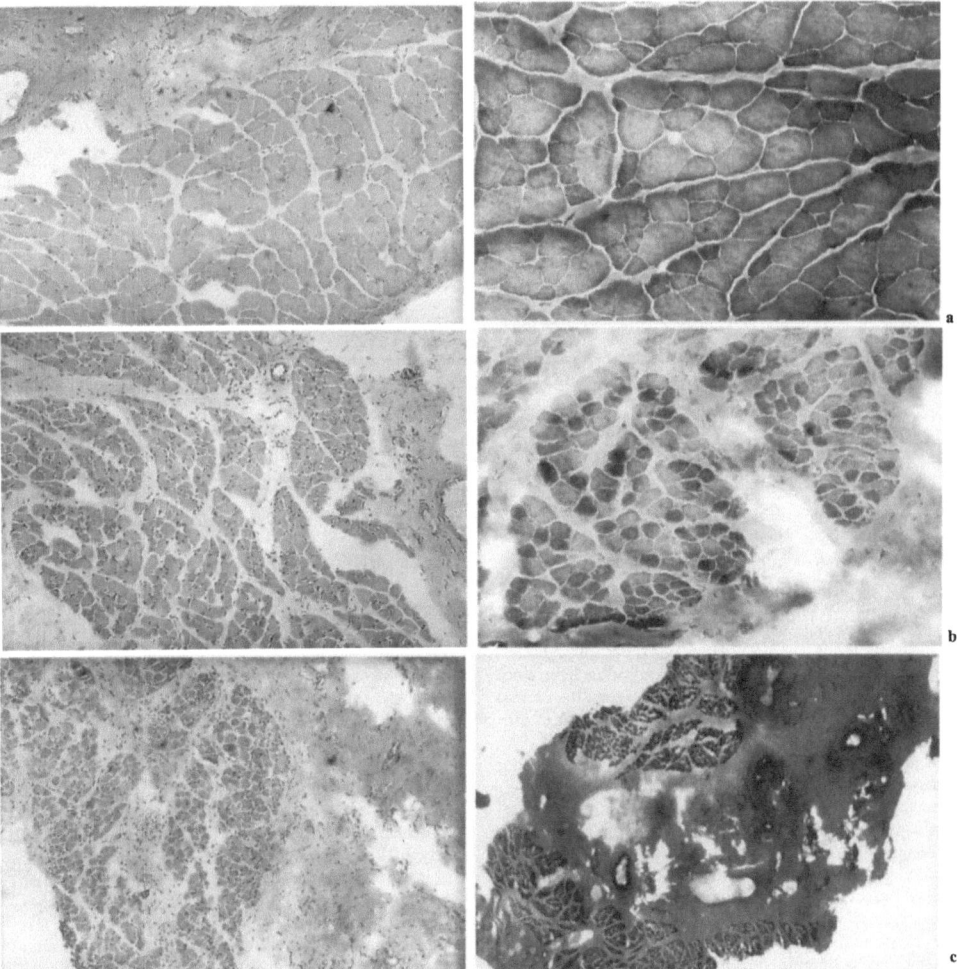

Fig. 1a–c Hematoxylin-eosin (HE) stain of cross-sectioned muscle fibers. **a** Normal muscle (control side). **b** Denervated/stimulated muscle. **c** Denervated/non-stimulated muscle

Fig. 2a–c Gomori Trichrome stain with differentiation into type I and type II fibers and estimation of mitochondrial activity. **a** Normal muscle (control side). **b** Denervated/stimulated muscle. **c** Denervated/non-stimulated muscle

Muscle Diameter

Histograms showed that the smallest diameter of muscle fibrils of unaffected levator labii superior muscles (control sides) was greater than that of denervated/stimulated muscles and the smallest diameter of the latter again greater than that of denervated/nonstimulated muscles (Figs. 3 and 4). Since a normal distribution of fibril dia-meters cannot be expected, we tested the values for significance using the U-test according to Mann and Whitney [26]. The difference of fibril diameters of type I and type II fibrils was highly significant between controls and both denervated muscle groups. Moreover, the diameters of type I as well as type II muscle fibers were significantly greater in the denervated/stimulated than in the denervated/nonstimulated group.

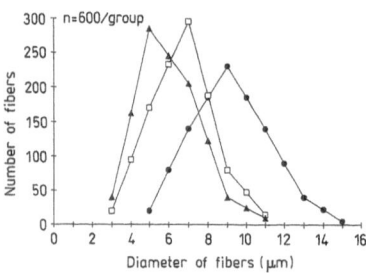

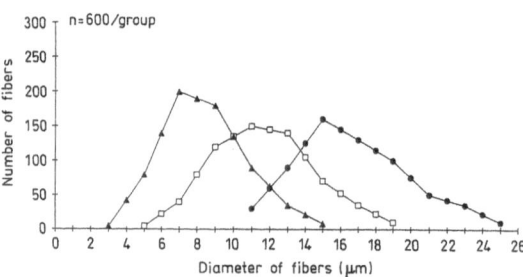

Fig. 3 Differences of type I fiber diameters are statistically highly significant between normal (control) sides (*circles*) and both denervated sides. Moreover the differences of fiber diameters between denervated/stimulated (*squares*) and denervated/non- stimulated (*triangles*) muscles are statistically significant

Fig. 4 Differences of type II fiber diameters are statistically highly significant between normal (control) sides (*circles*) and both denervated sides. Moreover, the differences of fiber diameters between denervated/stimulated (*squares*) and denervated/non- stimulated (*triangles*) muscles are statistically significant

Discussion

Previous experiments with denervated striated skeletal muscles indicated that a necessary prerequisite for the effectiveness of electrostimulation treatment are isometric muscle contractions and a certain muscle tension prior to the application of electric current [5, 7, 11, 13, 16, 17, 18]. These results suggested that electrostimulation therapy can only have limited or no effect at all on mimic muscles, because they cannot perform isometric contractions since they do not insert in bone. To our knowledge, the present investigation is the first to examine this hypothesis experimentally.

As expected, denervation of the levator labii superior muscle led to muscular atrophy with a reduction in muscle weight and muscle fiber diameter. But the extent of atrophy was statistically significantly less in denervated/stimulated muscles than in denervated/nonstimulated muscles (Figs. 3, 4). However, in comparison with controls, the extent of muscular atrophy was still great in both denervated muscle groups. Thus, electrostimulation therapy could be shown to be effective but could only partially prevent atrophy. This is in accordance with findings on skeletal muscles [11, 13, 24, 25].

Since muscle weight is not a very conclusive parameter for muscle function and physiology other parameters were tested in addition. Quantitation of CK and LDH confirmed the above findings. Both enzymes were reduced after denervation as compared to the controls but the reduction was less pronounced after electrostimulation (Table 1). This tendency is also in accordance with the literature [11, 13, 20]. Direct comparison of absolute values is not possible because the former experiments were conducted on skeletal muscles. Morphology of the muscles after HE staining again confirmed these results. The rounded muscle fibrils, central nuclei and great number of aggregated nuclei in the denervated/nonstimulated muscles

reflect the extent of the pathological changes in these muscles. It could be demonstrated that all these pathological changes were less pronounced in the denervated/stimulated muscles (Fig. 1). Histochemical staining for ACE showed only a few motoric endplates in the control muscles. No ACE activity could be shown in the denervated muscles. Surprisingly, two muscles in the denervated/stimulated group showed an increased number of motoric endplates in the ACE stain. Since reinnervation was excluded during surgery and in the NADH stain, which in the case of reinnervation would show a grouping of type I and type II fibrils in contrast to their normally random distribution, the only explanation of this phenomenon is a reconcentration of ACE at the motor endplates due to electrostimulation. Usually ACE diffuses all over the muscle surface after denervation [1, 17, 18].

With respect to "typing" histochemical staining for myofibrillar ATPase allowed no differentiation into type I and type II muscle fibrils on the levator labii superior muscle of our rats. Modification of the standard method of Padycula and Herman by changing the pH or preincubation at an alkaline pH of 10.5 did not give better results nor did the method of Pearse [2, 23]; thus, a subtyping of type II muscle fibers was impossible. At present we have no explanation for this striking fact, but it is known that histochemical staining of myofibrillar actomyosin ATPase is a very sensitive method markedly influenced by many factors including time, temperature, pH, type of buffer and ionic composition of the preincubation medium [15, 19, 22, 23]. Due to this fact we used the NADH-reductase stain for determination of muscle fiber diameter of type I and II fibers which differ considerably in size in the rat in contrast to humans. Apart from the presented study we have also investigated human denervated facial muscles by histochemical, lightmicroscopy and ultrastructural methods to get comparative data on the human [2, 27, 28].

Bearing in mind that conditions of the electrostimulation treatment were not necessarily ideal with regard to frequency of the electric current and interval between the application and duration of each stimulation period, all measured parameters show that mimic muscles do not in principle react any differently to denervation and subsequent electrostimulation than skeletal muscles, i. e. electrostimulation therapy after denervation can retard but not prevent muscular atrophy. Further experiments will have to investigate (a) the ideal conditions for electrostimulation treatment and (b) whether the above results can be applied to humans.

References

1. Axelsson J, Thesleff S (1959) A study of supersensitivity in denervated mammalian skeletal muscle. J Physiol [Lond] 149:178–193
2. Bardosi A, Goebel HH, Stennert E (1987) The ultrastructure of normal and denervated human facial muscles. Plast Reconstruct Surg 79:171–176
3. Brooke MH, Engel WK (1969) The histographic analysis of human muscle biopsies with regard to fiber types. Neurology (Minneap) 19:221–233, 469–477
4. Brown MD, Cotter M, Hudlicka ME, Smith G, Vroba A (1973) The effect of long term stimulation of fast muscles on their ability to withstand fatigue. J Physiol [Lond] 238:47–48
5. Dubowitz V, Brooke MH (1973) Muscle biopsy: a modern approach. Saunders, London
6. Duchenne GD (1872) De l'electrisation localisée, 3rd edition. Baillère, Paris, pp 864–870
7. Eccles JC (1944) Investigations on muscle atrophies arising from disuse and tenotomy. J Physiol [Lond] 103:253–266
8. Empfehlungen der Deutschen Gesellschaft für Klinische Chemie (1970) Z Klin Chemie 8:658–660
9. Empfehlungen der Deutschen Gesellschaft für Klinische Chemie (1972) Z Klin Chemie 10:182–192
10. Engel WK, Cunningham GG (1963) Rapid examination of muscle tissue. An improved trichrome method for fresh-frozen biopsy sections. Neurology (Minneap) 13:919–923
11. Erbslöh F, Hager H (1972) Sekundäre Muskelveränderungen bei peripheren Nervenläsionen. Melsunger Med Mitt 46:59–83
12. Farber E, Sternberg WH, Dunlap CD (1959) Histochemical localization of specific oxidative enzymes. I. Tetrazolium stains for diphosphopyridine nucleotide diaphorase and triphosphopyridine nucleotide diaphorase. J Histochem Cytochem 4:254–265
13. Fischer E, Ramsey VW (1945) The effect of daily electrical stimulation of normal and denervated muscles upon their protein content and upon some of the physicochemical properties of the protein. Am J Physiol 145:583–586
14. Gerebtzoff MA (1953) Recherches histochemiques sur les acetylcholine et choline-esterase. Acta Anat 19:366–379
15. Gollnick PD, Parsons D, Oakley CR (1983) Differentiation of fiber types in skeletal muscle from the sequential inactivation of myofibrillar actomyosin ATPase during acid preincubation. Histochemistry 77:543–555
16. Hopf HC (1974) Konservative Therapie und Rehabilitation der Lokalerkrankungen peripherer Nerven. Akt Neurol 1:38–45
17. Lomo T, Westgaard RH, Dahl HA (1974) Contractile properties of muscle: Control by pattern of muscle activity in the rat. Proc R Soc B 187:99–103
18. Lomo T, Westgard RH (1975) Further studies on the control of ACH sensitivity by activity in the rat. J Physiol 252:603–626
19. Matoba H, Allen JR, Bayla WM, Oakley CR, Gollnick PD (1985) Comparison of fiber types in skeletal muscles from ten animal species based on sensitivity of the myofibrillar actomyosin ATPase to acid or copper. Histochemistry 82:175–183
20. Melichna JE, Gutmann E (1974) Stimulation and immobilisation effects on contractile and histochemical properties of denervated muscle. Pflügers Arch 352:165–178
21. Nachlas MM, Walker DG, Seligman AM (1958) Histochemical method for the demonstration of DPN-diaphorase. J Biophys Biochem Cytol 4 (29):169
22. Padycula HA, Herman E (1955) The specificity of the histochemical method for adenosine triphosphatase. J Histochem Cytochem 3:170–183
23. Pearse AGE (1961) Histochemistry, theoretical and applied. 2nd edition. Churchill Livingstone, London
24. Pette D, Ramirez BU, Müller W, Simon R (1975) Influence of intermittent long-term stimulation on contractile, histochemical and metabolic properties of fiber populations in fast and slow rabbit muscles. Pflügers Arch 361:1–7
25. Pette D, Smith ME, Staudte HW, Vrbova G (1973) Effects of long-term electrical stimulation on some contractile and metabolic characteristic of fast rabbit muscles. Pflügers Arch 338:257–272
26. Sachs L (1974) Angewandte Statistik. Springer, Berlin Heidelberg New York, SS 230–238
27. Schwarting S, Schröder M, Stennert E, Goebell HH (1982) Enzyme histochemical and histographic data on normal human facial muscles. ORL 44:51–59
28. Schwarting S, Schröder M, Stennert E, Goebell HH (1984) Morphology of denervated human facial muscles. ORL 46:248–256

Eur Arch Otorhinolaryngology (1994) [Suppl]: S42–S43

INVITED LECTURES

P. P. Devriese

Rehabilitation of Facial Expression ("Mime Therapy")

The movements of expression in the face and the body, whatever their origin may have been, are in themselves of much importance for our welfare (Charles Darwin [4])

When the facial nerve degenerates for some reason, recovery of voluntary and involuntary (emotional) motor function will not be complete. This means that facial expression will be limited for the rest of the patient's life. The face will also remain asymmetrical to some degree, and the patient will have to learn to live with this handicap.

Unfortunately, it is not always possible to prevent denervation by medical or surgical treatment. If the nerve is not severed, e.g. by a trauma or a fracture of the temporal bone, it will regenerate from the central part to the facial musculature. Recovery will be more or less complete depending on the degree of degeneration [11]. The quantity and the quality of the outgrowth of the nerve fibres may be insufficient for facial expression to recover completely. Moreover, misdirection of fibres will take place and, for that reason, associated movements (synkineses) will appear. This phenomenon is particularly disturbing during eating, speaking etc., as the muscles of the eyelids will be activated at the same time as those of the mouth and jaw. So-called mass reinnervation will be directed to all muscles in the face and the neck, resulting in a feeling of contracture for the patient and a more or less asymmetrical face seen by the outside world. Finally, the direction of the muscular activity may be disturbed (autoparalytic syndrome [10]).

In about 15% of patients with Bell's palsy this situation will arise [7, 9]. After herpes zoster [6] and injuries involving the facial nerve (either extratemporal or endotemporal), this percentage will certainly be higher. This means that after other methods of treatment have been exhausted,

including reconstructive surgery of the nerve and face, about 45 patients a year in our department will need treatment to be able to resume their professional and social life. This problem compelled us to look for another non-conventional approach. In the early, 1970s we happened to meet a man named Jan Bronk, a professional mime actor and teacher, interested in applying mime in education and in rehabilitation of neurological patients. Being a master of facial and bodily expression par excellence, we asked him if he could use his expertise to help our unfortunate patients. Their contracted posture, face and respiration proved indeed to be a clue to the solution of the problem. He started with exercises to gain control of respiration and muscular tension. Once this control had been achieved, it proved possible to re-educate the face in order to restore facial expression as far as possible. The foundation of expression proved to be a better control of the body in general. Only after achieving that, was it possible to rehabilitate the face itself. In fact, the basic principles of mime were applied to the distorted face. The interrelation between respiration and expression is not surprising. The facial nerve was originally described by Charles Bell as "the respiratory nerve of the face" [1]. Charles Darwin himself wrote: "With man the respiratory organs are of especial importance in expression, not only in a direct, but a still higher degree in an indirect manner" [4]. Via mime, emotional control can be improved. This control is conducted by afferences from the thalamus and the globus pallidus via interneurons in the reticular formation [8].

This method was presented at the Third International Symposium in Zürich in 1976 [5]. The first results were presented at the symposium in Rio de Janeiro [3] and published in the literature [2, 12].

Mime therapy can be summarized as follows:

1. The aim of treatment is to help the patient accept his handicap.
2. The basic principles include the following:
   - Interrelation between respiration and expression.
   - Tension increases the abnormal movements, spasm and contracture.

P. P. Devriese
Academisch Ziekenhuis bij de Universiteit van Amsterdam,
Academisch Medisch Centrum, Meibergdreef 9,
1105 AZ Amsterdam, The Netherlands

- Facial expression is the result of the working of body and mind. Mastery of expression is only possible through control of the whole body and mind (the foundation of mime).
3. The method consists in:
   - Gaining control of the body.
   - Becoming conscious of the emotions.
   - Relating bodily expression to emotion.
   - Relating bodily movements to facial expression.
4. The stages of treatment are as follows:
   - Learning to control respiration to improve relaxation and coordination.
   - Becoming conscious of the whole body.
   - Exercising to remove tension in co-ordination with respiration to achieve complete relaxation.
   - Reactivating from the toes up to the face.
   - Mastering a new pattern of expression in the face and achieving co-ordination between the diseased and the healthy side.
5. The desired result of treatment consists in regaining control of the face, which restores confidence and results in fewer abnormal movements and less tension in the face.

Since 1974, 758 patients have been treated in the Netherlands in 5568 sessions by ten physiotherapists familiar with the method. On average, 7.5 treatment sessions of about 40 min once a week were needed (Table 1). The patient should exercise daily at home with a description and photographs of the exercises to achieve control of the face.

Table 1 Mime therapy in the Netherlands (1974–1991)

Institutions	Number of patients	Number of sessions	
		Total	Mean
Academic Medical Centre, Amsterdam (1974–1991)	544	4093	7.5
Amsterdam, Nijmegen, Groningen, Oss (1985–1991)	214	1475	6.9
Total	758	5568	7.3

As this is absolutely necessary, the patient must be well motivated before starting this kind of therapy. We wait a sufficient period of time to start the treatment, usually about 12 months, because spontaneous recovery should first be completed. If patients started earlier, frequent adjustments of the training would be necessary. Finally, rehabilitation of expression should also be offered after reconstructive surgery of the face, especially after dynamic procedures. The patient should not only be given the instrument for expression, but he also should learn to use it for that purpose.

References

1. Bell C (1821) On the nerves; giving an account of some experiments in their structure and function which leads to a new arrangement of the system. Philos R Soc [B] 109:398–424
2. Beurskens C, Bots I, Devriese PP (1987) Resultaten van mimetherapie bij patienten met een perifere facialisverlamming. Ned T Fysiother 97:140–145
3. Beurskens C (1989) The functional rehabilitation of facial muscles and facial expression. In: Castro D (ed) The facial nerve. Kugler and Ghedini, Amsterdam, pp 509–510
4. Darwin C (1965) The expression of the emotions in man and animals (1872). Reprint with a preface by Konrad Lorenz. University of Chicago Press, Chicago
5. Devriese PP, Bronk J (1977) Non-surgical rehabilitation of facial expression. In: Fisch U (ed) Facial nerve surgery. Kugler Medical, Amstelveen, The Netherlands, pp 290–294
6. Devriese PP, Moesker WH (1988) The natural history of facial paralysis in herpes zoster. Clin Otolaryngol 13:289–298
7. Devriese PP, Schumacher T, Scheide A, de Jongh RH, Houtkooper JM (1990) Incidence, prognosis and recovery of Bell's palsy. A survey of about 1000 patients. Clin Otolaryngol 115:15–27
8. Miehlke A (1973) Surgery of the facial nerve. Saunders, Philadelphia
9. Peitersen E (1982) The natural history of Bell's palsy. Am J Otol 4:107–111
10. Stennert E (1982) Das autoparalytische Syndrom – ein Leitsymptom der postparetischen Fazialisfunktion. Arch Otorhinolaryngol 236:97–114
11. Sunderland S (1951) A classification of peripheral nerve injuries producing loss of function. Brain 74:491–516
12. Van Gelder RS, Philippart SMM, Bernard BGES, Devriese PP, Whiting HTA, van Wieringen PCW (1990) Effects of myofeedback and mime-therapy on peripheral facial paralysis. Int J Psychol 25:140–145

Eur Arch Otorhinolaryngology (1994) [Suppl]: S44–S45

INVITED LECTURES

R. Balliet, J. Diels and T. J. Balliet

Facial Assessment Scales: Defining Selective Movement

Introduction

Gross facial grading systems, such as the commonly used House grading system [1], do not provide the detailed functional information that is required by the surgeon who is performing a procedure affecting a specific area or areas of the face or by the therapist who must be concerned with selective motor retraining. The present functional assessment scales (FAS) have been developed over the past 15 years by the first author to regionally assess retraining of postsurgical and other types of facial paralysis patients (e.g., cancer, trauma, acoustic neuroma, Bell's palsy, herpes zoster, congenital defects). The FAS have been used with up to 23 movements and gestures on hundreds of facial retraining patients. The methodology of facial retraining has been published elsewhere [2, 3].

The FAS are designed to be similar to the basic categories of standardized muscle testing, originated by Lovett in 1932 [4], which are used in various forms to subjectively grade the range of motion of various types of disabled patients involved in rehabilitation. Therapists commonly use the grades normal, good, fair, poor, trace, and zero with finer gradations being indicated by a "+" or a "–" between levels to categorize functional abilities (see "Using the Functional Assessment Scale Kinesis", below). They also use the grades mild, moderate, and severe to designate the degree of dysfunction (see "Using the Functional Assessment Scales: Hyperkinesis", below). The application of these terms to facial patients has not occurred until now, partly because selective motor retraining methods have only recently become available to therapists.

Using the Functional Assessment Scales: Kinesis

The FAS for kinesis (f') requires the user to rate on an ordinal scale the relative range of motion for any aspect of functional movement (f); f' would therefore include hypo-

kinesis, but not hyperkinesis, whereas, f is defined as any desired/voluntary movement or gesture. However, "usable" f must include a sufficient range of motion to be recognized as a significant portion of the required movement at a normal conversational distance (i.e., less than 1 m; see f' scores 3–10, below). The affected side's f is referenced for asymmetry to the f of the unaffected side producing the same movement. Table 1 describes the grading categories for the FAS for kinesis (f'), including the percentage of normal kinesis (f') for each score.

The f' scores of 10, 9, and 8 are within the normal limits (WNL, GENf column) of asymmetry found in subjects without pathology. A score of 10 is reserved for the rare individual who has perfect motor control and symmetry. Scores of 9 and 8 are the upper and lower limits of normal asymmetry. Scores of 0, 1, and 2 indicate no usable function (NO, GENf column). A score of 1 equals a just perceptible change in only resting tone. A score of 2 indicates a just perceptible change in both tone and movement.

Scores of 3–7 describe levels of usable movement that are more than just perceptible (MIN, GENf column) and

Table 1 Functional assessment scale (FAS), to rate functional movement (kinesis)

Score	Genf	Condition	f (%)
10		Excellent	100
9		Good +	90–99
8	WNL	Good –	80–89
7	LNL	Fair +	70–79
6		Fair –	60–69
5		Half	50–59
4		Poor +	40–49
3	MIN	Poor–	30–39
2	NO	Trace +	20–29
1		Trace –	10–19
0		None	0–9

f, functional movement.

that are less than the normal limits (LNL, GENf column) of asymmetry for normals without pathology. A score of 5 indicates a functional ability that is approximately half that of normal. Scores of 7 and 6 or 4 and 3 represent the two steps of functional ability between half (score 5) and the lowest of normal limits (score 8) or the highest level of no usable function (score 2), respectively.

Using the Functional Assessment Scales: Hyperkinesis

The vast majority of facial paralysis patients have excessive and/or undesired movement in a defined area (df) which is often not well correlated to their ability to produce voluntary facial movement (f). Therefore, the FAS for hyperkinesis (df') has been devised to estimate facial dysfunction (df) of various types of hyperkinesis. As seen in Table 2, the FAS for hyperkinesis (df') uses the same $0-10$ number scaling as the FAS for kinesis, i.e., a score of 0 is the lowest obtainable score, while a score of 10 is the highest.

Since the FAS for kinesis (df') rates asymmetry due to involuntary movement (df), separate df' scores can be determined for any, of three types of hyperkinesis. These are: (1) synkinesis, i.e., dysfunctional movement (df) in-

Table 2 Functional assessment scale (FAS) to rate dysfunctional movement (hyperkinesis)

Score	Condition	df (%)
10	None	0–9
9	Very mild	10–19
8	Mild	20–29
7	Mild/moderate	30–39
6	Moderate	40–49
5	Half	50–59
4	Moderate/severe	60–69
3	Severe/moderate	70–79
2	Severe	80–89
1	Very severe	90–99
0	Maximum	100

df, dysfunctional movement.

voluntarily accompanying functional movement (f); (2) associated movements, i.e., bilateral, nonpathological, patterned functional movements (f) triggered by the same or another functional movement or movements, (f); and (3) hypertonicity, i.e., dysfunctional movement (df) in the form of excessive tone.

Initially, the FAS for hyperkinesis is most easily used with just the even-numbered grades. With practice, the clinician will also want to use the odd-numbered grades when the two adjoining even-numbered grades seem too high or too low.

Discussion

The efficacy of the FAS has been studied [5] with 32 post-acute (average, 7.1 years post) patients of varying diagnoses (including Bell's palsy, acoustic neuroma, and trauma) and an average House grade of V. Preliminary results found that when the sum of FAS scores of each patient were rank ordered for treatment effects, their correlation to the House scale was high (r, 0.93). It was also found that with only 3 h of practice, interrator reliability averaged $r = 0.90$.

Although seemingly time consuming, we can rate most patients on both parts of the FAS for 16 different facial movement and gestures in less than 20 min. We use the FAS as a "language" by which many facial rehabilitative procedures can be simply documented, discussed, and modified.

References

1. House JW (1983) Facial nerve grading systems. Laryngoscope 93:1056–1069
2. Balliet R, Schinn J, Bach-Y-Rita P (1982) Facial paralysis rehabilitation: retraining selective motor control. Int Rehabil Med 4:67–74
3. Balliet R (1989) Facial paralysis and other neuromuscular dysfunction of the peripheral nervous system. In: Payton O (ed) Manual of physical therapy. Churchill Livingston, New York, pp 175–213
4. Kendal FP, McCreary EK (1991) Muscle testing and function. Williams and Wilkins, Baltimore
5. Balliet R, Diels J, Bednarek C. Refining a model for the retraining of facial paralysis (in preparation)

The Injured Nerve

Eur Arch Otorhinolaryngology (1994) [Suppl]: S49–S50

J.M. Schröder

Fine Structure of Degeneration and Regeneration of Peripheral Nerve Fibers

Introduction

Following peripheral nerve fiber degeneration, regeneration in general tends to be vigorous, although it depends to a large extent on blood vessels and blood supply, the surrounding connective tissue elements, including specialized fibroblasts and perineurial cells, and on various other conditions such as the type of the lesion (see [11, 17]), the species [7], and the age of the individual [18]. A number of local and distant, distal (peripheral) and proximal (central), factors are also of importance, e.g., nerve growth factors (see [6]), increased polyamines [15], local receptors, and the availability of adequate end organs and central synaptic connections (see [19]).

Differences in Regenerating Motor, Sensory, and Autonomous Nerves

The conditions for regeneration of peripheral, extrafusal, and intrafusal motoneurons differ considerably from those of peripheral sensory and autonomic ganglia. Motoneurons have a striking capacity to develop colateral branches for innervating large numbers of muscle fibers (muscle fiber type grouping; see [9]). On the other hand, sensory neurons innervate only few or single end organs. During regeneration multiple sprouts of individual axons ("clusters") enhance the chance of reestablishing connection to an appropriate end organ. This, however, can only be achieved over distances longer than approximately 3 cm if contact guidance is available.

Although there are numerous studies on the outcome of regeneration in experimental animals, only very few fine structural, morphometric data are available on human nerves at late stages of regeneration when the final success

J.M. Schröder
Institut für Neuropathologie der Medizinischen Fakultät
der RWTH Aachen,
Pauwellsstrasse 30, 52057 Aachen, Germany

of regeneration can be evaluated. We analyzed several examples of recovering human nerves: (a) a single sural nerve in a 12.9-month-old boy after a fascicular, diagnostic sural nerve biopsy at the age of 3 months [11]; (b) a spontaneously reinnervated dorsal branch of a cervical nerve, 22 months after excision of a 11-mm segment of this nerve for surgical treatment of spasmodic torticollis in a 39-year-old woman [12]; (c) an ineffective cross-facial anastomosis of a facial nerve with only very few regenerated nerve fibers (unpublished observations); (d) a sural nerve biopsy weeks after an attack of Guillain Barré syndrome with facial paralysis, showing scattered remyelinated nerve fibers with disproportionately thin myelin sheaths in relation to axonal caliber; and (e) other, usually less well defined conditions of peripheral nerve restitution in a series of more than 2500 sural nerve biopsies.

Dimensions of Regenerated Nerve Fibers

Following experimental nerve grafting in dogs [13, 14], experimental severance or crush injuries in rats [3, 5, 7], and surgical severance of dorsal branches of cervical nerves in man (for treatment of torticollis spasmodicus; [12]), dimensions of the largest regenerated nerve fibers were determined by measuring axonal diameters and myelin sheath thickness of individual nerve fibers at the light and electron microscopic level.

The main deficiency of regenerated nerve fibers in these and other conditions even long periods after the lesion (12–24 months after surgery) consisted in a disproportion between axon caliber and myelin sheath thickness [1, 7, 8, 10, 16]. The myelin sheaths were thinner in the largest regenerated than in normal nerve fibers, and where measured, internodal length was also reduced, although not to the same degree. Axonal calibers reached better values in rats than in dogs or man, indicating clear species differences [7]. It is suggested that reduced myelin sheath thickness and internodal length cause permanently reduced maximal conduction velocity of regenerated nerve fibers even many months or years after severance.

Peripheral Complications of Axonal Regeneration

Supernumerary axons and Schwann cells, aberrant axons, formation of minifascicles ("compartmentalization") in ischemic nerves, neuromas, nerve grafts ("isomorphous neuromatous reinnervation"), and other changes are well-known complications of peripheral nerve regeneration which largely depend on the type of the lesion studied [11, 17].

Recent transmission and scanning electron microscopic examination of muscle spindles revealed supernumerary nerve sprouts, abnormal contact relationships between axonal sprouts, between axonal sprouts and Schwannn cells, and between Schwann cells or axons and intrafusal muscle fibers [3, 5]. It appears likely that abnormal contact relationships between axonal sprouts and innervated end organs may represent abnormal impulse generators, (see [2]), causing a variety of sensory disturbances.

In addition, a striking increase of elastic fibers was observed in muscle spindles following various types of peripheral nerve lesions with or without reinnervation [4], whereas in peripheral nerve trunks there is usually only an increase of collagen and oxytalan fibers, but not of elastin.

Influencing Peripheral Nerve Regeneration

Attempts to influence the outcome of regeneration in the peripheral nervous system by using a tubulation system and by implanting peripheral nerves, muscle, or fat tissue into the distal end of a silicon tube about 11 mm in length [20] revealed optimal results in a nerve-nerve system and somewhat later, still optimal regeneration in the nerve-muscle system, but nearly no effective regeneration in the nerve-fat system. On the other hand, use of fat tissue in situ to prevent neuroma formation after experimental severance of the sciatic nerve in rats [21] resulted in minor inhibition of the outgrowth of regenerating nerve fibers and less reduction of neuroma formation than would have been expected from the silicon tube experiment. The fat tissue cuff around the severed proximal nerve stump, however, might not have been tight enough in situ, so that the fat tissue could not exert its inhibitory effects to a similar degree as in the tubulation system.

The fat tissue in the silicon chamber system did not prevent some initial, pioneer fibers from growing into the distal part of the silicon chamber, but the so-called second-stage of regeneration, clearly seen in the nerve-nerve and the nerve-muscle system, did not develop in the nerve-fat system [20]. This second stage of regeneration does not start before about 3–4 weeks after surgery, when the bulk of regenerating nerve fibers begins to grow, at a time when local growth factors at the site of the lesion have already decreased; it is obviously inhibited, or not induced, by fat tissue.

Many attempts are presently being undertaken to improve peripheral nerve regeneration, and it is hoped that more precise surgical techniques and new pharmaceutical approaches will finally lead to a better handling of motor, sensory, and autonomous disturbances following peripheral nerve lesions and neuropathy.

References

1. Beuche W, Friede RL (1985) A new approach toward analyzing peripheral nerve fiber populations. II. Foreshortening of regenerated internodes corresponds to reduced sheath thickness. J Neuropathol Exp Neurol 44:73–84
2. Culp WJ, Ochoa J (1982) Abnormal nerves and muscles as impulse generators. Oxford University Press, Oxford
3. Dieler R, Schröder JM (1990a) Abnormal sensory and motor reinnervation of muscle spindles following nerve transection and suture. Acta Neuropathol (Berl) 80:163–171
4. Dieler R, Schröder JM (1990b) Increase of elastic fibres in muscle spindles of rats following single or repeated denervation with or without reinnervation. Virchows Arch [A] Pathol Anat 417:213–221
5. Dieler R, Völker A, Schröder JM (1992) Scanning electron microscopic study of denervated and reinnervated intrafusal muscle fibers in rats. Muscle Nerve 15:433–441
6. Lindholm D, Thoenen H (1990) Role of neurotrophic factors in peripheral nerve regeneration. In: Samii M (ed) Peripheral nerve lesions. Springer, Berlin Heidelberg New York, pp 29–31
7. Schröder JM (1972) Altered ratio between axon diameter and myelin sheath thickness in regenerated nerve fibers. Brain Res 45:49–65
8. Schröder JM (1974) Two-dimensional reconstruction of Schwann cell changes following remyelination of regenerated nerve fibers. In: Hausmanova-Petrusewicz I, Jedrzejowska H (eds) Proceedings of the symposium on structure and function of normal and diseased muscle and peripheral nerve. Kazimierz upon Vistula, Poland, May 18–20, Polish Medical Publ. pp 299–304
9. Schröder JM (1982) Von Doerr W, Seifert G, Uehlinger E (eds) Spezielle pathologische Anatomie. Springer, Berlin Heidelberg New York (Pathologie der Muskulatur, vol 15)
10. Schröder JM (1987) Pathomorphologie der peripheren Nerven. In: Neundörfer B, Schimrigk K, Soyka D (eds) Praktische Neurologie, vol 2. Edition Medizin. VCH, Weinheim, pp 11–104
11. Schröder JM (1990) Pathomorphology of regenerating peripheral nerves. In: Samii M (ed) Peripheral nerve lesions. Springer, Berlin Heidelberg New York, pp 22–28
12. Schröder JM, Huffmann B, Braun V, Richter HP (1992) Spasmodic torticollis: severe compression neuropathy in rami dorsales of cervical nerves C1-6. Acta Neuropathol 84:416–424
13. Schröder JM, Seiffert KE (1970) Die Feinstruktur der neuromatösen Neurotisation von Nerventransplantaten. Virchows Arch [B] Zellpathol 5:219–235
14. Schröder JM, Seiffert KE (1972) Untersuchungen zur homologen Nerventransplantation. Morphologische Ergebnisse. Zentralbl Neurochir 53:103–118
15. Seiler N, Schröder JM (1970) Beziehungen zwischen Polyaminen und Nucleinsäuren. II. Biochemische und feinstrukturelle Untersuchungen am peripheren Nerven während der Wallerschen Degeneration. Brain Res 22:82–103
16. Smith KJ, Blakemore WF, Murray JA, Patterson RC (1982) Internodal myelin volume and axon surface area. J Neurol Sci 55:231–245
17. Sunderland S (1978) Nerves and nerve injuries. 2nd edn. Churchill Livingstone Edinburgh, p 1046
18. Tanaka K, Zhang QL, Webster HdeF (1992) Myelinated fiber regeneration after sciatic nerve crush: morphometric observations in young adult and aging mice and the effects of macrophage suppression and conditioning lesions. Exp Neurol 118:53–61
19. Wall PD, Devor M (1978) In: Waxman SG (ed) Physiology and pathobiology of axons. Raven, New York, pp 377–388
20. Weis J, Schröder JM (1989a) Muscle Nerve 12:723–734
21. Weis J, Schröder JM (1989b) J Neurosurg 71:588–593

Eur Arch Otorhinolaryngology (1994) [Suppl]: S51–S54

G. Raivich, M. Graeber, J. Gehrmann, M. T. Moreno-Flores, and G. W. Kreutzberg

Regulation of Transferrin Receptors and Iron Uptake in Normal and Injured Nervous System

Introduction

Iron is an essential requirement for many metabolic reactions occurring in living organisms. Iron-containing proteins play a crucial part in energy metabolism, DNA synthesis, and enzymatic production of reactive radicals (for a review see [5]). Particularly high requirements for iron are present in rapidly growing cells and tissues during development, including development of the nervous system [3, 7]. Iron deficiency is known to interfere with these processes [16, 24].

One problem associated with direct iron uptake into an iron-requiring cell is the very low solubility of iron (III) salts in physiological fluids [32]. To overcome this problem and provide iron to the dependent cells, the vertebrates have developed a very versatile transport system for a specific iron complex consisting of transferrin, an 80-kDa serum protein, and two ferric ions [2]. This uptake of iron-transferrin complex and the ensuing internalization is mediated by specific binding sites or transferrin receptors on the cell membrane of the iron-dependent cells. Although empty, iron-free transferrin also binds to these receptors, iron-saturated transferrin has a much higher receptor affinity, ensuring the preferential uptake of the iron-carrying moiety [18]. Both transferrin and transferrin receptors play a critical role in this iron uptake system [15]. Furthermore, induction of transferrin receptors appears to be an essential part of the common pathway preceding cell proliferation [20], and mitogens rapidly upregulate the expression of transferrin receptors on the cell membrane in vitro [6, 31]. Recent studies have also begun to unveil the regulation of transferrin receptors expression under in vivo conditions associated with cell growth and proliferation.

G. Raivich, M. Graeber, J. Gehrmann, M. T. Moreno-Flores, G. W. Kreutzberg (✉)
Department of Neuromorphology,
Max-Planck-Institute for Psychiatry,
82152 Planegg-Martinsried, Germany

In the present article we will review the data on transferrin receptor expression and associated changes in iron uptake occurring following injury and during regeneration in the central (CNS) and peripheral nervous system.

Central Nervous System

In the adult CNS, high levels of transferrin receptors are observed throughout the brain capillary network on endothelial cells, on large neuronal perikarya in the brain stem reticular formation, and in the neuropil of many different CNS regions, with particularly high expression in the medial habenula [12, 13]. There is moderate, but rapid, iron uptake from the blood circulation in eminentia mediana, discrete periventricular hypothalamic nuclei and subfornical organ, i.e., in CNS regions lacking a blood-brain barrier (Raivich et al., manuscript in preparation). Compared to these regions, iron uptake in all other parts of the CNS with the intact blood-brain barrier is very low. In addition, there is regional variation in CNS iron uptake which appears to reflect the density of transferrin receptors. For example, there is considerably more iron uptake into the gray than white matter, which corresponds with the level of receptor expression.

Transferrin receptors on blood capillary endothelia have been shown to mediate the transport of iron from blood circulation into the CNS tissue, thus circumventing the blood-brain barrier [8]. Although the apparent efficiency of iron uptake via endothelial transferrin receptors is considerably lower than that due to free diffusion in fenestrated endothelia, a number of studies have described a gradual increase in brain iron content after maturation of the blood-brain barrier, pointing to an efficient accumulation of this essential nutrient in the brain tissue. Interestingly, there is a very good correlation between the brain distribution of iron and ferritin, a 500-kDa iron-storage protein [12]. Biochemical data have also shown that brain ferritin is a major CNS iron-containing component [11]. Ferritin has been localized in a variety of different cell types, including brain microglia [10], and it is possible that these cells play a role similar to that of the reticuloendothelial macrophages [1] by scavenging iron-containing proteins and releasing iron into the extracellular space in a form that can be taken up by the neighboring cells.

There are different changes in transferrin receptor expression after direct and indirect injury. Direct trauma, e. g., by a short-term application of dry ice onto parietal skull, causes necrosis in the directly underlying part of the cerebral cortex. This type of injury leads to expression of transferrin receptors on two cell types: on brain vessels sprouting around the site of trauma and on a subpopulation of blood-borne macrophages invading the necrotic CNS tissue [27 a]. Since direct trauma leads to a rapid blood-brain barrier breakdown [28], blood proteins, including the iron-carrying transferrin, may gain access to the injured brain tissue and become available to these transferrin receptor-positive cells. A similar pathway of iron uptake has been demonstrated in the injured peripheral nerve (see below).

Indirect injury following transection of axonal pathways (axotomy) also leads to an induction of transferrin receptors, although this has not been observed in all axotomy models. Axotomy of the facial nerve caused an approximately four fold increase in transferrin receptors on the neuronal perikarya in the facial motor nucleus. This induction was also accompanied by a diffuse and approximately two fold receptor increase in the facial motor nucleus neuropil and relatively moderate iron uptake [9]. This relatively moderate iron uptake is in agreement with data showing no breakdown in the blood-brain barrier during retrograde reaction to axotomy [30] and suggests that a sizeable portion of iron-saturated transferrin in the axotomized facial nucleus may come from local stores and not from blood circulation.

In contrast to the facial motor nucleus, there was no change in transferrin receptor expression, for example, in the retinal ganglion cells following axotomy of the optic nerve. Although it is attractive to speculate that this difference could be due to the fact that under normal conditions axotomized retinal ganglion cells do not regenerate whereas the facial motoneurons do, it is also possible that this discrepancy in transferrin receptor expression may reflect the different pathways involved in the response to axotomy of different neurons. For example, sensory and sympathetic neurons regenerate vigorously after axotomy, but do not show an increase in neuronal transferrin receptors (see below).

Peripheral Nervous System

In the adult peripheral nervous system, transferrin receptors are present both on neurons and on non-neuronal cells. There is a clear and strong expression of transferrin recep-

tors on a subpopulation of neuronal perikarya in the sensory and sympathetic ganglia, which is accompanied by a rapid uptake of circulating iron. In peripheral nerves, there is moderate receptor expression restricted to the perinuclear cytoplasm of the myelinating Schwann cells [27]. Unlike brain capillaries, capillaries in the peripheral nervous system do not bear transferrin receptors, and only very modest immunoreactivity is present on the larger blood vessels. It should be noted, however, that the metabolically active sensory and sympathetic ganglia lie outside the blood-nervous system barrier [22] and may therefore not need a specific system of endothelial iron transport. In peripheral nerves, there is massive anterograde axonal transport of transferrin [14], suggesting that under normal conditions most transferrin found there may be of neuronal origin and not directly provided via circulation. This view is also supported by the extremely low levels in the endoneural uptake of circulating iron into the peripheral nerves [27].

Peripheral axotomy leads to distinct sets of changes in the axotomized ganglia and the injured peripheral nerve. In the axotomized sensory and sympathetic ganglia, there is no clear change in receptor expression and a moderate, approximately 30% – 40% decrease in iron uptake (G. Raivich et al., unpublished observations). In contrast, axotomy of a peripheral nerve leads to a massive, five- to tenfold increase in transferrin receptor expression and an even stronger, 20-fold increase in iron uptake [26]. Although the blood-nerve barrier normally prevents most molecules, including serum proteins, from entering the endoneural interstitium, this barrier rapidly disappears at the site of trauma and in the distal of the injured peripheral nerve [17, 21]. This breakdown of the blood-nerve barrier may explain the rapid entry of iron-saturated transferrin into the injured nerve, where iron then becomes available to the transferrin-dependent cells.

The massive upregulation in transferrin receptor expression is observed more or less simultaneously on two different cell types: on blood-borne macrophages invading the injured peripheral nerve and on resident Schwann cells. On both cell types, receptor expression is, however, only transient and regionally restricted. Although axotomy leads to infiltration of macrophages throughout the whole distal part of the injured peripheral nerve [4, 23], the macrophage transferrin receptors are preferentially expressed at the site of direct trauma [27]. This regionally selective receptor expression is of considerable interest since the trauma site is the region with particularly heavy cellular proliferation [29]. Activated macrophages contain and secrete a panoply of different growth factors [19] which may contribute to the cellular hyperplasia at the injury site. Clinically, this cellular reaction to nerve injury is frequently overactive and may compromise full neurological recovery.

Transferrin receptor expression on Schwann cells is observed throughout the distal part of the injured nerve [26] and corresponds closely to the biphasic pattern of

Schwann cell proliferation following axotomy. There is a transient, though massive increase in receptor expression in the denervated part of the injured peripheral nerve (maximum at day 4); this precedes the maximum of Schwann cell proliferation during Wallerian degeneration by about 24–48 h [29]. A second transient increase is observed during nerve regeneration and coincides with the ensuing reinnervation of the previously denervated Schwann cells. In a model of delayed reinnervation, this second part of receptor expression is observed on a distally moving 5- to 10-mm-wide nerve region which follows the most rapidly growing neurites [27]. As during Wallerian degeneration, this second part of transferrin receptor expression appears to precede slightly the temporal pattern of proliferation on the reinnervated Schwann cells [25]. In vitro experiments have shown that the induction of transferrin receptors and the associated iron uptake are a crucial step preceding cell proliferation [15, 20]. The present data on the regulation of Schwann cell transferrin receptors and cell proliferation after peripheral nerve injury strongly support a similar role for iron under in vivo conditions associated with cell proliferation.

Conclusion

The data summarized in this article describe an effective system of iron uptake in the nervous system, based on transferrin receptor-mediated endothelial transport across the blood-brain barrier, rapid diffusion in regions outside this barrier, anterograde transport of transferrin in peripheral nerves, and, finally, on the uptake of the iron-transferrin complex by the iron-dependent cells. This quite effective system is in line with the importance of iron as an essential nutrient for this normally metabolically active tissue. The availability of iron chelators and blocking antibodies against transferrin receptor may also provide an interesting opportunity to modulate the extent of iron delivery to the nervous tissue and to test its effects on the long-term clinical recovery following injury to the nervous system.

References

1. Aisen P (1990) Iron metabolism in the reticuloendothelial system. In: Ponka P, Schulman HM, Woodworth RC (eds) Iron transport and storage. CRC Press, Boca Raton, Florida, pp 281–295
2. Aisen P, Listowski I (1980) Iron transport and storage proteins. Annu Rev Biochem 49:357–393
3. Bothwell TH, Charlton RW, Cook JD, Finch CA (1979) Iron nutrition. In: Bothwell TH, Charlton RW, Cook JD, Finch CA (eds) Iron metabolism in man. Blackwell Scientific, London, p 15
4. Brown MC, Perry VH, Lunn ER, Gordon S, Heumann H (1991) Macrophage dependence of peripheral sensory nerve regeneration: possible involvement of nerve growth factor. Neuron 6:359–370
5. Cammack R, Wrigglesworth JM, Baum H (1990) Iron dependent enzymes in mammalian systems. In: Ponka P, Schulman HM, Woodworth RC (eds) Iron transport and storage. CRC Press, Boca Raton, Florida, pp 17–39
6. Castagnola J, Macleod C, Sunada H, Mendelsohn J, Taetle R (1987) Effects of epidermal growth factor on transferrin receptor phosphorylation and surface expression in malignant epithelial cells. J Cell Physiol 132:289–293
7. Dallman PR, Siimes MA, Manies EC (1975) Brain iron: persistent deficiency following short-term iron deprivation in the young rat. Br J Hematol 31:209–215
8. Fishman JB, Rubin JB, Handrahan JV, Connor JR, Fine RE (1987) Receptor-mediated transcytosis of transferrin across the blood-brain barrier. J Neurosci Res 18:299–304
9. Graeber MB, Raivich G, Kreutzberg GW (1989) Increase of transferrin receptors and iron uptake in regenerating motor neurons. J Neurosci Res 23:342–345
10. Grundke-Iqbal I, Fleming J, Tung YC, Lassmann H, Iqbal I, Joshi JG (1990) Ferritin is a component of the neuritic (senile) plaque in Alzheimer dementia. Acta Neuropathol 81:105–110
11. Hallgren B, Sourander P (1958) The effect of age on nonhaem iron in the human brain. J Neurochem 3:41–51
12. Hill JM (1990) Iron and proteins of iron metabolism in the central nervous system. In: Ponka P, Schulman HM, Woodworth RC (eds) Iron transport and storage. CRC Press, Boca Raton, Florida, pp 315–330
13. Jeffries WA, Brandon MR, Hunt SV, Williams AF, Gatter KC, Mason DY (1984) Transferrin receptors on endothelium of brain capillaries. Nature 312:162–163
14. Kiffmeyer WR, Tomusk EV, Mescher AL (1991) Axonal transport and release of transferrin in regenerating amphibian lims. Dev Biol 147:392–402
15. Laskey J, Webb I, Schulman HM, Ponka P (1988) Evidence that transferrin supports cell proliferation by supplying iron for DNA synthesis. Exp Cell Res 176:87–95
16. Lozoff B, Brittenham GM (1986) Behavioral of iron deficiency. Prog Hematol 14:23–53
17. Mellick RS, Cavanagh JB (1968) Changes in blood vessel permeability during degeneration and regeneration in peripheral nerves. Brain 91:141–160
18. Morgan EH (1983) Effect of pH and iron content of transferrin on its binding to reticulocyte receptors. Biochim Biophys Acta 762:498–502
19. Nathan C (1987) Secretory products of macrophages. J Clin Invest 79:319–326
20. Neckers LM, Cosman J (1983) Transferrin receptor induction in mitogen-stimulated human T-cells is required for DNA synthesis and cell division and is stimulated by interleukin 2. Proc Natl Acad Sci USA 80:3494–3498
21. Olsson Y (1966) Studies on vascular permeability in peripheral nerves. Distribution of circulating fluorescent serum albumin in normal, crushed and sectioned rat sciatic nerve. Acta Neuropathol 7:1–15
22. Olsson Y (1968) Topographical differences in the vascular permeability of the peripheral nervous system. Acta Neuropathol 10:26–33
23. Olsson Y, Sjöstrand J (1969) Origin of macrophages in Wallerian degeneration of peripheral nerves demonstrated autoradiographically. Exp Neurol 23:102–112
24. Oski FA (1979) The nonhematologic manifestations of iron deficiency. Am J Dis Child 133:315–322
25. Pellegrino RG, Spencer P (1985) Schwann cell mitosis in response to regenerating peripheral axons in vivo. Brain Res 341:16–25
26. Raivich G, Hellweg R, Graeber MB, Kreutzberg GW (1990) The expression of growth factor receptors during nerve regeneration. Restor Neurol Neurosci 1:217–223
27. Raivich G, Graeber MB, Gehrmann J, Kreutzberg GW (1991) Transferrin receptor expression and iron uptake in the injured and regenerating rat sciatic nerve. Eur J Neurosci 3:919–927

27a. Raivich G, Kreutzberg GW (1994) Pathophysiology of glial growth factor receptors. Glia 11:129–146

28. Rinder L, Olsson Y (1968) Studies on vascular permeability changes in experimental brain concussion. Acta Neuropathol 11:183–200

29. Sjöberg G, Kanje M, Edström A (1988) Influence of non-neuronal cells on regeneration in the rat sciatic nerve. Brain Res 453:221–226

30. Streit WJ, Graeber MB, Kreutzberg GW (1988) Functional plasticity of microglia. A review. Glia 1:301–307

31. Ward DM, Kaplan J (1986) Mitogenic agents induce redistribution of transferrin receptors from internal pools to the cell surface. Biochem J 238:721–728

32. Williams RJP (1990) An introduction to the nature of iron transport and storage. In: Ponka P, HM Schulman, RC Woodworth (eds) Iron transport and storage. CRC Press, Boca Raton, Florida, pp 1–16

Eur Arch Otorhinolaryngology (1994) [Suppl]: S55–S56

INVITED LECTURES

T.L. Eby

Clinical Experience in Nerve Grafting

The microsurgical techniques developed over the past 30 years have enabled nerve grafting techniques to become standardized to a large extent. Although some variations exist, there is agreement on the basic principles. In fact, it has been said that the surgical technique may have reached an optimal level, even though the results often remain disappointing.

A cable graft is utilized only when direct end-to-end anastomosis of the injured nerve cannot be performed. Obviously, a graft requires an additional anastomosis and clinical recovery of facial function is generally not as good. This is true even if rerouting of the facial nerve is required to achieve the end-to-end anastomosis [1]. Although devascularization of the rerouted nerve may slightly diminish the final clinical result, it is generally preferable to a long nerve graft.

The surgical technique of nerve grafting is well described and has changed little in recent years [2]. Best results are obtained using delicate tissue handling technique under the microscope [1]. It is important that the proximal stump be trimmed back to a viable region free of disease or injury. This may be difficult to judge clinically at the time of surgery, so a frozen section of the nerve stump may be useful, especially in cases of malignancy. More extensive proximal stump damage was found on electron microscopy than was clinically obvious in facial nerve injury from temporal bone fractures [3].

The nerve graft is most often obtained from sacrifice of the greater auricular or sural nerves. These make suitable donors because the loss of sensation in the areas they supply is usually not troublesome to the patient. The sural nerve should provide enough length for even intracranial to extratemporal facial nerve grafts. The graft length and diameter must be matched to the neural defect. A double graft may be used if the diameter of the graft is smaller than the facial nerve. Experimental studies have shown that cutting

the nerve ends obliquely will increase the surface area for anastomosis and increase the number of axons regenerating through it [4]. Cutting the facial stumps into a "fish-mouth" may also increase the surface area available for anastomosis to the graft. Branching of the sural nerve may be utilized if a graft between the main facial trunk and several division stumps is required.

The anastomosis of the grafted nerve must ensure complete apposition of the nerve ends without tension. Usually this is achieved by placing 9-0 or 10-0 nylon sutures in the perineurium after the outer epineurium has been trimmed back. Since sutures at an anastomosis can produce a foreign body reaction and interrupt axon progression, the number of sutures should be minimized. Sutureless anastomosis can also be useful in grafting. This is especially true for intracranial grafting, where limited exposure and lack of an epineurium make suturing difficult or impossible [5]. In this case, a collagen nerve guide often supplemented with fibrin glue has been successful in completing the anastomosis. Fisch has suggested that the collagen nerve guide should not be a complete tube, but a rolled tube with a window removed on top to allow for swelling. Within the fallopian canal, the anastomosis may be stable and require neither sutures nor nerve guide. The use of fibrin glue has been advocated as an adjunct to sutureless anastomosis [6]. Histoacryl glue has been largely abandoned because of the likelihood of toxic effects on the nerve [7].

Recovery of facial function after a nerve graft may require more time in some patients, but the same pattern is usually followed in all [1]. Initially the patient may perceive a tingling or tightening in the face, which is not seen by an observer. This usually occurs 6 weeks to 3 months after repair. Improvement in facial symmetry and muscle tone (usually at about 3 months) is the first change noted by an observer, followed by fine voluntary movements in the nasolabial fold, upper lip, or lower eyelid. This is usually present by 6 months. The strength of voluntary contractions then increases, first in the circumoral muscles followed by the circumorbicularis (at 9 months). The temporalis branch innervating the frontalis muscle is least

T.L. Eby
The University of Alabama at Birmingham, Hospital Annex 2,
Birmingham, AL 35233-6889, USA

likely to recover function. The ramus mandibularis also rarely recovers function to the lower lip. Maximum recovery of function is complete between 9 and 18 months in most patients, but delays of several years are possible.

Good facial tone at rest and facial movement with improved eye closure and oral competence are routinely achieved with current nerve graft techniques. However, synkinesis and loss of fine motor control of facial muscles inevitably accompany the return of function. Synkinesis may worsen up to 4 years after complete recovery of movement and an diminish initial good results. The cause for this disturbing progression of synkinesis is not understood.

Although many variables contribute to the differences seen in clinical results, several factors appear to have a significant effect. Graft length and the length of rerouting of the facial nerve before grafting probably reduce the clinical outcome. Although the outcome may not be strictly inversely proportional to length, it is clear that patients with the longest, intracranial to extratemporal, facial nerve grafts have a worse outcome than those with short grafts. The lack of revascularization and viability in long grafts may limit their effectiveness. Similarly, extensive rerouting of the facial nerve may lead to devascularization and increased fibrosis, causing a somewhat poorer clinical outcome. When segmental repair of the facial nerve in its extratemporal course is possible, results are better and synkinesis less pronounced. However, fascicular repair of the main trunk is unrewarding.

The timing of facial nerve repair continues to be subject to much discussion. Research has shown that early repair of facial nerve injury is technically easier and not associated with a worse outcome than delayed repair [8]. A delay in repair to await the height of axon regenerative activity does not appear to be justified. Unfortunately, delayed repair often occurs because of delayed referral. Regenerating axons from the proximal facial nerve stump can be found for at least 2 years after injury [3]. However, clinical results of grafting after a delay of 1 year or more are often disappointing.

The cause of facial nerve injury may also influence the outcome of nerve grafting. Large neoplastic lesions such as hemangiomas may compromise facial nerve blood supply and cause ischemia and poorer clinical recovery [9]. Traction injuries, e.g., from longitudinal temporal bone fractures, result in longer areas of nerve injury than can be easily recognised at surgery and may have worse clinical outcomes than transection injuries [3].

When the results of nerve grafting are poor, the cause is not always apparent. Histological examination may show extensive fibrosis at the anastomosis and a lack of myelinated axons transversing to the distal stump [7]. Misdirection of regenerating axons has been demonstrated and may result in neuroma formation. The role of unmyelinated and myelinated axons which remain outside fascicles has been questioned in patients who develop severe synkinesis [1].

In order to improve axon regeneration and ultimately clinical results of nerve grafting, entubulation repairs have become very popular for experimental study. The idea of protecting the microenvironment of regenerating nerves by placing the nerve stumps into some type of tube is not new. Initially, autogenous vein and arterial grafts were employed as a clinical method to protect the anastomosis. More recently it has become a research tool to study, promote, and control nerve regeneration.

Numerous materials have been employed as tubes to bridge gaps between nerve stumps, including silicone, collagen, polyglactin mesh, polypropylene mesh, and polytetrafluoroethylene (goretex). Much attention has focused on the bioresorbable materials as potentially more clinically useful. As a result of numerous studies, a common sequence of events can be described for regeneration of nerves through these tubes [10]. In the first week the chamber fills with fluid rich in neuronotrophic factors. This is then replaced by an acellular fibrinous matrix. By the second week there is ingrowth of fibroblasts, endothelial cells, and Schwann cells to form a cellular bridge. Only then to axons from the proximal stump enter and transverse the tube.

The distal nerve stump appears to have an important role in the regeneration process. Experiments with Y-shaped tubes clearly demonstrate preferential growth of axons to the limb with the distal stump. Schwann cells in the distal stump produce nerve growth factor and probably respond to cues from the axons to produce a favorable environment for further axon growth.

Many experimental manipulations enhance the regeneration process. The tube can be prefilled with fluid containing nerve growth factor, laminin, gangliosides, or other factors to shorten the first step. Alternatively, an artificial matrix such as oriented fibrin or nitrocellulose partitions can shorten the second step. Hope has been raised that nerve regeneration may be more effectively promoted and directed using entubulation repair in the future.

References

1. Spector GJ, Lee P, Peterein J, Roufa D (1991) Facial nerve regeneration through autologous nerve grafts: a clinical and experimental study. Laryngoscope 101:537–553
2. Fisch U (1974) Facial nerve grafting. Otolaryngol Clin North Am 7:517–529
3. Felix H, Eby TL, Fisch U (1991) New aspects of facial nerve pathology in temporal bone fractures. Acta Otolaryngol (Stockh) 111:332–336
4. Yamamoto E, Fisch U (1974) Experiments on facial nerve suturing. J Oto Rhinol-Laryngol 36:193–204
5. Fisch U, Dobie RA, Gmur A, Felix H (1987) Intracranial facial nerve anastomosis. Am J Otol 8:23–29
6. Meddars G, Mattox DE, Lyles A (1989) Effects of fibrin glue on rat facial nerve regeneration. Otolaryngol Head Neck Surg 100 (2):106–109
7. Eby TL, Pollak A, Fisch U (1990) Intratemporal facial nerve anastomosis: a temporal bone study. Laryngoscope 100(6):623–626
8. Barrs DM (1991) Facial nerve trauma: optimal timing for repair. Laryngoscope 101:835–848
9. Eby TL, Fisch U, Makek MS (1992) Facial nerve management in temporal bone hemangiomas. Am J Otol 13 (3):223–232
10. Hall SM (1989) Regeneration in the peripheral nervous system. Neuropathol Appl Neuobiol 15:513–529

Eur Arch Otorhinolaryngology (1994) [Suppl]: S 57 – S 59

INVITED LECTURES

J. Gavilán and C. Gavilán

Prognostic Value of Electroneurography in Bell's Palsy

Introduction

Prognosis is one of the most challenging problems concerning idiopothic facial paralysis. Electrodiagnostic tests in Bell's palsy are traditionally used to predict prognosis and determine the need for possible surgery. The most widely used electrodiagnostic tests are minimal nerve excitability, maximal nerve excitability, and electroneurography (ENoG). ENoG is currently considered the most sensitive prognostic tool for evaluation of patients with Bell's palsy. However, some technical deficiencies are still unresolved and the methodology of testing is not fully standardized.

Facial Nerve Neurophysiology

According to Seddon's classification [10], facial paralysis may be the consequence of three different pathologic situations: conduction block (neuropraxia), axonotmesis, and neurotmesis. Since most facial palsies have an intratemporal origin, direct evaluation of the damaged nerve segment is impossible. Electrodiagnostic tests are only indirect indicators of facial nerve neurophysiology. All electrodiagnostic tests attempt to determine the degree of distal axonal degeneration.

It is important to note that only neuropraxic nerves can propagate action potentials. Stimulatory electrical tests, therefore, can stimulate only neuropraxic fibers. Thus, the compound action potential (CAP) recorded by ENoG is a reflection of nerve fibers that have not degenerated. Electrical tests cannot distinguish between axonotmesis and neurotmesis [2].

Indirect distal assessment of a proximal intratemporal injury has an important delay in evaluation of nerve damage as axonal degeneration progresses distal to the stylo-

J. Gavilán (✉), C. Gavilán
La Vina, 2–4°D–Urb. Baymar,
28220 Majadahonda, Madrid, Spain

mastoid foramen. Thus, all electric tests show abnormal results days to weeks after degeneration has taken place.

Finally, nerve excitability, once lost, does not return even after recovery of voluntary movement. ENoG, therefore, is no longer useful in predicting prognosis after the facial nerve is denervated.

Technical Variables in Electroneurography

ENoG was described in 1973 by Esslen [3]. The test has also been named neuromyography by Adour [1], electroneuronography by Fisch [4], and evoked electromyography by May [8]. Despite the popularity reached by ENoG during the last 20 years, the technique is not completely standardized and some questions affecting the reproducibility of the test still remain unanswered.

The size and intercenter distance of stimulating and recording electrodes have been subject to controversy in the literature [1, 3]. The same can be said of the placement of the electrodes. Two techniques have been proposed for positioning the electrodes: the standard placement technique and the optimized placement technique. The use of optimized lead placement improves the qualitiy of the recording, producing a more reliable CAP.

The muscle response recorded by ENoG must be elicited by supramaximal stimulation. A supramaximal stimulus is a level of current above the minimum required to just depolarize all axons. However, the ideal stimulus intensity to obtain a reliable CAP is not always possible.

Other factors that can affect the outcome of ENoG are the pressure applied to the electrodes, the skin impedance, and the stimulus frequency.

Critical Points in the Interpretation of Electroneurography

ENoG has become one of the most widely used electrical tests to assess the early prognosis of patients with Bell's

Table 1 Side-to-side differences for amplitude and latency in 24 normal subjects

	Amplitude (%)	Latency
Mean	25.15	0.5 ms
SD	11.4	0.4 ms
CV	63	88%
Range	2 – 50	0 – 1.7 ms
TRV	3.15	1.9%

Amplitude is expressed as a percentage of the compound action potential (CAP) of greatest amplitude.
SD, standard deviation; CV, coefficient of variation; TRV, test-retest variability.

palsy. However, some clinical assumptions deduced from the results of ENoG are not easily acceptable.

The result of ENoG, expressed as a percentage, is presumed to reflect the number of degenerated fibers [4]. However, in 1985, we performed a study in normal subjects [5] in which a mean $25.15\% \pm 2.38\%$ side-to-side difference in the recorded CAP was obtained (Table 1). This side-to-side difference in normal subjects is in contradiction with the aforementioned hypothesis. It is difficult to accept that there are 25% degenerated nerve fibers in normal facial nerves. The most important clinical application of this finding is that differences smaller than 25% in patients with Bell's palsy are meaningless, since they are normally present in healthy subjects.

Our test-retest variability (TRV) was 3.15% (Table 1), ranging from 0.9% to 10.5%. Only one subject had a TRV greater than 10%. This low TRV suggests that computer averaging of responses is not necessary.

It has also been mentioned that the lack of reproducibility of ENoG may be due to the desynchronization of the motor unit volley [4]. Therefore, it is recommended that

Table 2 Predictor variables selected by stepwise discriminant analysis ($n = 313$)

Factor	Variable name	Coding procedure
X_1	ENoG amplitude	$X_1 > 50\% = 1$ $25\% < X_1 \leq 50\% = 2$ $10\% < X_1 \leq 25\% = 3$ $X_1 \leq 10\% = 4$
X_2	Stapedial reflex	Absent = 1 Present = 0
X_3	Family history	Present = 1 Absent = 0
X_4	Hilger test	$X_4 \leq 2$ ma = 1 2 ma $< X_4 \leq 3.5$ ma = 2 $X_4 > 3.5$ ma = 3
X_5	Degree of palsy	Minimal function reached [7]
X_6	Previous ipsilateral palsy	Yes = 1 No = 0
X_7	Facial pain	Yes = 1 No = 0
X_8	Hyperacusis	Yes = 1 No = 0

ENoG, electroneurography.

several stimuli be applied before the final CAP is recorded [4]. Our results show no difference between the first five and the last five CAP obtained after 25 successive stimuli [5]. These findings indicate that stimulus repetition before registering the definitive CAP is not justified.

Electroneurography as a Prognostic Indicator

The previous technical considerations stress the limitations and deficiencies of ENoG. To ascertain the weight of each one of the multiple methods currently used in the prognostic evaluation of Bell's palsy, we performed a prospective statistical study by means of discriminant analysis (DA) [6]. A coding procedure was used for the amplitude of ENoG, creating four different categories (Table 2). According to facial recovery, two groups were created: (1) patients with facial recovery of 100% and (2) patients with facial recovery of less than 100%.

Eight variables were defined by stepwise DA as having maximum weight in determining the prognosis of patients with Bell's palsy (Table 2). The linear discriminant function determined by these variables is

$$12.48 - 3.82 X_1 - 3.44 X_2 - 5.46 X_3 - 2.81 X_4 + 0.04 X_5 \\ - 3.69 X_6 - 1.99 X_7 + 1.73 X_8 = 0$$

The code to develop this function is shown in Table 2. If the resulting figure is greater than 0, the patient should be included in the 100% facial recovery group. If the resulting figure is less than 0, the patient has an expected facial recovery of less than 100%.

The discriminant function has an overall accuracy of 95%. The rate of correct prediction for good prognosis (100% recovery) is 95.8% and for bad prognosis (less than 100% recovery) is 90.9%.

Conclusions

Even with its deficiencies, ENoG remains an important predictor variable in determining the prognosis of patients with Bell's palsy. However, if the treatment goal is to prevent denervation, it may be futile to use electrical tests for patient selection, because electrodiagnosis can only detect denervation 3 days after the damaging lesion has occurred [2].

The decreasing trend toward surgery makes questionable the need for prognostic testing. What, then is, the current role of electrodiagnostic tests for the clinician who does not believe in surgery for Bell's palsy?

Prognostic information is worthwhile for planning purposes, clinical documentation, and peace of mind when the results indicate good prognosis. Peace of mind is an important argument when the severity of the disease compromises the life of the patient. However, the natural history of Bell's palsy shows that 84% of untreated patients have good recovery without steroids or surgery [9]. When the treatment does not depend on the results of prognostic tests, ENoG is useful only for clinical documentation. In such instances, prognostic tests are meaningful only from an academic standpoint. Currently, we believe that electrodiagnosis is not helpful if the clinician makes no changes to the treatment plan on the basis of prognostic tests.

References

1. Adour KK, Sheldon MI, Kahn ZM (1980) Maximal nerve excitability testing versus neuromyography: prognostic value in patients with facial paralysis. Laryngoscope 90:1540–1547
2. Adour KK (1994) Facial nerve testing. In: Tackler RK, Brakmann DE (eds) Textbook of neurotology. Mosby, St Louis (in press)
3. Esslen E (1973) Electrodiagnosis of facial palsy. In: Miehlke A (ed) Surgery of the facial nerve. Saunders, Philadelphia, pp 45–51
4. Fisch U (1980) Maximal nerve excitability testing versus electroneuronography. Arch Otolaryngol 106:352–357
5. Gavilán J, Gavilán C, Sarriá MJ (1985) Facial electroneurography: results on normal humans. J Laryngol Otol 99:1085–1088
6. Gavilán C, Gavilán J, Rashad M, Gavilán M (1988) Discriminant analysis in predicting prognosis of Bell's palsy. Acta Otolaryngol (Stockh) 106:276–280
7. Janssen FP (1963) Over de postoperative facialisverlamming. Thesis, University of Amsterdam
8. May M, Blumenthal F, Taylor FH (1981) Bell's palsy: surgery based upon prognostic indicators and results. Laryngoscope 91:2092–2103
9. Peitersen E (1982) The natural history of Bell's palsy. Am J Otol 4:107–111
10. Seddon HJ (1943) Three types of nerve injury. Brain 66:237–288

Eur Arch Otorhinolaryngology (1994) [Suppl]: S 60–S 61

D. Edgar, J. Carter, S. Runswick, and P. Ybot

Role of Laminin for Axonal Growth

Introduction

The basement membrane glycoprotein laminin has been shown in vitro to stimulate the growth or regeneration of neuronal processes [2], to act together with neurotrophic factors to promote neuronal survival [8] and to stimulate the proliferation of glial cells [23]. Furthermore, experiments after lesion in vivo indicate that laminin is required for the survival of neural cells [17] and is involved in the regeneration of axons peripheral nerves [27].

Location of Laminin in the Nervous System

The transitory appearance of laminin immunoreactivity has been observed in the developing central nervous system at the time of axonal growth [4, 5, 24]. Similarly, in the developing peripheral nervous system, laminin immunoreactivity has been shown associated with axonal membranes [18]. An indication that the normal expression of laminin is necessary for the correct development of the nervous system is provided by the observations on the ls/ls lethal spotted mouse mutant and in Hirschsprung's disease in humans [25]. In both examples, the presence of abnormal basement membranes and the corresponding abnormal distribution of laminin have been correlated with the inability of migrating neural crest cells to colonise the distal gut, and in the case of the mouse mutant, abnormal migration was shown to be the consequence of the abnormal microenvironment provided by the gut wall [16]. Contact between laminin and neurons during development is facilitated because the laminin is not restricted to a basement membrane, but rather is in direct contact with neural cells,

being seen as patchy deposits on their membranes [13, 18]. This situation is in contrast to that in the adult, where laminin is confined to basement membranes on the exterior of the axon-Schwann cell units and absent from the central nervous system. Thus, the roles of laminin during development are likely to be more diverse and widespread than they are in the adult.

The reason for the developmental redistribution of laminin within the nervous system remains unknown. However, the fact that there are high levels of expression of laminin mRNA in developing peripheral nerves at the time when there is much soluble laminin indicates that the rate of laminin synthesis exceeds that with which it may be incorporated into basement membranes [19]. The rate-limiting step in basement membrane deposition in the nervous system and elsewhere remains to be established.

Expression of Laminin in the Nervous system

Reports describing laminin immunoreactivity in neurons of the central nervous system [12, 29] and laminin mRNA in retinal ganglion cells [28] remain controversial. It is, however, well established that laminin is expressed by at least some neuroepithelial and glial cells of both central and peripheral nervous systems during embryogenesis and sometimes also in the adult by reactive astrocytes after lesion [4, 6, 21, 22, 24].

In the peripheral nerve, Schwann cells, fibroblasts and perineurial cells have been shown to express laminin [15, 26]. Additionally, cultures of cells derived from peripheral nerves have been shown to synthesise the laminin-associated protein nidogen/entactin [1, 7]. It is not, however, clear whether different cells contribute individual components to the endoneurial basement membrane.

The crucial roles and interactions mediated by the basement membrane of peripheral nerve have been demonstrated in a series of experiments carried out by Bunge and co-workers [3]. Although isolated Schwann cells express

D. Edgar, J. Carter, S. Runswick, and P. Ybot
Department of Human Anatomy and Cell Biology,
University of Liverpool, U.K.

laminin, axon-Schwann cell contact is necessary for basement membrane formation, which is itself necessary for myelination of large-diameter axons by Schwann cells [9, 10]. These workers went on to show that optimal synthesis of collagen type IV together with fibroblasts and/or the interstitial extracellular matrix were normally necessary for basement membrane formation. However, addition of exogenous laminin to cultured Schwann cells was able to stimulate the appearance of basement membrane-like structures [3, 10]. These observations indicate that basement membrane deposition depends upon the provision of the appropriate cellular and extracellular matrix environment and that the stoichiometry of available basement membrane components is critical.

Recent observations indicate that the ratio of nidogen/entactin to laminin expression increases during peripheral nerve development (unpublished observations). Given that laminin can only bind to basement membrane (type IV) collagen via nidogen/entactin [11], then this basement membrane glycoprotein is a prime candidate to be the rate-limiting factor in basement membrane deposition in the developing nervous system.

Acknowledgement This work is supported by the Wellcome Trust, the Anatomical Society of Great Britain and Ireland, and the European Community.

References

1. Baron-Van Evercooren A, Gansmueller A, Gumpel M, Baumann N, Kleinman HK (1986) Schwann cell differentiation in vitro: extracellular matrix deposition and interaction. Dev Neurosci 8:182–196
2. Baron-Van Evercooren A, Kleinman HK, Ohno S, Marangos P, Schwarz JP, Dubois-Dalq ME (1982) Nerve growth factor, laminin and fibronectin promote neurite growth in human fetal sensory ganglion cultures. J Neurosci Res 8:179–194
3. Bunge MB, Clark MB, Dean AC, Eldridge CF, Bunge RP (1990) Schwann cell function depends upon axonal signals and basal lamina components. Ann NY Acad Sci 580:281–287
4. Cohen J, Burne JF, McKinlay C, Winter J (1987) The role of laminin and the laminin/fibronectin receptor complex in the outgrowth of retinal ganglion cell axons. Dev Biol 122:407–418
5. Cohen J, Nurcombe V, Jeffrey P, Edgar D (1989) Developmental loss of functional laminin receptors on retinal ganglion cells is regulated by their target tissue, the optic tectum. Development 107:381–387
6. Drago J, Nurcombe V, Bartlett PF (1991) Laminin through its long arm E8 fragment promotes the proliferation and differentiation of murine neuroepithelial cells in vitro. Exp Cell Res 192:256–265
7. Dziadek M, Edgar D, Paulsson M, Timpl R, Fleischmajer R (1986) Basement membrane proteins produced by Schwann Cells and in neurofibromatosis. Ann NY Acad Sci 486:248–259
8. Edgar D, Timpl R, Thoenen H (1984) The heparin-binding domain of laminin is responsible for its effects on neurite outgrowth and neuronal survival. EMBO J 3:1463–1468
9. Eldridge CF, Bunge MB, Bunge RP, Rigamonti L, Procacci P, Ledda M (1989) Differentiation of axon-related Schwann cells in vitro. II. Control of myelin formation by basal lamina. J Neurosci 9:625–638
10. Eldridge CF, Bunge MB, Bunge RP, Wood PM (1987) Differentiation of axon-related Schwann cells in vitro. I. Ascorbic acid regulates basal lamina assembly and myelin formation. J Cell Biol 105:1023–1034
11. Fox JW, Mayer U, Nischt R, Aumailley M, Reinhardt D, Wiedemann H, Mann K, Timpl R, Krieg T, Engel J, Chu M-L (1991) Recombinant nidogen consists of three globular domains and mediated binding of laminin to collagen type IV. EMBO J 10:3137–3146
12. Hagg T, Muir D, Engvall E, Varon S, Manthorpe M (1989) Laminin-like antigen in rat CNS neurons: distribution and changes upon brain injury and nerve growth factor treatment. Neuron 3:721–732
13. Halfter W, Song-Fua C (1987) Immunohistochemical localization of laminin, neural cell adhesion molecule, collagen type IV and T-61 antigen in the embryonic retina of the Japanese quail by in vivo injection of antibodies. Cell Tissue Res 249:487–496
14. Ide C, Tohyama K, Yokota R, Nitatori T, Onodera S (1983) Schwann cell basal lamina and nerve regeneration. Brain Res 288:61–75
15. Jaakkola S, Peltonen J, Uitto JJ (1989) Perineurial cells co-express genes encoding interstitial collagens and basement membrane zone components. J Cell Biol 108:1157–1163
16. Jacobs-Cohen RJ, Payette RF, Gershon MD, Rothman TP (1987) Inability of neural crest cells to colonize the presumptive aganglionic bowel of ls/ls mice: requirement for a permisive local microenvironment. J Comp Neurol 255:425–428
17. Kalcheim C, Barde Y-A, Thoenen H, LeDouarin NM (1987) In vivo effect of brain-derived neurotrophic factor on the survival of developing dorsal root ganglion cells. EMBO J 6:2871–2873
18. Kücherer-Ehret A, Graeber M, Edgar D, Thoenen H, Kreutzberg GW (1990) Immunoelectron microscopical localisation of laminin in normal and regenerating mouse sciatic nerve. J Neurocytol 19:101–109
19. Kücherer-Ehret A, Pottgiesser J, Kreutzberg GW, Thoenen H, Edgar D (1990) Developmental loss of laminin from the interstitial extracellular matrix correlates with decreased laminin gene expression. Development 110:1285–1293
20. Liesi P (1985) Laminin-immunoreactive glia distinguish regenerative adult CNS systems from non-regenerative ones. EMBO J 4:2505–2511
21. Liesi P (1985) Do neurons in the vertebrate CNS migrate on laminin? EMBO J 4:1163–1170
22. Liesi P, Kaakkola S, Dahl D, Vaheri A (1984) Laminin is induced in astrocytes of adult brain by injury. EMBO J 3:683–686
23. McGarvey ML, Baron-Van Evercooren A, Kleinman HK, Dubois-Dalcq M (1984) Synthesis and effects of basement membrane components in cultured rat Schwann cells. Dev Biol 105:18–28
24. McLoon SC, McLoon LK, Palm SL, Furcht LT (1988) Transient expression of laminin in the optic nerve of the developing rat. J Neurosci 8:1981–1990
25. Parikh DH, Tam PKH, van Velzen D, Edgar D (1992) Abnormalities in the distribution of laminin and collagen type IV in Hirschsprung's disease. Gastroenterology 102:1236–1241
26. Peltonen J, Jaakkola S, Chu M-L, Uitto J (1990) Selective expression of extracellular matrix genes encoding type VI collagen and laminin by Schwann cells, perineurial cells, and fibroblasts from normal nerve and neurofibromas. Ann NY Acad Sci 580:501–504
27. Sandrock AW Jr, Matthew WD (1987) An in vitro neurite-promoting antigen functions in axonal regeneration in vivo. Science 237:1605–1608
28. Sarthy PV, Fu M (1990) Localization of laminin B1 mRNA in retinal ganglion cells by in situ hybridization. J Cell Biol 110:2099–2108
29. Suzuki H, Yamamoto T, Yamamoto H, Konno H, Iwasaki Y, Ohara Y, Terunuma H (1990) Intraneuronal laminin-like immunoreactivity in the human central nervous system. Brain Res 520:324–329

Eur Arch Otorhinolaryngology (1994) [Suppl]: S 62–S 65

K.K. Adour

Bell's Palsy: Synopsis by an Otologist

Introduction

Prior to 1931, patients with Bell's palsy were most often evaluated and treated in the Departments of Neurology and Physical Medicine. Treatments were empiric and usually reserved for those with delayed recovery. In 1931, Arthur Duel, based on collaborative work with Sir Charles Ballance, performed the first facial nerve decompression for Bell's palsy [2]. The operation suggested by Ney in 1922 [24] and Martin in 1931 [16] was based on the assumption that entrapment of the facial nerve in the temporal bone caused the paralysis. The primary ischemic theory of pathogenesis postulated dysfunction of the autonomic nervous system, producing arteriolar spasm and thrombosis in the vessels supplying the nerve within the rigid bony fallopian canal. Later a secondary ischemic hypothesis suggested a primary inflammatory, viral, or immunologic edema causing disturbances of the microcirculation, leading to loss of nerve conductivity. Both concepts suggest that these processes lead to anoxia, followed by compensatory dilation of the vessels and transudation, further increasing the vascular compression effect. The goal of treatment would be to reduce the compressive effect and break the vicious cycle damaging the facial nerve. Bell's palsy became a "surgical disease".

Bell's palsy became synonymus with the term idiopathic facial paralysis, defined as a unilateral facial paralysis of unknown cause. Since other diseases of the temporal bone such as acute and chronic otitis media and primary and secondary tumors were known to cause facial paralysis, Bell's palsy was a diagnosis of exclusion. Now that there was a possible surgical treatment for Bell's palsy, otologists became more interested in the disease, stating they were qualified to make accurate diagnosis and could institute appropriate treatment. Gradually, more articles

K.K. Adour
1000 Green Street #1203, San Francisco, CA 94133, USA

began to appear in the otolaryngology literature, and today a cursory review of the Index Medicus confirms that the majority of published Bell's palsy articles are written by otologists. Even though otologists were highly qualified to make the exclusionary diagnosis of Bell's palsy, serious questions arose about patient selection, timing, and extent of surgical facial nerve decompression.

Patient Selection

The natural history of Bell's palsy was such that the majority of patients recovered without treatment. Thus, selection of patients for surgical treatment became a major dilemma for otologists. It became necessary to devise methods for determining which patients were at risk for nerve degeneration (denervation) and subsequent delayed poor recovery. In the early years, the decision to perform facial nerve decompression was based on faradic-galvanic muscle stimulation tests. The loss of brisk response to faradic stimulation and its replacement by prolonged, sluggish response to galvanism was labeled the "reaction of degeneration". Lack of galvanic response was a contraindication for surgery.

In the 1950s it was suggested that clinical testing based on the differential of the faradic-galvanic response might not be reliable. As a result of the lack of reliability of electrical testing, the decision to operate was based upon clinical experience (empirical indication). Factors such as the presence of pain at onset and poor muscle tone were stressed as indicators of poor prognosis. Patients with these clinical signs were considered for facial nerve decompression.

The 1960s were influenced by Richardson's and Wynn Parry's work in 1957 on electrodiagnosis [26, 27]. Campbell and Lauman [13] standardized facial nerve testing using nerve excitability, and Hilger [6, 7] designed the portable facial nerve stimulator. For facial nerve testing, the stimulating electrode producing a square wave measured in volts (V) or milliamperes (ma) was placed over the facial nerve trunk and threshold intensity producing a visible muscle contraction was recorded. This was the minimal nerve excitability test (NET). Per cutaneous nerve excitability testing became the standard for patient selection for surgery, although there was disagreement about interpretation. Campbell stated that a difference of 2 ma between the affected and unaffected side should be used as the criterion for decompression. Alford [1] suggested 3 ma and Jongkees [9–11] used a 3.5-ma difference to select patients for treatment. Because of this lack of agreement in interpretation, a modification was suggested using maximal stimulation (MST) of the peripheral facial nerve branches to yield a more accurate and earlier assessment of denervation.

Salivary flow testing as a predictor of prognosis was heralded by Magielski and Blatt as a "practical and invincible guide to deciding for or against surgical decompression of the facial nerve" [15]. Performing the test was technically difficult, time consuming, and uncomfortable for the patient and never gained popularity.

The determination of denervation by nerve excitability tests relied on visual assessment of muscle motion and was considered to be only partially reliable. To obviate interpretation errors, Fisch and Esslen devised electroneurography (ENoG) to produce a recorded measurement of facial muscle compound summation action potentials (CAP) [5]. ENoG became the gold standard electrical test for patient selection for surgery.

Timing of Surgery

Although there was some agreement that electrical testing was a good method of patient selection for surgery, there was wide disagreement on when to perform surgery. Ballance and Deul [2] operated when there was persistent absence of faradic response, but did not define "persistent" within a time frame. Lack of galvanic response was a contraindication for surgery.

Morris defined "persistent" as 3–4 weeks after faradic response was lost [22]. He added that decompression was indicated when faradic response was lost and there was cessation of voluntary improvement. He further suggested operating between 6 and 12 weeks after onset of the palsy when there was no evidence of voluntary motion and reaction of degeneration was present. Tumarkin advised "early" surgery, but did not specifically define "early", which we can deduce to mean before 2 months [33]. In the 1940s, Lathrop, suggested decompression in any patient after 3 months without recovery and response to faradic stimulation.

In the 1950s, Cawthorne, who became a leading advocate of facial nerve decompression, operated 1 month after onset of the palsy when there was loss of faradic stimulation [4]. Jongkess stressed decompression within 12 weeks

of onset when the reaction of degeneration was present. Kettle summarized the philosophies of his contemporaries and avoided strict guidelines for timing of decompression [12].

In the 1960s, the results of per cutaneous nerve excitability tests continued to determine the timing of surgery. The role of surgery was to prevent denervation of the facial nerve and to operate on those patients who had "impending denervation". Prediction of impending denervation was based on the test differential between affected and unaffected sides and daily electrical tests were advocated. Performing a decompression became a "surgical emergency" when the test became abnormal.

The concept of "impending denervation" has carried over through the 1970s and the 1980s and it was agreed that surgical intervention after complete loss of electrical excitability was not indicated. At the present time, the most popular concept for the timing of surgery is based on a differential of 90 % in the recorded ENoG compound muscle action potential (CAP) of the affected and unaffected side occuring with 2 weeks of onset of the paralysis.

Extent of Surgery

The intratemporal facial nerve is divided into five segments:

1. The *meatal portion* is that portion which traverses the internal auditory meatus.
2. The *labyrinthine segment* begins as the nerve enters the falloplian canal, then extends to and includes the geniculate ganglion.
3. The *horizontal segment* begins just posterior to the geniculate ganglion and extends to the ampullary end of the horizontal semicircular canal.
4. The *pyramidal segment* lies between the horizontal segment and the vertical segment, intimately related to the inferior surface of the horizontal semicircular canal and the superior-posterior wall of the middle ear.
5. The *vertical segment* begins below the posterior end of the horizontal semicircular canal, ending at the stylomastoid foramen.

Another portion of the facial nerve, the *iter chordae posterius*, represents the bony passages surrounding the facial nerve where the chorda tympani nerve enters the middle ear space. Over the past six decades, each of these segments has been implicated as a crucial area causing entrapment of the facial nerve in Bell's palsy.

When the operative treatment of Bell's palsy was first introduced in 1932, Ballance and Duel [2] proposed decompression of the distal 1 cm at the stylomastoid foramen. They emphasized that removal of less than half of the outer bony wall was sufficient and that no effective decompression occurred until the fibrous sheath was slit. Tumarkin disagreed with the concept of unroofing the fallopian canal and performed a simple mastoidectomy, he ablated the stylomastoid artery to diminish tympanic vascular compression [34]. In 1936, Morris suggested that the entire lower half of the facial nerve should be decompressed [22] and in 1939 Tickle performed decompression of the entire vertical segment [31].

With the advent of the acoustic impedance measurement of Metz [20], the operating microscope, and of Tschiassny's [32] topographic diagnosis, otologists were theoretically able to pinpoint the site of the compression: surgery should only be undertaken when the site of the lesion was surgically accessible. For Cawthorne, surgical treatment was permissible in the area from the face to the geniculate ganglion [4]. In contrast to Ballance and Duel, Sullivan and Smith advocated removal of two thirds of the circumferential bony canal "as far as surgically possible" and posterior incision of the sheath to protect arcading arterioles [29]. Lewis developed the facial recess approach to the horizontal and geniculate portion of the facial nerve and questioned the reliability of accurate localization of the site of the lesion [14]. Lewis also advised the endaural approach, used copious irrigation to cool the nerve, removed the thin bone from the perineurium with a pick and dental excavator, and slit the sheath of the posterior surface to protect the arterioles. Shambaugh insisted that only the vertical segment be decompressed and that the ossicles should not be disturbed [29]. Jongkees stressed decompression of the vertical and pyramidal segments [10, 11].

The middle cranial fossae approach to the internal auditory canal was devised by House in 1961 [8], making it possible to decompress the entire facial nerve. Early in 1970, Fisch advocated total facial nerve decompression and demonstrated swelling in the meatal and labyrinthine segments [5]. Later in 1970, Fisch, based on these surgical findings, believed that decompression of *only* the meatal and labyrinthine segments was necessary and began the facial nerve decompression at the internal auditory canal through the middle cranial fossa approach. This concept persisted throughout the 1980s until the advent of magnetic resonance imaging (MRI), which using gadolinium enhancement showed inflammatory response in multiple areas of the facial nerve in the fallopian canal. Studies are underway to determine whether the extent and location for surgery can be improved using these MRI findings.

Present Status of Surgery

Laboratory and clinical studies have established that Bell's palsy is a viral, autoimmune, demyelinating disease probably caused by the herpes simplex virus, and a recent study demonstrated the efficacy of treatment with the antiviral agent acyclovir (Zovirax). The selection of patients, timing of surgery, and the extent of surgical decompression may become only footnotes of history. Jongkees' statement in the 1960s that surgery cannot benefit a viral disease gains further validity in the 1990s. The wheel has come full turn. The primary role of the otologist in the treatment of Bell's palsy is again, as it was in the 1930s, relegated to ruling out other diseases as a cause for paralysis.

References

1. Alford BR (1967) Electrodiagnostic studies in facial paralysis. Arch Otolaryngol 85:259–264
2. Ballance C, Duel AB (1932) The operative treatment of facial palsy by the introduction of nerve grafts into the fallopian canal and by other methods. Arch Otolaryngol 15:1–70
3. Blatt IM, Freeman JA (1969) Bell's palsy III. Further observations on the pathogenesis of Bell's palsy and the results of chorda tympani neurectomy. Trans Am Acad Ophthalmol Otolaryngol 73:420–438
4. Cawthorne T (1951) The pathology and surgical treatment of Bell's palsy. Proc R Soc Med 44:565–568
5. Fisch U, Esslen E (1972) Total intratemporal exposure of the facial nerve. Arch Otolaryngol 95:335–341
6. Hilger JA (1949) The true nature of Bell's palsy. Laryngoscope 59:228–235
7. Hilger JA (1984) Facial nerve stimulator. Trans Am Acad Ophthalmol Otolaryngol 68:74–76
8. House WF (1961) Surgical exposure of the internal auditory canal and its contents through the middle cranial fossae. Laryngoscope 71:1363–1385
9. Jongkees LBW (1957) Treatment of Bell's palsy. Neurology 7:697–702
10. Jongkees LBW (1965) Bell's palsy: a surgical emergency. Arch Otolaryngol 81:497–501
11. Jongkees LBW (1969) The timing of surgery in intratemporal facial paralysis. Laryngoscope 79:1557–1561
12. Kettel K (1959) Peripheral facial palsy: pathology and surgery. Thomas, Copenhagen
13. Laumans EPJ (1965) Nerve excitability tests in facial paralysis. Arch Otolaryngol 81:478–488
14. Lewis ML Jr (1956) A variation in technique of facial nerve decompression. Laryngoscope 66:1451–1463
15. Magaleski WF, Blatt IM (1958) Submaxillary salivary flow: a test of chorda tympani nerve function as an aid in diagnosis and prognosis of facial nerve paralysis. Laryngoscope 68: 1770– 1789
16. Martin RC (1931) Intratemporal suture of the surgical repair of the facial nerve. Arch Otolaryngol 259–264
17. May M et al. (1971) The prognostic accuracy of the maximal stimulation test compared with nerve excitability test in Bell's palsy. Laryngoscope 81:931–938
18. May M, Hawkins CD (1972 Bell's palsy: results for surgery: salivation tests versus nerve excitability test as a basis of treatment. Laryngoscope 82:1337–1662
19. May M (1978) Progressive ascending paralysis, therapeutic implications. Laryngoscope 88:61–72
20. Metz O (1946) The acoustic impedance measured on normal and pathological ears. Acta Otolaryngol [Suppl] 63:1–254
21. Meurman OH (1958) Endaural tympanic approach to the facial nerve. Acta Otolaryngol 49:495–498
22. Morris WM (1938) Surgical treatment of Bell's palsy. Lancet 1:429–431
23. Morris WM (1939) Surgical treatment of facial paralysis: review of 46 cases. Lancet 2:558–561
24. Ney KW (1922) Facial paralysis and the surgical repair of the facial nerve. Laryngoscope 32:327–347
25. Peitersen E (1982) The natural history of Bell's palsy. Am J Otolaryngol 4:107–111

26. Richardson AT, Wynn Parry CB (1957a) The theory and practice of electrodiagnosis. Ann Phys Med 4:3–16
27. Richardson AT, Wynn Parry CB (1957b) The theory and practice of electrodiagnosis. Ann Phys Med 4:41–58
28. Shambaugh GE Jr (1959) Surgery of the ear. Saunders, Philadelphia, pp 543–571
29. Sullivan JA, Smith JB (1950) The otological concept of Bell's palsy and its treatment. Ann Otol Rhinol Laryngol
30. Thomander L, Stalberg E (1981) Electroneurography in the prognostication of Bell's palsy. Acta Otolaryngol 92:221–237
31. Tickle TG (1939) Nerve graft operation for facial paralysis. Laryngoscope 49:475–481
32. Tschiassny K (1946) The site of the facial nerve lesion in cases of Ramsay Hunt's syndrome. Ann Otol Rhinol Laryngol 55:152–174
33. Tumarkin IA (1936) Some aspects of the problem of facial paralysis. Proc R Soc Med 29:1685–1691
34. Tumarkin IA (1951) (Discussion). In: Cawthorn T, The pathology and surgical treatment of Bell's palsy. Proc R Soc Med 44–565

Eur Arch Otorhinolaryngology (1994) [Suppl]: S66

ABSTRACT

R. Heumann, B. Hengerer, M. Brown, H. Perry, A. Markus, and G. D. Borasio

Role of Oncogenes in Neural Regeneration

In the intact rat sciatic nerve the nonneuronal cells surrounding the axons synthesize very low amounts of nerve growth factor (NGF). After cutting the nerve there is a biphasic increase in levels of NGF-mRNA in the distal nerve segment and in the tip of the proximal stump where axonal regrowth is initiated. The rapid transient increase of NGF-mRNA (first phase) is preceded by an almost immediate elevation in the levels of the mRNAs coding for the nuclear protooncogenes c-*fos* and c-*jun*. A *trans*-activating effect of *FOS* on the NGF-promoter was demonstrated by using sciatic nerve derived fibroblasts carrying an exogenous inducible *fos* gene. Further analysis shows that an AP-1 consensus sequence located in the first intron of the *NGF* gene is essential for the *fos*-mediated increase of NGF-mRNA levels.

Unlike the initial transient increase of NGF-mRNA, the second persistent phase of increase in NGF synthesis after nerve cut is mediated by macrophages which synthesize interleukin-1. The role of lesion-induced macrophage recruitment in regulating NGF synthesis and sensory axon regrowth in vivo was investigated in mutant mice (strain C57/Ola). In these mice the lesion-induced recruitment of macrophages and the onset of Wallerian degeneration is delayed. The results suggest that macrophages are not only responsible for the degradation of severed axons and of myelin debris but in addition direct the synthesis of NGF and sensory (but not motor) axon regrowth.

Lesion-induced retrograde degeneration of sensory axons and cell bodies is observed expecially during development. After sciatic nerve lesion functional regeneration depends on the capacity of the damaged neurons to survive the axotomy. Mechanisms of survival were investigated using chick embryonic sensory neurons as a model. Intracellular application of purified recombinant protooncogene p21*ras* proteins prevented neuronal cell death in cultured sensory neurons that are dependent on the presence of the appropriate neurotrophic factor. Conversely, intracellular application of affinity purified F_{ab} fragments derived from the function-blocking monoclonal antibody Y13-259 against p21*ras* specifically interfered with nerve growth factor (NGF) mediated survival action. The results implicate that the intracellular signal transduction of NGF in neural crest derived sensory neurons is mediated by p21*ras* protein.

R. Heumann (✉), B. Hengerer, M. Brown, H. Perry, A. Markus, and G. D. Borasio
Ruhr-University, Molecular Neurobiochemistry,
44780 Bochum, Germany

The Facial Nucleus
and Its Cellular Environment

Eur Arch Otorhinolaryngology (1994) [Suppl]: S69–S70

INVITED LECTURES

W. J. Streit

The Role of Microglia in Regeneration

Introduction

Injury to the facial nerve results in a regenerative response of facial motor neurons (FMN) in the facial nucleus. The complex metabolic events that develop in injured FMN as a direct consequence of the nerve lesion affect not only the motor neurons themselves, but also exert consequential influences on their immediate microenvironment. Located throughout the neuropil of the facial nucleus are glial cells, among them microglia, which react sensitively to any disturbance affecting FMN. Following is a summary of some of the known microglial reactions that occur in response to lesions affecting FMN, as well as discussion on how microglial reactivity might play a role in regeneration.

Early Response of Microglial Cells to Axotomy

The facial nerve system of the rat has provided a very useful experimental model for studying microglial reactions, because it allows the generation of the same reproducible neuronal lesion each time by performing a simple axotomy. As a consequence, the microglial response has become standardized and much easier to study. The first observations regarding microglial activation in the rat facial nucleus were made by Kreutzberg [12], who showed with light microscopic autoradiography that microglia undergo vigorous proliferation within 3–4 days after nerve transection. At the time no microglia-specific markers were available, and definitive identity of the proliferating cells as microglia was established some 20 years later by Graeber et al. [9] using electron microscopic autoradiography. Microglia typically proliferate in the immediate vicinity of axotomized motor neurons, which results in the

W. J. Streit
Department of Neuroscience, U of F Health Service Center,
University of Florida College of Medicine,
Gainesville, FL 32610-0244, USA

tight ensheathment of the neuronal perikarya by microglial cytoplasmic processes. Blinzinger and Kreutzberg [2] showed that such perineuronal microglia were capable of interposing their cytoplasmic processes in between the neuronal surface membrane and axosomatic boutons, thereby effectively deafferenting the FMN. It is unknown whether the stripping away of synapses by microglial processes is selective in removing either excitatory or inhibitory inputs; however, in addition to the possible electrophysiological significance of synaptic stripping, it is conceivable that the close microglial ensheathment of injured neurons could serve a neuronotrophic function in helping the neuron to recover from injury. The fact that microglia in tissue culture can be stimulated to release high amounts of nerve growth factor (NGF) [14] would support such a hypothesis, although synthesis of NGF by microglia has not been shown to occur in vivo. It has also been shown that blood monocytes, to which microglia are undoubtedly related, can produce neuronotrophic activity following stimulation with colony-stimulating factors [3]. Since the receptors for both macrophage colony-stimulating factor and granulocyte-macrophage colony-stimulating factors are known to be expressed by reactive microglia in the regenerating facial nucleus [16], one could speculate that those reactive microglia can be stimulated to produce neuronotrophic action. NGF may not play a major role in this process, since FMN do not express NGF receptors, but instead increase their expression of the transferrin receptor after axotomy [10]. Future studies should therefore examine the possible involvement of other known neurotrophic factors, and the possibility certainly remains that a neurotrophic role of microglia could be mediated via a yet unknown trophic agent.

Neuroimmunological Considerations of Microglial Activity

While the investigation of microglia during FMN regeneration with regard to neuronotrophic activity is still in its infancy, considerable progress has been made in recent years on the immunological aspects of microglial reactivity in response to axotomy. These studies have led to the conclusion that microglia act as representatives of the immune system in the CNS. The concept of an indigenous microglial neuroimmune network has its roots in del Rio-Hortega's astute observations in the 1920s and 1930s, which led him to regard microglia as components of the reticuloendothelial system invading the developing brain [4]. For much of the following decades, microglial research was intensely focused on the possible monocytic origin of these cells, which was never really proven. The availability and application of antibodies directed against leukocyte antigens in the late 1980s resulted in the observation that antigens of the major histocompatibility complex (MHC), formerly thought to be completely absent from brain tissue, are expressed by reactive microglial cells in the facial nucleus after axotomy [17, 18]. Early during the axon reaction, microglia rapidly increase the expression of MHC class I molecules, reaching maximal levels after about 5–7 days. In parallel with class I expression, a much more gradual upregulation of class II (Ia) antigens is observed, which differs in two respects from class I expression: the cell types involved and the time course of expression. Both parenchymal microglia and extraparenchymal perivascular cells (for a definition of these cell types, see [11] demonstrate increased Ia expression, which is limited to only a selected fraction of all the cells present in a given area. This is in contrast to the expression of class I antigens, which are upregulated by all microglia in the area of the facial nucleus. Unlike class I expression, which happens readily and rapidly during the retrograde response, the appearance of class II antigens follows a protracted time course lasting up to several months after axotomy. Although the significance of MHC expression of microglia is understood in terms of the immunological implications, i.e., that the CNS contains indigenous immunocompetent cells that are capable of antigen presentation, its relevance for a role of microglia in supporting regenerative response of FMN is not readily apparent. One could reasonably suspect, however, that immunological activation in terms of phenotypic changes in accompanied by a similar stimulation of secretory activity. Microglia are known to be highly secretory cells in tissue culture [6, 8, 15], and cytokine immunoreactivity has been demonstrated in situ on human microglia in encephalitis and Alzheimer's disease [5]. Among the known microglial secretory products are cytokines, such as the interleukins and tumor necrosis factor, which are known to have multiple effects, including specific actions related to nervous system regeneration, for example, the induction of NGF mRNA by interleukin-1 (IL-1) [13]. In addition to IL-1, a number of other proinflammatory agents have been shown to increase NGF expression in vitro, whereas anti-inflammatory drugs such as dexamethasone suppress NGF production [7]. The converse situation that neurotrophic agents have neuroimmunomodulatory activity is also supported by some

studies [1, 19]. In concluding this discussion, it is apparent that a systematic in situ study of microglial cytokine/growth factor production would aid tremendously in illuminating a possible interplay between immunological and neuronotrophic activity.

References

1. Abramchik GV, Yermakova SS, Kaliunov VN, Tanina RM, Tumilovich MK (1988) The immunomodulatory effect of nerve growth factor. J Neurosci Res 19:349–356
2. Blinzinger K, Kreutzberg G (1968) Displacement of synaptic terminals from regenerating motoneurons by microglial cells. Z Zellforsch 85:145–157
3. Bryant HU, Burgess SK, Gendelman HE, Meltzer MS, Holaday JW, Bernton EW (1991) Neuronotrophic activity associated with monocyte growth factors and products of stimulated monocytes. In: Fredrickson RCA, McGaugh JL, Felten DL (eds) Peripheral signalling of the brain. Hogrefe and Huber, Toronto, pp 83–99
4. Del Rio-Hortega R (1932) Microglia. In: Penfield W (ed) Cytology and cellular pathology of the nervous system, vol 2. Hoeber, New York, p 481
5. Dickson DW, Lee SC, Mattiace L, Yen SHC, Brosnan C (1993) Microglia and cytokines in neurological disease, with special reference to AIDS and Alzheimer's disease. GLIA 7:75–83
6. Frei K, Siepl C, Groscurth P, Bodmer S, Fontana A (1988) Immunobiology of microglial cells. Ann NY Acad Sci 540:218–227
7. Friedman WJ, Lärkfors L, Ayer-LeLievre C, Ebendal T, Olson L, Persson H (1990) Regulation of β-nerve growth factor expression by inflammatory mediators in hippocampal cultures. J Neurosci Res 27:374–382
8. Giulian D (1987) Ameboid microglia as effectors of inflammation in the central nervous system. J Neurosci Res 18:155–171
9. Graeber MB, Tetzlaff W, Streit WJ, Kreutzberg GW (1988) Microglial cells but not astrocytes undergo mitosis following facial nerve axotomy. Neurosci Lett 85:317–321
10. Graeber MB, Raivich G, Kreutzberg GW (1989) Increase of transferrin receptors and iron uptake in the regenerating facial facial motoneurones. J Neurosci Res 23:342–345
11. Graeber MB, Streit WJ (1990) Perivascular microglia defined. Trends Neurosci 13:366
12. Kreutzberg GW (1966) Autoradiographische Untersuchungen über die Beteiligung von Gliazellen an der axonalen Reaktion im Facialiskern der Ratte. Acta Neuropathol (Berl) 7:149–161
13. Lindholm D, Heumann R, Meyer M, Thoenen H (1987) Interleukin-1 regulates synthesis of nerve growth factor in non-neuronal cells of rat sciatic nerve. Nature 330:658–659
14. Mallat M, Houlgatte R, Brachet P, Prochiantz A (1989) Lipopolysaccharide-stimulated rat brain macrophages release NGF in vitro. Dev Biol 133:309–311
15. Merrill JE (1987) Macroglia: neural cells responsive to lymphokines and growth factors. Immunol Today 8:146–150
16. Raivich G, Gehrmann J, Kreutzberg GW (1991) Increase of macrophage colony-stimulating factor and granulocyte-macrophage colony-stimulating factor receptors in the regenerating rat facial nucleus. J Neurosci Res 30:682–686
17. Streit WJ, Graeber MB, Kreutzberg GW (1989) Peripheral nerve lesion produces increased levels of major histocompatibility complex antigens in the central nervous system. J Neuroimmunol 21:117–123
18. Streit WJ, Graeber MB, Kreutzberg GW (1989) Expression of Ia antigen on perivascular and microglial cells after sublethal and lethal motor neuron injury. Exp Neurol 105:115–126
19. Thorpe LW, Stach RW, Hashim GA, Marchetti D, Perez-Polo JR (1987) Receptors for nerve growth factor on rat spleen mononuclear cells. J Neurosci Res 17:128–134

Eur Arch Otorhinolaryngology (1994) [Suppl]: S 71 – S 74

INVITED LECTURES

C. A. Haas, F. L. Dumoulin, P. Lazar, G. Raivich, M. Reddington, W. J. Streit, and G. W. Kreutzberg

The Role of Calcitonin Gene-Related Peptide in the Regenerating Facial Nucleus

Introduction

Neuronal injury is known to induce characteristic changes in axotomised neurons [2, 15, 20, 25] that are accompanied by a perineuronal glial reaction [22]. These alterations are thought to enable the neuron to initiate neurite outgrowth and to successfully regenerate its peripheral axon [9]. The complex cellular interactions and their regulation during neuronal regeneration are as yet poorly understood. Insight into the mechanisms regulating this process might also provide important clues for the treatment of neurological disease. The recent discovery of neuropeptides with trophic and differentiation-inducing effects has provided a new approach to this problem.

Calcitonin gene-related peptide (CGRP) is a neuropeptide of 37 amino acids generated by alternative splicing of the calcitonin gene primary transcript [1]. CGRP is widely distributed in the peripheral and central nervous systems, including sensory and motor systems of the spinal cord (reviewed by Ishida-Yamamoto and Tohyama [19]). CGRP is most abundantly present in sensory neurons, but it has also been found in motoneurons and neurons of the autonomic nervous system. Apart from its neuromodulatory action, CGRP exerts various differentiation-inducing and trophic actions on neurons [5, 31]. Therefore, interest has focused on a possible involvement of this neuropeptide in neuronal regeneration.

This paper will review the currently available in vivo and in vitro data on CGRP expression during motoneuron regeneration and CGRP effects on cultured glial cells.

C. A. Haas (✉)
Anatomical Institute I, University of Freiburg,
Albertstrasse 17, 79001 Freiburg, Germany

F. L. Dumoulin, P. Lazar, G. Raivich, M. Reddington,
W. J. Streit, and G. W. Kreutzberg
Department of Neuromorphology,
Max-Planck-Institute for Psychiatry,
82152 Martinsried, Germany

Calcitonin Gene-Related Peptide in Regenerating Motor Neurons

Axotomy of the rat facial nerve leads to an increase in CGRP immunoreactivity in facial motoneurons [26, 29]. An initial increase was noted as early as 15 h after axotomy; enhanced CGRP immunoreactivity (IR) was seen up to 39 days after injury [29]. In addition, a redistribution of CGRP-IR in axotomised motoneurons was observed: in normal motoneurons, faint CGRP-IR is confined to perikarya; however, after axotomy CGRP-IR is seen to extend prominently into dendrites [26, 29]. An increase of CGRP-IR in lesioned motoneurons seems to be a general phenomenon, since it has been observed in axotomized motoneurons of the rat hypoglossal and oculomotor nerves [26] as well as in axotomized rat cervical and lumbar motoneurons [3, 26–28].

In the regenerating rat facial nucleus, a change occurred from a low CGRP content to peak levels, reaching a five-fold increase 3 days after axotomy. CGRP levels returned to control levels 9 days after injury [8]. The increase in CGRP occurring after facial nerve lesion was accompanied by an increase in CGRP mRNA: quantitative measurement of CGRP mRNA revealed a peak at postoperative day 1 [8]. With in situ hybridization histochemistry, an increased number of CGRP mRNA-positive facial motoneurons was demonstrated as early as 15 h, reaching a peak during the first day after injury [16]. The lesion-induced expression of CGRP mRNA clearly precedes the increase of the peptide, indicating a de novo synthesis of CGRP in axotomized facial motoneurons.

Long-term studies on CGRP peptide and CGRP mRNA expression in the regenerating rat facial nucleus revealed a second peak (approximately 500% of control) 21 days after axotomy [8]. This second increase in CGRP mRNA did not occur if reinnervation was prevented, whereas the first peak was unaffected [8]; this suggests that the second peak could be induced by reinnervation of the peripheral target tissue. It is possible that neurotrophic factors that are normally retrogradely transported accumulate during long-term denervation in the denervated peripheral tissue and induce a short, but massive, rebound in the level of CGRP synthesis in the motoneurons immediately following reinnervation of the peripheral target.

In contrast to the observed changes in CGRP expression in injured motoneurons, no alterations in specific, high-affinity CGRP binding to the facial nucleus is seen during regeneration. Studies on the cellular localization of CGRP binding also showed it to be unaffected by selective destruction of motoneurons with the toxic lectin ricin [7]. These data suggest that most of the CGRP binding sites are extraneuronal and could be present on glial cells within the normal and regenerating facial motor nucleus.

In addition to alterations in gene expression, metabolism, and structure that occur in the perikarya of injured neurons, a perineuronal glial reaction also occurs that is thought to support neuronal regeneration [22]. In view of the data on the regulation of CGRP and the distribution of CGRP binding in the facial motor nucleus, it has been suggested that perineuronal glial cells might be the primary target of neuronal CGRP and that CGRP might be a mediator in the neuronal-glial interactions [8, 16, 29] taking place during regeneration. Indeed, the temporal pattern of CGRP expression in regeneration facial motoneurons corresponds well to that of the early and delayed astrocyte reactions [13, 14] in the regenerating facial nucleus, slightly preceding the glial changes. Moreover, a redistribution of CGRP immunoreactivity predominantly into dendrites is observed, which could be indicative of a local release of the peptide, possible by dendritic secretion [21]. Further support for this hypothesis that newly synthesized neuronal CGRP might interact with glial receptors in the facial nucleus to initiate and regulate astrocytic responses accompanying motoneuron regeneration also comes from in vitro data on the effects of CGRP on astrocytes, which are presented below.

In Vitro Effects of Calcitonin Gene-Related Peptide on Glial Cells of the Central Nervous System

Addition of CGRP to primary astrocyte cultures resulted in a rapid morphological change of these cells, identified immunocytochemically using antibodies against the astrocyte marker glial acidic fibrillary protein (GFAP) [24]. They changed from a flat, polygonal appearance to a multipolar form bearing many processes. This effect was rapid, being observed 20–30 min after additon of 1 μM CGRP. The appearance of the cells after addition of CGRP was very similar to that produced by treatment of astrocytes with dibutyryl cyclic adenosine monophosphate (AMP) [10]. An identical change in astrocyte morphology was observed after treating the cultures with forskolin, which directly stimulates adenylate cyclase. The resulting stellate astrocyte form has been likened to that of reactive astrocytes found in the vicinity of neurons after a wide variety of pathological insults in vivo [10]. The morphological action of CGRP on identified astrocytes indicates the presence of CGRP receptors on these cells and supports a role for CGRP as a mediator of neuron-glia interaction.

The apparent similarity between the actions of CGRP and cyclic AMP derivatives on astrocyte morphology in vitro suggested that cyclic AMP might be a second messenger mediating the CGRP effect. Indeed, an association of CGRP receptors with the stimulation of cyclic AMP synthesis has been reported on cells from various sources [12, 18, 23]. Astrocyte cultures also responded to addition of CGRP with an increase in their cyclic AMP content [24]. The pharmacological properties of this response are characteristic of a CGRP-specific receptor rather than being mediated via an interaction between CGRP and a calcitonin receptor. Thus, calcitonin showed only a small stimulation of cyclic AMP accumulation over the peptide concentration range studied. In addition, the CGRP fragment CGRP(8-37), which has been reported to be an antagonist at CGRP receptors [4, 6], blocked the stimulatory action of CGRP on cyclic AMP. These data indicated the presence of CGRP receptors coupled to adenylate cyclase in astrocyte cultures. This observation, together with the similarity between the morphological actions of CGRP and cyclic AMP derivatives on GFAP-positive cells, suggests a role for CGRP receptors coupled to adenylate cyclase in controlling the state of differentiation and activation of astrocytes.

In contrast to the rapid morphological action of CGRP in vitro, which probably involves rapid rearrangements of cytoskeletal elements [11], the hypertrophy of astrocytes observed in the vicinity of damaged neurons in vivo is a long-term phenomenon involving an increased synthesis of GFAP [13, 30]. It is therefore important to establish to what extent CGRP might exert an effect at the level of gene expression. This problem was approached by studying the activation of the *fos* proto-oncogene. This gene is rapidly activated by a variety of stimuli in mammalian cells and serves, together with other so-called primary response genes, to mediate the long-term activation of target genes. It therefore provides a convenient model for establishing the ability of CGRP to stimulate transcriptional events.

Addition of CGRP at concentrations similar to those that increase cyclic AMP accumulation led to a rapid increase in the amount of c-*fos* mRNA in astrocyte cultures [17]. The response reached a maximum after 30 min and declined within 1 h to basal levels. Half maximal stimulation of c-*fos* mRNA was observed with 100 nM CGRP, but significant induction was already evident with only 30 nM. As in the case of the increase in cyclic AMP accumulation, calcitonin had only a weak effect on c-*fos* induction, indicating mediaton by a CGRP-specific receptor. These observations raise the question as to the mechanisms mediating the action of CGRP on c-*fos*. One obvious candidate as a second messenger is cyclic AMP. Indeed, c-*fos* was also induced in astrocyte cultures by incubation with forskolin or the inhibitor of cyclic nucleotide phosphodiesterase, Ro 20-174. Further, the action of CGRP on c-*fos* mRNA accumulation was potentiated in the presence of Ro 20-174. These data strongly suggest that activation of astrocytic CGRP receptors leads to a cyclic AMP-mediated activation of the c-*fos* gene, the product of which would, in turn, act to stimulate the induction of as yet unidentified target genes.

Conclusions

Axotomized motor neurons display characteristic changes in CGRP expression following injury, suggesting a role for CGRP in neuronal regeneration. This is supported by the presence of specific, high-affinity, non-neuronal CGRP binding in the regenerating motor nuclei. Furtermore, data from in vitro experiments also show that CGRP induces changes in gene expression and production of second messengers in cultured astrocytes. These data support the hypothesis that CGRP might be a mediator of the interaction between neurons and non-neuronal cells taking place during the process of nerve regeneration. In addition, CGRP could also be involved in the regeneration of neuromuscular synapses as well as acting as a regulatory antisprouting factor. However, further investigations, both in vivo and in vitro, are necessary to throw light on the exact functional role of CGRP in neuronal regeneration. It is to be hoped that these new data will contribute to a better understanding of the regulation of the complex cellular interactions that finally leads to successful regeneration.

References

1. Amara SG, Jonas V, Rosenfeld MG, Ong SE, Evans RM (1982) Alternative RNA processing in calcitonin gene expression generates mRNAs encoding different polypeptide products. Nature 298:240–244
2. Anderson HJ, Aguayo AJ, Blackshaw SE, Bray D, Gilliatt RW, Grinnell AD, Kreutzberg GW, Parnas I, Purves D, Rothshenker S, Schwab ME, Willard MB (1982) Early responses to neural injury. In: Nicholls JG (ed) Repair and regeneration of the nervous system. Report of the Dahlem workshop on repair and regeneration of the nervous system, Berlin, 29. Nov-4. Dec 1981, Springer, Berlin Heidelberg New York, pp 315–339
3. Arvidsson U, Johnson H, Piel F, Cullheim S, Hökfelt T, Risling M, Terenius L, Ulfhake B (1990) Peripheral nerve section induces increased levels of calcitonin gene-related peptide (CGRP)-like immunoreactivity in axotomized motoneurons. Exp Brain Res 79:212–216
4. Chiba T, Yamaguchi A, Yamanati T, Nakamura A, Morishita T, Inui T, Fukase M, Noda T, Fujita T (1989) Calcitonin gene-related peptide receptor antagonist human CGRP(8-37). Am J Physiol 256:E331–E334
5. Denis-Donini S (1989) Expression of dopaminergic phenotypes in the mouse olfactory bulb induced by the calcitonin gene-related peptide. Nature 339:701–703
6. Dennis T, Fournier A, Cadieux A, Pomerleau F, Jolicouer FB, StPierre S, Quirion R (1990) hCGRP$_{8-37}$, a calcitonin gene-related peptide antagonist revealing calcitonin gene-related peptide heterogeneity in brain and periphery. J Pharmacol Exp Ther 254:123–128
7. Dumoulin FL (1991) Calcitonin gene-related peptide in der Regeneration motorischer und sensorischer Neurone der Ratte. MD thesis, Technical University of Munich
8. Dumoulin FL, Raivich G, Streit WJ, Kreutzberg GW (1991) Differential regulation of calcitonin gene-related peptide (CGRP) in regenerating rat facial nucleus and dorsal root ganglion. Eur J Neurosci 3:338–342
9. Fawcett JW, Keynes RJ (1990) Peripheral nerve regeneration. Annu Rev Neurosci 13:43–60
10. Fedoroff S, McAuley AJ, Houle JD, Devon RM (1984) Astrocyte cell lineage. V. Similarity of astrocytes that form in the presence of dbcAMP in cultures to reactive astrocytes in vivo. J Neurosci Res 12:15–27
11. Goldman JE, Abramson B (1990) Cyclic AMP-induced shape changes in astrocytes are accompanied by rapid depolymerization of actin. Brain Res 528:189–196
12. Goltzmann D, Mitchell J (1985) Interaction of calcitonin and calcitonin gene-related peptide at receptor sites in target tissue. Science 227:1343–1345
13. Graeber MB, Kreutzberg GW (1986) Astrocytes increase in glial fibrillary acidic protein during retrograde changes of facial motor neurons. J Neurocytol 15:363–373
14. Graeber MB, Kreutzberg GW (1988) Delayed astrocyte reaction following facial nerve axotomy. J Neurocytol 17:209–220
15. Grafstein B, McQuarrie IG (1978) Role of the nerve cell body in axonal regeneration. In: Cotman CW (ed) Neuronal plasticity. Raven, New York, pp 155–195
16. Haas CA, Streit WJ, Kreutzberg GW (1990) Rat facial motor neurons express increased levels of calcitonin gene-related peptide mRNA in response to axotomy. J Neurosci Res 27:270–275
17. Haas CA, Reddington M, Kreutzberg GW (1991) Calcitonin gene-related peptide stimulates the induction of c-fos gene expression in rat astrocyte cultures. Eur J Neurosci 3:708–712
18. Hirata Y, Takagi Y, Takata S, Fukuda Y, Yoshimi H, Fujita T (1988) Calcitonin gene-related peptide receptor in cultured vascular smooth muscle cells and endothelial cells. Biochem Biophys Res Commun 151:1113–1121
19. Ishida-Yamamoto A, Tohyama M (1989) Calcitonin gene-related peptide in the nervous system. Prog Neurobiol 33:335–386
20. Kreutzberg GW (1982) Acute neural reaction to injury. In: Nicholls JG (ed) Repair and regeneration of the nervous system. Report of the Dahlem workshop on repair and regeneration of the nervous system, Berlin, 29. Nov-4. Dec. 1981, Springer, Berlin Heidelberg New York, pp 57–69
21. Kreutzberg GW, Toth L (1974) Dendritic secretion: a way for the neuron to communicate with the vasculature. Naturwissenschaften 61:37
22. Kreutzberg GW, Graeber MB, Streit WJ (1989) Neuron-glial relationship during regeneration of motoneurons. Metab Brain Dis 4:81–85
23. Laufer R, Changeux JP (1987) Calcitonin gene-related peptide elevates cyclic AMP levels in chick skeletal muscle: possible neurotrophic role for a coexisting neuronal messenger. EMBO J 6:901–906
24. Lazar P, Reddington M, Streit WJ, Raivich G, Kreutzberg GW (1991) Stimulation of adenosine 3',5'-monophosphate accumulation by calcitonin gene-related peptide in astrocyte cultures from neonatal rat brain. Neurosci Lett 130:99–102
25. Lieberman AR (1971) The axon reaction: a review of the principal features of perikaryal responses to axon injury. In: Pfeiffer CC, Smythies JR (eds) International review of neurobiology, vol 14. Academic, New York, pp 49–124

26. Moore RY (1989) Cranial motor neurons contain either galanin- or calcitonin gene-related peptide-like immunoreactivity. J Comp Neurol 282:512–522

27. Noguchi K, Senba E, Morita Y, Sato M, Tohyama M (1990) α-CGRP and β-CGRP mRNAs are differentially regulated in the rat spinal cord and dorsal root ganglion. Mol Brain Res 7: 299–304

28. Piel F, Arvidsson U, Johnson H, Cullheim S, Villar M, Dagerlind A, Terenius L, Hökfelt T, Ulfhake B (1991) Calcitonin gene-related peptide (CGRP)-like immunoreactivity and CGRP mRNA in rat spinal cord motoneurons after different types of lesions. Eur J Neurosci 3:737–757

29. Streit WJ, Dumoulin FL, Raivich G, Kreutzberg GW (1989) Calcitonin gene-related peptide increases in rat facial motoneurons after peripheral nerve transection. Neurosci Lett 101:143–148

30. Tetzlaff W, Graeber MB, Bisby MA, Kreutzberg GW (1988) Increased glial fibrillary acidic protein synthesis in astrocytes during retrograde reaction of rat facial nucleus. GLIA 1:90–95

31. Tsujimoto T, Kuno M (1988) Calcitonin gene-related peptide prevents disuse-induced sprouting of rat motor nerve teriminals. J Neurosci 8:3951–3957

Eur Arch Otorhinolaryngology (1994) [Suppl]: S75 – S77

M. B. Graeber

The Role of Astrocytes in Facial Nerve Regeneration

Introduction

Traumatic injury to a peripheral nerve is seldom followed by complete recovery of function. It seems likely that local changes at the site of direct lesioning, e.g., misguided outgrowth of axons and neuroma formation, represent a major cause underlying this clinical problem. Yet little is known about whether cellular and/or molecular alterations occurring within the central nervous system (CNS) could also be involved. A classical and well-studied experimental model to approach this question is the central nucleus of origin of the rat facial motor nerve [13]. Following crush or cut of the facial nerve, the affected motor neurons respond with highly reproducible alterations in their metabolism, morphology, and electrophysiology. This "axonal reaction" is considered to form part of an inherent neuronal "regeneration program" which is triggered by axotomy [21]. Importantly, adult rat facial motor neurons not only survive, but regenerate following axotomy. In addition to changes in the motor neurons, a glial reaction is radily apparent soon after facial nerve injury. Microglial cells proliferate [10–12], engage in the early detachment and displacement ("stripping") of synaptic terminals from the surface of regenerating motor neurons [1], and express de novo a number of molecules which support their role as intrinsic CNS scavenger and immune effector cells [6, 7, 17, 18]. Microglia are not the only glial cell type which responds to axotomy. Probably through direct signaling from the injured motor neurons, astrocytes are also stimulated to react.

M. B. Graeber
Institute of Neuropathology,
Ludwig Maximilians University,
80337 München, Germany

Glial Fibrillary Acidic Protein Synthesis Marks the Early Response of Astrocytes to Axotomy

Astrocytic synthesis of the glial fibrillary acidic protein (GFAP) is one of the first non-neuronal changes known to occur following axotomy [20]. GFAP is a major cytoskeletal constituent and a cell type-specific marker for astrocytes, where it can be localized to 8- to 9-nm glial filaments [2]. With the arrival of immunocytochemical techniques and of antibodies specific for GFAP, identification of astrocytes in tissue sections has been greatly facilitated. In addition, increased GFAP expression by astrocytes can be regarded as a sensitive indicator of tissue pathology [22]. This also holds true for the regenerating facial nucleus, where an increase in GFAP immunoreactivity can be detected as early as 2 days after axotomy [3]. Interestingly, only very few astrocytic profiles can be labeled in the normal facial nucleus, while there is a massive increase in this intermediate filament antigen following facial nerve transection. This increase is not only rapid and extensive in that it affects the ipsilateral facial nucleus as well as its surroundings [3], but also long-lasting, i.e., GFAP expression remains upregulated for at least 3 months after facial nerve transection (M. B. Graeber and G. W. Kreutzberg, unpublished observations). Electron microscopy reveals ultrastructural signs of astrocytic hypertrophy [3]. Thus, during the retrograde neuronal response to axotomy, GFAP-negative, "protoplasmic" astrocytes which predominate in the normal rat facial nucleus develop into the GFAP-positive, "fibrous" type. Using [35S] methionine incorporation, two-dimensional polyacrylamide gel electrophoresis, and in situ hybridization experiments, it has been shown that GFAP is newly synthesized by the reactive astrocytes [20]. There appears to be an inverse relationship between the amount of GFAP synthesized and the success of neuronal regeneration. For example, there is a stronger and more sustained increase in GFAP expression following facial nerve resection as compared with simple crush lesioning [20]. This indicates a direct relationship between the severity of neuronal injury and the intensity of astrocytic activation.

Astrocytes Responding to Facial Nerve Axotomy Do Not Proliferate

[³H] Thymidine autoradiography in combination with electron microscopy clearly shows that it is only microglia, and not astrocytes, which undergo mitosis following rat facial nerve axotomy [10], i.e., there is astrocytic hypertrophy without hyperplasia. Similarly, microglia, but not astrocytes, acquire vimentin immunoreactivity in the regenerating rat facial nucleus [8, 9]. This situation contrasts astroglial behavior in direct or degeneration-type CNS lesions, where astrocytes may proliferate, acquire vimentin immunoreactivity, and exhibit increased histochemical oxidative enzyme activity [5]. An explanation for these differences may be provided by the fact that a typical astroglial scar does not form in the regenerating facial nucleus, and microglia do not turn into phagocytes. Therefore, during regeneration, glial responses appear to be well controlled and help provide appropriate conditions for neuronal survival. Signaling pathways involved in this regulation are just beginning to be explored [15, 16]. Interestingly, microglia leave their perineuronal positions about 2 weeks after axotomy and migrate into the neuropil. The reason for this behavior could be related to a second, delayed response in the astrocytes which we observed beginning about 2–3 weeks after facial nerve transection.

The Delayed Astrocytic "Lamellar Reaction"

Studying the time course of the reactive GFAP expression, we found that the astrocytes, in addition to synthesizing GFAP and reorganizing their cytoskeleton, also reshape their cell processes. These cell processes grow in length, cross the neuropil, and come in close contact with neuronal somatic and dendritic surface membranes [4]. During the second to third week after axotomy, they eventually take over the perineuronal positions of the microglia. Three weeks after facial nerve transection, the regenerating motor neurons are almost completely surrounded by GFAP-positive astrocytic cell processes [3]. Electron microscopy reveals that the astrocytes have additionally formed stacks of extremely thin, sheet-like or lamellar cell processes which cover most neuronal surfaces with the apparent exception of small dendrites. These astrocytic lamellar processes exhibit strong activity for the ectoenzyme 5'-nucleotidase, and we have used this enzymatic activity to depict the contours of the astrocytic lamellar processes as they touch the neurons [4]. Very few intact synaptic contacts are preserved as the result of this lamellar insulation. It may be important to note in this context that microglia are potentially cytotoxic cells which have the capacity to develop into full-blown macrophages [19].

A dichotomy of glial behavior becomes apparent under conditions of neuronal degeneration with microglia phagocytosing neuronal debris [9, 19]. In contrast, there is no phagocytosis taking place under conditions of neuronal regeneration where astrocyte processes interpose between neurons and microglial cells. Thus, it is tempting to speculate that neuronal ensheathment by astrocytes may serve to protect the regenerating motor neuron against microglial cytotoxicity. This hypothesis is supported by the observation that in the degenerating facial nucleus neurons wrapped by astrocytic cell processes are not as readily phagocytosed [19]. Yet, the astrocytic "lamellar reaction" may represent a bi-edged sword with regard to functional recovery. We have observed astrocytic lamellar cell processes interposed between neuronal surfaces and afferent axonal endings later than 300 days after cut lesioning. This is paralleled by an abnormal, i.e., reduced density of afferent axosomatic and axodendritic synaptic contacts on the surface of the regenerating motor neurons. Therefore, reactive astrocytes maintain the state of synaptic deafferentation of the regenerating motor neuron which is initially associated with the microglial response [1]. Peripheral reinnervation of the facial musculature recommences at about 4 weeks after facial nerve transection, but a discrete deficit in complex whisker movements is still present 1 year after the operation. Obviously, if applicable to human biology, these findings could to be of clinical importance. This possibility is currently being explored [14].

Conclusions

Our findings demonstrate that there are profound, long-term changes in the synaptic organization of a regenerating motor nucleus and that astrocytes may play an active role in this process. The astrocytic lamellar reaction may serve a twofold function in both insulating and at the same time protecting the motor neuron during regeneration. Our findings could help to explain why patients suffering from a prolonged period of functional recovery after peripheral nerve trauma may be unable to regain full control over fine motor movements although peripheral reinnervation of the musculature has been achieved. We suggest an involvement of CNS glia to be considered when a post-traumatic "nuclear syndrome" of impaired functional recovery is discussed in the context of facial or other peripheral nerve injuries.

Acknowledgement I would like to thank Dr. G. W. Kreutzberg for his support during these studies.

References

1. Blinzinger K, Kreutzberg G (1968) Displacement of synaptic terminals from regenerating motoneurons by microglial cells. Z Zellforsch 85:145–157
2. Eng LF (1985) Glial fibrillary acidic protein (GFAP): the major protein of glial intermediate filaments in differentiated astrocytes. J Neuroimmunol 8:203–214

3. Graeber MB, Kreutzberg GW (1986) Astrocytes increase in glial fibrillary acidic protein during retrograde changes of facial motor neurons. J Neurocytol 15:363–373

4. Graeber MB, Kreutzberg GW (1988) Delayed astrocyte reaction following facial nerve axotomy. J Neurocytol 17:209–220

5. Graeber MB, Kreutzberg GW (1990) Astrocytic reactions accompanying motor neuron regeneration. In: Seil FJ (ed) Advances in neural regeneration research. Wiley-Liss, New York, pp 215–224

6. Graeber MB, Streit WJ, Kiefer R, Schoen SW, Kreutzberg GW (1990) New expression of myelomonocytic antigens by microglia and perivascular cells following lethal motor neuron injury. J Neuroimmunol 27:121–132

7. Graeber MB, Streit WJ, Kreutzberg GW (1988) Axotomy of the rat facial nerve leads to increased CR3 complement receptor expression by activated microglial cells. J Neurosci Res 21:18–24

8. Graeber MB, Streit WJ, Kreutzberg GW (1988) The microglial cytoskeleton: vimentin is localized within activated cells in situ. J Neurocytol 17:573–580

9. Graeber MB, Streit WJ, Kreutzberg GW (1989) Formation of microglia-derived brain macrophages is blocked by adriamycin. Acta Neuropathol 78:348–358

10. Graeber MB, Tetzlaff W, Streit WJ, Kreutzberg GW (1988) Microglial cells but not astrocytes undergo mitosis following rat facial nerve axotomy. Neurosci Lett 85:317–321

11. Kreutzberg GW (1966) Autoradiographische Untersuchung über die Beteiligung von Gliazellen an der axonalen Reaktion im Facialiskern der Ratte. Acta Neuropathol 7:149–161

12. Kreutzberg GW (1968) Über perineuronale Mikrogliazellen (autoradiographische Untersuchungen). Acta Neuropathol [Suppl] 4:141–145

13. Kreutzberg GW (1982) Acute neural reaction to injury. In: Nicholls JG (ed) Repair and regeneration of the nervous system. Springer, Berlin Heidelberg New York, pp 57–69

14. Nacimiento W, Podoll K, Graeber MB, Töpper R, Ostermann H, Noth J, Kreutzberg GW (1992) Contralateral early blink reflex in patients with facial nerve palsy: indication for synaptic reorganization in the facial nucleus during regeneration. J Neurol Sci (in press)

15. Raivich G, Gehrmann J, Kreutzberg GW (1991) Increase of macrophage colony-stimulating factor and granulocyte-macrophage colony-stimulating factor receptors in the regenerating rat facial nucleus. J Neurosci Res 30:682–686

16. Streit WJ, Dumoulin FL, Raivich G, Kreutzberg GW (1989) Calcitonin gene-related peptide increases in rat facial motoneurons after peripheral nerve transection. Neurosci Lett 101:143–148

17. Streit WJ, Graeber MB, Kreutzberg GW (1989) Peripheral nerve lesion produces increased levels of major histocompatibility complex antigens in the central nervous system. J Neuroimmunol 21:117–123

18. Streit WJ, Graeber MB, Kreutzberg GW (1989) Expression of Ia antigen on perivascular and microglial cells after sublethal and lethal motor neuron injury. Exp Neurol 105:115–126

19. Streit WJ, Kreutzberg GW (1988) Response of endogenous glial cells to motor neuron degeneration induced by toxic ricin. J Comp Neurol 268:248–263

20. Tetzlaff W, Graeber MB, Bisby MA, Kreutzberg GW (1988) Increased glial fibrillary acidic protein synthesis in astrocytes during retrograde reaction of the rat facial nucleus. GLIA 1:90–95

21. Tetzlaff W, Graeber MB, Kreutzberg GW (1986) Reactions of motoneurons and their microenvironment to axotomy. Exp Brain Res [Suppl] 13:3–8

22. Vijayan VK, Lee YL, Eng LF (1990) Increase in glial fibrillary acidic protein following neural trauma. Mol Chem Neuropathol 13:107–118

Note added in proof

Post-traumatic synaptic stripping also occurs in the human facial nucleus: Graeber MB, Bise K, Mehraein P (1993) Synaptic stripping in the human facial nucleus. Acta Neuropathologica 86:179–181

Eur Arch Otorhinolaryngology (1994) [Suppl]: S 78 – S 81

A. R. Møller

Pathophysiology of Hemifacial Spasm

Introduction

Hemifacial spasm (HFS) is characterized by attacks of
spasm on one side of the face that usually begin as small
contractions around the eye and that over several years
increase in intensity while progressing down the face as the
intensity of the spasm increases [4, 5]. The attacks also
occur during sleep and can be precipitated by emotional
factors. Between attacks, the facial muscles seem to function normally, except for synkinesis of facial muscles and
maybe a slight weakness of facial muscles in individuals
who have had HFS for a long time [4, 5]. The incidence of
HFS is very low (0.74 per 100000 in white men in the USA
and 0.81 per 100000 in white women) [3]. HFS is believed to be caused by vascular compression of the intracranial portion of the facial nerve at its root exit zone
(REZ). Microvascular decompression (MVD) of the facial
nerve offers a high rate of success for total cure [16, 17, 19]
with little side effects, but there is no known medical treatment effective in curing HFS [34]. The beneficial effects of
various kinds of destructive procedures to the peripheral
branches of the facial nerve [10, 11, 39] and blockage of
the facial nerve [5, 6, 22] are often short-term, but the side
effects are considerable.

Two hypotheses have been presented regarding the
pathophysiology of HFS. One postulates that the spasm
and synkinesis of HFS are caused by an abnormal facilitation of (ephaptic) cross-transmission between nerve fibers
of the facial nerve at the location of the vascular compression [12, 13, 45]; the other hypothesis explains the
symptoms of HFS as being caused by a hyperactive facial
motor nucleus ([9, 44]; for a recent review see [24]).

The abnormal, or delayed, muscle respone [7] that can
be demonstrated in patients with HFS by stimulating one
branch of the facial nerve by recording electromyographic

A. R. Møller
Department of Neurological Surgery, School of Medicine,
University of Pittsburgh, Pittsburgh, PA 15213-2582, USA

potentials from muscles innervated by another branch of
the facial nerve [26, 35] is a sign of an abnormal cross-
transmission; it is probably specific to HFS and is absent
postoperatively following successful MVD for HFS [2]; in
fact, it disappears immediately when the offending vessel
is lifted off the facial nerve (and it returns if the vessel is
again allowed to make contact with the facial nerve [27]).

The abnormal muscle response has been used by several investigators to study the pathophysiology of HFS and
has been interpreted as favoring the ephaptic hypothesis
[35, 40] or being in favor of the nucleus hypothesis [23,
25 – 31, 38].

The R_1 component of the blink reflex [30, 36, 42] is present in recordings from muscles in the lower face in patients with HFS and is a sign of synkinesis in these patients
[36].

The Nucleus Hypothesis

In intraoperative recordings of abnormal muscle contraction made in patients undergoing MVD operations for
HFS, the latency of the abnormal muscle contraction was
consistently longer (2.2 ms [27]) than the sum of the conduction times in the facial nerve that would have been
involved if the location of the cross-transmission upon
which the abnormal muscle contraction relies was the site
of vascular contact; this finding indicates that the facial
motonucleus is the anatomical location of the physiological anomaly that gives rise to the other symptoms and
signs that are characteristic of HFS. The subsequent
findings that the blink reflex could be elicited intraoperatively in patients undergoing MVD operations on the side
of HFS (but not on the other side; Fig. 1) [30] further support the assumption that the facial motonucleus is hyperactive, as do the results of preoperative studies that showed
that the latency of the R_2 component of the blink reflex is
shorter when elicited from the affected side [8, 42]. The
fact that the spasm in patients with HFS normally begins
around the eye indicates that the trigeminal system may

Fig. 1 Results of stimulating the supraorbital nerve (*top*) and the zygomatic branch of the facial nerve (*bottom*) in a patient undergoing micro-vascular depression (*MVD*) to relieve hemifacial spasm (HFS) before (*A*) and after (*B*) the offending blood vessel had been moved off the facial nerve. *Left*, responses from the mentalis muscle to stimulation of the supraorbital nerve (to elicit the blink reflex) before and after MVD of the facial nerve. *Right*, compound action potential (CAP) recorded simultaneously from the intracranial portion of the facial nerve before and after MVD of the facial nerve in response to stimulation of the supraorbital nerve (from [30])

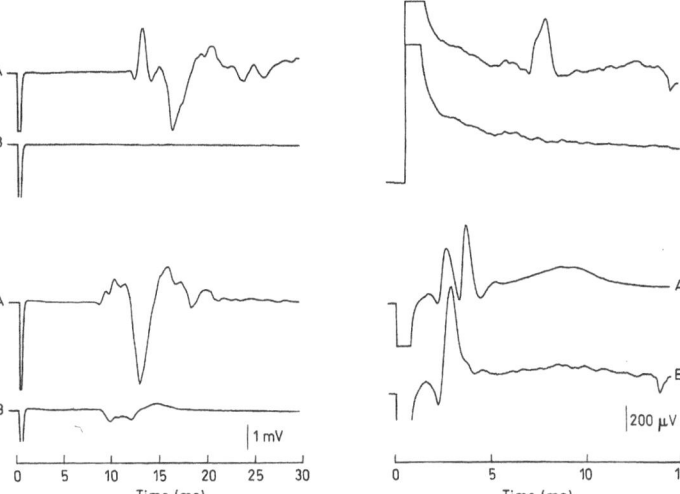

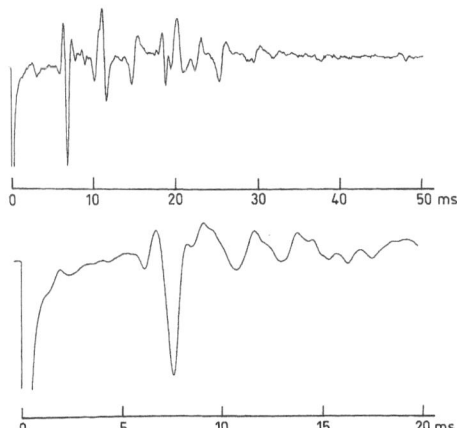

Fig. 2 Recordings of the abnormal muscle response in a rat, the facial nerve of which had been electrically stimulated daily for 4 weeks. *Top*, response to a single stimulus showing afterdischarges in addition to the initial response. *Bottom*, average of 256 responses similar to those above, but shown on a shorter time scale. Note that because the later discharges do not appear synchronously with the stimulus, they cancel out when many responses are summed (from [41])

facial motonucleus that connect neurons innervating different parts of the face could be activated as a result of hyperactivity, as has been suggested in other areas such as pain [43].

We believe that antidromic stimulation of the facial nerve can influence facial motoneurons to the degree where they become hyperactive [23, 25, 26, 30, 31], and recently [15, 32] it has become possible to identify the vessel that specifically causes the abnormal muscle response by observing this response intraoperatively. This has confirmed that small arteries of a few hundred micrometers in diameter and even veins can cause HFS [18, 21], suggesting that it is the actual contact with a vessel affecting the facial nerve that can cause the development of HFS and that pulsatile pressure does not seem to be a prerequisite for the development of HFS. The suggestion that the irritation of the facial nerve by a blood vessel may influence the facial motoneurons to become hyperactive [23, 26, 32], similar to that of the kindling phenomenon [14], is supported by the finding that chronic electrical stimulation of the facial nerve in animals over a period of time can render the facial motonucleus hyperactive ([33, 41]; S. Saito and A.R. Møller, unpublished observations; Fig. 2).

It has recently been proposed that it is the interaction between a hyperactive facial motonucleus and ephaptic transmission at the site of the vascular compression that causes the signs of HFS [38].

make the facial motoneurons that innervate the facial muscles around the eye more excitable.

Synkinesis in HFS could be caused by an abnormal cross-transmission between facial motoneurons innervating different facial muscles, and dormant synapses in the

The Ephaptic Hypothesis

Ephaptic transmission depends on direct contact between denuded axons of the facial nerve and on a slowing of neural conduction so that reexcitation can occur after the end of the refractory period [37], but the lack of evidence for a slowing of neural conduction speaks against this hypothesis [1, 8, 20, 42], because it opposes the hypothesis that extensive demyelination occurs at the site of vascular compression. It has also been found unlikely that a sufficient number of denuded nerve fibers would be in contact with each other to cause the massive contractions that are seen in patients with HFS [8].

Single muscle fiber recordings of the abnormal muscle response in patients with HFS [40] were interpreted as being in favor of the ephaptic hypothesis because of the low jitter, but these results may rather support the hypothesis that the abnormal muscle response is an exaggerated F response, thus indicating hyperactivity of the facial motonucleus.

Conclusions

Although the ephaptic hypothesis was most favored by investigators in the past, recent electrophysiological evidence obtained from patients with HFS before, during, and after MVD operations to relieve HFS has created doubt about this hypothesis and instead has supported the more complex nucleus hypothesis.

We are, however, far from being able to explain the pathophysiology of HFS, and it may seem unnecessary to spend research efforts on a disease in which there already exists very good methods of treatment. However, HFS may be a model for other diseases that cannot be studied experimentally and as extensively as HFS and for which there are fewer treatments available, because HFS is one of the few disorders in which quantitative electrophysiological recordings can be made that can provide results that are important in explaining its pathophysiology. We are therefore convinced that HFS is worthy of further study.

References

1. Auger RG (1979) Hemifacial spasm: clinical and electrophysiological observations. Neurology 29:1261–1272
2. Auger RG, Piepgras DG, Laws ER Jr, Miller RH (1981) Microvascular decompression of the facial nerve for hemifacial spasm: clinical and electrophysiologic observations. Neurology 31:346–350
3. Auger RG, Whisnant JP (1990) Hemifacial spasm in Rochester and Olmsted County, Minnesota, 1960 to 1984. Arch Neurol 47:1233–1234
4. Digre K, Corbett JJ (1988) Hemifacial spasm: differential diagnosis, mechanism, and treatment. In: Tolosa E (ed) Facial dyskinesia. Raven, New York, pp 151–176 (Advances in neurology, vol 39)
5. Ehni G, Woltman HW (1945) Hemifacial spasm. Arch Neurol Psychiatry 53:205–211
6. Elmquist D, Toremalm NG, Elmer A, Mercke U (1982) Hemifacial spasm and electrophysiological findings and the therapeutic effect of facial nerve block (Special Lambert Symposium). Muscle Nerve 5:589–594

7. Esslen E (1957) Der Spasmus facialis eine Parabiosserscheinung: elektrophysiologische Untersuchungen zum Entstehungsmechanismus des Facialisspasmus. Dtsch Z Nervenheilkd 176:149–172
8. Esteban A, Molina-Negro P (1986) Primary hemifacial spasm: a neurophysiological study. J Neurol Neurosurg Psychiatry 49:58–63
9. Ferguson JH (1978) Hemifacial spasm and the facial nerve nucleus. Ann Neurol 4:97–103
10. Fisch U (1986) Extracranial surgery for facial hyperkinesis. In: May M (ed) The facial nerve. Thieme, New York, pp 509–523
11. Fisch U, Esslen E (1972) The surgial treatment of facial hyperkinesia. Arch Otolaryngol 95:400–405
12. Gardner WJ (1962) Concerning the mechanism of trigeminal neuralgia and hemifacial spasm. J Neurosurg 19:947–958
13. Gardner WJ, Sava GA (1962) Hemifacial spasm – a reversible pathophysiologic. J Neurosurg 19:240–247
14. Goddard GV (1964) Amygdaloid stimulation and learning in the rat. J Comp Physiol Psychol 58:23–30
15. Haines SJ, Torres F (1991) Intraoperative monitoring of the facial nerve during decompressive surgery for hemifacial spasm. J Neurosurg 74:254–257
16. Jannetta PJ (1970) Microsurgical exploration and decompression of the facial nerve in hemifacial spasm. Curr Top Surg Res 2:217–220
17. Jannetta PJ (1981) Hemifacial spasm. In: Samii M, Jannetta PJ (eds) The cranial nerves. Springer, Berlin Heidelberg New York, pp 484–493
18. Jannetta PJ (1984) Hemifacial spasm caused by a venule: case report. Neurosurgery 14:89–92
19. Jannetta PJ, Abbasy M, Maroon JC, Ramos FM, Albin MS (1977) Etiology and definite microsurgical treatment of hemifacial spasm: operative technique and results in 47 patients. J Neurosurg 47:321–328
20. Kim P, Fukushima T (1984) Observations on synkinesis in patients with hemifacial spasm. J Neurosurg 60:821–827
21. Kondo A, Ishikawa J, Yamasaki T, Konishi T (1980) Microvascular decompression of cranial nerves, particularly of the seventh cranial nerve. Neurol Med Chir (Tokyo) 20:739–751
22. Kraft SP, Lang AE (1988) Cranial dystonia blepharospasm and hemifacial spasm: clinical features and treatment, including the use of botulinum toxin. Can Med Assoc J 139:837–846
23. Møller AR (1987) Hemifacial spasm: ephaptic transmission or hyperexcitability of the facial motor nucleus? Exp Neurol 98:110–119
24. Møller AR (1991) The cranial nerve vascular compression syndrome. II. A review of pathophysiology. Acta Neurochir (Wien) 113:24–30
25. Møller AR (1991) Interaction between the blink reflex and the abnormal muscle response in patients with hemifacial spasm: results of intraoperative recordings. J Neurol Sci 101:114–123
26. Møller AR, Jannetta PJ (1984) On the origin of synkinesis in hemifacial spasm: results of intracranial recordings. J Neurosurg 61:569–576
27. Møller AR, Jannetta PJ (1985) Microvascular decompression in hemifacial spasm: intraoperative electrophysiological observations. Neurosurgery 16:612–618
28. Møller AR, Jannetta PJ (1985) Hemifacial spasm: results of electrophysiologic recording during microvascular decompression operations. Neurology 35:969–974
29. Møller AR, Jannetta PJ (1985) Synkinesis in hemifacial spasm: results of recording intracranially from the facial nerve. Experientia 41:415–417
30. Møller AR, Jannetta PJ (1986) Blink reflex in patients with hemifacial spasm: observations during microvascular decompression operations. J Neurol Sci 72:171–182
31. Møller AR, Jannetta PJ (1986) Physiological abnormalities in hemifacial spasm studied during microvascular decompression operations. Exp Neurol 93:584–600

32. Møller AR, Jannetta PJ (1987) Monitoring facial EMG responses during microvascular decompression operations for hemifacial spasm. J Neurosurg 66:681–685
33. Møller AR, Sen CN (1990) Recordings from the facial nucleus in the rat: signs of abnormal facial muscle response. Exp Brain Res 91:18–24
34. Moses H, Alexander GE (1982) Carbamazepine for hemifacial spasm. Neurology 32:286–287
35. Nielsen VK (1984) Pathophysiological aspects of hemifacial spasm, part I. Evidence of ectopic excitation and ephaptic transmission. Neurology 34:418–426
36. Nielsen VK (1984) Pathophysiological aspects of hemifacial spasm, part II. Lateral spread of the supraorbital nerve reflex. Neurology 34:427–431
37. Rasminsky M (1980) Ephaptic transmission between single nerve fibers in the spinal nerve roots of dystrophic mice. J Physiol (Lond) 305:151–169
38. Roth G, Magistris MR, Pinelli P, Rilliet B (1990) Cryptogenic hemifacial spasm. A neurophysiological study. Electromyogr Clin Neurophysiol 30:361–370
39. Samii M (1981) Surgical treatment of hemifacial spasm. In: Samii M, Jannetta PJ (eds) The cranial nerves. Springer, Berlin Heidelberg New York, pp 502–504
40. Sanders DB (1989) Ephaptic transmission in hemifacial spasm: a single-fiber EMG study. Muscle Nerve 12:690–694
41. Sen CN, Møller AR (1987) Signs of hemifacial spasm created by chronic periodic stimulation of the facial nerve in the rat. Exp Neurol 98:336–349
42. Valls-Sole J, Tolosa ES (1989) Blink reflex excitability cycle in hemifacial spasm. Neurology 39:1061–1066
43. Wall PD (1977) The presence of ineffective synapses and the circumstances which unmask them. Philos Trans R Soc Lond Biol 278:361–372
44. Wartenberg R (1952) Hemifacial spasm. A clinical and pathophysiological study. University Park Press, New York
45. Williams HL, Lambert EH, Woltman HW (1952) The problem of synkinesis and contracture in cases of hemifacial spasm and Bell's palsy. Ann Otol Rhinol Laryngol 61:850–870

Anatomy and The Denervated Muscle

Eur Arch Otorhinolaryngology (1994) [Suppl]: S 85 – S 86

W. Happak, G. Burggasser, J. Liu, H. Gruber, and G. Freilinger

Anatomy and Histology of the Mimic Muscles and the Supplying Facial Nerve

Introduction

For several years now free muscle transplantation has been the treatment of choice for dynamic reanimation of the paralysed face. Different skeletal muscles such as the m. gracilis and the m. pectoralis minor are used. However, despite the fact that the skeletal muscles showed good voluntary contraction after transplantation in many cases, they are not capable of producing emotional expressions. Skeletal muscles have been extensively investigated [4], but few data have been published about the mimic muscle system [1 – 3], in addition, the mimic muscles were cited in the same group as skeletal muscles [6]. This study was done to get more information about the delicate mimic muscle system.

Material and Methods

More than 100 human cadavers were dissected within 3 – 6 days after death. All human subjects investigated had died of acute disease. The facial nerve or the mimic muscles were dissected in each head.

The facial nerve was prepared carefully under the OP microscope to determine multiple anastomoses and the branching pattern before entering the mimic muscles. The mimic muscles were dissected and prepared for histological (H.E.), histochemical (alkaline and acid ATPase) and

W. Happak (✉)
Department of Plastic and Reconstructive Surgery,
Surgical University Clinic,
Währinger Gürtel 18 – 20, 1090 Vienna, Austria

G. Burggasser, H. Gruber and G. Freilinger
Department of Plastic Surgery at the Second Surgical Clinic and
III. Department of Anatomy of the University of Vienna, Austria

J. Liu
Department of Plastic Surgery at the Zhong Shan Hospital
University Shanghai, China

end-plate (cholinesterase, CHE) staining. Each specimen was evaluated under the microscope. The muscles stained for the end plates were teased to obtain single muscle fibres prior to embedding.

Results

After division into its four branches (r. frontalis, r. zygomaticus, r. buccalis, r. marg. mandibulae), the facial nerve showed, an elaborate network of anastomoses. Four to eight anastomoses were found between the zygomatic and buccal branch, and two to four branches were found between the frontal and zygomatic and between the buccal and the marginal mandibulae branches in a great number of the cadavers. After forming the plexus, the different branches of each motor branch divides into its fascicles to innervate the corresponding mimic muscles. No well-defined entrance of the fascicles into the muscles was observed. The entrance of the fascicles is spread all over the different mimic muscles. The muscles stained with CHE to determine the end-plates showed no definite motor zone. Several motor zones are spread in excentric positions all over the muscles at the point of entrance of the fascicles. Between two and four large motor zones were evaluated at each mimic muscle as well as several small zones. After teasing the muscles, up to five end-plates were found on a single muscle fibre. Multiply innervated muscle fibres were found in each of the prepared mimic muscles. The distance between the end-plates varied from 10 to 200 μm (Fig. 1).

H.E.-stained muscles were evaluated for connective tissue. No typical epimysial tissue was detected surrounding the different mimic muscles. The perimysial septa were loose and fat cells were intermingled. The endomysium was thickened and fat cells were also detected (Fig. 2).

The histochemically stained specimens for alkaline and acid ATPase showed dramatic differences between the

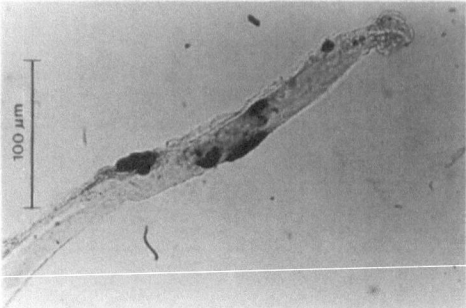

Fig. 1 Teased single mimic muscle fibre with four end-plates (stained for cholinesterase, CHE, after Koelle and Friedwald) within a distance of 100 μm

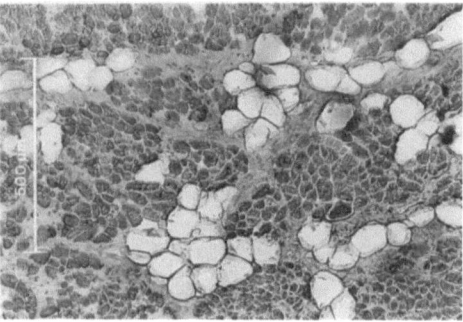

Fig. 2 H.E.-staiend section of a mimic muscle showing the loose epimysial, perimysial and endomysial connective tissue

individual muscles. The content of slowly contracting type I fibres varied from 15% (m. orbicularis oculi) to 67% (m. buccinator). Three groups of mimic muscles could be differentiated (Table 1): (1) the phasic group with only 15% slowly contracting type I fibres; (2) the intermediate group with 28%–37% type I fibres; (3) the tonic group with 41%–67% type I fibres.

Conclusion and Discussion

The structure of the skeletal muscles has been well investigated [4]. Most muscles have one well-defined supplying nerve, one motor zone and a peri-, epi- and endomysium. Each muscle fibre is innervated by only one motor end-plate positioned centrally on the fibre. All these characteristics are typical of skeletal muscles, but could not be detected in the mimic muscles. The plexus of the facial nerve, the innervation pattern of different mimic muscles, the multiple innervation of each single muscle fibre, the different muscle architecture and the histochemical characteristics show a highly differentiated muscle-nerve system. Only few muscles in the human body, such as the extraocular and laryngeal muscles, show similar characteristics to the mimic muscles. It has been postulated that the laryngeal muscles [5] have a independent innervation and contraction mechanism. We can assume the same to be true for the mimic muscle system. These results provide further support for our postulation that better corresponding donor muscles should be used for reconstruction of the paralysed face, to enable a better emotional expression. Therefore, it appears necessary for us to search for those muscles or muscle groups which are more compatible to the mimic muscle system than those already in use.

Table 1 The three groups of mimic muscles

Group	Muscles	Percentage of type I fibres
Phasic	M. orbicularis oculi M. procerus M. nasalis	14–15
Intermediate	M. zygomaticus major M. orbicularis oris M. mentalis M. levator labii superioris Platysma M. levator anguli oris M. lev. lab. sup. alaequi nasi M. depressor labii inferioris	28–37
Tonic	M. corrugator supercilii M. depressor anguli oris M. occipitofrantalis M. buccinator	41–67

References

1. Freilinger G, Gruber H, Happak W, Pechmann U (1987) Surgical anatomy of the mimic muscle system and facial nerve: importance for reconstructive and aesthetic surgery. Plast Reconstr Surg 80 (5):686–690
2. Freilinger G, Happak W, Burggasser G, Gruber H (1990) Histochemical mapping and fiber size analysis of mimic muscles. Plast Reconstr Surg 86 (3):422–428
3. Happak W, Burggasser G, Gruber H (1988) Histochemical characteristics of human mimic muscles. J Neurol Sci 83: 25–35
4. Peachy LD (1983) Skeletal muscle. American Physiological Society, Bethesda, (Handbook of physiology, section 10)
5. Rossi G (1990) From the pattern of human vocal muscle fibre innervation to funtional remarks. Acta Otolaryngol Suppl (Stockh) 90 (413):2–10
6. Polgar J, Johnson MA, Weightman D, Appleton D (1973) Data and fibre size in thirty-six human muscles. An autopsy study. J Neurol Sci 19:307–318

Eur Arch Otorhinolaryngology (1994) [Suppl]:S87–S90

T. Kozawa, S. Murakami and N. Yanagihara

Motor Innervation Pattern of the Orbicularis Oris Muscle in Guinea Pig

Introduction

Using evoked electromyography, Nishimura and Yanagihara [2] found that the orbicularis oris muscle in the vicinity of the midline was innervated by bilateral facial nerves. Figure 1a shows the evoked electromyograms (EMG) of the orbicularis oris muscle in a normal adult.

The evoked EMG potential can be elicited beyond the midline, although the latency is prolonged and the amplitude decreases, as Nishimura and Yanagihara reported. The findings agree with previous descriptions.

However, there are no detailed studies about the innervation pattern and muscle fiber arrangement of the orbicularis oris muscle. The aim of the present study is to clarify the motor innervation pattern and muscle fiber arrangement of this muscle.

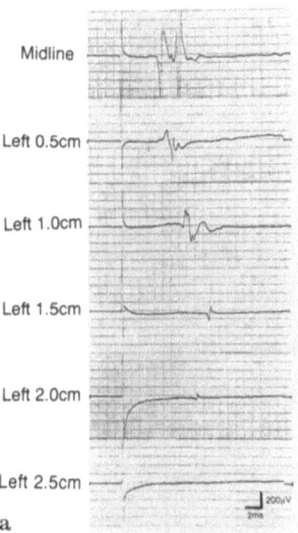

Fig. 1 a Evoked electromyogram (EMG) of orbicularis oris muscle in a normal adult; while the right extratemporal facial nerve trunk was stimulated, the evoked EMG potential can be elicited on the left side

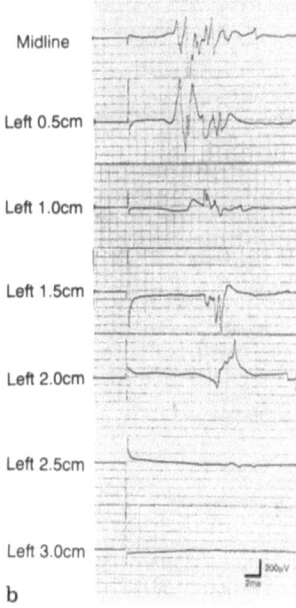

Fig. 1 b Evoked EMG of orbicularis oris muscle in a patient; the evoked EMG potential can be elicited on the left side more laterally

T. Kozawa, S. Murakami, and N. Yanagihara
Department of Otolaryngology, Ehime University School
of Medicine, Shigenobu-cho, Onsen-gun, Ehime, 791-02, Japan

Methods

Female guinea pig weighing from 350 to 600 g were used for this study.

Evoked Electromyograms

The extratemporal facial nerve trunk was exposed and stimulted by a bipolar electrode. A supramaximal square-wave stimulation lasting for 0.1 ms was given and the evoked EMG was recorded through a bipolar needle electrode from the lower lip. The evoked EMG was elicited at seven points on the lower lip: 0, 2, 4, and 6 mm bilaterally from the midline.

Glycogen Depletion Method

The extratemporal facial nerve trunk was stimulated repeatedly for 2 h with square-wave stimulus; intensity ranged from 7 to 10 V, the width was 1 ms and the frequency ranged from 50 to 100 Hz with an interval of 0.5 s. After the stimulation was finished, the muscle in the lower lip was dissected. Sixteen-micrometer-thick frozen serial sections were made and stained by periodic acid-schiff (PAS staining. Unstimulated muscle fiber was positively stained with PAS because of its rich glycogen content, while after repeated muscle contraction by electrical nerve stimulations, glycogen in the muscle fibers was consumed and muscle fibers were unstained by PAS (PAS-negative) [1]. The fibers that were PAS-negative after electrical stimulation were thought to be innervated by that nerve.

Results

Evoked Electromyograms

Figure 2 shows the evoked muscle responses. On the stimulated side, triphasic muscle action potential with a latency of 2.5 ms was recorded. On the nonstimulated side, the amplitude declined and the latency was prolonged concomitant with the distance from the midline. No evoked response was elicited beyond 4 mm contralateral from the midline.

Glycogen Depletion Experiment

Figure 3 shows PAS-stained specimens obtained from the lower lip. At 6 mm lateral from the midline on the stimulated side, most muscle fibers were PAS negative (Fig. 3a). At the midline, about 50% of the muscle fibers became PAS negative (Fig. 3b). Figure 3c, d shows the nonstimulated side 2 mm lateral from the midpoint. Forty percent of the

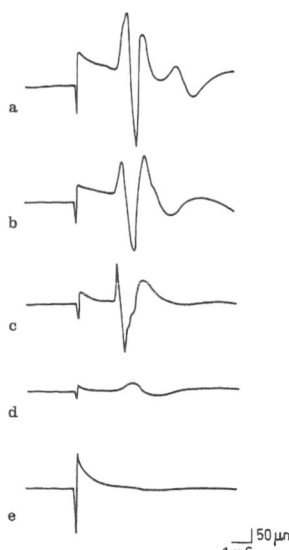

Fig. 2a–e Evoked electromyogram (EMG; guinea pig) 4 mm lateral from the midline on the stimulated side (**a**), 2 mm lateral from the midline on the stimulated side (**b**), at the midline (**c**), 2 mm lateral from the midline on the nonstimulated side (**d**), and 4 mm lateral from the midline on the nonstimulated side (**e**)

muscle fibers were PAS negative. In this specimen, there were two different distribution patterns of PAS-negative fibers: one was a concentrated type, like islands (Fig. 3c), and the other was a scattered type among the PAS-positive fibers (Fig. 3d). At a point 4 mm from the midline on the nonstimulated side, about 30% of the muscle fibers became PAS negative (Fig. 3e). Figure 3f shows the section 6 mm lateral from the midline on the nonstimulated side. Most muscle fibers were PAS positive, i.e., there was no innervation of nerve fiber.

Discussion

The results of glycogen depetion experiments were well correlated with those of evoked EMG; as the amplitude of evoked EMG decreased, the number of PAS-negative fibers also decreased.

There are two possible motor innervation patterns of the orbicularis oris muscle: (1) nerve fibers extend beyond the midline and innervate the other side of muscle fibers or (2) each muscle fiber is innervated by unilateral facial nerves, while muscle fibers intermingle on the other side. In the present study, the glycogen depletion method revealed that there were two different distribution patterns of PAS-

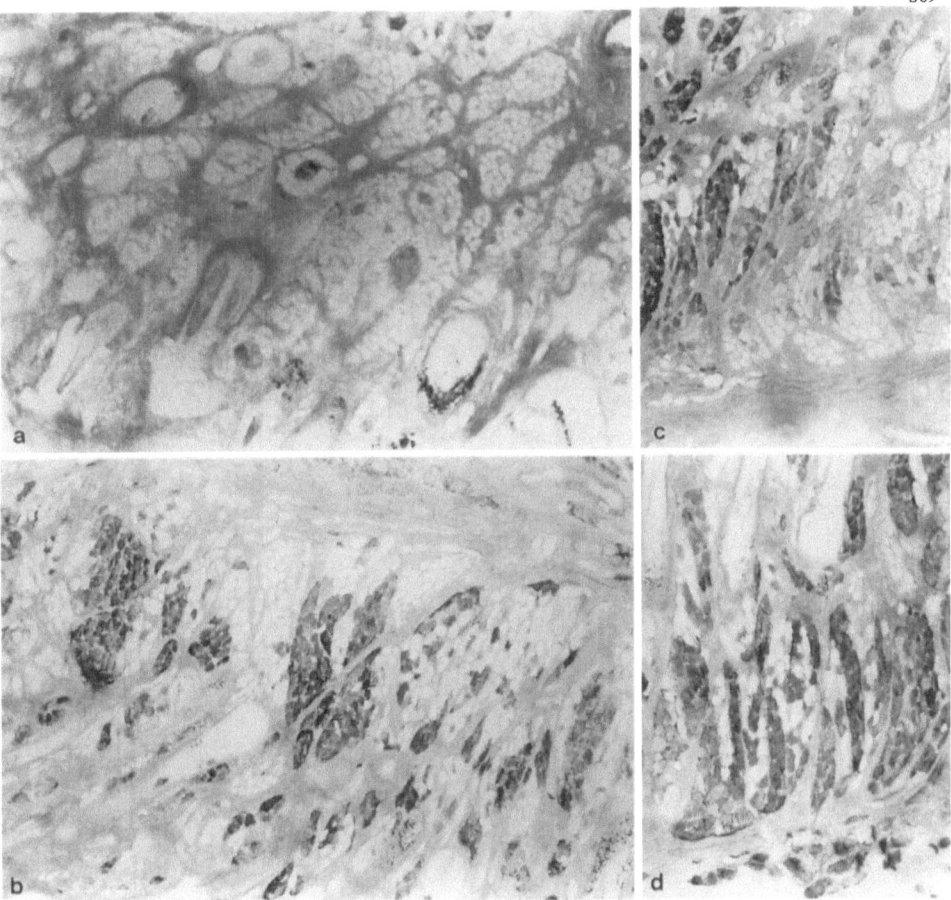

Fig. 3a–f Periodic acid-Schiff (PAS)-stained specimen obtained from the lower lip (×25). **a** 6 mm lateral from the midline on the stimulated side. **b** Midline. **c, d** 2 mm lateral from the midline on the nonstimulated side (**c** concentrated type; **d** scattered type). **e** 4 mm lateral from the midline on the nonstimulated side. **f** 6 mm lateral from the midline on the nonstimulated side. For **e** and **f** see p. S 90

negative fibers in the specimen of nonstimulted side the concentrated and the scattered type (Fig. 3c, d). We presume that the scattered type corresponds to the pattern 1 above and the concentrated type to pattern 2.

In some patients whose facial nerve were totally sectioned following acoustic neurinoma surgery, circumoral disfigurement improved without any repair procedure. The evoked EMG shown in Fig. 1b was obtained from one of these patients 10 months after acoustic neurinoma surgery.

The evoked EMG demonstrates that the orbicularis oris muscle in the paralyzed side is innervated beyond the midline to a point 2.5 cm contralaterally. Nerve sprouting from the healthy side to the paralyzed side is thought to develop.

Further studies will be needed to clarify the innervation pattern more clearly and to determine how the nerve fibers sprout from the other side of orbicularis oris muscle after the facial nerve is sectioned.

Fig. 3 (Cont.)

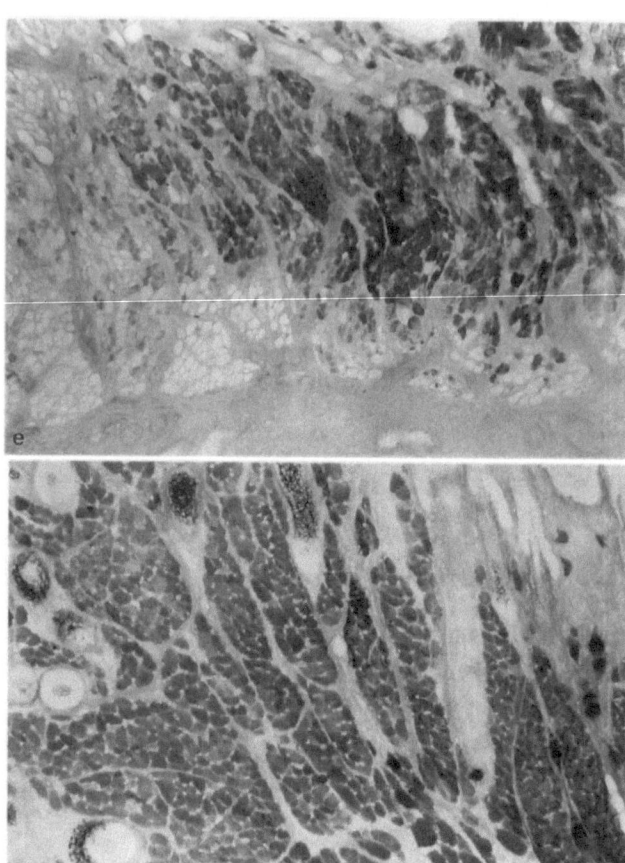

References

1. Edström L, Kugelberg E (1968) Histochemical composition, distribution of fibers and fatiguability of single motor units. Anterior tibial muscle of the rat. J Neurol Psychiatry 31:424–433
2. Nishimura H, Yanagihara N (1967) Evoked electromyographic investigation of the facial muscles (I). Pract Otol (Kyoto) 85:453–464

Eur Arch Otorhinolaryngology (1994) [Suppl]: S91–S95

FREE PAPERS AND POSTERS

E. Stennert

Why Does the Frontalis Muscle "Never Come Back"? Functional Organization of the Mimic Musculature

Introduction

The normal function of the forehead muscle after severe damage to the facial nerve, and especially after nerve reconstruction in the trunk region, cannot be regained. This striking phenomenon was described as early as in 1936 by Martin and in 1948 by Tickle [1, 5]. Miehlke (1973), in his classical monograph [2] on the "Surgery of the Facial Nerve" summarized this fact as follows: "Every expert in the surgery of the facial nerve knows about the repeatedly mentioned experience that, after a lesion of the facial nerve, recovery of the frontal part of the occipito-frontal muscle is either incomplete or non-existent. This is almost the rule after neurotmesis... The peculiar behavior of this muscle is not yet explained", and he continued: "One might be permitted to think that the frontal part of the occipito-frontal muscle has some special tendency toward atrophy and fibrosis" (p. 239).

This clinical experience of a permanent loss of function of the frontalis muscle, however, is in a strong contrast to electromyographic (EMG) findings, which can be recorded from the obviously paralyzed muscles.

Method

The data were gained from a selected group of 55 patients who all suffered from a complete disruption of the facial nerve stump, either in its tympanic or mastoidal portion due to an iatrogenic injury during middle ear surgery. Moreover, in all patients the nerve lesion had been reconstructed by the implantation of a free nerve graft from the greater auricular nerve. The patients ranged in age from 6 to 65 years; their mean age was 38 years.

E. Stennert
Klinik und Poliklinik für Hals-, Nasen- und Ohrenheilkunde
der Universität zu Köln, Joseph-Stelzmann-Strasse 9,
50924 Köln, Germany

All patients were followed up to at least 12 months postoperatively. The function of the involved frontalis muscle was investigated by clinical observation and by needle EMG. The clinical determination of the degree of functinal recovery was gained by measuring the extent of the contraction of the frontalis muscle, during the intentional movement "frowning", exactly above the middle of the pupil, in comparison to the healthy side, thus grouping the differences into 25% steps. This clinical recovery of function was related to the needle EMG, recorded from the involved side and classified into silence, single oscillations, single discharge pattern, transitory pattern and interference pattern.

Results

The results can briefly be summarized as follows (Table 1):

1. In all 55 patients at least some reinnervation of the frontalis muscle could be proved by EMG.
2. The vast majority of patients showed an excellent muscle reactivation on EMG, with proof of a transitory pattern or even an interference pattern ($n = 38$; 69%).
3. In reality, the degree of reinnervation is even better due to *false sprouting* of regenerating axons, so that additional motor units can be activated in the frontalis muscle by other mimic movements.
4. In contrast, 42 patients, i.e., 77%, were not able to frown and only 13 patients had a slight visible contraction of the forehead.

Discussion

What is the reason for the discrepancy between poor clinical function and EMG findings which prove a successful reinnervation of the frontalis muscle? The answer lies in the *functional organization of the mimic musculature* of

Table 1 Electrophysiological and clinical findings after facial nerve reconstruction

EMG pattern	Number of cases	Contraction of frontalis muscle compared to healthy side (number of cases within 25% steps)			
		0%	25%	50%	100%
Silent	0	–	–	–	–
Single oscillations	4	4	–	–	–
Single discharge pattern	13	11	2	–	–
Transitory pattern	31	24	7	–	–
Interference pattern	7	3	4	–	–
Total	55	42	13	–	–
Percentage	100	77	23	–	–

Activity of the frontalis muscle established by EMG recording and by clinical observation during the intentional movement "frowning" (i.e. lifting the eyebrows)

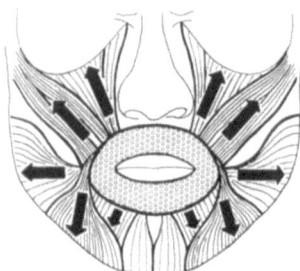

Fig. 1 Diagram of the oral sphincter system. A centrally located ringshaped sphincter muscle (orbicularis oris muscle) with radially attached expander muscles (perioral muscles). The orbicularis oris muscle and the perioral muscles are real antagonists

It is recommended that the term *"mass movements"* should only be used if this border line is crossed by nerve fiber aberration from the cranial to the caudal sphincter system and vice versa, thus leading to a loss of the above-mentioned functional autonomy. However, fiber aberration within a sphincter system is no less disturbing: normal function of any sphincter system is based on the natural antagonism of expanders and constrictors. The best example for this is given by the perioral muscle-system: the most important muscle for stretching the mouth is the zygomatic muscle, and, for pursing the lips, the orbicularis oris muscle is contracted. Since activation of one of these muscles requires the relaxation of the other, both movements are of an antagonistic nature: showing the teeth and pursing the lips simultaneously is not possible. Or in other words: whistling and laughing are mutually exclusive.

the human face. Although the architecture of the mimic muscles looks rather complex, the muscles can be divided into three *muscle groups,* belonging to two *separate sphincter systems*:

In the *lower half of the face* this structural principle is realized in an ideal fashion: the orbicularis oris muscle, as a constrictor, is located centrally in the midline of the face and is attached by the perioral muscles all together acting as expanders and thereby as antagonists to the orbicularis oris muscle (Fig. 1). In the *upper part of the face* the realization of a sphincter is generally identical, but modified due to the binate arrangement around the eyes (Fig. 2). The analysis of movement patterns shows clearly that the innervation of the *oral sphincter system* in the lower half of the face is distinctly separate from the innervaton of the *ocular sphincter system* in the upper part. One of these two parts of the face with their sphincter and expander muscles can be moved without the other. The anatomical organization into the ocular and the oral sphincter system (marked by line A in Fig. 3) explains and helps us to understand the functional autonomy of both innervatoric units.

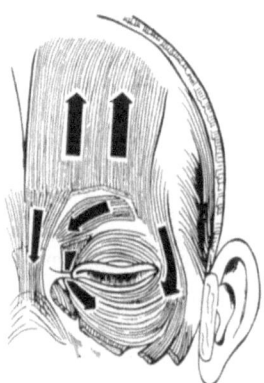

Fig. 2 Diagram of the ocular sphincter system. The depressor supercilii, corrugator supercilii, and procerus muscles are synergists to the orbicularis oculi muscle and pull the eyebrow caudally and medially. All these muscles together are antagonists to the occipitofrontalis muscle, which lifts the eyebrow up

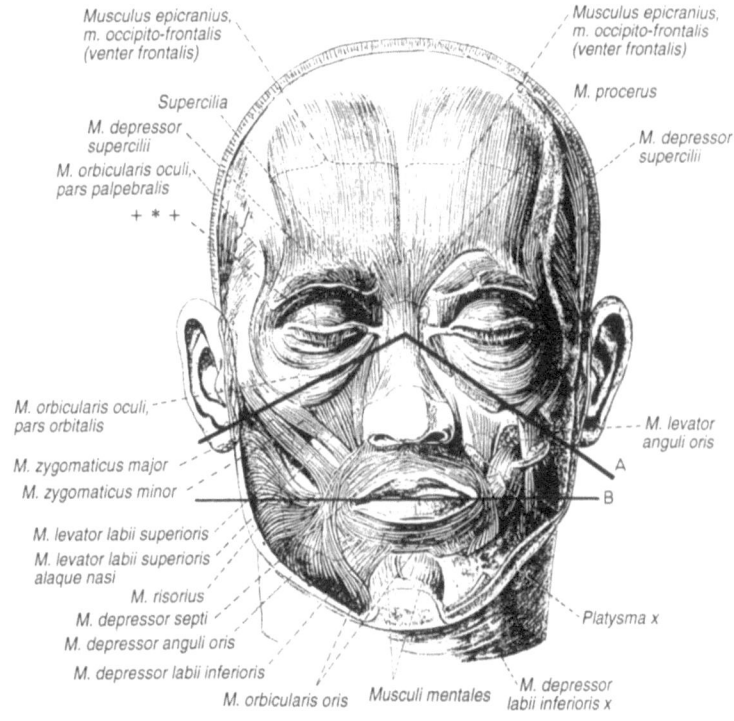

Fig. 3 The mimic muscles are divided into two sphincter systems. *Line A* indicates the borderline between the oral and the ocular sphincter system. Both systems are functionally independent of each other. If this functional autonomy is lost due to nerve fiber aberration, mass movements develop. *Line B* marks the borderline between upwardly and downwardly directed perioral muscles. (Anatomical drawing by courtesy of Sobotta-Becher [3])

Fiber aberration due to false sprouting necessarily always results in *a crosswise innervation of the antagonists within the same sphincter system* and thus makes a mutual blocking of the antagonistic muscle movements unavoidable. Since the organism in effect "paralyzes" itself, the term "*autoparalytic syndrome*" is suggested as a description of this pathophysiological mechanism [4]. Clinically, the autoparalytic syndrome appears as a partial paresis, which is generally described in the literature as "*weakness*", but in fact, this phenomenon would be better classified as "*pseudo-paresis*". The understanding of this pathomechanism and the analysis of *the functional anatomy of the ocular sphincter system* gives us the answer to the question why the frontalis muscle "never comes back" after severe nerve injury (Fig. 2):

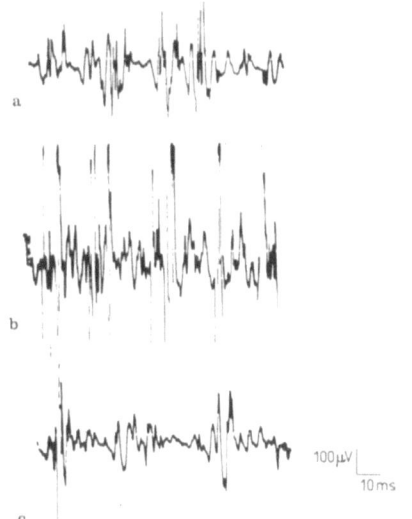

Fig. 4a–c EMG recordings from the *frontalis muscle* with identical positioning of the electrodes during testing all of the following mimic functions: lifting the eyebrow (**a**), closing the eyes (**b**), pulling the eyebrows together (**c**). Due to fiber aberration the activation of the antagonistic muscles (orbicularis oculi muscle and corrugator supercilii muscle) leads to a "paradoxical" ("crosswise") innervation of the frontalis muscle

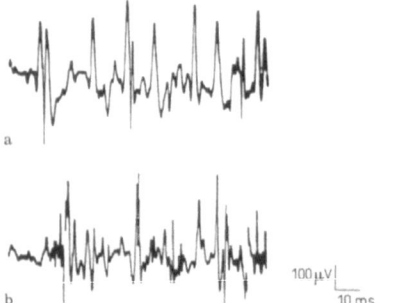

Fig. 5a, b EMG recordings from the corrugator supercilii muscle (**a**) and the orbicularis oculi muscle (**b**) during frowning. Both muscles, as well as the depressor supercilii muscle and the procerus muscle, pull down the eyebrow during frowning, thus counteracting the frontalis muscle and thereby simulating a "paresis" of the frontalis muscle. Normally these muscles should show no activation during frowning

The depressor supercilii muscle as the medial part of the orbicularis oculi muscle together with the corrugator supercilii muscle, the procerus muscle and the lateral part of the orbicularis oculi muscle are mutual antagonists of the occipitofrontalis muscle. The former group of muscles lowers the eyebrows and pulls them towards the nose; the latter muscle, which is attached to the galea aponeurotica, lifts the eyebrows up.

As we demonstrated previously [4], the crossinnervation of these antagonists can clearly be demonstrated and proved electromyographically. After recovery following severe damage to the facial nerve, EMG recordings from the different muscles belonging to the ocular sphincter system demonstrate the obligatory reinnervation of all muscles belonging to the system (Fig. 4). With respect to function, this means a simultaneous activation of antagonists. On the other hand, the intention "frowning", i.e. lifting the eyebrow, (frontalis muscle) leads to a simultaneous activation of all its antagonists (depressor supercilii muscle, corrugator supercilii muscle and procerus muscle)

Fig. 6a–d *Left*, clinical example of a patient with a complex "paradoxical" innervation of the ocular sphincter system. **a** During rest the tone of the muscles is equal on both sides due to the good reinnervation. **b** When frowning, the left frontalis muscle (operated side) keeps "paretic", but the eyelid loses partially. **c** During eye closure, in contrast, an obvious lifting of the eyebrow happens. *Right* EMG recordings in the frontalis muscle of the patient on the left trying to frown (**b**), closing the eyes (**c**) and pulling the eyebrows together (**d**). The pattern of the muscle action potentials (MAP) shows fewer spikes during the natural movement intention (**b**) than with the antagonistic movement functions (**c** and **d**)

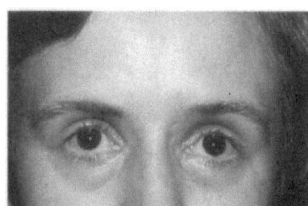

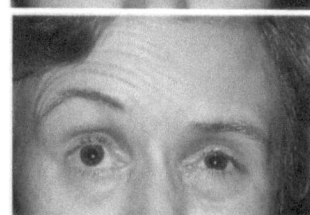

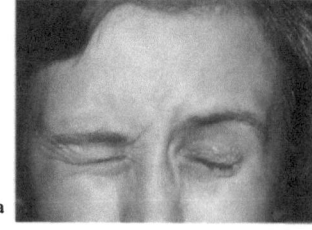

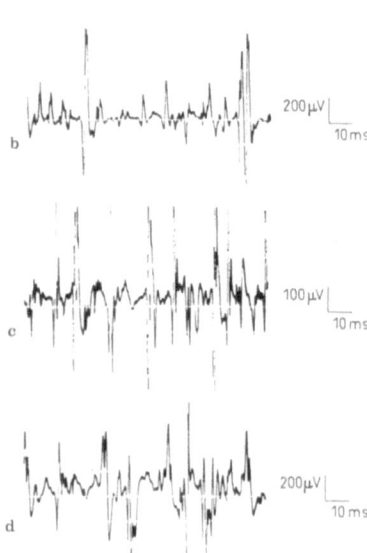

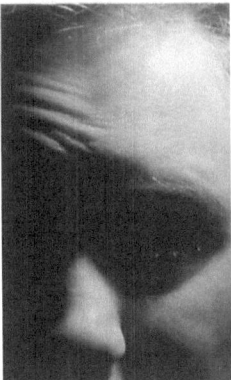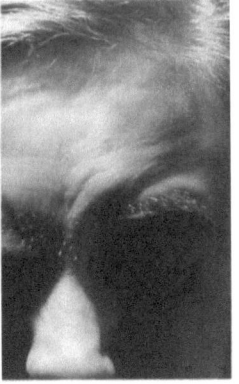

Fig. 7 Clinical example of the "paradoxical" innervation of the sphincter and expander muscles of the ocular sphincter system. *Left*; In frowning, the affected side remains "paretic". *Right;* Powerful closure of the eyelids leads to frowning

(Fig. 5), thus stimulating "paresis" of the frontalis muscle. Although the frontalis muscle is *reinnervated* very well by *electrophysiological* criteria, its *clinical function* due to the autoparalytic syndrome almost *"never comes back"*. This so-called weakness is, therefore, not the result of a missed reinnervation causing a paresis or paralysis, but is the consequence of a misdirected reinnervation, causing a

crosswise ("paradoxical") innervation of antagonists, and thus leading to a "functional paresis", i.e. "autoparalysis" (Fig. 6).

This pathomechanism may be recognized even clinically by carefully observing the eye region. As demonstrated in Fig. 7, the forehead muscle seems to be completely "paretic" while frowning (left). On the other hand, powerful closure of the eyes leads in the medial part of the ocular sphincter system to the physiological synergistic contraction of the depressor supercilii muscle, corrugator supercilii muscle and procerus muscle, but at the same time at the lateral part of the ocular sphincter system to the pathological antagonistic contraction of the frontalis muscle with elevation of the lateral part of the eyebrow, where the influence of the above-mentioned antagonists is only minimal.

References

1. Martin RC (1936) Surgical repair of the facial nerve. Arch Otolaryngol 23:458
2. Miehlke A (1973) Surgery of the Facial Nerve. Urban and Schwarzenberg, Munich
3. Sobotta-Becher J (1957) Atlas der deskriptiven Anatomie des Menschen, Teil 1, Urban and Schwarzenberg, Munich
4. Stennert E (1982) Das Autoparalytische Syndrom – ein Leitsymptom der postparetischen Fazialisfunktion. Arch Otorhinolaryngol 236:97–114
5. Tickle TG (1948) Surgery of the seventh nerve. JAMA 136: 969–972

Eur Arch Otorhinolaryngology (1994) [Suppl]: S 96 – S 101

FREE PAPERS AND POSTERS

V.M. Kazakov

Affection of Mimic Muscles, Simulating Damage of the Facial Nerve in Patients with Facioscapulohumeral Muscular Dystrophy

Introduction

In facioscapulohumeral muscular dystrophy (FSHMD) patients, the mimic muscles can be involved asymmetrically and isolatedly or the weakness of these muscles can predominate in the clinical picture for a long period. In connection with this, difficulties can arise in differentiating between myogenic affections and neurogenic ones, due to damage of facial nerve. The purpose of the present paper is to analyze the peculiarities of clinical affection of mimic muscles for early diagnosis in FSHMD patients.

Patients and Methods

A total of 214 patients with affection of mimic muscles aged from 4 to 85 years and duration of disease from 1 to 46 years were chosen for clinical analysis; 69 cases (63 hereditary and six "sporadic") were under personal observation and 145 cases (110 hereditary and 35 "sporadic") were taken from the literature [3]. The investigation of function and strength of the individual mimic muscles was conducted by special methods [1, 4] and following Duchenne's recommendations [2]. The results of the manual testing of 12 pairs of muscles in each patient were coded on the punch card K-5. Motor nerve conduction velocity tests, electromyograms (EMG) of the limb muscles, and analysis of some serum enzymes were performed for confirmation of myodystrophy in some patients from each pedigree and in each "sporadic" case.

V.M. Kazakov (✉)
Department of Neurology, Pavlov's Medical Institute,
L. Tolstoy Str. 6/8, 197089 St. Petersburg, Russia

Results

In the majority of patients (52%) FSHMD began during the first 10 years of life with affection of mimic muscles. However, only 59 patients said directly that the disease began with changes in their facial expression. The other 155 patients considered that in the earlier period shoulder girdle muscles were affected, and they did not complain of weak mimic muscles. Nevertheless, at the first medical examination the facial muscles already were involved, and in 31 patients there was even myopathic facies; thus we can assume that in all these patients the face was affected simultaneously with shoulder girdle muscles or even earlier.

Although some patients did not complain of weak mimic muscles, by asking parents or relatives the existence of definite symptoms dating back to childhood that indicated weakness of some mimic muscles was discovered. For example, some patients always slept with their eyes half open, and when washing their face and hair they often got soap in their eyes in spite of screwing them up (weakness of orbicularis oculi muscles); they always had "a crying-like face", they could not use certain toys (pipe, whistle) and could not learn to whistle (weakness of orbicularis oris muscle); they always smiled weakly and had pouting lips (weakness of zygomaticus muscles). Sometimes, relatives commented that the patient had had an unexpressive face since childhood. A total of 25 patients taken from the literature had different degrees of weakness of the mimic muscles on the right and left sides of the face, and 15 patients had mimic muscle weakness mostly on one side.

In my personal observations, asymmetry of affected mimic muscles was observed more frequently (in 47 out of 69 cases). Many patients had different degrees of weakness of the same mimic muscles on either side of the face; in other patients, certain muscles were involved on one side of the face and other muscles on the other side. Orbicularis oris, zygomaticus, orbicularis oculi, levator anguli oris,

Table 1 Frequency and degree of weakness of the mimic muscles in 214 patients with facioscapulohumeral muscular dystrophy

Muscles	Right side					Left side				
	Frequency	Degree of weakness				Frequency	Degree of weakness			
		Mild	Moderate	Severe	No function		Mild	Moderate	Severe	No function
Frontalis	83	25	–	24	34	78	24	–	20	34
Corrugator supercilii	50	13	–	15	22	46	13	–	11	22
Orbicularis oculi	140	32	–	30	78	138	33	–	32	73
Nasalis	6	–	–	2	4	6	–	–	2	4
Procerus	21	8	–	5	8	22	10	–	4	8
Zygomaticus	149	59	–	45	45	148	60	–	44	44
Risorius	2	–	–	1	1	2	–	–	1	1
Orbicularis oris	178	39	34	56	49	176	39	33	53	51
Levator labii superioris	77	16	–	35	26	73	13	–	33	27
Levator anguli oris	83	14	–	35	34	75	13	–	28	34
Depressor labii inferioris	6	3	–	2	1	6	3	–	1	2
Depressor anguli oris	8	–	–	4	4	9	–	–	4	5

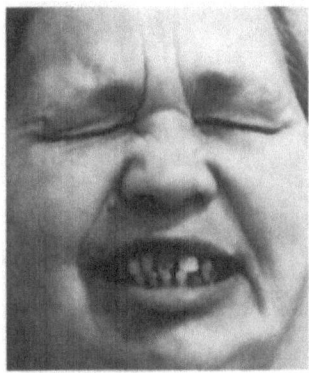

Fig. 1 A 60-year-old woman slight weakness of the orbicularis oculi muscles; orbital parts seen more clearly on the left side. On screwing up the eyes, the eyelashes were not fully concealed in the depths of the eyelids, the radial wrinkles are absent in the external angle of the left orbit, and the synergistic muscles (corrugator and procerus) contract very weakly on the left side. Severe weakness of zygomaticus muscles is seen more clearly on the left side. The patient can show her teeth by contracting the levator labii superioris muscle (note straight, deep nasolabial folds in upper parts) and contracting the depressor labii inferioris and depressor anguli oris (note the additional folds going from external angles of mouth downwards and outwards)

levator labii superioris, frontalis, and corrugator supercilii muscles were involved most often (Table 1).

The degree of affection of the individual mimic muscles varied from slight affection to absence of function (loss of the muscle). Wide-eye splits are a sign of weakness of the orbicularis oculi muscles. If patients had a slight weakness of these muscles, when screwing up their eyes the eyelashes were not fully concealed in the depths of the eyelids (Figs. 1–3). If patients had a severe weakness of the orbicularis oculi muscles, in attempting to screw up their eyes their eyelids only touched due to the action of palpebral parts of the orbicularis oculi muscles (Figs. 4–6). Inability to close the eyes and lagophthalmos were signs of loss the orbital and palpebral parts of the orbicularis oculi muscles (Fig. 7).

"Crying" expression of the face is a sign of weakness of the orbicularis oris muscle. If patients had a slight weakness of this muscle, in puckering their lips to whistle or in attempting to puff out the cheeks asymmetry of the lips or mouth was seen (Figs. 8–10). If patients had severe weakness of the orbicularis oris muscle, they could not pucker their lips to whistle and or puff out their cheeks (Figs. 11, 12). Inability to stretch out the lips is a sign of loss of the orbicularis oris muscle (Fig. 13).

Pouting lips is a sign of weakness of the zygomaticus muscles and predominant action of the orbicularis oris muscle. Transversely bearing teeth is a sign of slight

S98

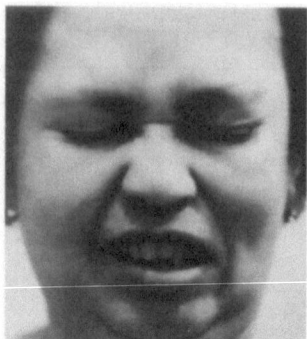

Fig. 2 A 39-year-old woman (the daughter of the patient in Fig. 1). Slight weakness of orbital parts of the orbicularis oris muscles. On screwing up the eyes, the eyelashes are not fully concealed in the depths of the eyelids, the radial wrinkles are absent in the external angles of orbits, and the corrugator muscles contract very weakly. Severe weakness of zygomaticus muscles is seen more clearly on the right side. The patient can show her teeth by contracting the muscles elevating the upper lip, more clearly visible on the right side (note straight, deep nasolabial folds) and contracting the depressor anguli oris and depressor labii inferioris muscles, more clearly visible on the left side (note the additional folds going from external angles of mouth downwards)

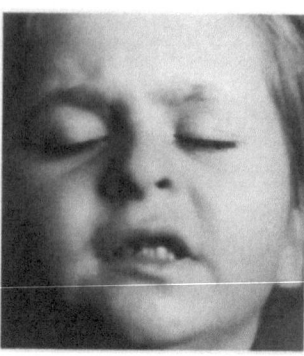

Fig. 4 A 7-year-old girl (the daughter of the patient in Fig. 2). Severe weakness of the orbital parts of the orbicularis oculi muscles. In attempting to screw up the eyes, eyelids only touch; there are no radial wrinkles in the external angles of the orbits, and corrugator and procerus muscles do not contract. Severe weakness of zygomaticus muscles on both sides and the levator labii superioris muscle on the right side. On attempting to show her teeth, the external angles of the mouth do not move outwards and upwards. The patient can show her teeth by contracting the levator labii superioris and levator anguli oris muscles on the left side only.

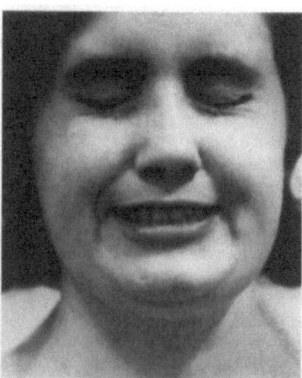

Fig. 3 A 29-year-old woman. Slight weakness of the orbital parts of the orbicularis oculi muscles. On screwing up the eyes, the eyelashes were not fully concealed in the depths of the eyelids and corrugator and procerus muscles do not contract. Slight weakness of zygomaticus muscles seen more clearly on the left side. The external angles of mouth go outwards, but not upwards; the left nasolabial fold is straight and does not form typical windings in upper and lower parts; the additional folds go from the external angles of the mouth downwards and outwards. The patient can show her teeth by contracting the risorius muscles and tensing the levator labii superioris and depressor anguli oris muscles

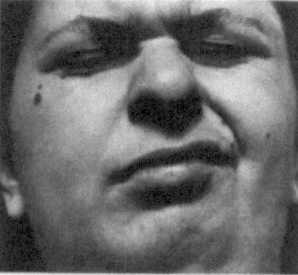

Fig. 5 A 29-year-old woman. Severe weakness of levator labii superioris and levator anguli oris muscles on the right side (the weak deepening of the right nasolabial fold confirms this), as well as the orbital parts of the orbicularis oris muscles. Same patient as in Fig. 4 reexamined after 22 years

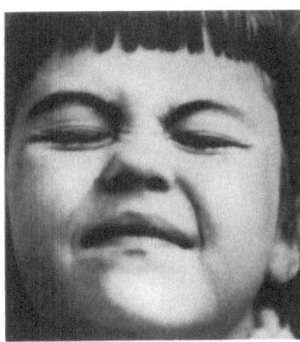

Fig. 6 A 6-year-old child. Severe weakness of the orbital parts of the orbicularis oculi muscles. On attempting to screw up the eyes, the eyelashes are not fully concealed in the depths of the eyelids, the radial wrinkles in the external angles of the orbits and wrinkles between brows are absent. Slight weakness of levator labii superioris on the right side (the weak deepening of the right nasolabial fold confirm this)

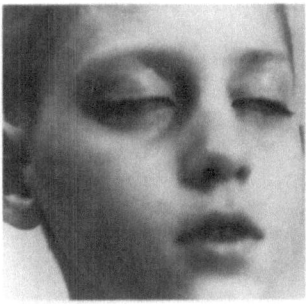

Fig. 7 A 10-year-old child with myopathic facies resembling facial diplegia. No function of mimic muscles. Slight displacement of the external angles of mouth outwards is due to tension of risorius muscles

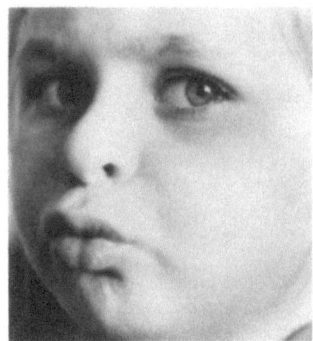

Fig. 8 Same patient as in Fig. 4. Slight weakness and atrophy of orbicularis oris muscle on the left side. Asymmetry of lips when puckering them to whistle

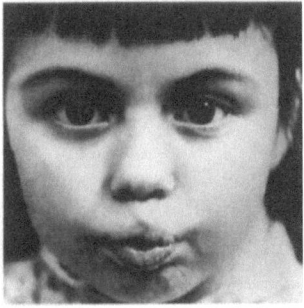

Fig. 9 Same patient as in Fig. 6. Slight weakness of orbicularis oris muscle on the right side. Asymmetry of the lips when puckering them to whistle

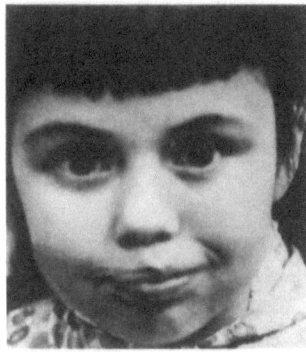

Fig. 10 Same patient as in Fig. 6. Inability to puff out cheeks, asymmetry of the mouth (slight weakness of orbicularis oris muscle seen more clearly on the right side)

weakness of the zygomaticus muscles (Fig. 3). If patients had severe weakness of these muscles, they were able to show their teeth due to contraction of the muscles elevating the upper lip and muscles depressing the lower lip, or due to contraction of the risorius muscles (Figs. 1, 2, 4, 14). Inability to bare teeth is a sign of loss of the zygomaticus muscles (Fig. 7).

In 31 patients (children and adults), almost total absence of function of mimic muscles on both sides of the face was observed. These patients had myopathic facies and the clinical picture suggested damage of the facial nerve on both sides. The patients had unexpressive faces and the facies of crying and laughter was absent or very weak (Figs. 7, 15).

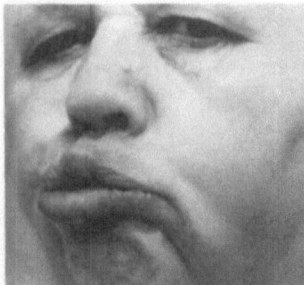

Fig. 11 Same patient as in Fig. 1. Severe weakness and atrophy of orbicularis oris muscle seen more clearly on the left side. On attempting to pucker lips to whistle, the mouth remains in the form of a transverse split. Asymmetry of the mouth also seen

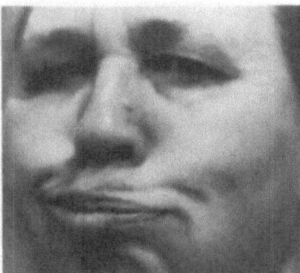

Fig. 12 Same patient as in Fig. 1. Inability to puff out the cheeks is due to severe weakness and atrophy of orbcularis oris muscle, seen more clearly on the left side

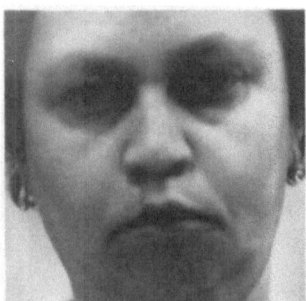

Fig. 13 Same patient as in Fig. 2. Loss of orbicularis oris muscle. Inability to stretch out the lips. Protrudence of the upper lip is due to tension of the levator labii superioris muscle

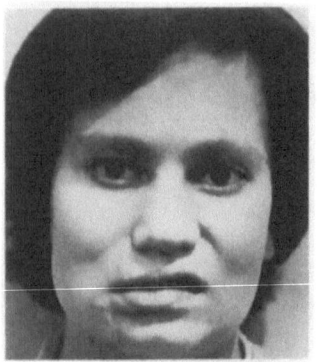

Fig. 14 A 12-year-old child. Severe weakness of zygomaticus muscles. On attempting to show the teeth, typical dimples are formed at the external angles of the mouth due to contraction of the risorius muscles. Deeping of nasolabial folds is due to tension of the muscles elevating the upper lip, seen more clearly on the left side

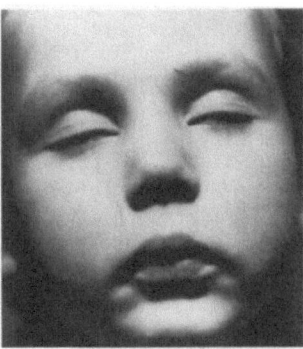

Fig. 15 A 4-year-old child with myopathic facies. Inability to close the eyes; the sclerae are seen (loss of the orbital and palpebral parts of the orbicularis oculi muscles). The nasolabial folds are absent as well as the wrinkles between brows and along bridge of nose (loss of dilatators of mouth muscles and corrugator and procerus muscles). The upper lip overhangs, reminiscent of the "tapir lip" (loss of muscles elevating the upper lip)

Conclusion

In FSHMD patients, asymmetrical affection of mimic muscles was observed, mostly in the lower parts of the face (orbicularis oris, zygomaticus, levator labii superioris, and levator anguli oris) and occasionally in the upper parts of the face (frontalis, orbicularis oculi). The clinical picture in some patients suggested damage of the facial nerve. However, detailed examination of individual mimic muscles using simple clinical tests and taking into consideration the actions of synergistic and antagonistic muscles helps to find more widespread involvement of mimic muscles on both sides of the face. More difficulties arise when the mimic muscles are affected mostly on one side of the face or the patient has myopathica facies" (resembling facial diplegia) with the shoulder girdle muscles relatively intact. In such cases, revealing an early pattern of muscle involvement (sternal portions of pectoralis major, brachioradialis, latissimus dorsi, and tibialis anterior), characteristic of FSHMD, could help to correct diagnosis.

Occasionally, acute neuritis of the facial nerve develops in FSHMD patients. Thus in two of our patients who thought that they were healthy and did not notice the weakness of their mimic muscles, neuritis of the facial nerve on the left side suddenly developed after acute respiratory infection.

On examining patients, weakness of mimic muscles on both sides of the face, more marked on the left side, and topography of weakness and atrophy of the shoulder girdle, arm, and lower leg muscles characteristic of FSHMD were found. EMG and genealogical investigation confirmed the diagnosis.

References

1. Daniels L, Williams M, Worthingham C (1956) Muscle testing. Techniques of manual examination, 2nd edn. Saunders, Philadelphia
2. Duchenne GBA (1872) De l'électrisation localisée, 3rd edn. Bailliére, Paris
3. Kazakov VM, Bogorodinsky DK, Znoyko ZV, Skorometz AA (1974) The facio-scapulo-limb (or the facioscapulohumeral) type of muscular dystrophy. Clinical and genetic study of 200 cases. Eur Neurol 11:236–260
4. Kendall HO, Kendall FM (1949) Muscles, testing and function. Williams and Wilkins, Baltimore

Eur Arch Otorhinolaryngology (1994) [Suppl]: S 102 – S 104

FREE PAPERS AND POSTERS

G. Ralli, E. Pafundi, R. Gradini, and E. Morgante

Muscle Ultrastructural Changes in Long-Standing Idiopathic Total Facial Nerve Palsy

Introduction

Total facial palsy may be idiopathic, iatrogenic, traumatic, or caused by inflammatory, viral, or tumoral diseases. In these cases, the loss of facial movements may be irreversible and the only possible chance for the patients is a surgical procedure. Facial muscle reinnervation procedures may be effective even when performed years after the onset of the paralysis. One of the factors that must be considered in planning this surgery is the capacity of the muscle fibers to regain their contractile action. In the present study, the ultrastructural changes of the denervated muscle (auricularis posterior muscle) in cases of long-standing idiopathic facial nerve paralysis are evaluated.

Material and Methods

Biopsies of auricularis posterior muscle and of sternocleidomastoid muscle were taken from three patients with long-standing (over 10 years) idiopathic total facial nerve palsy. The samples (1 × 1 cm) were straightened and left to dry for 2 min to avoid excessive contraction in the fixative. Part of the tissue was fixed in formalin, embedded in paraffin, sectioned, and stained with hematoxylin and eosin for light microscopy. The remaining tissue was processed for transmission electron microscopy as follows: fixation in glutaraldehyde 2.5% in phosphate buffer 0.1 M, pH 7.2 (for at least 4 h at 4 °C); washing in buffer solution for 2 h and postfixation in OsO_4 (1.33%) for 2 h; dehydration in

graded ethanol solutions and toluene; Epon 812 (4 h at room temperature), followed by polymerization of the resin (24 – 36 h at 60 °C). The blocks were oriented to obtain both transverse and longitudinal sections. Sections (2 – 3 µm) stained with toluidine blue were used for light microscopy. Ultrathin sections (obtained by Ultramicrotome Reichert E), after adequate staining with uranyl acetate and lead hydroxyde, were examined with a CEM-10 Philips transmission electron microscope (TEM).

Results and Discussion

A reduction of the myofibril diameter of the affected muscle was noted at the light microscopy. In addition, an increase of endomysial and perimysial connective tissue was evident.

The TEM sections showed ultrastructural pathological changes, compatible with muscle denervation. Sections from sternocleidomastoid muscle (used as a control) showed normal skeletal muscle: sarcomeres were well organized and oriented, and mitochondria had a normal strucutre (Fig. 1). Biopsies taken from the auricularis posterior muscle showed large group atrophy of muscle cells, increased connective and adipose tissue, disruption of sarcomeres, large and abnormal mitochondria, vacuolar degeneration, and mitochondria-laden outpouchings of the sarcolemma. Motor end plates were absent. The nuclei of the myocytes showed no major changes (Fig. 2 – 4). Long-standing facial paralysis is a challenging clinical and surgical problem, especially when the possibility of facial reanimation is considered. The role of biopsy in long-standing facial nerve palsy is controversial. A correlation between clinical, morphological, and instrumental findings is not always present, especially in cases of long-standing facial paralysis [1 – 3]. A biopsy of the denervated muscles may be helpful in deciding the treatment. A severe atrophy or a fibrosis of the myocytes would not allow a reinnervation surgical procedure. In such a case, the myo-

G. Ralli (✉) and E. Pafundi
II ENT Department, University of Rome "La Sapienza", Policlinico Umberto I, Viale Regina Elena, 324, 00161 Rome, Italy

R. Gradini and E. Morgante
Department of Experimental Medicine,
University of Rome "La Sapienza", Policlinico Umberto I,
Viale Regina Elena, 324, 00161 Rome, Italy

Fig. 1 Section of sterno-cleidomastoid muscle showing the ultrastructure of normal muscle. (Transmission electron microscopy, TEM; original magnification, ×2000)

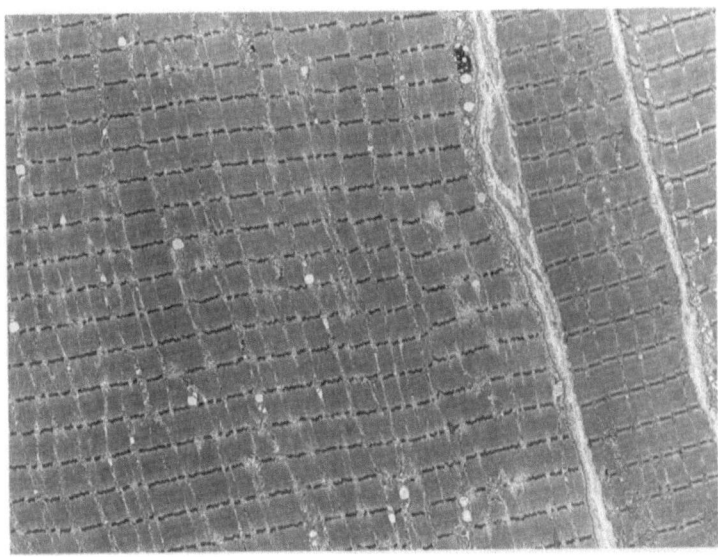

Fig. 2 Section of retroauri-cularis muscle in long-standing facial nerve palsy. Vacuolar degeneration and disruption of sarcomeres are seen. (Transmission electron microscopy, TEM; original magnification, ×4000)

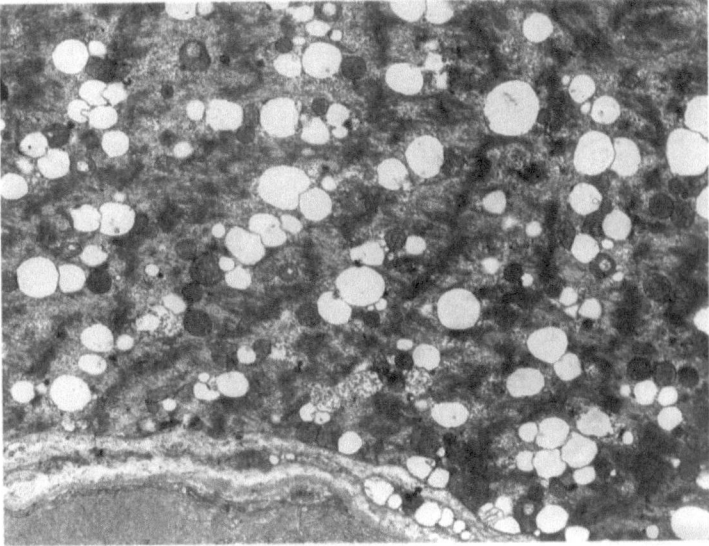

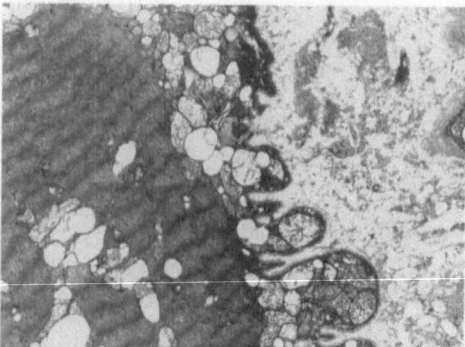

Fig. 3 Section of retroauricularis muscle in long-standing facial nerve palsy, showing mitochondria-laden outpouchings of the sarcolemma and large and abnormal mitochondria. (Transmission electron microscopy, TEM; original magnification, ×4000)

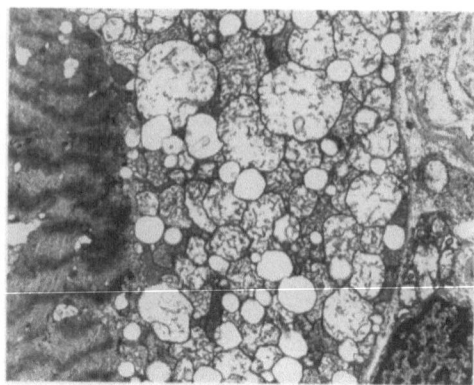

Fig. 4 Section of retroauricularis muscle in long-standing facial nerve palsy, showing large and abnormal mitochondria and partial disruption of the sarcomeres. (Transmission electron microscopy, TEM; original magnification, ×6000)

cytes would not be able to regain their function and a muscle graft or a passive suspension technique may be the only practicable surgical procedure. On the other hand, less extensive changes occurring in denervated muscles should be compatible with a functional recovery. In this case, a procedure such as facial decompression, nerve graft, facio-facial or hypoglossal-facial anastomosis may be indicated. Muscle ultrastructural changes due to denervation increase progressively according to the time of biopsy. However, a strict correlation between the duration of the denervation and the severity of the atrophy is not sufficently demonstrated. Our cases showed ultrastructural changes confined to the cytoplasm, whereas the nuclei were free of obvious pathology. These findings, even if obtained in a limited number of patients, show that the nuclei of the muscle cells are still intact after long-standing denervation. Therefore, a reinnervation surgical procedure might be useful even many years after the onset of facial nerve paralysis.

References

1. Belal A (1982) Postdenervation muscular changes in facial paralysis: a histopathological and electron microscopic study. In: Graham MD, House WF (eds) Disorders of the facial nerve. Raven, New York, pp 137–146
2. Belal A (1984) Muscle biopsy in facial palsy. In: Portmann M (ed) Facial nerve. Masson, New York, pp 194–197
3. Schwarting S, Schroder M, Stennert E, Goebel HH (1984) Morphology of denervated human facial muscles. ORL 46: 248–256

Eur Arch Otorhinolaryngology (1994) [Suppl]: S 105 – S 106

FREE PAPERS AND POSTERS

A. Jakubiec-Puka and J. Szczepanowska

Comparison of Myosin in Denervated and Immobilized Muscles

Introduction

Striated muscles differ in respect to velocity, power of contraction and resistence to fatigue. The striated muscle is a
very plastic and adaptable tissue [8]; transformation of
fibre types, muscle hypertrophy or atrophy can appear
within a short time [3, 4, 6]. Alterations occur as a result of
functional or anatomical demands, hormonal influence etc.
Both denervation and immobilization bring about muscle
atrophy and diminishing of the contractile apparatus (references in [3, 4, 7, 9]), but differences between the effect
of inactivity and that of lack of innervation are not fully
understood. The type-dependent differences in muscle reaction are also unclear. All these issues are of practical
importance.

Myosin, the major component of myosin filaments in
the contractile apparatus, is composed of six subunits: four
light chains and two heavy chains. Maximum velocity and
power of muscle contraction are correlated with the
myosin heavy chains (MHC type, which can be adjusted
according to muscle functional demands (references in
[4, 6]). In the present paper, changes in the MHC content in
the denervated or immobilized muscle are compared. The
results are discussed and compared with previous ones.

Materials and Methods

Slow-twitch (soleus) and fast-twitch (gastrocnemius) rat
leg muscles were denervated [3] or immobilized in a
neutral or in a shortened position [9]. The methods used
were described previously: examination of muscle ultrastructure [5], estimation of the total MHC content [6] and

A. Jakubiec-Puka (✉) and J. Sczepanowska
Department of Cell Biochemistry, Nencki Institute of Experimental
Biology, ul. Pasteura 3, 02-093 Warsaw, Poland

separaration [1], identification [2] and quantitative evaluation [9] of the individual MHC isoforms – 1, 2A(S) and 2B
[2] – which are present in the slow-twitch oxidative, the
fast-twitch oxidative-glycolytic and the fast-twitch glycolytic fibres, respectively.

Results and Discussion

The striated muscle atrophied following both inactivity
and denervation. Early reaction to denervation, immobilization or tenotomy was stronger in the slow than in the
fast muscle [4, 6, 7, 9]. A shortened position of the immobilized muscle increased its atrophy [9]; the fast muscle
immobilized in a neutral position for a short time did not
atrophied [9].

In the denervated muscle, the myosin filaments disappeared before the actin filaments. The proportion of myosin to actin filaments decreased (Fig. 1), as did the ratio
of MHC to actin [3, 7]. During the first month after denervation, such changes were very pronounced in the slow
muscle, whereas in the fast one they were negligible [7].
The loss of the total MHC content was much higher in the
slow than in the fast muscle (Fig. 2a). Thus, the response of
the contractile apparatus to early denervation is quite different in the slow and in the fast muscle. Both muscles
became similar only in the later stage of denervation atrophy [7]. In the slow and fast muscles immobilized for a
short time, the ratio of MHC to actin and the proportion of
the corresponding filaments were the same as in the controls. In contrasts after tenotomy the MHC to actin ratio
decreased, especially in the slow muscle [6].

Susceptibility of the individual MHC isoforms to
muscle denervation and immobilization was not uniform.
After denervation, the proportion of the MHC-1 and
MHC-2B and the amount of fibres of corresponding types
decreased, whereas those of the type 2A increased [2, 4].
Though the content of each MHC isoform decreased, their
decreases differed in degree (Fig. 2a). In the immobilized
muscles, the content of MHC isoforms characteristic for

Fig. 1a, b Electron micrographs of slow muscle (soleus), transverse sections through the A-band. **a** Denervated muscle. Lack of hexagonal arrangement of filaments and decreased proportion of myosin to actin filaments. **b** control muscle. Filaments in a regular, hexagonal arrangement

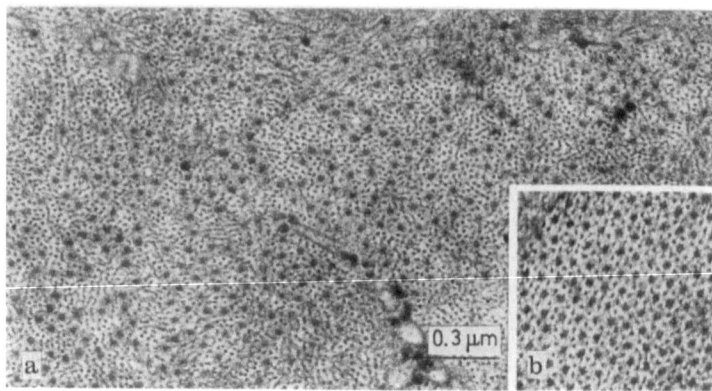

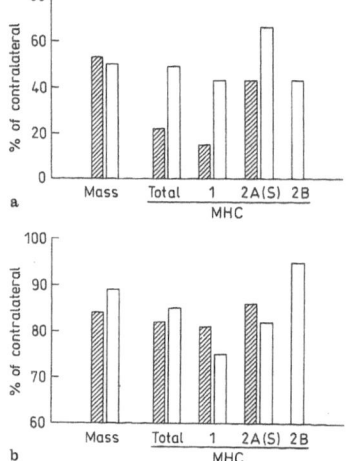

Fig. 2a, b Changes in the content of myosin heavy chains (MHC) in slow (soleus, *shaded bars*) and fast (gastrocnemius, *white bars*) muscles. Contents of the *MHC* total and of the particular MHC isoforms were evaluated as described [6, 9]. **a** 16 days after denervation. **b** 4 days after immobilization in shortened position

2. The content of MHC-1 is controlled mainly by muscle activity.
3. The content of MHC-2A(S) is controlled by muscle activity; in the denervated muscle it remains comparatively high.
4. The MHC-2B is relatively unsusceptible to inactivity, while it is supressed by the increased "slow" muscle activity; this isoform is susceptible to denervation.
5. The same rules seem to apply to the MHC isoforms and to the muscle fibre types.

References

1. Carraro U, Catani C (1983) A sensitive SDS-PAGE method separating myosin heavy chain isoforms of rat skeletal muscles reveals the heterogeneous nature of the embryonic myosin. Biochem Biophys Res Commun 116: 793–802
2. Carraro U, Catani C, Degani A, Rizzi C (1990) Myosin expression in denervated fast- and slow-twitch muscles: fiber modulation and substitution. In: Pette D (ed) The dynamic state of muscle fibres. De Gruyter, Berlin, pp 247–261
3. Jakubiec-Puka A, Kulesza-Lipka D, Krajewski K (1981) The contractile apparatus of striated muscle in the course of atrophy and regeneration. I. Myosin and actin filaments in the denervated rat soleus. Cell Tissue Res 220: 651–663
4. Jakubiec-Puka A, Kordowska J, Catani C, Carraro U (1990) Myosin heavy chain isoform composition in striated muscle after denervation and self-reinnervation. Eur J Biochem 193: 623–628
5. Jakubiec-Puka A, Carraro U (1991) Remodelling of the contractile apparatus of striated muscle stimulated electrically in a shortened position. J Anat 178: 83–100
6. Jakubiec-Puka A, Catani C, Carraro U (1992) Myosin heavy chain composition in striated muscle after tenotomy. Biochem J 282: 237–242
7. Jakubiec-Puka A (1992) Changes in myosin and actin filaments in fast skeletal muscle after denervation and self-reinnervation. Comp Biochem Physiol 102A: 93–98
8. Pette D, Staron RS (1990) Cellular and molecular diversities of mammalian skeletal muscle fibers. Rev Physiol Biochem Pharmacol 116: 1–76
9. Szczepanowska J, Jakubiec-Puka A (1992) Myosin heavy chains in striated muscle after immobilization. Basic Appl Myol 2: 97–105

fatigue-resistent fibres (1, 2A and 2S) decreased, whereas that of MHC-2B virtually did not change (Fig. 2b). The MHC isoforme react similarly to tenotomy [6]. Thus, it seems that both the muscle-nerve junction and muscle activity are very important here.

The results presented here and previous ones allow us to conclude as follows:

1. The myosin filaments and the MHC are, in general, less stable in the slow than in the fast muscle; they are less stable than the actin filaments and the actin.

Eur Arch Otorhinolaryngology (1994) [Suppl]: S 107 – S 108

INVITED LECTURES

H. Strenge, B. Benz, and H. Weber

Respiratory-Related Electromyographic Activity of Facial Muscles

Introduction

In the course of extensive electrophysiological examinations following peripheral paresis of the facial nerve, we unexpectedly observed an activation of different facial muscles in relation to breathing. As we are not aware of any previous studies of this phenomenon, we report some details of our electromyographic (EMG) findings.

Materials and Methods

A total of 19 men and 22 women, aged 11 – 76 years, who had suffered a one-sided peripheral paresis of the facial nerve, were studied between 17 months and 6 years following the illness. The paresis had been complete in 18 and incomplete in 23 cases; 33 of the patients were diagnosed has having Bell's palsy, seven suffered from herpes zoster cephalicus, and the paralysis in one patient was due to the operative removal of an acoustic neuroma.

The examinations performed were standardized according to clinical and neurophysiological aspects, including EMG, electroneurography, and the electrically elicited blink reflex [7]. The inferior part of the orbicularis oculi muscles and the orbicularis oris muscles of both sides were recorded simultaneously using coaxial needle electrodes. Spontaneous activity, the recruiting effect of voluntary innervation, and the degree of uncontrollable coactivation by isolated face muscle contraction were assessed. Moreover, abnormal excitability was evaluated by allowing the patients to breathe deeply for 2 min. Acoustic feedback was used to control muscle relaxation during this maneuver.

H. Strenge (✉), B. Benz and H. Weber
Clinics of Neurology and Otolaryngology, University of Kiel, Niemannsweg 147, 24105 Kiel, Germany

Results

Figure 1 shows the discharge pattern of single motor unit (SMU) potentials of orbicularis muscles in relation to respiration recorded in a 49-year-old male 2 years after removal of an acoustic neuroma with a resulting left-sided facial paresis. During deep breathing (Fig. 1A), the left orbicularis oris muscle shows block discharges of SMU beginning 2 – 3 s before maximal diaphragm activity (top trace) and ending approximately 1 – 2 s thereafter. Orbicularis oris unit activity is almost totally absent during the Valsalva maneuver (Fig. 1B) and quiet expiration (Fig. 1C). When ventilation returned to normal, the familiar discharge (Fig. 1A) of SMU in the orbicularis oris with distinct temporal relationship to the forced inspiration regularly reappeared.

These spontaneous discharges are exemplary for the findings in ten out of a total of 41 patients. This subpopulation (six men and four women, aged between 29 and 73 years) suffered from six left-sided and four right-sided complete and incomplete pareses with the etiology ratio corresponding to the total sample.

It is conspicious that the respiratory-related EMG activity of the orbicularis oris was only present on the affected side, whereas in the orbicularis oculi, activity was also observed on the clinically nonaffected side in three cases. The discharge phenomena occurred in all ten patients within seconds following the start of hyperventilation.

With increased ventilation either new SMU were recruited or previously active SMU with continuous (tonic) activity increased the frequency of their discharge (three patients).

The average firing rates ranged from 9 to 26/s and peak rates from 26 to 40/s. In eight out of the ten patients there was an additional presence of involuntary coactivation of the respective muscle, and in six of these there was an aberrant blink reflex response to the m. orbicularis oris.

Fig. 1A–C Discharge patterns of facial motor units during deep breathing (**A**), Valsalva maneuver (**B**), and quiet expiration (**C**). Top trace in each panel (ICS 5–6 R): surface diaphragm electromyogram (*EMG*) from the 5–6 intercostal space along the right midclavicular line. Recordings from a 49-year-old man 2 years after left-sided peripheral facial paresis. *OCL*, left m. orbicularis oculi; *ORR*, right m. orbicularis oris; *ORL*, left m. orbicularis oris

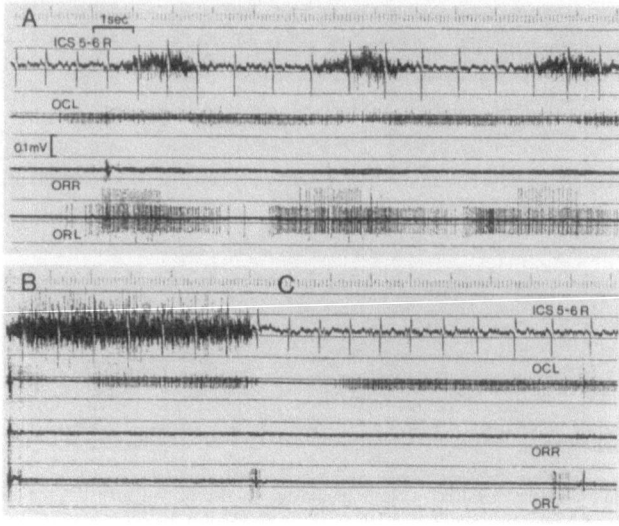

Discussion

The occurrence of respiratory-linked discharges in cranial nerves is not new. There are few results available from animal experiments with description of an inspiratory activation in the glossopharyngeal, vagal, and hypoglossal nerves as well as in the inferior alveolar branch of the trigeminal nerve [4, 6]. Smith et al. [5] reported that the facial nucleus of the cat receives bilateral afferent projections from the rostral division of the ventral respiratory neurons in the area of the nucleus ambiguous. These predominantly inspiratory neurons innervate by preference the ventral and lateral areas of the facial nucleus in which the motor neurons for the buccolabial muscles are located [2].

Our results suggest that facial afferents from inspiratory brain stem neurons also exist in humans and that this respiratory drive can become apparent by altered nuclear excitability after facial nerve regeneration [1]. It is also possible, however, that misconducted, regenerated axons of the nasal muscles, known to show respiratory-related discharges [3], are partially involved in this phenomenon.

References

1. Bratzlavsky M, van der Eecken H (1977) Altered synaptic organization in facial nucleus following facial nerve regeneration: an electrophysiological study in man. Ann Neurol 2:71–73
2. Jenny AB, Saper CB (1987) Organization of the facial nucleus and corticofacial projection in the monkey: a reconsideration of the upper motor neuron facial palsy. Neurology 37:930–939
3. Lansing RW, Solomon NP, Kossev AR, Andersen AB (1991) Recording single motor unit activity of human nasal muscles with surface electrodes: applications for respiration and speech. Electroencephalogr Clin Neurophysiol 81:167–175
4. Smith JC, Feldman JL (1987) In vitro brainstem-spinal cord preparations for study of motor systems for mammalian respiration and locomotion. J Neurosci Methods 21:321–333
5. Smith JC, Morrison DE, Ellenberger HH, Otto MR, Feldman JL (1989) Brainstem projections to the major respiratory neuron populations in the medulla of the cat. J Comp Neurol 281:69–96
6. St John WM (1987) Pneumotaxic mechanisms influence phrenic, hypoglossal, and trigeminal activities. Exp Neurol 97:301–314
7. Strenge H, Benz B, Weber H (1990) Electrophysiological features of residual nerve deficits following peripheral facial palsy. In: Castro D (ed) The facial nerve. Kugler and Ghedini, Amsterdam, pp 97–99

Eur Arch Otorhinolaryngology (1994) [Suppl]: S 109

POSTERS

M. Popova

Stimulation of the Regeneration Process in Denervated Muscle

As is well known regeneration is the most important capability of different organisms. One problem faced by researchers in biology and medicine is the difficulty of investigating nerves and skeletal muscle. In this study the regeneration process in denervated skeletal muscle was stimulated by the implantation of autogenous minced muscle.

In a second series of experiments the posterior extremity of rats was irradiated with a dose of 20 Gy. The musculus gastrocnemius was completely cut across, and the minced muscle tissue taken from the left nonirradiated extremity was autotransplantated into the defect of the irradiated muscle. In 1 week in the intensive regeneration process had developed in the transplanted minced tissue. The muscular fibers of the proximal and distal stumps showed significant regeneration activity despite the radiation damage. After 2 months the defect was filled with young muscular fibers. The integrity and functional activity of the irradiated muscle was restored.

M. Popova
Institute of Evolutionary Animal Morphology and Ecology,
Leninsky prospect, 33 117071 Moscow, Russia

Eur Arch Otorhinolaryngology (1994) [Suppl]:S110–S112

POSTERS

K. Shimada, H. Moriyama, M. Ikeda, H. Tomita, S. Shigihara, and R. F. Gasser

Peripheral Communication of the Facial Nerve at the Angle of the Mouth

Introduction

The detailed, peripheral locations of the facial nerve communications with the terminal branches of the trigeminal nerve have not been described thoroughly in anatomical textbooks. In a percentage of clinical cases, there is evidence of functional recovery of portions of the facial musculature following surgical section of the main trunk of the facial nerve. For example, there can be spontaneous recovery of function near the angle of the mouth.

This phenomenon was observed by Martin and Halsper [3] in 28.5% of their cases. Our interest in an anatomical reexamination of the communications was stimulated when a patient, who had undergone a parotidectomy with severance of the contained facial nerve branches, had spontaneous recovery of facial muscle function near the angle of the mouth.

Materials and Methods

The facial skin and underlying tissues were removed in mass from the anterior and lateral surface of the skull. The three specimens were preserved in a absolute ethyl alcohol solution containing 0.001% alizarin red prior to and also during dissection. This method more easily distinguished

K. Shimada (✉) and H. Moriyama
Present address: Showa University, School of Medicine,
5-8, Hatanodai 1, Shinagawa-ku, Tokyo 142, Japan

M. Ikeda and H. Tomita
Nihon University School of Medicine,
Department of Otolaryngology 30-1, Kami-machi Oyaguchi,
Itabashi-ku, Tokyo 173, Japan

S. Shigihara and R. F. Gasser
Louisiana State University Medical Center, Department of Anatomy
1901 Perdido Street, New Orleans, Louisiana 70112, USA

the fine-caliber nerve branches from the adjacent connective tissues, which were stained deep red [5]. The dissections were performed with needle forceps under a stereomicroscope (Wild M630) at ×6 magnification.

Observations

Communications were observed in six areas between the following branches:

1. The auriculotemporal branch of the mandibular nerve and branches of the facial nerve in the parotid gland.
2. The zygomaticotemporal branches of the maxillary nerve and temporal branches of the facial nerve.
3. The infratrochlear branch of the opthalmic nerve and zygomatic branches of the facial nerve.
4. The zygomaticofacial branch of the maxillary nerve and zygomatic branches of the facial nerve.
5. The infraorbital branch of the maxillary nerve and zygomatic branches of the facial nerve in the orbicularis oculi muscle.
6. The buccal branch of the mandibular nerve and buccal branches of the facial nerve in the buccinator and orbicularis oris muscle.
7. The mental branch of the inferior alveolar nerve and the buccal and marginal mandibular branches of the facial nerve (Figs. 1, 2).

In the elaborate communications or plexuses between the peripheral branches of the facial nerve and trigeminal nerves, the most delicate and complex plexuses were found in areas 6 and 7. In the previous two areas, the communications were most complex and variable in area 6.

Discussion

At the angle of the mouth many facial muscles come together. The muscles in this area are very complex and

Fig. 1A Example of communications in the dissected material. *White arrows*, facial nerve. **B** The higher magnification of the angle of mouth. *Black arrow* heads indicate the communication area. **E**, Eye; **FA**, facial artery; **MM**, masseter muscle; **MN**, mental nerve (the third branch of trigeminal nerve); **PG**, parotid gland; **SG**, submandibular gland

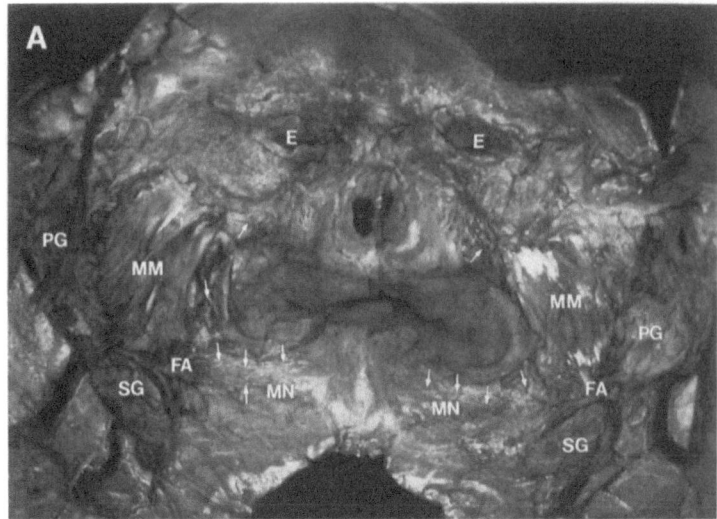

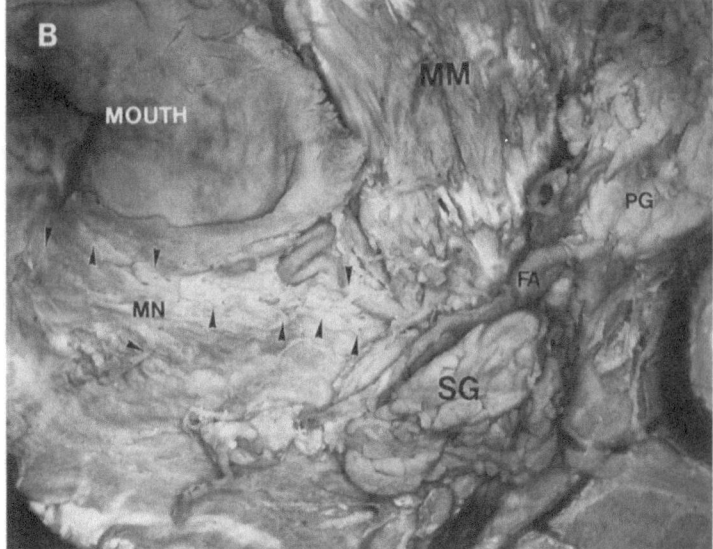

variable [1, 2, 4]. Based on our observations, these muscles were innervated by the zygomatic, buccal and marginal mandibular branches of the facial nerve. Most communications were located in three general areas: infraorbital, buccal and mental. The communications in the angle of the mouth and mental area were more variable and complex than in the other two areas. Communications in the mental foramen area, where sensory mental branches of the trigeminal nerve intermingle with terminal motor fibres of the facial nerve, may provide a pathway for trigeminal motor fibres to reinnervate facial muscles at the angle of the mouth. The extablishment of such a nerve fibre pathway may explain the spontaneous recovery of muscle function observed clinically.

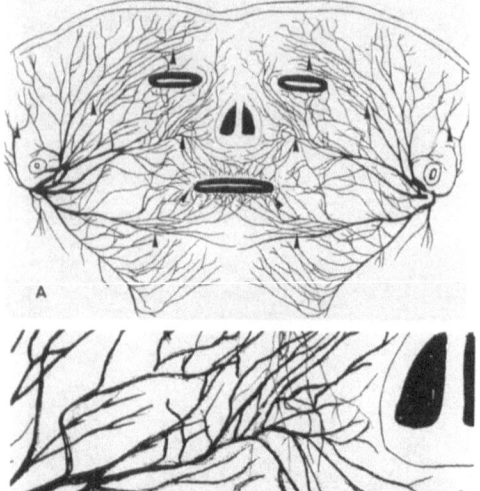

References

1. Greyling LM, Meiring JH (1992) Morphological study on the convergence of the facial muscles at the angle of the mouth. Acta Anat 143:127–129
2. Lightoller GHS (1925) Facial muscles: the modiolus and muscles surrounding the rima oris with some remarks about the panniculus adiposis. J Anat 60:1–84
3. Martin H, Helsper JT (1957) Spontanuous return of function following surgical section or excision of the seventh cranial nerve in the surgery of parotid tumors. Ann Surg 146:715–727
4. Shimada K, Gasser RF (1989) Variations in the facial muscles at the angle of the mouth. Clin Anat 2:129–134
5. Tanaka S, Mizukami S (1991) Vagal communicating branches between the facial and glossopharyngeal nerves, with references to their occurrence from the embryological point of view. Acta Anat 142:25–32

Fig. 2A Communications between the peripheral branches of the facial and trigeminal nerves (*arrowheads*). **B** Large magnification of the angle of the mouth area. *Arrowheads* as in **A**

Eur Arch Otorhinolaryngology (1994) [Suppl]:S113

POSTERS

E. I. Maksimenko

Development and Reinnervation of Rat Muscle Grafts in Interspecific Transplantations

Using the method of Prof. A. N. Studitski, it was possible to obtain viable muscle grafts under interspecific transplantation in rodents. Albino rat gastrocnemius muscles were kept wrapped in a cellophane film for 10–12 months and then their whole or minced fragments were placed on the site of the same removed muscles of Mongolian gerbils. Within 60 days after the operation the donor's muscle survived and developed from myoblasts to young striated myofibers in the recipient's muscle bed. There were many basophilic myosimplasts with a great number of nuclei and myotubes. Nuclear chains appeared in myofibers. Ultrastructural examination revealed many satellite cells and myoblasts under a basal membrane of young myofibers in groups of two to four cells side by side. The characteristic feature of such myofibers was their sprouting and the presence of narrow parallel rows of long membranes with glycogen granules packed regularly; these structures often formed the concentric figures. In spite of the fact that the myogenic processes ran more slowly and inertly than the same ones in autotransplantation (only 10–14 days after xenotransplantation myogenic effects appeared and myogenesis proceeded for a long time; nevertheless in 2 months we had 20% of the muscle grafts (2.5 times less than in autotransplantation); here the best results were obtained under minced muscle xenotransplantation. It is well known that innervation of the rat skeletal muscle grafts was complete 30–60 days after autotransplantation, but with the xenotransplantation specific neuromuscle contacts were not found. The regenerating nerve fibers grew from the stumps in the transplant's periphery only. This reason may be the decisive one in the dystrophy and destruction of the xenografts with in 4 months after the operation. The connective tissue can show strong development, fully replacing the young muscle tissue.

E. Maksimenko
A. N. Severtzov Institute of Evol. Animal Morphology & Ecology, Moscow, Russia, 117071

Eur Arch Otorhinolaryngology (1994) [Suppl]: S 114 – S 116

POSTERS

H. Tanaka

Trigeminal-Facial Nerve Communication and Its Clinical Application

Introduction

Weakly coordinated movement between the masseter muscle and the facial musculature is sometimes observed in patients whose facial nerve has been dissected or shows severe denervation. If this group of patients receives long-term training that is well planned and based on logical knowledge, spontaneous facial movement can be restored in most patients.

Training Program

Our training program is made up of the following components:

1. Heat therapy two to three times a day.
2. Low-frequency therapy for a short time.
3. Powerful massage of the masseter muscle [1], particularly the anterior part, at a high frequency.
4. Training in mastication [2] in which the entire muscle is sufficiently contracted while applying the finger to the masseter muscle.
5. Training in pulling the corner of the mouth in the superolateral direction and closing the lips during the above-mentioned mastication.
6. The above-mentioned training cycle is repeated more than ten times daily (about 5 min per cycle).

Case Presentation

Two typical clinical cases are presented in Figs. 1 and 2 to show the results of this training.

H. Tanaka
Tanaka ENT Hospital, 6–7 Toyooka-cho, Tsurumi-ku, Yokohama 230, Japan

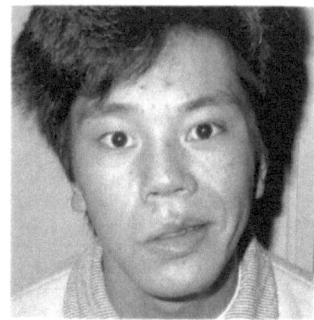

Fig. 1 Traumatic facial nerve palsy (left). A small bone fragment was removed 1 month after the onset and rehabilitation was also started 1 month after the onset of palsy. Coordinated movement was achieved 2 months after the onset of palsy

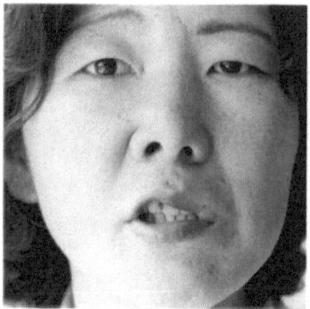

Fig. 2 Acoustic tumor (left). Facial nerve grafting during surgery with no effect. Rehabilitation was started 5 years after surgery and coordinated movement was achieved 7 years after surgery

Discussion

It is important to know how and where coordinated movement between the masseter muscle and the corner of the mouth occurs and to find a method that maximizes this movement. The cross-over of nerves may occur at any of the points from the nerve nucleus to the peripheral nerve end. If the fiber leading from the facil nucleus enters the facial muscle after passing through the trigeminal nerve, patients should show some degree of facial movement after dissection of the facial nerve. The buccal nerve of the trigeminal nerve is in contact with the buccal rami of the facial nerve. Cross-over in this region would explain the regional confinement of movement, although the buccal nerve is primarily a sensory nerve [3]. Some investigators consider a motor nerve to be included [4, 5], but this view is not widely endorsed. The hypothesis that sprouting penetrates through a nerve fascicle or that the sprouting reaches the periphery after traveling a long distance is unreasonable and unlikely. When coordinated movement was observed more carefully, we found that the nasolabial groove was more marked in the lower half, that the angle of the mouth is pulled laterally and is not raised upwards, and that the lips are closed. These features of coordinated

movement can be produced only by the buccal muscle. This muscle is wide and is in direct contact with the masseter muscle in a sufficiently wide area. On electromyograms, all other muscles were electrically silent; only the buccal muscle showed spikes synchronous with the masseter muscle. It seems most reasonable to think that this coordinated movement occurred because the buccal muscle was innervated by the collateral sprouting of the masseter nerve or the terminal sprouting of the masseter.

The limitations of this therapy include the following:

1. In rare cases, no effect is obtained despite maximum efforts.
2. This method is not effective in the upper half of the face.
3. Unless it is based on a well-devised plan, this method does not produce any noteworthy effect.

However, the therapy does offer certain advantages:

1. In cases in which rehabilitation was initiated at an early stage, about the same level as on the normal side was reached in young patients and about 50% of the normal side in elderly patients.
2. In cases in which rehabilitation was initiated 5–6 years after surgery, about 50% of the normal side was reached in patients with little muscle atrophy; the symmetric oral angle was restored in patients with muscle atrophy.
3. The time when movement was restored was after 2 months at the earliest and more than 2 years at the latest.

Because sprouting withdraws when the original nerve is regenerated [6] (Fig. 3), some characteristics of clinical applications are as follows:

1. No surgery is required.
2. It does not prevent the regeneration of denervated nerves.
3. It is suitable for cases with nerve reconstruction.
4. It is suitable for cases in which nerve reconstruction was unsuccessful.
5. Both normal movement and coordinated movement can be used.

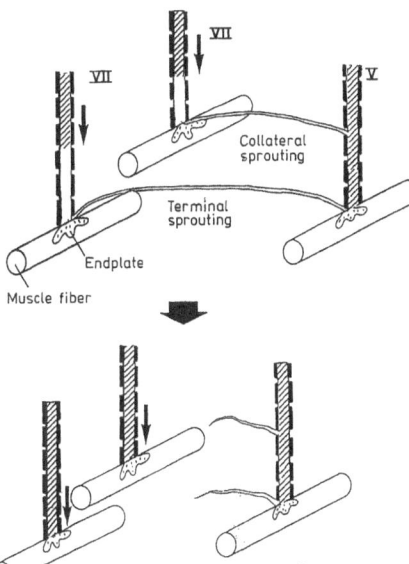

Fig. 3 Sprouting withdraws when the original nerve is regenerated. *VII*, seventh cranial nerve

Conclusion

As one of the mechanisms of spontaneous recovery of the facial nerve after dissection or denervation, the sprouting of the masseter nerve or the masseter muscle is thought to innervate the buccal muscle to cause coordinated movement. The maximal practical use of this mechanism may be applied to the therapy of various types of facial nerve palsy.

References

1. Frederick JN, Kosman AJ (1948) Effect of "Neurotripsy" on the partially denervated muscle of the dog. Proc Soc Exp Biol Med 69:605–607
2. Norris CW, Proud GO (1981) Spontaneous return of facial motion following seventh cranial nerve resection. Laryngoscope 91:211–214
3. Banfai P (1976) Die angewandte klinische Anatomie des Nervus facialis. II. Anastomosen. HNO 24:280–294
4. Huber E (1930) Evolution of facial musculature and cutaneous field of trigeminus. Q Rev Biol 5:133–188
5. Baumel JJ (1974) Trigeminal-facial nerve communications: their function in facial muscle innervation and reinnervation. Arch Otolaryngol 99:34–44
6. Thompsen W (1978) Reinnervation of partially denervated rat soleus muscle. Acta Physiol Scand 103:81–91

Eur Arch Otorhinolaryngology (1994) [Suppl]: S 117–S 119

POSTERS

H. Moriyama, K. Shimada, N. Goto, S. Shigihara, and R. F. Gasser

Observations on the Geniculate Ganglion in Adult Human Dissections

Introduction

The geniculate ganglion is of clinical importance because it is the site of the nerve cell bodies for the special sense of taste. Its location has been described in anatomy textbooks as being on the facial nerve at the point in the facial canal where the nerve bends sharply backwards laterally making a right angle. The name "geniculate" is derived from the shape of the ganglion described above. None of the textbooks give a detailed account of the shape of the ganglion or of the ramus that arises in the vicinity of the ganglion and communicates with tympanic nerve and tympanic plexus. We made detailed dissections of the ganglion in Japanese adults and found that the communicating ramus with tympanic nerve and tympanic plexus was usually not a single branch, but several branches that arose in all of the regions described in the literature. The ganglion often had an outer S or sigmoid shape that varied with the number and region of origin of the branches. Regarding the three dissections, we counted neurons in the geniculate ganglion.

Material and Methods

Twenty head halves from the cadavers were used. After decalcification of these dissections by Plank-Rychlo fluid; we dissected facial nerves and their surrounding struc-

tures in detail under an operation microscope (WILD 630). Regarding the three dissections, we counted neurons in the geniculate ganglion by the following procedures:

1. Fixation: Primary fixative: 10% solution of formalin (3.7%–4.0% formalhyde). Secondary fixative: mixture of 5% potassium dichromate and 5% potassium chromate (1:4 in volume) for 3 weeks (2 weeks at room temperature and 1 week at 37 °C) [7].
2. Washing in running water.
3. Dehydration and celloidin embedding.
4. Cutting sections 30 μm thick, serial sections, numbering.
5. Staining. Every fifth section was stained by the luxol fast blue plus periodic acid-Schiff plus hematoxylin triple stain (LPH stain) method [7].
6. Counting (systemic sampling method, quasi-random sampling). The neurons having a distinct nucleolus were counted under the microscope (Abercrombie's counting method [1]).

H. Moriyama (✉), K. Shimada, and N. Goto
Showa University School of Medicine, Department of Anatomy, 5-8, Hatanodai 1, Shinagawa-ku, Tokyo 142, Japan

S. Shigihara and R. F. Gasser
Louisiana State University Medical Center, Department of Anatomy, 1901 Perdido Street, New Orleans, Louisiana 70112, USA

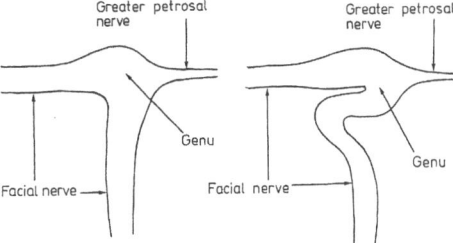

Fig. 1 Two types of the genu of the facial nerve. *Left*, L-shaped; *right*, S-shaped

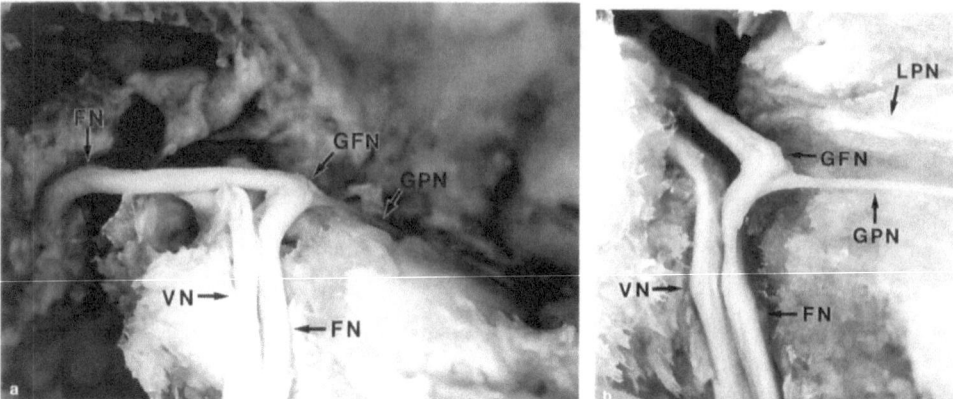

Fig. 2a, b Dissection of L-shaped genu. *GPN*, greater petrosal nerve; *GFN*, genu of the facial nerve; *FN*, facial nerve; *VN*, vestibular nerve; *LPN*, lesser petrosal nerve

Observations and Discussion

Classification of the Shape of the Genu of the Facial Nerve

We classified the shape of the genu of the facial nerve into two types: (1) L-shape type – the facial nerve bends backwards laterally making a right angle at the genu of the facial nerve; this type has been described in the literature [2, 5, 6, 8, 9] (Figs. 1, 2). (2) S-shape type – the facial nerve bends sharply forwards in an acute angle just before the genu of the facial nerve; this type has an outer S or sigmoid shape (Figs. 1, 3). A total of 11 L-shape and nine S-shape types were observed in our dissections.

Communicating Ramus Between the Facial Nerve and the Tympanic Nerve or Tympanic Plexus

We obtained some interesting findings of the communicating ramus between the facial nerve and the tympanic nerve or tympanic plexus. Regarding this communicating ramus, anatomy textbooks describe the presence of the communicating ramus [2, 3, 5, 8, 9], but not the region and numbers of rami or nerve fibers. As far as we know, Vidic and Young first described the communicating ramus [11]. The site of the communicating ramus varies as follows: (a) the second part of the facial nerve adjacent to the geniculate ganglion, (b) the surface of the geniculate ganglion, (c) the greater petrosal nerve. In our observations, a single communicating ramus was present in one head half, dual rami in one, triple in one, and including an absence in 17 heads examined.

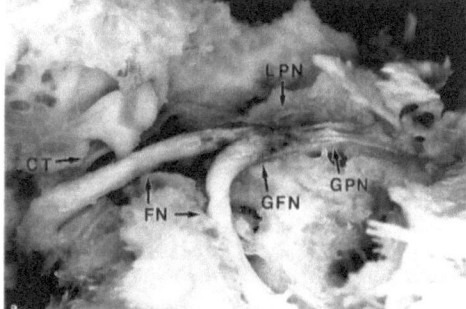

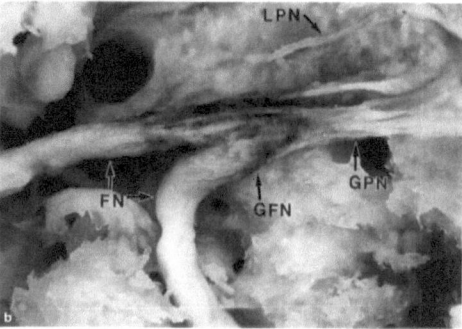

Fig. 3a, b Dissection of S-shaped genu. *CT*, chorda tympani; *FN*, facial nerve; *LPN*, lesser petrosal nerve; *GPN*, greater petrosal nerve; *GFN*, genu of the facial nerve

Neuronal Numbers of the Geniculate Ganglion

According to Schimert [10], the number of neurons in the geniculate ganglion was 1400; however, Buskirk [4] stated that the average number was 2129, with a range of 1462 to 3682. Our data were as follows:

- Cadaver No. 337 (93-year-old man, right side): 1818
- Cadaver No. 521 (77-year-old man, left side): 2163
- Cadaver No. 528 (49-year-old woman, right side): 1810

The average number is thus 1930.

References

1. Abercrombie M (1946) Estimation of nuclear population from microtome sections. Anat Rec 94:239–247
2. Aqur AMR (1991) Grant's atlas of anatomy, 9th edn. Williams and Wilkins, Baltimore, p 544
3. Bean RB (1913) The cephalic nerves: suggestions. Anat Rec 7:221–235
4. Buskirk CV (1945) The seventh nerve complex. J Comp Neurol 82:303–333
5. Clara M (1959) Das Nervensystem des Menschen. Barth, Leipzig, pp 374–383
6. Fisch V (1977) Facial nerve surgery. Kugler, Amstelveen/Aesculapius, Birmingham, pp 16–17
7. Goto N (1987) Discriminative staining methods for the nervous system: luxol fast blue + periodic acid-Schiff + hematoxylin triple stain and subsidiary staining methods. Stain Technol 62/5:305–315
8. Kopsch FR (1923) Lehrbuch und Atlas der Anatomie des Menschen, Sects. 5 and 6. Thieme, Leipzig, pp 279–285
9. Schaeffer JP (1942) Morris' human anatomy, 10th edn. Blakiston, Philadelphia, pp 1063–1065
10. Schimert J (1936) Der Nervus intermedius und das Ganglion geniculi nervi facialis. Mikrosk Anat Forsch 39:35–44
11. Vidic B, Young PA (1966) Gross and microscopic observations on the geniculo-tympanic nerve in man. Anat Rec 154:436

Eur Arch Otorhinolaryngology (1994) [Suppl]: S 120

ABSTRACT

A. Pollak, R. Ruan, and U. Fisch

Spatial Occupancy of the Facial Nerve in the Fallopian Canal

The purpose of this study was to investigate the spatial relationship of the facial nerve throughout its course within the fallopian canal by measuring the cross-sectional surface area from the labyrinthine to the mastoid segment on 20 normal human temporal bones, all sectioned serially in the horizontal plane. The average occupancy of the facial nerve in the fallopian canal was found to be 63% in the labyrinthine segment, 41% in the tympanic segment, and 33% in the mastoid segment. The restricted space surrounding the facial nerve in the labyrinthine segment of the fallopian canal may lead to entrapment of the facial nerve in the presence of edema.

A. Pollak (✉), R. Ruan, and U. Fisch
ENT Department, University Hospital, 8091 Zürich, Switzerland

Eur Arch Otorhinolaryngology (1994) [Suppl]:S121

ABSTRACT

M. Asai, S. Murakami, and N. Yanagihara

Funicular Structure and Nerve Fiber Topography in the Extratemporal Facial Nerve

The facial nerve has a specific funicular structure. The nerve has multiple funiculi only in the extratemporal portion. It has remained controversial whether each funiculus in a nerve has a topographic organization of nerve fibers. The problem has not yet been investigated in the facial nerve. Using guinea pigs, the experiment was conducted to find the relationship between funicular structure and nerve fiber topography by anterograde degeneration technique.

At the extratemporal trunk just below the ramification of the inferior labial branch, one funiculus was dissected and transected using microscissors under the operating microscope. After 4–6 days, the nerve trunk peripheral to the section and each of the main peripheral branches, i.e., anterior auricular, zygomatico-orbital, superior labial, were dissected out and examined histologically.

In the facial nerve trunk, all the degenerated nerve fibers were confined in the one funiculus, while in the multifunicular peripheral branches the degenerated fibers were found in several funiculi in one main branch. The result indicates a loose topographic organization of the nerve fibers is present in the funiculus of the facial nerve trunk.

M. Asai (✉), S. Murakami, and N. Yanagihara
Department of Otolaryngology,
Ehime University School of Medicine,
Shigenobu-cho, Onsen-gun, Ehime 791-02, Japan

Physical Training

Eur Arch Otorhinolaryngology (1994) [Suppl]: S 125 – S 126

C.H.G. Beurskens, J. Oosterhof, J.W.H. Elvers, R.A.B. Oostendorp, and M.E.J. Herraets

The Role of Physical Therapy in Patients with Facial Paralysis: State of the Art

Introduction

Although there have been several reports indicating the success of physical therapy, few scientific data seem to be available. To assess the efficacy of physical therapy, a so-called criteria-based meta-analysis was conducted [1].

Materials and Methods

Using the keywords facial paralysis, physical therapy, rehabilitation, facial expression, and biofeedback we carried out a literature research from the following sources:

- On-line search Index Medicus (1966-medio 1991).
- Documentation center of the National Institute for Research and Postgraduate Education in Physical Therapy.
- Reference search of collected articles and books.
- Screening from abstracts and proceedings.

The 70 articles found were divided according to the languages, as shown in Fig. 1.

However, only 17 (24%) of the 70 articles turned out to be effect research. Therefore, we had to split the research into two parts: effect research and descriptive research. This chapter will only discuss the effect research. (References for the descriptive research are available on request.) A criteria list was made for the methodological assessment of the effect research, and the list was divided into 127 items. All articles were reviewed by two independent reviewers. For statistical data analysis, only the descriptive statistics are used [4, 8].

C.H.G. Beurskens, J. Oosterhof, J.W.H. Elvers, R.A.B. Oostendorp, and M.E.J. Herraets
University Hospital Nijmegen, Department Physical Therapy, Postbus 9101, 6500 HB Nijmegen, The Netherlands

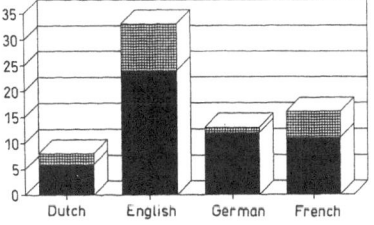

Fig. 1 Descriptive (*black bars*) and effect (*shaded bars*) research ($n = 70$)

Results

In the collected articles, the effect research was divided into one randomized clinical trial (RCT) [14] two quasi-experimental designs [10, 16], and 14 pre-experimental designs [2, 3, 5–7, 9, 11–13, 15, 17–20].

Concerning the population of the studies, they were not comparable, because of the large differences in numbers of patients, differences in causes, duration of causes, and ages of the patients.

The form of intervention in these studies was:

- Exercise therapy [2, 3, 5–7, 9–11, 15–17, 19, 20]
- Physical applications [6, 7, 9–14, 16–20]
- Massage [2, 3, 11, 14, 17, 19, 20]

These interventions were mostly (71%) given as combination therapy. The most frequently given combination was exercise therapy with biofeedback.

It turned out to be even more difficult to make a comparison between the studies because there were six different forms of physical applications: biofeedback [4, 6, 7, 10, 19], ultrasound [12, 13, 18], low-frequency electrotherapy [11, 14, 16, 20], short-wave diathermy [16], infrared [17, 19] and heat application [14, 17, 20].

Most of the studies do not discuss the method of intervention, and most interventions are executed in a different way concerning the number of treatments (10–216), the duration (5 min to several hours), and the frequency (one per week to 14 per week).

For the measurement of the effects (i.e., more symmetry in rest and during movement, less synkinesis, and a better well-being), ten different measuring instruments are used:

- House grading scale [6, 10, 18]
- House-Brackman facial nerve grading system [5]
- Portmann's classification [3]
- Photographs [2, 3, 5, 6, 9, 11, 14]
- Video [6, 10]
- Lines drawn on the face [7]
- Psychological questionaire [19]
- Granger's evaluation method [11]
- Seven-grade scale [11]
- Nerve excitability test [16]

As an effective intervention the following were mentioned: exercise therapy [2, 3, 7, 11, 17, 19, 20], biofeedback [5–7, 10], massage [2, 3, 11, 17, 20] low-frequency electrotherapy [11, 20], ultrasound [13, 18], heat application [20], and magneto-therapy [9].

Conclusions and Discussion

In view of the fact that there is only one RCT, we have to be very careful about drawing conclusions. In addition, some articles did not reckon with the possibility of a spontaneous recovery of the facial nerve. Therefore, in studies with patients having a facial paralysis shorter than 1 year and without a control group, it cannot be determined whether the effect is due to the intervention or due to spontaneous recovery.

As a final conclusion we can say that exercise therapy, massage, and biofeedback tend to have a positive effect. Exercise therapy and massage resulted in more symmetry during movement and a better well-being, while biofeedback resulted in less synkinesis. As a guideline for future experimental research, controlled studies on the effect of exercise therapy and biofeedback are recommended.

References

1. Beckerman H, Bouter L (1991) Effectiviteit van Fysiotherapie. Een literatuurstudie. Rijksuniversiteit Limburg, Vakgroep Epidemiologie en Biostatistiek, Maastricht
2. Beurskens C, Bots I, Devriese PP (1987) Resultaten van mimetherapie bij patienten met een perifere facialisverlamming. Ned Tijd Fysiother 97 : 140–145
3. Beurskens C (1988) The functional rehabilitation of facial muscles and facial expression. Castro D (ed) Facial nerve, Proceedings of the 6th international symposium on the facial nerve. pp 509–511
4. Bland M (1991) An Introduction in medial statistics. Oxford Medical Publications, Oxford
5. Brudny J, Hammerschlag PE, Cohen NL et al. (1988) Electromyographic rehabilitation of facial function and introduction of a facial paralysis grading scale for hypoglossus-facial nerve anastomosis. Laryngoscope 98 : 405–410
6. Brudny J (1991) Biofeedback in facial paralysis: electromyographic rehabilitation. In: Rubin L (ed) The paralysed face, vol 30. Mosby, St Louis, pp 247–264
7. Corral-Romero MA, Bustamante-Balcarcel A (1982) Biofeedback rehabilitation in seventh nerve paralysis. Ann Otol 91: 166–168
8. Elvers JWH (1989) Inleiding tot de beschrijvende statistiek. Uitgave SWSF
9. Fombeur JP, Koubbi G, Chevalier AM et al. (1988) De l'apport des aimants dans les séquelles des paralysies faciales. Ann Chir Plast 105 : 397–402
10. Hammerschlag PE, Brudny J, Cusumano R et al. (1987) Hypoglossal facial nerve anastomosis and electromyographic feedback rehabilitation. Laryngoscope 97 : 705–709
11. Hwang LL, Lien IN (1975) The effect of physical therapy for peripheral facial palsy. J Form Med Assoc 74 : 345–352
12. Jébéjian R (1985) Résultats du traitement précoce de la paralysie faciale périphérique par les ultrasons. Bull Memm S F.O 96: 287–291
13. Jébéjian R (1984) Traitement de la paralysie faciale périphérique par les ultrasons. Ann Otol Laryngol (Paris) 101 : 471–479
14. Mosforth J, Taverner D (1958) Physiotherapy for Bell's palsy. Br Med J 13 : 675–677
15. Peitersen E, Andersen P (1966) Spontaneous course of 220 peripheral non-traumatic facial palsies. Acta Otolaryng [Suppl] 224 : 296–300
16. Salam EA, Elyahky WS (1968) Evaluation of prognosis and treatment in Bell's palsy in children. Acta Paediatr Scand 57 : 468–472
17. Sigwald J, Barrié M, Jonvelle A et al. (1969) La rééducation kinésithérapique de la paralysie faciale périphérique primitive ou secondaire. La semaine des hopitaux/therapeutique 45 : 913–920
18. Talmi YP, Finkelstein Y, Shem-Tov Y et al. (1989) Is ultrasound treatment beneficial in Bell's palsy? Ear Nose Throat J 68: 722–726
19. van Gelder RS, Philipart SMM, Bernard BGES et al. (1988) Effecten van myofeedback en mimetherapie. Logopedie en Foniatrie 60 : 120–126
20. von Jaster H (1969) Klinische Aspekte zur katarrhalischen Form der peripheren Fazialisparese. Z Arztl Fortbild 63 : 497–499

Eur Arch Otorhinolaryngology (1994) [Suppl]: S 127 – S 128

POSTERS

E. Dalla Toffola, S. Ricotti, L. Petrucci, G. Carenzio, E. Bilucaglia, G. Salvini, C. Zandrini, and A. Moglia

Functional Recovery and Electromyographic/Electroneurography Evaluation in Bell's and Ramsay-Hunt's Palsy Patients Undergoing Physical Training

Introduction

In a previous study [3] we showed the course of Bell's palsy in patients undergoing rehabilitation treatment; in this study, we compare Bell's to Ramsay-Hunt's palsy (R-H).

Materials and Methods

The Following criteria were applied in selecting patients for this study:

1. Bell's palsy or R-H at onset.
2. Clinical evaluation within 30 days after onset.
3. Electrophysiological evaluation 30 ± 7 days after onset.
4. Rehabilitation program carried out at our institute.
5. Clinical control at the end of the rehabilitation treatment.
6. Clinical follow-up a minimum period of 6 months after the end of the treatment.

From 1978 to 1990, we examined 136 patients with facial nerve palsies: 65 patients with Bell's (42 men, 23 women) and 11 with R-H (three men, eight women) met our inclusion criteria. The mean age of the Bell's palsy patients was 43.12 years (range, 18 – 78 years) and of the R-H patients 47.36 (range, 26 – 75 years). A total of 33 Bell's palsy patients and six R-H patients had plegia (MRCR = 0) and 32 Bell's palsy patients and five R-H patients had paresis (MRCR > 1). The duration of outpatient rehabilitation treatment in Bell's palsy patients was 1 – 7 months and in R-H patients 4 – 16 months. The patients were discharged from the treatment further to recovery or stabilization of

E. Dalla Toffola (✉), S. Ricotti, L. Petrucci, G. Carenzio,
E. Bilucaglia, G. Salvini, C. Zandrini, and A. Moglia
Cattedra di Medicina Fisica e Riabilitazione, Università di Pavia
Policlinico S. Matteo, P. le Golgi 2, 27100 Pavia, Italia

the neurological deficit ascertained during at least two subsequent controls with a 2-week interval; clinical follow-up was carried out at least 7 months after discharge.

We evaluated the following according to our previous work [3]: (a) muscle strength; (b) electromyogram/electroneurography (EMG/ENG); (c) motor recovery; and (d) mimicry, voluntary motility, and synkinesis.

In order to allot a single quantitative value to the clinical evaluation of muscular strength and to the many parameters of the neurophysiological test, we calculated the DE of the muscular and EMG/ENG test. (The DE corresponds to the square root of the sum of the square differences from the normal value of each parameter). Thus, we obtained a single numerical value "summing up" the performed test, which expresses how far each patient is from the healthy subject (whose value is equal to zero). As for the DE of the EMG/ENG, we took into consideration activity at rest, M latency, and M amplitude. As for the DE of the muscle test, we took into consideration muscular strength of the examined muscles. The rehabilitation treatment was carried out through BFB-EMG (bio-feed-back electromyographic).

Results

The muscle strength recovery results for Bell's palsy patients were as follows: absent in one (1.5%), scarce in 20 (30.8%), good in 17 (26.1%), and very good in 27 (41.6%) patients. In the R-H patients, muscle strength recovery was scarce in seven (63.7%) and good in four (36.3%) patients (X_2, 7.954; $p < 0.05$).

The follow-up was carried out for an average of 29 months (range, 7 – 144 months; median, 26 months) after discharge in Bell's palsy patients and for an average period of 36 months (range, 6 – 72 months; median, 22 months) in R-H patients.

The results of analysis of objective synkinesis for Bell's palsy patients were: absent in 38 (58.4%), slight in 21

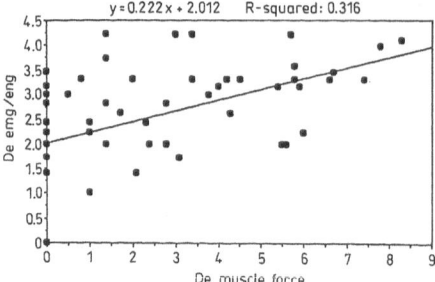

Fig. 1 Regression line between Euclid's distance (ED) of neurophysiological test and ED of muscular strength evaluated during follow-up in patients affected by Bell's syndrome. *DE*, square root of the sum of the square differences from the normal value of each parameter. *EMG*, electromyogram; *ENG*, electroneurography. Correlation coefficient (CC) 0.562; $p < 0.001$

(32.3%), and serious in six (9.3%) patients. In R-H patients, objective synkinesis was absent in two (18.2%), slight in two (18.2%), and serious in seven (63.6%) patients (X_2, 19.8; $p < 0.001$). As far as subjective synkinesis was concerned, it was absent in 31 (47.4%), slight in 21 (32.3%), and serious in 13 (20%) Bell's palsy patients. In R-H patients, it was absent in three (9%), slight in six (54.6%) and serious in four (36.4%) patients (X_2, 5.765; not significant). The initial recovery time, i.e., the appearance of voluntary activity, was an average of 54.9 days (range, 7–164 days; median, 32 days) in Bell's palsy patients – in particular, 30 days (range, 7–90 days; median, 30 days) in those without synkinesis, and 76.48 days (range, 19–146 days; median, 85 days) in those with synkineses – and of 91 days (range, 30–180 days; median, 90 days) in R-H patients. In order to evaluate the seriousness of the initial neurological damage in the two groups, we compared the averages of the DE of the EMG/ENG test (Bell's: mean, 2.497; SD, 0.988; R-H; mean, 3.801: SD, 1.195; t test, 3.927; $p < 0.001$), thus showing the presence of a more serious neurological damage in R-H. We calculated the correlation coefficient (CC) between the DE of the EMG/ENG test 30 days after onset of palsy and: (a) clinical picture on admittance to treatment (palsy or paresis); (b) DE of muscle strength at the end of rehabilitation treatment; (c) DE of muscle strength during the follow-up. In Bell's palsy, there was a significant correlation between the EMG/ENG picture and the objective examination either on admittance to treatment in paralysed patients (CC, 0.278; $p \leq 0.05$), at the end of treatment (CC, 0.505; $p \leq 0.001$), or during follow-up (CC, 0.562; $p \leq 0.001$; Fig. 1). In the R-H, no CC was statistically re-

levant. Muscle strength at the end of rehabilitation treatment was evaluated during different timespans (about 4 months in Bell's palsy patients and 14 months in R-H), according to the different times needed to reach clinical stabilisation. In Bell's palsy, the average DE was 3.51, in R-H, 6.24 (t, 2.965; $p \leq 0.01$), thus proving a better short-term prognosis in Bell's palsy. This difference was consistently significant also during follow-up (mean DE, 2.18 in Bell's palsy, 5.05 in R-H; t, 3.48; $p \leq 0.01$). Being aware that in Bell's palsy the development of synkinesis is more likely the more serious the clinical and neurophysiological injury, we compared the mean of the DE of EMG/ENG of Bell's patients who developed synkinesis and those who did not: mean DE for patients with synkinesis, 2.918 (SD, 0.841); mean DE for patients without, 1.865 (SD, 0.854, t, 4.915; $p \leq 0.01$).

Discussion and Conclusions

When considering muscle strength recovery in Bell's palsy and R-H patients we noticed a better recovery in Bell's patients. When we compared the recovery quality by grouping together patients who developed moderate or serious synkinesis, we noticed that in Bell's patients the incidence was 41.6%, in R-H 81.8%. The EMG/ENG test carried out on the 30th day showed that all patients developing synkinesis suffered from serious nerve injuries and had a high DE EMG/ENG. The comparison between the DE EMG/ENG showed that the picture in R-H is much more serious than in Bell's palsy. In Bell's palsy, we noticed significant differences in the neurophysiological test between patients who recovered very well and those who developed synkinesis and had a partial recovery, while all R-H patients showed problems in motor recovery.

The EMG/ENG test is valuable to evaluate the neurological deficit, to plan times and best techniques for recovery, and to prognosticate the quality of recovery (synkinesis), especially for Bell's palsies. Treatment with BFB-EMG suggests at an early stage a rehabilitation exercise program for patients which finely modulates the activity of motor units, which are reinnervated step by step in order to revive full facial mimicry [1, 2, 4].

References

1. Baillet R (1982) Facial paralysis rehabilitation and retraining selective muscle control. Int Rehab Med 4:67–74
2. Basmajian JV (1975) Biofeedback training. Ann J Occup Ther 29:469–470
3. Dalla Toffola E et al. (1988) Il recupero dopo paralisi di facciale. Valutazione Clinica ed elettrofisiologica. Eur Medicophys 24/2:75–81
4. Jonkel WR (1978) Bell palsy, muscle reeducation by electromyograph feed-back. Arch Phys Med Rehabil 59:240–242

Eur Arch Otorhinolaryngology (1994) [Suppl]: S 129–S 132

POSTERS

H. J. Diels

Treatment of Facial Paralysis Using Electromyographic Feedback – A Case Study

Introduction

Facial expression is our primary means of nonverbal communication. It is how we present ourselves to the world and the way in which other distinguish our emotions. Impairment of facial function may limit expressive movements as well as produce a variety of functional deficits. Facial paralysis is not only physically disabling, but can be psychologically disabling as well. The effectiveness of neuromuscular retraining for postacute facial paralysis is well documented [1, 2, 3, 4, 5, 6] and is a growing field of practice. The neuromuscular Retraining Clinic (NMRC), Facial Retraining Program, at the University of Wisconsin Hospital and Clinics, Madison, has applied this research to an active clinical practice since 1983. Over 350 individuals with diagnoses such as postsurgical removal of acoustic neuroma and other tumors, Bell's palsy, traumatic injury, cancer, congenital abnormalities, postanastomosis, and muscle transfers have been treated. Patients with paralysis, paresis, and/or synkinesis resulting from a peripheral injury to the seventh cranial nerve (C. N. VII) have effectively learned to improve facial motor control using specific neuromuscular retraining techniques and augmented feedback, including electromyographic (EMG) biofeedback.

The patient presented is an 8-year-old girl with congenital palsy of the marginal mandibular branch of the left facial nerve resulting in paralysis of the left lip depressor masculature. Relative hyperactivity of the right depressors was present. Referral for facial retraining was made by a plastic surgeon after consulting with the parents, who reported a decrease in the patient's self-esteem which corresponded with unkind remarks from her schoolmates

H. J. Diels
Neuromuscular Retraining Clinic, Department of Rehabilitation Medicine, University of Wisconsin Hospital and Clinics, 2710 Marshall Ct., Madison, WI 53705, USA

about her appearance. There was evidence that the patient was beginning to inhibit her normal emotional affect in order to hide her "crooked smile". The parents were concerned about the long-term psychological effect of this disability. It was decided to attempt facial neuromuscular retraining to improve symmetry during smile before consideration of more invasive surgical procedures.

Method

The patient was scheduled for a 2-day outpatient evaluation and treatment session at NMRC. Initial evaluation was completed on the first day, including videotape and photographic documentation of all facial nerve muscle groups as well as a clinical evaluation using the University of Wisconsin facial paralysis clinical assessment scale [7]. All facial muscle groups were found to function within normal limits, with the exception of the left depressor musculature, in which no response could be elicited. The patient received a diagram of the facial muscles and the function of each group was described, demonstrated, and attempted by the patient. She was also instructed to color the chart using different colored markers in order to enhance her learning. The patient demonstrated good understanding of the facial muscle functions and understood the area of deficit. On the second day of treatment, four-channel EMG and mirror feedback were employed. Using the Therapeutic Technologies Incorporated neuroEDUCATOR II system, surface electrodes were placed over the zygomatic and depressor areas bilaterally. Due to the patient's etiology, it was felt that the best approach to attain symmetry was to inhibit the contralateral (right), relatively hyperactive, depressor muscles. The patient and her parents were oriented to the EMG monitor. Initially, the patient was asked to produce her "normal" smile without attempts at control (Fig. 1). After analyzing the results she was instructed to attempt to produce equal responses utilizing the EMG feedback (Fig. 2). Several trials were attempted. Threshold levels

Fig. 1 Bilateral smile initial trial. Note relative hyperactivity of right depressors

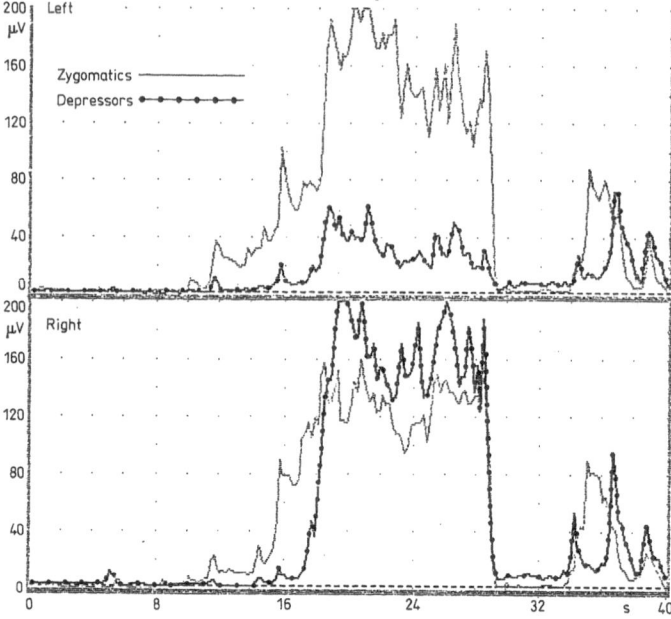

Fig. 2 Bilateral smile trial 2. Note beginning inhibition of right depressors

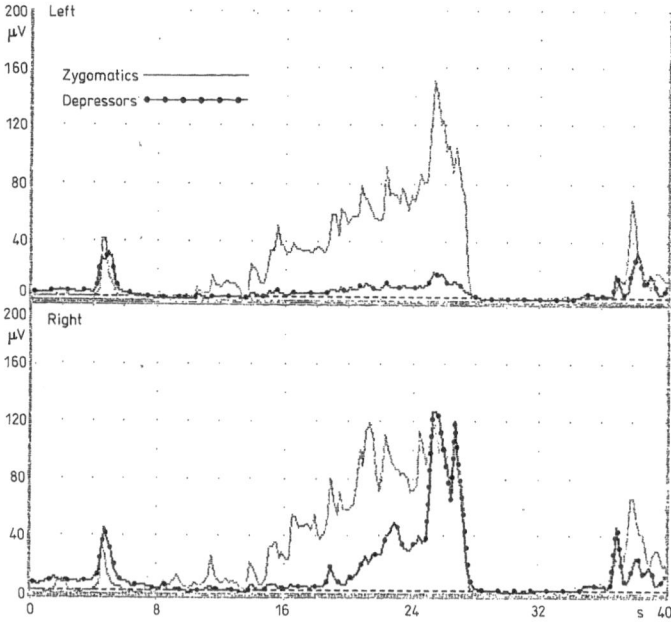

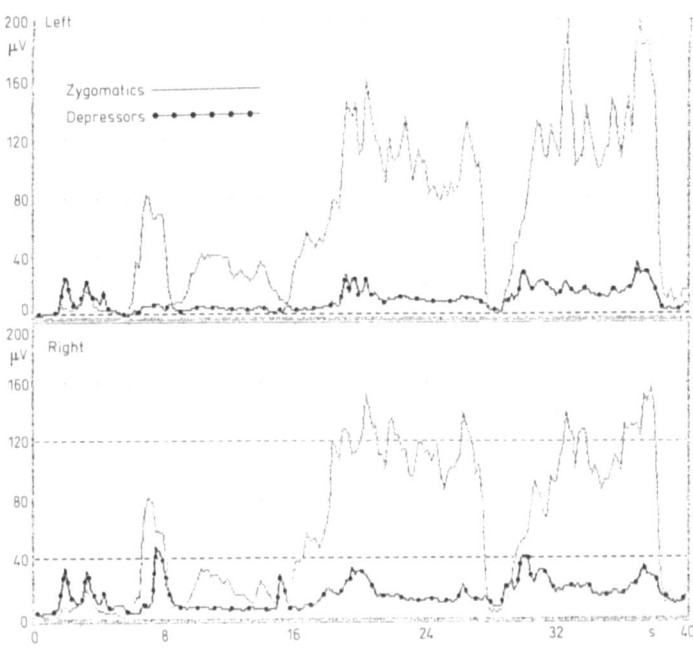

Fig. 3 Bilateral smile after 20 min. Note symmetry of depressors bilaterally

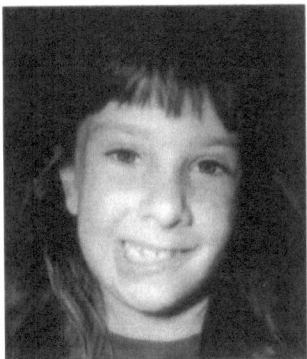

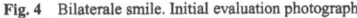

Fig. 4 Bilaterale smile. Initial evaluation photograph

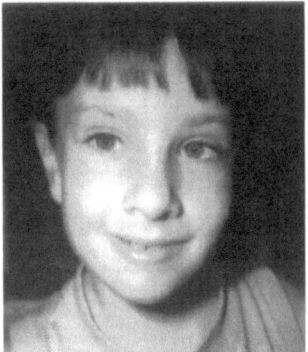

Fig. 5 Bilateral smile. Post-treatment photograph

were added to provide additional reference and facilitate the desired response, which the patient achieved after approximately 20 min (Fig. 3). After demonstrating consistency of response, the patient was asked to rehearse the movement without the EMG feedback, using only the mirror. She again consistently demonstrated the correct response. She was also able to duplicate the movement with no external feedback source. Photographic reevaluation was completed and comparison made between the initial and post-training photographs (Fig. 4, 5). The patient and her parents were pleased with the results. A daily home program using mirror feedback was developed to promote consistent practice of new skills and generalization into spontaneous expression. The patient was instructed to perform the new movement pattern several times during the day both with and without mirror feedback and with occasional verbal feedback from her parents. No further EMG feedback or formal therapeutic sessions were employed.

Results

This patient demonstrated excellent consistency of response both with external feedback (EMG, mirror) and without, following approximately 1 h of training. Equal EMG values correlated clinically with symmetrical facial expression during smile. In a follow-up telephone conversation 6 months after treatment, the patient was reported to be compliant with the home retraining program. She demonstrated success using the new pattern voluntarily and, according to her parents, her self-esteem had improved. At 18 months post-treatment, it was reported that the movement had generalized into all spontaneous activities, except when crying, at which time the asymmetry was apparent. Surgical intervention is no longer being considered.

Discussion

This case demonstrates rapid acquisition of new motor skills using surface electrode EMG and appropriate neuromuscular reeducation techniques. EMG feedback facilitated the learning of a more desirable motor pattern. EMG is only one of many techniques used in facial neuromuscular

retraining. These techniques are applied to patients on an individualized basis in an optimal treatment environment and generalized through home programs. Neuromuscular retraining may be a cost-effective alternative to surgical intervention for appropriate patients with facial paralysis. Patients must be highly motivated and have good cognition to follow through with the home program. It is an extremely effective technique for treatment of postacute patients who have facial paralysis as the result of a peripheral C. N. VII injury.

References

1. Balliet R, Shinn J, Bach-y-Rita P (1982) Facial paralysis rehabilitation: re-training selective muscle control. Int Rehab Med 4(I):67–74
2. Brown M, Nahai F, Wolf S, Basmajian J (1978) Electromyographic biofeedback in the reduction of facial palsy. Am J Phys Med 57:183–190
3. Brudny J, Hammerschlag P, Cohen N, Ransohoff J (1988) Electromyographic rehabilitation of facial function and intraduction of a facial paralysis grading scale for hypoglossal-facial nerve anastomosis. Laryngoscope 98:405–410
4. Jankel W (1978) Bell's palsy: muscle re-education by electromyograph feedback. Arch Phys Med Rehabil 59:240–242
5. May M, Croison G, Kleins (1989) Bell's palsy: management of sequelae using EMG rehabilitation, botulinum toxin, and surgery. Am J Otol 3:220–229
6. Ross B, Nedzelski J, McLean J (July 1991) Efficacy of feedback training in long-standing facial nerve paresis. Laryngoscope 101:744–750
7. Balliet R (1989) Facial paralysis and other neuromuscular dysfunctions of the peripheral nervous system. In: Payton OD (ed) Manual of physical therapy, 1st edn. Churchill Livingstone, New York, pp 175–213

Eur Arch Otorhinolaryngology (1994) [Suppl]: S133–S134

POSTERS

S.S.M. Hussain, S.J. Winterburn, and A.R.H. Grace

Eutrophic Electrical Stimulation in Long-Standing Facial Palsy

Introduction

The use of electrical stimulation in the treatment of facial palsy has previously been shown to offer no significant advantage [1].

However, with increased knowledge of the physiology of facial muscles [2] it has been shown that electrical stimulation with characteristics of frequency and pattern corresponding to those that occur in a normal facial muscle would, if reproduced and applied in the form of stimuli to a damaged motor unit, encourage restoration of normal structure and function [3]. This study aims to assess the effect of the application of such electrical stimulation in patients with long-standing facial palsy.

Materials, Methods and Results

Eutrophic electrical stimulation was applied by means of a dual-channel battery-operated stimulator with a frequency of 8 Hz and pulse width of 80 ms.

Five patients were included; all had facial palsy of at least 12 months duration (mean, 59 months; Table 1).

Table 1 Patients' details

Patient no.	Age (years)	Sex	Diagnosis	Operation	Time since onset of palsy	Status at commence-ment of treatment [a]	Present state
1	60	M	Right parotid carcinoma	Excision of tumour Resuturing of severed facial nerve	12 months	FPRI 0 FPRP 1	5 6
2	52	M	Right acoustic neuroma	Translabyrinthine excision Tumour was vascular and adherent to nerve Nerve divided in medial third and resutured	18 months	FPRI 1 FPRP 4	6 7
3	66	M	Left acoustic neuroma	Translabyrinthine excision VII nerve in continuity	12 months	FPRI 5 FPFP 5	8 8
4	22	F	Right cholesteatoma CSOM	Modified radial mastoidectomy Damage to VII nerve	20 years	FPRI 5 FPFP 6	7 8
5	64	F	Right Ramsay-Hunt syndrome		12 months	FRPI 2 FPRP 3	8 9

FPRI, facial paralysis recovery index; FPRP, facial paralysis recovery profile.
[a] Assessments based on Adour facial paralysis recovery index and facial paralysis recovery profile.

S.S.M. Hussain, S.J. Winterburn, and A.R.H. Grace
Departments of Otolaryngology and Physiotherapy,
York District Hospital, York, England, U.K.

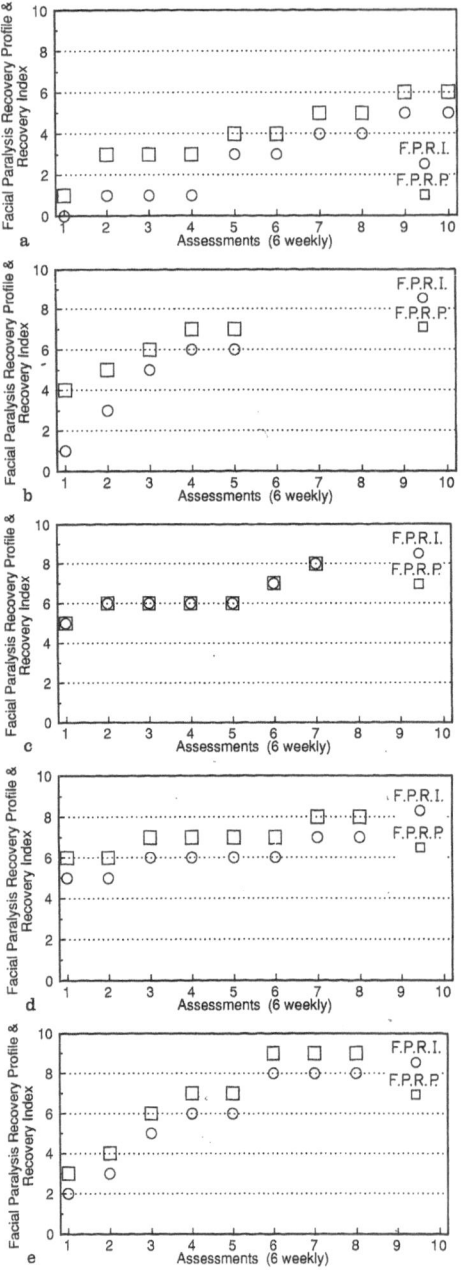

Fig. 1a–e Six-weekly assessment of patients 1 (**a**), 2 (**b**), 3 (**c**), 4 (**d**) and 5 (**e**) for details of diagnosis and treatment see Table 1. *FPRI*, facial paralysis recovery index; *FPRP*, facial paralysis recovery profile

Pre- and post-treatment assessments were based on Adour facial paralysis recovery profile and recovery index [4], photographs and the patients' own assessment.

All patients were given a facial stimulator for home use and were instructed on the placement of the electrodes at their initial physiotherapy assessment. Treatment was gradually increased each day up to 8 h a day. Patients were assessed every 6 weeks (Fig. 1).

Gradual improvement was noted in all five cases. These findings were in agreement with patient's own assessments and their photographs.

Conclusions

Eutrophic electrical stimulation has restored an appreciable degree of function in a small group of patients with long-standing facial palsy. However, further work is needed to support the concept of eutrophic electrical stimulation and to evaluate its effectiveness.

References

1. Mosforth J, Taverner D (1958) Physiotherapy for Bell's palsy BMJ 9 : 675–679
2. Kidd GL (1984) An analysis of the firing characteristics of motor units in facial muscles of expression. J Physiol (Lond) 354 : 55
3. Farragher D, Kidd GL, Tallis R (1987) Eutrophic electrical stimulation for Bell's palsy. Clin Rehabil 1 : 265–271
4. Adour KK, Byl FM, Hilsinger RL, Kahn ZM, Sheldon MI (1983) The true nature of Bell's palsy: an analysis of 1000 consecutive patients. Laryngoscope 88 : 787–801

Plastic Surgery

Eur Arch Otorhinolaryngology (1994) [Suppl]: S137–S139

P. E. Hammerschlag, N. L. Cohen, R. Palu, and J. J. Brudny

Management of Facial Paralysis with Jump Interposition Graft Hypoglossal-Facial Anastomosis with Gold Lid Weight

Introduction

Until 1990, we managed irreversible facial nerve paralysis with "classical" hypoglossal-facial anastomosis, lateral canthoplasty, and electromyographic (EMG) biofeedback rehabilitation [1–4]. The classical or standard hypoglossal-facial anastomosis utilized a completely transected ipsilateral hypoglossal nerve for facial reinnervation. Substantial facial rehabilitation in 48 patients was achieved, especially in terms of strong facial muscle tone and symmetry at rest exclusive of the forehead region.

While there is improvement in facial function with the classical hypoglossal-facial anastomosis, problematic rehabilitation deficits persist. Involuntary (blinking) eye closure frequently does not occur and synkinesis is common with eye closure, whether it is volitional or spontaneous. Lower facial mimetic movement and involuntary smile are usually diminished compared to those associated with volitional efforts. Hypertonus and facial spasms are common, particularly with fatigue, and active rehabilitation strategies are required to control these symptoms [4].

Hemilingual dysfunction and atrophy associated with complete transection of the hypoglossal nerve impairs ipsilateral intraoral manipulation of food and its mastication. Patients also infrequently encounter difficulties with speech and drooling. The authors believe that these difficulties are due to synergistic deficits of both the facial and hypoglossal nerve. It is not possible to delineate precisely which of these two impaired cranial nerves is predominantly responsible for the aforementioned deficiencies. In over half the patients rehabilitated with the standard hypoglossal-facial anastomosis technique, transient drooling occurred with certain activities such as eating, talking, and osculation.

Resultant total ipsilateral tongue (hypoglossal) deinnervation also precludes the classical hypoglossal-facial anastomosis procedure for patients with concomitant lower cranial (IX, X) dysfunction: iatrogenic transection of the hypoglossal nerve in these functionally compensated individuals can potentially produce an uncompensated patient with intractable dysphagia and/or aspiration.

In 1990, May presented a modification of the classical hypoglossal-facial nerve anastomosis technique which addressed the above shortcomings [5]. An interpositional jump graft was placed between the distal facial nerve trunk or branches and a partially transected proximal hypoglossal nerve, preserving ipsilateral lingual function, to eliminate the sequelae of ipsilateral tongue deinnervation. A gold weight was implanted in the upper eye lid to allow involuntary eye closure in synchrony with the contralateral eye [6, 7]. We present our results with the jump interpositional graft between a partially transected hypoglossal nerve and the facial nerve, upper eyelid gold weight implantation, and lateral canthoplasty in 12 patients.

Materials

Facial nerve paralysis was secondary to acoustic neuroma resection in eight patients, all of whom had tumors larger than 3 cm (Table 1). In the remaining four cases, facial nerve paralysis were caused by a facial neuroma, glomus jugulare tumor, medulloblastoma, and cerebellar astrocytoma (Table 2). This presentation updates a previous report in six patients [8].

A series of 48 patients with the standard hypoglossal nerve anastomosis and lateral canthoplasty was retrospec-

P. E. Hammerschlag (✉) and N. L. Cohen
Department of Otolaryngology, New York University School of Medicine, 550 First Avenue, New York, NY 10016, USA

R. Palu
Department of Ophthalmology, New York University School of Medicine, 550 First Avenue, New York, NY 10016, USA

J. J. Brudny
Department of Rehabilitation Medicine, New York University School of Medicine, 550 First Avenue, New York, NY 10016, USA

Table 1 Results of the jump interposition graft hypoglossal-facial anastomosis (JIGHFA) procedure in eight patients with facial paralysis secondary to acoustic nerve resection

Age	Time interval between onset of paralysis and JIGHFA	Time interval between JIGHFA and first evidence of facial reinnervation (months)	Follow-up (months)	Result I/VI[a]
16	2	4	24	II/VI
50	0	8	19	II/VI[b]
53	0	5	18	II/VI[b]
16	0	8	14	III/VI
42	2	5	14	III/VI[b]
65	3	10	12	IV/VI
15	0	5	12	III/VI
17	4	6	6	III/VI[c]

[a] Degree of facial innervation based on the Brudny modification of the House-Brackman scale [4].
[b] Gold weight removed.
[c] Concomitant deficit of the lower tenth cranial nerve.

Table 2 Result of the jump interpositon graft hypoglossal-facial anastomosis (JIGHFA) procedure in four patients with facial paralysis secondary to etiology other than acoustic neuroma

Age	DX	Time interval between onset of paralysis and JIGHFA (months)	Time interval between JIGHFA and first evidence of facial reinnervation (months)	Follow-up (months)	Result I/VI[a]
19	Cerebellar Astrocytoma	24	13	19	III/VI[b, c]
9	Medulloblastoma	16	< 13	8	III/VI[b]
68	VII Neuroma	0	5	14	III/VI
72	HZO	11	18	24	III/VI

[a] Degree of facial innervation based on the Brudny modification of the House-Brackman scale [4].
[b] Concomitant deficit of the lower tenth cranial nerve.
[c] Concomitant deficit of the lower ninth cranial nerve.

tively reviewed with a questionnaire and/or chart analysis. Twenty-two patients returned the questionnaire.

Methods

The ipsilateral hypoglossal nerve trunk was partially and obliquely transected just distal to the hypoglossal descendens branch. Half the hypoglossal nerve trunk was preserved after partial transection. An interpositional jump nerve graft, either ipsilateral greater auricular or sural nerve, was placed between the partially transected proximal hypoglossal nerve and the transected facial nerve trunk. The nerves were anastomosed without tension with interrupted perineural 9-0 or 10-0 nylon sutures.

The eye was managed with a gold weight placed in the upper lid and, if indicated, a lower lid lateral canthoplasty.

Results

In seven of the eight patients with facial paralysis secondary to acoustic neuroma resection, facial reinnervation was visible within 8 months after the jump interpostional facial hypoglossal anastomosis (JIGFHA) surgery. The eighth patient's reinnervation appeared within 10 months following her reanimation surgery. Facial reinnervation was present within 5 months for the patient with the facial neuroma; within 13 months for the patients with the cerebellar astrocytoma and medulloblastoma; and within 18 months for the patient with herpes zoster oticus. In summary, all patients with facial paralysis have achieved facial reinnervation with this procedure.

All patients had their reanimation surgery performed within 4 months after the advent of facial paralysis, except in patients with etiologies other than neuroma: medulloblastoma (16 months), astrocytoma (24 months), and herpes zoster oticus (11 months). Eight of the ten patients with reinnervation are undergoing EMG biofeedback rehabilitation.

The acoustic neuroma patients were followed for 6–24 months after facial reanimation surgery with seven out of nine patients with follow-up periods of at least 12 months. Preliminary observation reveals voluntary movement and strong facial tone at rest. Observation by the authors suggest that in three of the eight patients, reinnervated facial tone and symmetry at rest is equal to the best results of

S 139

those rehabilitated with the classical hypoglossal facial anastomosis. Improvement of variable degree in facial tone symmetry has occurred in the five patients who participated in EMG biofeedback.

Voluntary movement is approximately equal following these two techniques of facial reinnervation, but hypertonus is considerably less than those with the JIGFHA procedure. Preliminary assessment suggest that synkinesis is less in the patients with JIGHFA.

With the gold weight implantation in the upper eye lid in conjunction with the JIGFHA technique, there is involuntary eye closure frequently in synchrony with contralateral blinking. The gold weight was rejected by one patient and removed in two patients. Since the orbicularis oculi muscles were sufficiently reinnervated, further oculoplastic rehabilitation was not warranted.

In all 12 patients, there was excellent preservation of lingual function without atrophy or impairment of speech, deglutition, and mastication. JIGFHA was performed in two patients with concomitant lower cranial nerve deficits, both with ipsilateral vocal cord paralysis and one also with partial ipsilateral glossopharyngeal paresthesia. Mild intermittent drooling from the ipsilateral oral commissure has occurred in three patients and this is comparable to those with the classical hypoglossal-facial anastomosis.

Discussion

Markedly reduced hypertonus and facial spasm in this series of 12 patients may be due to the reduced axonal supply from the partially transected hypoglossal nerve. Synkinesis initially may be less apparent because facial movement may be less vigorous due to diminished axonal supply. Deglutition, mastication, and speech have not been problematic in the group of 12 patients with preserved lingual function. Continued long-term observation is required to determine whether the JIGFHA technique avoids problems of speech, drooling, and mastication in contrast to the classical hypoglossal-facial anastomosis.

JIGFHA allows for dynamic reinnervation in those with concomitant lower cranial nerve deficits, unlike the hypoglossal-facial anastomosis, as demonstrated in two of our patients with such deficits.

Initial management of eyelid closure and protection is superior with the gold weight in the upper eyelid, since its success is dependent upon inhibition of the levator palpebrae superioris muscle and not on facial innervation. Subsequent facial reinnervation allows for long-term ocular protection, especially if the gold weight is rejected or removed, as in two cases. For this reason we anastomose the facial nerve trunk instead of only the lower facial branches as in other reports [9].

References

1. Baker DC, Conley J (1979) Facial nerve grafting: a thirty year retrospective review. Saunders, Philadelphia (Clinics plastic surgery, vol 6)
2. Hammerschlag PE (1987) Hypoglossal-facial nerve anastomosis for correction of facial paralysis. Futura, Mount Kisco (Modern technic in surgery, vol 37)
3. Hammerschlag PE, Brudny J, Cusumano R, Cohen NL (1987) Hypoglossal-facial nerve anastomosis and electromyographic feedback rehabilitation. Laryngoscope 97:705–709
4. Brudny J, Hammerschlag PE, Ransohoff J, Cohen NL (1988) Electromyographic rehabilitation for facial function and introduction of a facial paralysis grading scale for hypoglossal-facial anastomosis. Laryngoscope 98:405–410
5. May M, Sokel SM, Mester SJ (1991) Hypoglossal-facial nerve interpositional jump graft for facial reanimation without tongue atrophy. Otolaryngol Head Neck Surg 104:818–825
6. Smellie GD (1966) Restoration of the blinking reflex in facial palsy by a simple lid-load operation. Br J Plast Surg 19:279–283
7. Jobe RP (1974) Technique for lid-loading in the management of lagophthalmos in facial palsy. Plast Reconstr Surg 53:29–31
8. Hammerschlag PE, Cohen NL, Brudny J (1992) Rehabilitation of facial paralysis following acoustic neuroma excision with jump interpostional graft hypoglossal-facial anastomosis and gold weight-lid implantation. Proceedings of the 1st international conference on acoustic neuroma. Kugler, Amsterdam
9. Kartush JM, Lundy L (1992) Facial nerve outcome in acustic neuroma surgery. Otolaryngol Clin North Am 25:3

Eur Arch Otorhinolaryngology (1994) [Suppl] : S 140

FREE PAPERS AND POSTERS

J.-P. A. Nicolai and J. J. Manni

Individually Adjusted Curvatures of Upper Eyelid Gold Implants: A Valuable Approach?

Several methods have been described to correct paralytic lagophthalmos. Lateral tarsorraphy, popularized in the 1950s, is in our opinion obsolete, because so many better methods now exist.

The methods described include magnets, elastomere wire inserted around the palpebral fissure, springs on the principle of the safety pin, and in particular gold weights. The technique of implantation of a gold weight as rehabilitation of long-standing facial paralysis has now become an established procedure. In our center, optimal results, i.e. minimal percentage of extrusion and of astigmatism, were aimed at by designing the implants individually for each patient using a mold technique [2].

In the Maxillo-facial prosthetics Department, an imprint of the patients eyelids was taken from which a plaster cast was made. The form and size of the implant was then drawn on this plaster cast. From this, the dental technician casts a gold implant of the desired weight, which was sterilized and inserted under local anesthesia, except in cases where other corrective surgery for the facial paralysis was performed. About 100 patients have been treated up to now, with a rate of extrusion of the implant of about 2%.

Commercially available gold implants have a standard curve and are not individually adjusted for each patient. The literature reports no more extrusions in this group.

Therefore, the curvature of the plaster mold impressions of 40 patients were measured. The distance of the curve to a fixed point was determined at five different locations on the plaster cast. The results showed wide variations, which could roughly be put into four categories, from very flat to more curved. The curve did not appear to be a segment of a circle. The greatest distance between the highest points of the flattest and most curved implants appeared to be several millimeters. Kelly [1] reported a long-term extrusion rate of 61% for 1-g 24-carat gold weights (inserted through a lateral skin incision). It remains unclear why prefabricated, commercially available gold implants with a standard curvature appear to have no more extrusions than custom-cast implants, unless they are not reported. For the time being, we will continue to implant custom-made gold implants, cast from individually taken molds.

References

1. Kelly SA (1992) Gold eyelid weights in patients with facial palsy. Plast Reconstr Surg 89 : 436–440
2. Nicolai J-PA, de Koomen H, Storm van Leeuwen JB, Sybrandy S (1986) Gold weights in upper eyelids for the correction of paralytic lagophthalmos. Eur J Plast Surg 9 : 66–68

J.-P. A. Nicolai and J. J. Manni
Regional Center of Plastic, Reconstructive and Hand Surgery,
Eusebiusbuitensingel 3, 6828 HS Arnhem, The Netherlands

Eur Arch Otorhinolaryngology (1994) [Suppl]: S141

FREE PAPERS AND POSTERS

J.-P. A. Nicolai and J. J. Manni

Static Suspension of Eyebrow with Gore-Tex

The ptotic eyebrow in facial paralysis is an underestimated problem in the patients afflicted. Several surgical techniques have been described in the past, such as "lemon-slice" skin excision above the eyebrow, several parallel skin excisions of the forehead skin, suspension with fascia lata sling, and even transposition of part of the nonafflicted frontal muscle.

In the Facial Paralysis Rehabilitation Center we have treated 34 patients with static suspension using a strip of stretched polytetrafluoroethylene (Gore-tex) subcutaneously [1]. There were 20 women and the mean age of the patients was 62.4 years. The mean follow-up was 11.6 months. In 14 patients, the strip was cranially sutured to the galea aponeurotica; in 13, it was hung on a ridge burred out of the frontal bone; and in 7, it was knotted to itself through a tunnel through the frontal bone. In 35% of the patients reoperation was necessary, because of recurring ptosis, early infection ($n = 1$) or late fistula ($n = 5$). Only one patient needed two reinterventions; he had had his Gore-tex strip suspended on a frontal bone ridge from which it had slipped. Late fistula occurred up to 9 months after operation and necessitated partial removal of the implant without generally needing resuspension, probably because of scar tissue having formed. Histologic examination of the removed specimens revealed no fibroblast ingrowth, despite the assumptions of the manufacturer. Including those who needed revision surgery, 70% of the patients expressed satisfaction with the result.

Reference

1. Steinkogler FJ (1987) Ein neues Material für die Frontalisschlingen Operation bei kongenitaler Ptose. Klin Monatsbl Augenheilkd 191: 361–363

J.-P. A. Nicolai and J. J. Manni
Regional Center of Plastic, Reconstructive and Hand Surgery,
Eusebiusbuitensingel 3, 6828 HS Arnhem, The Netherlands

Eur Arch Otorhinolaryngology (1994) [Suppl] : S 142 – S 144

FREE PAPERS AND POSTERS

M. Deutinger and G. Freilinger

Temporalis Transfer for Correction of Lagophthalmos

Introduction

The inability to close the eyelid in orbicularis oculi palsy decreases protection of the eye. In order to prevent corneal and conjunctival irritation, operative treatment is often necessary. Different methods have been described such as gold weight, palpebral spring, lid magnets, and the implantation of silastic rods. Lateral tarsorrhaphy and medial and lateral canthoplasty are other methods used for eye protection in the management of lagophthalmos. Gillies [6] described a dynamic method for correction of lagophthalmos without foreign material. Transposition of the temporalis muscle is superior to implantation of foreign material. We used the Gillies' method, which combines static support of the eyelid with dynamic function, for correction of lagophthalmos. All patients were examined postoperatively in order to prove the efficiency of this method.

Patients and Methods

The operation was performed in 21 patients during the last 10 years, and 17 patients were reexamined. The youngest patient was 4.5 years old when the operation was performed, and the oldest patient was 68 years old. The shortest follow-up time was 2 months. The ability of lid closure and conjunctival and corneal irritation were evaluated clinically, as was scar formation and the donor defect. In all but one patient the orbicularis oculi palsy resulted from long-standing facial paralysis. Table 1 shows the reasons for facial paralysis and lagophthalmos in our patients. In ten patients the temporalis muscle transposi-

M. Deutinger (✉) and G. Freilinger
2nd Department of Plastic Surgery, University of Vienna,
Spitalgasse 23, A-1090 Wien, Austria

Table 1 Causes of lagophthalmos

Cause	No. of patients
Cranial trauma	5
Operation of cranial tumor	4
Idiopathic facial paralysis	9
Congenital facial paralysis	2
Lupus vulgaris	1

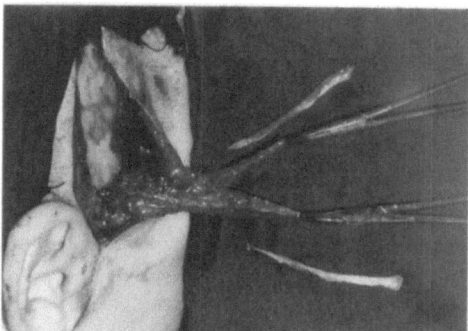

Fig. 1 Preparation of the temporalis muscle

tion was part of reanimation of the face with free muscle transfer and was executed at the time of cross-face nerve transplantation. The temporalis fascia was exposed through a longitudinal incision in the temporal region. A strip of 2 – 3 cm in width was outlined from the cygomatic arch to the parietal bone. The muscle with attached pericranium and overlying fascia was then stripped down to the zygomatic arch and divided into two parts (Fig. 1). If these strips of tissue did not reach the medial canthal region, a prolongation with a fascial strip was necessary (Fig. 2). From a horizontal lateral canthal incision, a tunnel was dissected through each lid, close to the eyelid margin. A

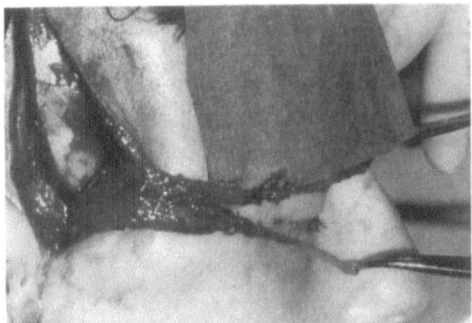

Fig. 2 After prolongation the temporalis muscle reaches the medial canthal region

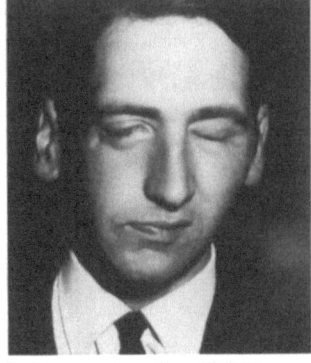

Fig. 4 Patient after correction of lagophthalmos

second, slightly curved incision was needed to expose the medial palpebral tendon. The two strips were threaded through the tunnels and fixed to the medial palpebral tendon and to themselves. This was done under tension so that the upper lid overlaps the lower lid by a few millimeters. Special training for lid closure and opening was performed postoperatively.

Results

In all patients epiphora was markedly reduced, even if a complete closure of the eyelid was not achieved. The application of ointments or eyedrops postoperatively was only necessary in one patient who suffered from a dry eye after a cerebral tumor exstirpation. Ten patients were able to close their eyelids completely (Figs. 3, 4). In seven of the examined patients, closure of the eyelid was not perfect;

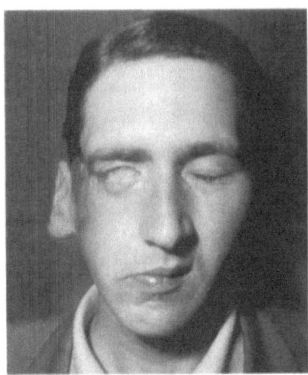

Fig. 3 Patient with lagophthalmos before surgery

however, the preoperative complaints were reduced, because the transposed temporalis muscle gives good support to a sagging lower lid and so epiphora is diminished. In two patients retightening was necessary due to stretching of the muscle strip.

Chewing was not impaired and the eyelid could be closed independently from chewing. The scars medially and laterally in the eye were inconspicuous and the scar in the temporal region was well disguised by hair growth. The muscle bulge in the lateral orbital rim disappeared in the course of time.

Discussion

For closure of the eye, a functioning orbicularis oculi muscle is necessary. The passage of tears into the lacrimal sac is assisted by the action of the orbicularis muscle. The lacrimal portion of the muscle is attached to the lacrimal sac. Contracture of the orbicularis muscle dilates the lacrimal sac and inverts the lacrimal punctum. This occurs each time the patient blinks. Therefore, it is evident that the lower lid plays an important role in providing normal tearflow. After transposition of the temporalis muscle, the lower lid gets so much support that the lacrimal punctum can be inverted even if the contraction force for the upper lid is not strong enough to close the eye completely. Corneal irritation diminishes as well and is independent from a complete closure of the eye, which is mainly a function of the upper lid. In cases of lagophthalmos and a sagging lower lid or ectropion, Gillies' procedure is a very helpful method of correction. There are static and dynamic operative methods used for correction of lagophthalmos. Lateral tarsorrhaphy [8], medial [5] and lateral canthoplasty [4], and the implantation of silastic rods [1] are described as static operative methods. In order to reconstruct a dynamic lid function, lid loading [2, 7, 13], lid springs [3, 9, 11], and lid magnets [12] can be used. Dynamic lid function without foreign material can be achieved by transposition of the temporalis muscle. As complications of foreign material are well known, the use of foreign material is limited in our department to cases in which the temporalis muscle is not available. Stretching of the muscle strip postoperatively may be a disadvantage of this method. It is also quite difficult even for an experienced surgeon to fix the muscle strip under appropriate tension [10]. The fascial strip of the lower lid provides contact of the lacrimal punctum with the medial conjunctival sac. This is important for decrease of epiphora and corneal irritation even if lagophthalmos is not completely corrected. Transposition of temporalis muscle is the method of choice when lagophthalmos is combined with a sagging lower lid or ectropion.

References

1. Arion HG (1972) Dynamic closure of the lids in paralysis of the orbicularis muscle. Int Surg 57 : 48 – 50
2. Barcqlay TL, Roberts AC (1969) Restoration of movement to the upper eyelid in facial palsy. Br J Plast Surg 22 : 257 – 261
3. Cary LG, Ranshoff J (1968) The palpebral spring for paralysis of the upper eyelid in facial nerve palsy. J Neurosurg 29 : 431 – 433
4. Freeman BS (1977) Facial palsy. In: Converse JM (ed) Reconstructive plastic surgery, 2nd edn, vol 3. Saunders, Philadelphia, p 1833
5. Edgerton MT (1967) Surgical correction of facial paralysis: a plea for better reconstruction. Ann Surg 165 : 985 – 989
6. Gillies HD (1934) Experiences with fascia lata grafts in the operative treatment of facial paralysis. Proc R Soc Med 2 : 1372 – 1384
7. Jobe RP (1974) A technique for lid loading in the management of lagophthalmos of facial palsy. Plast Reconstr Surg 53 : 29 – 32
8. Mc Laughlin CR (1974) Surgical support in permanent facial paralysis. Plast Reconstr Surg 2 : 25 – 29
9. Levine RE (1974) Management of the eye in facial paralysis. Otolaryngol Clin North Am 7 : 531 – 544
10. Masters FW, Robinson DW et al. (1965) Temporalis transfer for lagophthalmos due to the seventh nerve palsy. Am J Surg 110 : 607 – 611
11. Morel Fatio D, Lalardrie JP (1964) Palliative surgical treatment of facial paralysis. The palpebral spring. Plast Reconstr Surg 33 : 446 – 456
12. Mühlbauer WD, Sageth H et al. (1973) Restoration of lid function in facial palsy with permanent magnets. Chir Plast (Berlin) 1 : 295 – 299
13. Nicolai JPA, de Koomen H et al. (1986) Gold weights in upper eyelids for the correction of paralytic lagophthalmos. Eur J Plast Surg 9 : 66 – 68

Eur Arch Otorhinolaryngology (1994) [Suppl]: S 145 – S 146

F. P. Stook, J.-P. Nicolai, W. Rijnders, and M. Kon

Pectoralis Minor Transplantation in the Netherlands

Introduction

In 1986 the plastic surgeons participating in the Facial Nerve Study Group in the Netherlands were not satisfied with the results of their muscle transplantations. At the beginning of the 1980s, the extensor digitorum brevis muscle [5, 6, 8 – 11] was used in the Netherlands for reanimation of the paralyzed face. The overall impression was that this muscle did not have enough force after it was transplanted. Some Dutch plastic surgeons had experience with the gracilis muscle [2, 4, 6], but found it rather bulky. Therefore, the members of the Facial Nerve Study Group agreed to use the pectoralis minor muscle as a study object in patients with an irreversible facial palsy. A multicenter project was started, including hospitals in Amsterdam, Arnhem, Ede, and Utrecht. The pectoralis minor transplantation was introduced to us by Douglas Harrison [3]. One of the goals was to create a large group of patients. Whether or not this type of muscle would give satisfactory reanimation of the face, as well as possible improvements, would be discussed at a later stage. One of the authors (FPS) participated in all of the pectoralis minor transfers and videotaped the patients at regular intervals before and after the operation.

Anatomy and Operative Technique

The pectoralis minor muscle is a flat, triangular-shaped muscle which arises from the second, thirth, fourth, and sometimes the fifth rib. It has a broad flat tendon which inserts into the coracoid process of the scapula. The main artery comes directly from the axillary artery and enters

F. P. Stook, J.-P. Nicolai, W. Rijnders, and M. Kon
Drechtsteden Hospital, van der Steenhovenplein 1,
3317 NM Dordrecht, The Netherlands

the hilus of the pectoralis minor. Superficial to the artery lies the medial pectoral nerve, which is considered to be the motor nerve. The venous drainage of this muscle is via a venous plexus at the base of the muscle, which goes to the axillary or the lateral thoracic vein.

With regard to the operative technique, the skin incision is made in the axilla just dorsal to the anterior axillary border. The pectoralis minor muscle can easily be found lying over the brachial plexus and the axillary vessels. The tendon is divided at the coracoid process and the muscle is pulled back. The nerve, vein, and artery belonging to the pectoralis minor muscle are identified. Before the muscle is transferred, a second team has prepared the face for the muscle and placed key sutures for fixation of the muscle near the mouth. The origin of the muscle can be fixed to the preauricular fascia under proper tension. The vessels are anastomosed end-to-end to the facial artery and vein. The nerve of the pectoralis minor is sutured to the cross-facial nerve graft using interfascicular technique [1]. The sural nerve graft was transfered in stage 1 of the operation, approximately 1 year before.

Preliminary Results

Between 1986 and 1992, 31 patients with an irreversible facial palsy were operated. The etiology of the facial paralysis varied. In fact, there were two large groups. One group of facial paralysis was caused by intracranial tumors and the other was of congenital origin. There was an equal distribution between left and right, male versus female, and age in both groups of patients. Because this report concerns preliminary results of the pectoralis minor muscle transplantation in the Netherlands in five patients (16.1%), it is too early to draw any conclusions about muscle activity. Of a total of 31 patients, seven (22.6%) have no muscle activity and are rated as failures. In 19 patients (61.3%), there is muscle activity of clinical relevance. The overall success percentage may still rise over 70% if the patients who are now in the "too early to draw any conclusions" group show muscle activity of clinical relevance. Whether there is muscle activity and the quality of such activity is primarily determined by axon growth through the cross-facial nerve graft.

Discussion

The progress of axon regeneration can be followed by recording Tinel's sign. If the length of the implanted nerve graft is known and the location of Tinel's sign is measured, axon regeneration speed can be calculated; the speed versus the age of the patient can be plotted on a graph (Fig. 1). There appears to be a negative correlation between the speed of axon regeneration and age. The older the patient, the longer the regeneration takes. This is a normal finding in peripheral nerve lesions, but has not been described before in cross-facial nerve grafts.

The time between muscle transplantation and the clinical observation of muscle activity in our group of patients ranges from 5 to 7 months. Figure 2 shows the correlation between age and the number of months needed to obtain

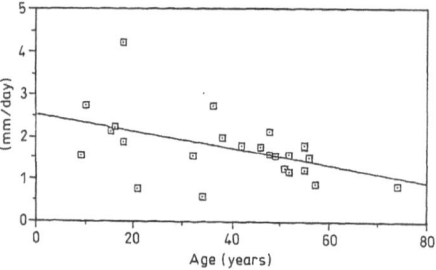

Fig. 1 Relationship between age and axon regeneration after cross-facial nerve grafts

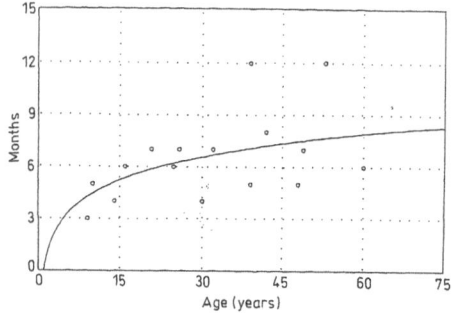

Fig. 2 Relationship between age and the beginning of muscle activity after pectoralis minor transplantation

clinical muscle activity after transplantation; the figure shows, the time needed for a transplanted pectoralis minor muscle to start moving after transplantation at a given age and a line of expectation which correlates the number of months needed for the beginning of muscle activity to a certain age. Muscle activity is expected sooner in children than in adults.

On the basis of these findings, we can find out whether it is better to abandon this type of operation at a certain age. Other procedures such as the temporalis muscle transposition advocated by Rubin [7] should be taken into consideration in these cases.

Conclusion

It is obviously too early to draw any definite conclusions from these preliminary findings. A certain number of patients will definitely improve with time. Although we found an important relation between age and axon regeneration, it does not give information about the quality of muscle activity.

Muscle excursion measurements will have to be done. These measurements will be done with a newly developed instrument from the International Registry for Neuromuscular Reconstruction in the Face to document muscle excursion and to make a valid comparison of results between national and international centers possible.

References

1. Anderl H (1973) Reconstruction of the face through crossfacial nerve transplantation in facial paralysis. Chir Plast 2 : 17
2. Harii K, Ohmori K, Torii S (1976) Free gracilis muscle transplantation with microvascular anastomoses for the treatment of facial paralysis. Plast Reconstr Surg 57 : 133
3. Harrison DH (1985) The pectoralis minor vascularised muscle graft for the treatment of unilateral facial palsy. Plast Reconstr Surg 75 : 206
4. Manktelow RT (1984) Free muscle transplantation for facial paralysis. Clin Plast Surg 11 : 215
5. Mayou BJ, Watson JS, Harrison DH (1981) Free microvascular and microneural transfer of the extensor digitorum brevis muscle for the treatment of unilateral facial palsy. Br J Plast Surg 34 : 362
6. O'Brien BM, Franklin JD, Morrison WA (1980) Cross facial nerve grafts and microvascular free muscle transfer for long established facial palsy. Br J Plast Surg 33 : 202
7. Rubin LR (1991) Reanimation of total unilateral facial paralysis by the contiguous facial muscle technique. The paralyzed face. Mosby, New York, p 156
8. Tolhurst DE, Boss KE (1982) Free vascularised muscle grafts in facial palsy. Plast Reconstr Surg 69 : 760
9. Nicolai JPA, Robinson PH (1981) Negative experiences with free muscle grafts. In: Freilinger G et al. (eds) Muscle transplantation. Springer, Vienna New York, pp 209–213
10. Nicolai JPA (1981) Free muscle grafting in facial paralysis. Br J Plast Surg 34 : 91–94
11. Nicolai JPA, Vingerkoets HM, Notermans SLH (1982) Our experience with Freilinger's method for dynamic correction of facial paralysis. Br J Plast Surg 35 : 483–488

Eur Arch Otorhinolaryngology (1994) [Suppl]: S 147 – S 148

FREE PAPERS AND POSTERS

M. Broniatowski, S. Grundfest-Broniatowski, C. R. Davies, G. B. Jacobs, Y. Nose, and H. M. Tucker

An Experimental Model for Complex Dynamic Control of the Reinnervated Face

Introduction and Background

None of the standard approaches to facial paralysis has been able to reinstate active dynamic symmetry. This ultimate goal can be now envisioned by using the intact side as a source of information for mobilization of the impaired musculature along physiological principles. Facial expression results from intricate relationships between forces along different vectors which are exquisitely integrated by the central nervous system. When, for whatever reason, connections are severed between the midbrain facial nucleus and the muscles under its command, these missing circuits must somehow be reestablished. This entails both afferent and efferent connections, in lieu of proprioceptive input and motor output, both of which are indispensable to normal facial motility.

Material and Methods

The direct availability of reinnervating material and the potential for some spontaneous facial expression designa-

M. Broniatowski (✉)
St. Vincent Charity Hospital, Cleveland Clinic Foundation, and Case Western University, Cleveland, OH 44155, USA

S. Grundfest-Broniatowski
Staff, Dept. of General Surgery, The Cleveland Clinic Foundation

R. Davies
Research Engineer, Department of Biomedical Engineering and Applied Therapeutics, The Cleveland Clinic Foundation

B. Jacobs
Project Staff, Department of Biomedical Engineering and Applied Therapeutics, The Cleveland Clinic Foundation

Y. Nose
Department of Surgery, Bayor College of Medicine, Houston, Texas

M. Tucker
Chairman, Department of Otolaryngology and Communicative Disorders, The Cleveland Clinic Foundation and the Cleveland Research Institute, Cleveland, Ohio

te the canine a good nonprimate model for facial experimentation. All branches of the facial nerve were cut on one side in four animals. Then, the ipsilateral orbicularis oculi and oris were reinnervated by "foreign" motor nerves, i.e., with temporal nerve and cervical nerve pedicles, respectively. Following a period of neurotization of 5 – 6 months, each region of the reinnervated face was electrically mobilized by means of an optoisolated pulse width stimulator modulated by information from the intact contralateral side. Displacement on the intact side around the eye or the mouth was picked up by a sensor resulting in single analog voltage input changes to the stimulator. The efferent dual output currents were distributed between the pedicles reinnervating the eye and the mouth to achieve synergistic and reciprocal contractions ([1], Fig. 1).

Results

As can be seen in Fig. 2, single input from the normal face was able to trigger contractions in two different territories on the reinnervated side. Moreover, they were induced by a normal central nervous system, thus restoring voluntary motion, and were also automatic and mimetic (Fig. 2). The delays separating initiation of motion on the good side and its implementation on the reinnervated side were of the same order of magnitude as with normal neuromuscular transmission between the brain and its effectors.

Justification and Discussion

The current approach to facial rehabilitation derives from the necessity of reestablishing dynamic symmetry abolished by unilateral peripheral paralysis (the most common type). One of the few nonprosthetic methods which comes close to satisfaction is the hypoglossal-facial transfer. However, this approach borrows information from a nucleus foreign to facial motion, sacrifices some tongue motion,

Fig. 1 In this block diagram of the study, a sensor placed on the right (intact) side detects ocular or oral displacement generated via stimulation of the facial nerve. The pacemaker then distributes the current in a synergistic or antagonist fashion to two different reinnervated territories on the left side. Reproduced from Otolaryngol Head Neck Surg, with permission

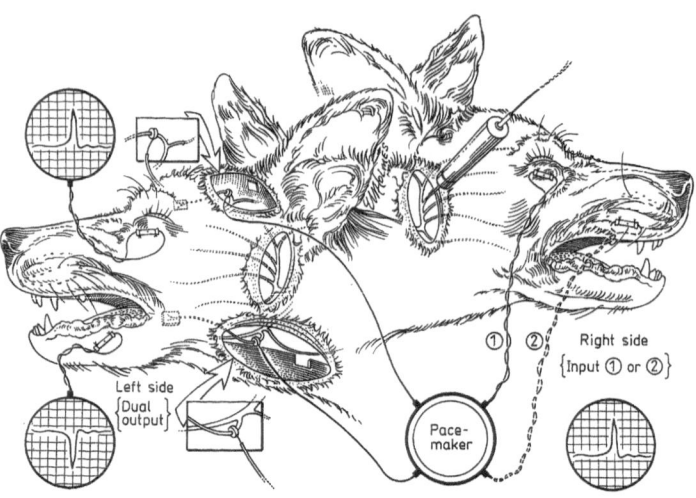

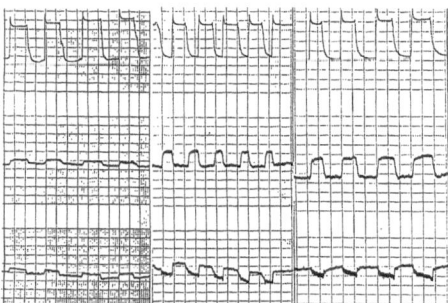

Fig. 2 These curves demonstrate that synergistic (*left*) and antagonistic (*middle* and *right*) motion can be reestablished on the reinnervated side (*bottom*, orbicularis oculi; *middle*, orbicularis oculi), from information originating on the intact face (*top*). Reproduced from Otolaryngol Head Neck Surg, with permission

and cannot be implemented in the absence of a central facial stump of appropriate length. Moreover, while it may achieve good symmetry at rest, it is plagued by mass motion. With these considerations in mind, the authors have proposed that one day we may well need to abandon surgical approaches which make use only of adjacent tissues for implantations of neuroprosthetic substitutes for the missing functions. In our opinion, there are definitely theoretical advantages to the latter. First, the normal facial nucleus stays in command of facial motion by using the good side as its source of information. Since symmetry is the goal, there cannot be any better source of information. Second, it encompasses the generally ignored, but paramount input of unconscious proprioceptive circuits in the genesis of coordinated facial motion. Finally, it does not alter the impaired CNS, which it only selectively supplements.

The practical advantages are no less important. In this age of electronics, technology widely outstrips medical indications. It may not be necessary to reanimate more than two levels, e.g., the eye and the mouth, to achieve tremendous progress. Finally, implantation techniques should be well within the capabilities of practitioners trained in the field of head and neck surgery. Obviously, more work will have to be done before standards can be set for long-term implantation in the human, but the authors remain confident that the current scheme will serve as an experimental model for further progress towards the rehabilitation of the paralyzed human face.

Reference

1. Broniatowski M, Grundfest-Broniatowski S, Davies CR, Jacobs GB, Tucker HM, Nose Y (1991) Dynamic rehabilitation of the paralysed face. III. Balanced coupling of oral and ocular musculature from the intact side in the canine. Otolaryngol Head Neck Surg 105 : 727–734

Eur Arch Otorhinolaryngology (1994) [Suppl]: S 149

ABSTRACTS

D. H. Harrison

Pectoralis Minor Muscle Graft for the Treatment of Unilateral Facial Palsy

Two groups of patients with unilateral facial palsy present themselves. The two groups can be categorized as either congenital or acquired and the acquired cause is most commonly due to acoustic neuromas. Congenital facial palsy is rarely due to birth trauma and the exact reason for the nerve damage is obscure. Whichever the cause of the facial palsy they most commonly present at least 1 year after the onset and therefore are unsuitable for crossed facial nerve grafts. In consequence, a new nerve and new muscle need to be inserted into the paralysed side of the face. We therefore extend the buccal branch of the functioning 7th nerve employing a 20-cm sural nerve graft. The nerve graft is left in place for 6 months and then the paralysed side of the face is elevated and a pectoralis minor muscle graft is harvested from the chest wall and inserted into the paralysed side of the face. The muscle is revascularised using the facial artery and vein and reinnervated using the distal end of the crossed facial sural nerve graft. The dissection of the pectoralis minor muscle graft will be demonstrated with the neurovascular variations. Postoperative monitoring of the flap in its subcutaneous position is achieved using an impedance monitor, which produces a wave pattern on the oscilloscope.

Over 70 of these transfers have been completed but we will demonstrate the results with our success rate in a large group. We feel the shape of the pectoralis minor is particularly suitable for reanimation of the face as its fan shape produces opening of the mouth on smiling in order to demonstrate the teeth and very little of it requires resection, as it is not overlong. It is probably the muscle of choice in this form of reconstruction.

References

Harrison DH (1990) Current trends in the treatment of established unilateral facial palsy. Ann R Coll Surg Engl 72 : 94 – 98
Harrison DH (1985) The pectoralis minor vascularised muscle graft for the treatment of unilateral facial palsy. Plast Reconstr Surg 75 : 206

D. H. Harrison
Plastic Surgery Centre, Mount Vernon Hospital, Northwood, Middx

Eur Arch Otorhinolaryngology (1994) [Suppl]:S 150

ABSTRACTS

K. Ueda, K. Harii, and A. Yamada

Extended Follow-up Study of Vascularized Muscle Transplantation for Treatment of Long-Standing Facial Palsy

In a case of facial paralysis where a facial nerve stump is not available at the recipient site, free vascularized muscle transplantation combined with a cross-face nerve graft can provide natural symmetrical contraction synchronous with contralateral facial movement. Since 1973, when this procedure was first reported by one of the authors (K. Harii), we have transplanted more than 150 skeletal muscles (usually the gracilis muscle) for the treatment of established facial paralysis.

While the fact that the grafted muscle undergoes functional recovery in a manner similar to that of a temporarily denervated muscle is known, the extent of this and when the grafted muscle will actually demonstrate improvement in function is not clearly recognized. For the purpose of elucidation, not only a long follow-up study but also a wide-ranging study from various angles were necessary.

In this presentation, the quantitative evaluation of muscle activity and analysis of muscle fatigue based on EMG findings are described, and action of the grafted muscle independent of facial movement of the nonaffected side is reported.

K. Ueda, K. Harii, and A. Yamada
Department of Plastic Surgery, University of Tokyo, Japan

Eur Arch Otorhinolaryngology (1994) [Suppl]:S151

ABSTRACTS

J.K. Terzis

Eye Sphincter Substitution Schemes

Purpose. To critically analyze microreconstructive schemes aiming at the functional substitution of the paralyzed eye sphincter.

Methods and Materials. Thirty patients with lagophthalmos have been treated with microneurosurgical techniques to restore coordinated eye closure. Each patient was studied extensively with preoperative videos, electromyographic studies, and appropriate neuroradiology. The patients' deficit was analyzed and a therapeutic reanimation plan instituted.

Neural microreconstructive procedures were used exclusively in cases where the muscle target was still present. These included: (a) ipsilateral crossovers with the facial, hypoglossal, and trigeminal cranial nerves as possible motor donors, and (b) contralateral VII, via cross-facial nerve grafts.

Autologous muscle was used in the form of free or pedicled microneurovascular muscle in long-standing cases or developmental facial paralysis. These transfers involved embryologically similar muscle, i.e., facial muscle such as frontalis, platysma, and occipitalis, or foreign muscle, such as gracilis, adductor longus, and temporalis. Alternative reconstructive regimes included a combination of the following procedures: (a) tendon grafts to suspend the paralyzed lower eyelid, (b) inversion of the lower punctum, (c) two types of eye springs, (d) wedge excision of the lower lid, (e) lateral canthoplasty, and (f) gold weight.

Patients were followed for up to 5 years. Autologous muscle substitution invariably required revisions at 1 year.

Summary of Results. Functional restoration of the missing orbicularis oculi muscle has been accomplished in 30 patients with facial paralysis. In all cases the functional status of the globe improved. A rewarding degree of reanimation and improved cosmesis resulted in the majority of cases.

Conclusions. Microsurgical substitution of the missing eye sphincter has yielded rewarding results in a population of 30 patients with lagophthalmos.

J.K. Terzis
Eastern Virgina Medical School – MRC, 700 Olney Road,
Norfolk, VA 23507, USA

Eur Arch Otorhinolaryngology (1994) [Suppl]: S 152

ABSTRACTS

J.K. Terzis

Reanimation Schemes for Partial Facial Palsies

Purpose. To study partial facial palsies, to understand the mechanism of the deformity, and to design therapeutic schemes to reverse the facial imbalance.

Methods. Thirty-five cases of incomplete facial paralysis were treated by the author over the past 7 years. Each case was individually assessed, and reconstructive goals established. The aims of microsurgery included the following: (1) preserve existing function; (2) eliminate synkinesis between upper and lower face; (3) strengthen electively motor territories to accomplish symmetry and coordination at extremes of facial animation; (4) use of aesthetic procedures such as "mini" face-lifts, blepharoplasty, revisions of the drooping alar base, or correction of associated eye deformities such as lower lid ectropion and lagophthalmos; (5) restore overall symmetry and dynamic coordination of the mimic musculature as well as try to achieve a pleasing aesthetic result.

The microsurgical procedures used in these cases included: (1) provision of new motor targets by local muscle transfer or use of free "mini" muscles; (2) pacing of old motor targets or newly transferred targets with ipsilateral or contralateral facial nerve motor fibers; (3) use of cross-facial nerve grafting for treatment of synkinesis and for restoration of coordinated facial animation; (4) "revisional" microsurgial procedures for the partially paralyzed eye sphincter, and nasal deformities; (5) "mini" face-lift and blepharoplasty, if needed, provide an additional "perk" to the patient with incomplete facial paralysis.

Results. The treatment of synkinesis remains a challenging problem. The use of cross-facial nerve grafting provides a long-term solution. Revisions of the partially paralyzed eye sphincter yield best results if carried out with the patient under sedation and cooperating with the surgeon. An incomplete smile has been effectively addressed by provision of new targets. "Revisional" aesthetic microsurgery invariably yields pleasing results. Experience with 35 clinical cases will be presented.

Conclusions. Our approach to partial facial palsies has been one of exact diagnosis of the lesion, and design of novel microsurgical therapeutic schemes that aim at functional restoration and pleasing aesthetics.

J. Terzis
Eastern Virginia Medical School – MRC, 700 Olney Road,
Norfolk, VA 23507, USA

Eur Arch Otorhinolaryngology (1994) [Suppl]: S 153

ABSTRACTS

R. E. Mountain, M. A. Glasby, J. A. M. Murray, and J. F. Sharp

Freeze-Thawed Skeletal Muscle Autografts:
Experimental Evaluation of These Grafts in Facial Nerve Repair

Freeze-thawed coaxially aligned skeletal muscle autografts provide an exciting new concept in peripheral nerve repair, and research has confirmed their potential clinical use in the repair of peripheral nerves. They can be easily harvested and then frozen in liquid nitrogen, thawed in distilled water and cut to appropriate size before insertion. A matrix of large myotubules is provided, through which regenerating axons can migrate.

Using the buccal branch of the rat facial nerve as a model, we compared five freeze-thawed muscle grafts with five interposed nerve grafts. Three hundred days after grafting, the nerves was evaluated by electrophysiological and morphological means. Nerve conduction velocities were significantly reduced in both grafted groups when compared to control nerves. But no significant difference in conduction velocity was noted between the nerve graft and muscle graft groups. Strength-duration curves and measurements of chronaxie suggest that the muscle grafted group are slightly less electrically excitable than nerve grafted and control groups. The histological assessment reveals a similar distribution profile of axon and fibre size for either graft. G-ratios comparing myelination of fibres were similar in both groups.

In another experiment, freeze-thawed grafts were used to repair the buccal branch of five sheep facial nerves. Conduction velocities and histological assessment of these grafts again show evidence of significant reinnervation and give support to their future clinical use in human facial nerve repair.

R. E. Mountain, M. A. Glasby, J. A. M. Murray, and J. F. Sharp
Department of Otolaryngology, Edingburgh University, Edingburgh, Scotland, U. K.

Eur Arch Otorhinolaryngology (1994) [Suppl]: S 154

ABSTRACTS

G. Oberascher and E. Alzner

Facial Nerve Paralysis: Gold Weight Implants as Alternative to Tarsorrhaphy

Facial nerve paresis or paralysis can be the result of infection, trauma, surgery in the temporal bone, malignant parotid gland tumors, or resection of skull base tumors. Serious functional and also aesthetic problems may result following eyelid paralysis.

The inability to blink and lubricate the eye can lead to exposure keratitis, corneal abrasions, and even blindness. Though tarsorrhaphy has been the classic method of providing adequate corneal coverage, this procedure has many disadvantages, e.g., cosmetically unsatisfactory results, limited vision, and sometimes pure corneal protection. This presentation demonstrates the surgical technique of gold weight implantation as well as lower lid procedures of horizontal lid shortening in patients with paralytic lower lid ectropion. The indications and results of this procedure are discussed.

G. Oberascher and E. Alzner
Department of Otolaryngology and Ophthalmology,
5020 Salzburg, Austria

Eur Arch Otorhinolaryngology (1994) [Suppl]: S 155

ABSTRACTS

G. Salimbeni

Facial Reanimation in Facial Paralysis

Results in the treatment of facial paralysis are presented. Cases were presented in which, according to the area of the nerve lesion and the time of the lesion, different techniques were used:

ipsilateral nerve grafts for interruption of the nerve in the soft tissues of the face, cross-face grafts, for intracranial facial nerve lesions, muscle microvascular transplants for long-standing facial paralysis. The less than satisfactory results are also presented for comparison with the results of others so that the techniques of facial reanimation can be discussed and improved.

G. Salimbeni
Divisione di Chirurgia Plastica, Ospedale Cisanello, 56124 Pisa, Italy

Facial Nerve Disorders in Children and Others

Eur Arch Otorhinolaryngology (1994) [Suppl]: S 159 – S 160

S. Koike, S. Hashimoto, M. Toshima, F. Shoji, M. Ishigaki, and T. Takasaka

Steroid Therapy for Facial Nerve Palsy in Children

Introduction

It is widely acceptd that the incidence of facial nerve palsy in children under 15 years is in the order of 15% – 20% of all facial nerve palsy [1]; their prognosis is good compared with adult cases.

Since 1989, we have treated children with facial nerve palsy using steroid therapy. In this paper, we report the results of steroid therapy in children with facial nerve palsy in our clinic and discuss its effectiveness.

Subjects

The subjects were 24 children under 15 years treated with steroid therapy within 10 days after the onset of facial nerve palsy. In this series, patients with congenital or traumatic facial nerve palsy were excluded. Age and sex distribution of the 24 patients is shown in Table 1. Eighteen out of 24 patients had Bell's palsy and four had Ramsay Hunt syndrome. As for the other two patients, one had infectious mononucleosis and the other recurrent facial nerve palsy of unknown aetiology. Twenty-three out of 24 patients were tested by nerve excitability test (NET) daily, if possible, before and during the treatment.

Evaluation of facial movement was performed by the 40-point grading scale method proposed by the Japan Society of Facial Nerve Research [2]. If the initial score of facial movement was less than 10 points, i.e. complete palsy, patients were treated by high-dose steroid therapy from an early stage. In contrast, if the initial score was better than 11 points, i.e. incomplete palsy, the patients

Table 1 Age and sex distribution of patients treated

Age (years)	Bell's palsy		Ramsay Hunt syndrome		Other		Total
	m	f	m	f	m	f	
0 – 4	1	4	0	0	1	1	7
5 – 9	0	3	0	1	0	0	4
10 – 15	5	5	3	0	0	0	13
Total	6	12	3	1	1	1	24

m, male; f, female.

were treated with conventional low-dose steroid therapy. The protocol of high-dose steroid therapy is summarized in Table 2. The initial dosage of predonisolone was 2.0 (or in some cases, 3.0) mg/kg per day, and the whole course of steroid therapy was completed in 10 – 14 days. The protocol of conventional low-dose steroid therapy is summarized in Table 3. The initial dosage of predonisolone was 1.0 mg/kg per day, and the whole course of steroid therapy was completed in 7 days. Hydroxyethyl starch, pentoxiyfylline and methylcobalamin were also added to the protocol. In cases of Ramsay Hunt syndrome, acyclovir was also used; 5 mg acyclovir/kg was infused intravenously every 8 h for 5 days at the early stage of the treatment.

Sixteen out of 24 cases were treated with high-dose steroid therapy. All four patients with Ramsay Hunt syndrome were treated with high-dose steroid therapy and acyclovir.

Results

Results and the clinical curse of the 24 cases are summarized in Table 4. Twenty-three patients recovered completely within 24 weeks after onset of facial nerve palsy; the recovery rate was 95.8%. Three quarters of the patients recovered completely within 16 weeks after onset of facial

S. Koike (✉), M. Toshima, F. Shoji, M. Ishigaki, and T. Takasaka
Department of Otolaryngology, Tohoku,
University School of Medicine, 1-1 Seiryo-cho, Aoba, Sendai 980, Japan

Table 2 Protocol of high-dose steroid therapy in children

Days of treatment	Hydroxyethyl starch (ml/day)	Solita T3 (ml/day)	Predonisolone (mg/kg per day)	Pentoxyfylline (mg/kg per day)	Vitamin B_{12} (µg/kg per day)
1, 2	250–500	–	2.0 i.v.	6 orally	30 orally
3, 4	250–500	–	1.5 i.v.	6 orally	30 orally
5, 6	–	250–500	1.0 i.v.	6 orally	30 orally
7	–	250–500	0.5 i.v.	6 orally	30 orally
8	–	–	0.4 orally	6 orally	30 orally
9	–	–	0.3 orally	6 orally	30 orally
10	–	–	0.2 orally	6 orally	30 orally

Acyclovir was added to the protocol in children with Ramsay Hunt syndrome.

Table 3 Protocol of conventional low-dose steroid therapy in children

Days of treatment	Predonisolone (mg/kg per day)	Pentoxyfylline (mg/kg per day)	Vitamin B_{12} (µg/kg per day)
1, 2	1.0 orally	6 orally	30 orally
3, 4	0.5 orally	6 orally	30 orally
5, 6	0.2 orally	6 orally	30 orally
7	0.1 orally	6 orally	30 orally

nerve palsy. As for the patients with Ramsay Hunt Syndrome, however, three needed more than 17 weeks to recover completely. The only one patient who showed incomplete recovery was a 3-year-old girl with recurrent facial nerve palsy of unknown aetiology. In this series, there have been no serious side-effects during or after steroid therapy.

Discussion

Although the prognosis of facial nerve palsy in children unter 15 years is good compared with adults cases, the reported recovery rate of facial nerve palsy in children was only 70%–80% [3, 4]. In our present series, the recovery rate was 95.8%. The treatment of facial nerve palsy is controversial, yet many papers have reported the effectiveness of steroid therapy from an early stage [5–7]. Stennernt reported the high recovery rate of 96% in patients with Bell's palsy treated with high-dose steroid therapy [8]. In our series, we treated children with complete facial nerve palsy with high-dose steroid therapy and achieved a high recovery rate. Out data show the effectiveness of steroid

therapy for children with facial nerve palsy. Steroid therapy resulted not only in a higher recovery rate, but also a shortening of recovery time. We have not experienced any serious side-effects of steroid therapy so far, though late-onset complications cannot yet be ruled out. Facial nerve palsy can progress from a mild, incomplete form to a severe, complete form and, at present, it is impossible to predict which cases will progress to a severe complete palsy. If the treatment is delayed until severity is determined, irreversible nerve damage may occur. This is why we recommend steroid therapy for children with facial nerve palsy an early stage, although we are trying to reduce the total dose of steroid used.

References

1. May M (1986) Facial nerve disorders in the new born and children. In: May M (ed) The facial nerve. Thieme, New York, pp 401–419
2. Yanagihara N (1977) Grading of facial palsy. In: Fisch U (ed) Facial nerve surgery. Aescalapius, Birmingham, Alabama, pp 533–535
3. Alberti PW, Biagioni E (1972) Facial paralysis in children. A review of 150 cases. Laryngoscope 82 : 1013–1020
4. Adour KK, Frederick MB (1978) The true nature of Bell's palsy: analysis of 1000 consecutive patients. Laryngoscope 88 : 787–801
5. Adour KK (1982) Current concepts in neurology: diagnosis and management of facial paralysis. N Engl J Med 307 : 348–351
6. Burgess LPA (1984) Bell's palsy: the steroid controversy revisited. Laryngoscope 94 : 1472–1476
7. May M (1985) Idiopathic (Bell's) facial palsy: natural history defies steroid or surgical treatment. Laryngoscope 95 : 406, 409
8. Stennert E (1982) New concept in the treatment of Bell's palsy. Disorders of the facial nerve. Raven, New York, pp 313–318

Table 4 Clinical course of the 24 cases

Time interval between onset of facial nerve palsy and recovery (weeks)	High-dose steroid therapy	Conventional low-dose steroid therapy	Total	Cumulative recovery rate (%)
≤ 4	6	2	8	33.3
≤ 8	9	4	13	54.2
≤ 12	9	6	15	62.5
≤ 16	11	7	18	75.0
≤ 20	15	7	22	91.7
≤ 24	15	8	23	95.8
Incomplete recovery	1	–	1	–

Eur Arch Otorhinolaryngology (1994) [Suppl]: S 161 – S 162

INVITED LECTURES

F. F. J. Declau, W. Jacob, S. Montoro, and P. Van de Heyning

Developmental Aspects of the Facial Canal: A Light and Scanning Electron Microscopic Study

Introduction

Most anatomy and embryology textbooks deal with the development of the facial canal with very brief and incomplete descriptions. Whereas dehiscences have been attributed to persistence of the stapedial artery [4] or middle ear infections in early childhood [1], most authors believe that the normal formation of a closed facial canal is entirely the result of otic capsule ossification. However, postmortem temporal bone studies by Marquet [5] have demonstrated preferential sites for facial canal dehiscences. Dehiscences were most frequently found in the vestibular region of the tympanic segment (12%). In contrast, dehiscences were very rare in the cochlear region of the tympanic segment (only 1%). In the labyrinthine segment, a prevalence of 7% was found. These observations suggest a more complex facial canal development which cannot be entirely explained by otic capsule ossification.

Materials and Method

In a series of 13 human fetuses, the course of the facial canal in the temporal bone was investigated by the use of light and scanning electron microscopy. The normal development of the facial canal was correlated to clinical aspects of facial nerve dehiscences. Details have been described elsewhere [3].

F. F. J. Declau (✉) and P. Van de Heyning
Departments of Otorhinolaryngology, University of Antwerp,
Universiteitsplein 1, 2610 Wilrijk, Belgium

W. Jacob and S. Montoro
Departments of Electron Microscopy and Chemistry,
University of Antwerp, Universiteitsplein 1, 2610 Wilrijk,
Belgium

Results and Discussion

Our observations confirm the physiologic presence of fetal dehiscences. Their location in fetuses is precisely circumscribed and depends on both their topographic relation with the otic capsule and its degree of maturation. The intratympanic part of the facial canal and the geniculate ganglion area were the last regions to be covered by bone. Our observations demonstrate a more complex facial canal development not limited simply to the ossification of the otic capsule, as previously descibed by other authors [2]. The time sequence of the histological development permitted us to distinguish three phases in facial canal development. Until 16 weeks gestational age (phase 1), the facial canal is merely an open sulcus within the cartilaginous otic capsule. The perichondrium forms a sort of connective tissue-like frame of condensed mesenchyme around the neural fiber bundle (Fig. 1). Phase 2 (16 – 21 weeks gestational age) is characterized by the endochondral ossification of the otic capsule. As compared to the previous cartilage stages, the primitive facial sulcus remains virtually completely dehiscent and only covered by a thin fibrous layer. The importance of the inner and outer connective tissue sheets around the facial canal is confirmed: these fibrous layers seem to be responsible for its final architecture and not the otic capsule ossification by itself. The periosteal ossification is delayed at the inner fibrous layer, while the side walls acquire a periosteal investment in continuity with the underlying endochondral bone. Consequently, the shpae of the facial sulcus is altered. During phase 3 (22 – 25 weeks gestational age), periosteal ossification starts in the inner sheet, while intramembranous bone is formed within the outer fibrous sheet and results in the final closure of the facial canal wall (Fig. 2).

Our findings show that those regions of the facial canal wall which are covered by intramembranous bone are the most susceptive to dehiscences, which is totally in agreement with the dehiscence rate found in adults [5, 6]. In

Fig. 1 Facial canal at the vestibular portion of the tympanic segment at 14 weeks gestation. The facial canal is merely a shallow sulcus at the tympanic side of the cartilaginous otic capsule. The facial nerve (*F*) is not covered by bone and is in close relation to the mesenchyme of the middle ear cleft (*M*). The perichondrium of the otic capsule (*P*) splits around the facial nerve as a connective tissue-like frame. HFS stain; *bar*, 100 μm

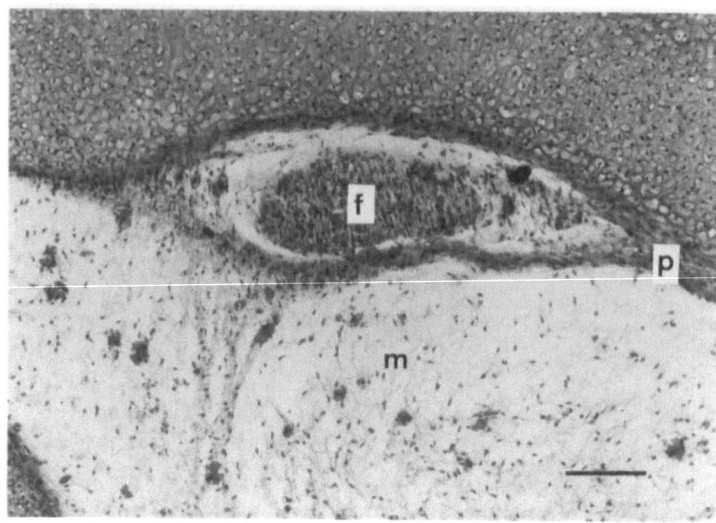

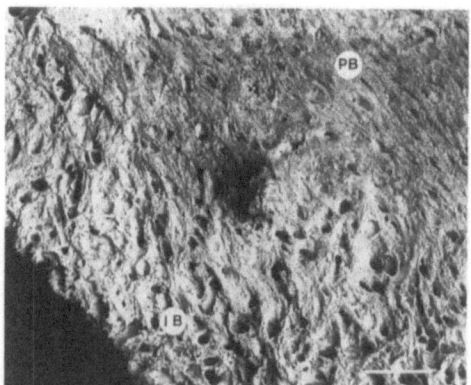

Fig. 2 Facial canal at the vestibular region of the tympanic segment at 22 weeks. Immature bone (*IB*) forms the tympanic border of the facial canal and is in continuity with the more organized layer of the periosteal layer of the otic capsule (*PB*). Scanning electron microscopy; *bar*, 100 μm

terms of time sequence, it is the type of bone which is the last to be formed in order to close the facial canal wall.

References

1. Albing W, Rauchfuss A (1987) Fetal development of the tympanic part of the facial canal. Arch Otolaryngol 243:374–377
2. Bast T (1930) Ossification of the otic capsule in human fetuses. Carneg Contr Embryol 121:53–82
3. Declau F, Jacob W, Montoro S, Marquet J (1991) Dehiscence of the facial canal: developmental aspects. Int J Pediatr Otorhinolaryngol 21:21–32
4. Kaplan S, Catlin F, Weavert T, Feigin R (1984) Onset of hearing loss in children with bacterial meningitis. Pediatrics 73:575–578
5. Marquet J (1981) Congenital malformations and middle ear surgery. J Soc Med 74:119–128
6. Marquet J, Declau F (eds) (1988) Congenital middle ear malformations. Acta Otolaryngol Belg 42 (2):123–302

Eur Arch Otorhinolaryngology (1994) [Suppl]: S 163 – S 164

FREE PAPERS AND POSTERS

H. Saito, T. Takeda, and S. Kishimoto

Vulnerability of the Facial Nerve in Entrapment Palsy: Comparative Study in Guinea Pigs and Humans

Introduction

The rationale for facial nerve decompression is to release the facial nerve and its vessels from entrapped compression. We have been investigating the possibility and timing of facial nerve entrapment in the facial canal in the early stages of its damage. We also studied differences between cross-sectional area ratios – facial nerve to facial canal (FN/FC) – of human adult and child temporal bones [1]. We revealed that the FN/FC ratio of children is significantly smaller than that of the adults. We report results of our experiments on the swelling changes of damaged facial nerves with time in guinea pigs [2]. We wanted to find out whether the experimental data of guinea pigs are applicable to human pathology. The aim of this paper is to measure the FN/FC ratios in guinea pigs and to show that the facial nerve of the guinea pigs is useful for an experimental model of entrapped facial palsy in humans.

Materials and Methods

Seventeen horizontally sectioned temporal bones from 17 guinea pigs were used in this study. Data were obtained from a section of each temporal bone immediately peripheral to the cochleariform process. As the facial nerve of guinea pigs has a straight course and the facial canal in the labyrinthine segment of horizontally sectioned specimens included the wide internal auditory meatus, only the horizontal segment was measured and analyzed.

The FN/FC ratios were calculated using a programmed computed planimeter. The cross-sectional areas were traced on magnified photocopies to the sections. The

H. Saito (✉), T. Takeda, and S. Kishimoto
Department of Otolaryngology, Kochi Medical School, Nankoku, 783 Kochi, Japan

means and standard deviations of sets of ratios were determined. The data were analyzed using the t test compared with our previous data on human adult and child temporal bones [1].

Results

The FN/FC ratios in guinea pigs in the horizontal segment ranged from 0.40 to 0.62. The average ratio was 0.47 and the SD was 0.05. Table 1 shows the ratios of each temporal bone and their numerical values of areas of the facial nerve and the facial canal traced on the magnified copies.

Comparison of data for guinea pigs with the previous data for human adult and child temporal bone specimens revealed that the FN/FC ratios of guinea pigs specimens were in between those in the tympanic segment of human

Table 1 Facial nerve (FN) and facial canal (FC) areas and FN/FC ratios (guinea pigs)

Case	FN ($$)	FC ($$)	FN/FC[a]
1	210.90	385.89	0.55
2	72.39	180.69	0.40
3	245.10	395.01	0.62
4	125.40	257.64	0.49
5	135.09	261.06	0.52
6	81.51	185.82	0.44
7	116.85	255.36	0.46
8	130.53	288.99	0.45
9	119.13	287.28	0.41
10	125.97	262.20	0.48
11	83.22	206.34	0.40
12	125.40	294.69	0.43
13	144.78	322.05	0.45
14	112.29	262.20	0.43
15	94.05	206.91	0.45
16	106.02	224.58	0.47
17	57.00	116.85	0.49

[a] Average ratio, 0.47; SD ± 0.05.

Table 2 Facial nerve to facial canal (FN/FC) ratios in humans and guinea pigs (mean + SD)

Segment	Adult humans	Children	Guinea pigs
Labyrinthine	0.46 ± 0.07 [a]	0.31 ± 0.08	–
Tympanic	0.52 ± 0.17 [b]	0.35 ± 0.10	0.47 ± 0.05 [a]
Mastoid	0.37 ± 0.04	0.18 ± 0.12	–

Data for humans quoted from [1].
[a] Entrapped at severe damage.
[b] Entrapped at mild damage.

adult and child specimens (Table 2). There was no statistically significant difference between the FN/FC ratios of guinea pigs and those of adults. Th FN/FC ratios of human pediatric specimens were significantly smaller than those of guinea pigs ($p < 0.01$).

Discussion

This study confirmed that the FN/FC ratios in guinea pigs were close to those of human adult temporal bones [1, 3]. Therefore, our previous data on nerve-swelling experiments are applicable to human adult pathology. However, the data for pediatric cases would be lower.

Our experimental study of guinea pigs showed that severely damaged facial nerves swell more than 2.14 times in the initial swelling stage of Wallerian degeneration and that in damaged nerves comparable to half-sectioned facial nerves the maximum swelling is 1.44 times [2].

Therefore, in guinea pigs, nerve to canal ratios greater than 0.47 and 0.69 may have chance to be entrapped in the canal in severely damaged cases and half-damaged cases, respectively. In clinical cases, totally damaged facial nerves at initial visit have no chance of recovery without pathologic synkinetic movement regardless of any treatment remedy. Therefore, data from partially damaged nerves in guinea pigs offer important information on the chance of entrapment in the clinical cases. For these cases, we must release nerve compression to avoid cure with synkinesis.

Presscott [4] reported that the overall recovery rate after facial palsy among children treated conservatively was a high as 96%. Applying the value of 0.69 in the damaged nerve comparable to half-sectioned facial nerves in guinea pigs to the data of pediatric specimens, no segment of the facial nerve becomes so swollen that it is entrapped in the canal in the maximum swelling stage, even when positive are added to the values. Even when applying the FN/FC ratio of 0.47 to the pediatric specimens, only 19.2% (five of 26) of the nerves are found to be swollen to the point that they are entrapped in the facial canal at the state of maximum swelling (Table 2). Taking into consideration the fact that the mean FN/FC ratio in pediatric specimens is significantly smaller than that of guinea pigs, the percentage might be far less.

Conclusion

This paper shows that he guinea pig is a suitable animal model for human adult facial nerve-swelling experiments. This study reinforced our previous speculation that the small FN/FC ratios in pediatric cases play an important role in the better recovery rate after facial palsy among children.

Acknowledgement. This work was supported by grant no. 01480407 from the Japanese Ministry of Education.

References

1. Saito H, Takeda T, Kishimoto S (1992) Facial nerve to facial canal cross-sectional area ratio in children. Laryngoscope 102 : 1172–1176
2. Saito H, Nakatani H, Kishimoto S (1990) Swelling of the degenerating facial nerve. In: Castro D (ed) The facial nerve. Kugler Ghedini, Amstelveen, pp 345–347
3. Ogawa A, Sando I (1982) Spatial occupancy of vessels and facial nerve in the facial canal. Ann Otol Rhinol Laryngol 91 : 14–19
4. Prescott CJA (1987) Idiopathic facial nerve palsy in children and the effect of treatment with steroids. Int J Pediatr Otolaryngol 13 : 257–264

Eur Arch Otorhinolaryngology (1994) [Suppl]: S 165 – 167

FREE PAPERS AND POSTERS

S. F. Mucci and A. Sismanis

Melkersson-Rosenthal Syndrome: Report of Two Cases and Review of Literature

Introduction

Melkersson-Rosenthal Syndrome (MRS) is a rare disorder; its classical presentation includes unilateral edema of the face and/or lips, relapsing unilateral facial paralysis, and fissured dorsum of tongue (lingua plicata). The incidence of this syndrome has been estimated to be 1:2100 [9]. The following two cases representative examples of MRS.

Cases 1

A 4-year-old black male was admitted to our medical center in October 1981 with sudden onset of a complete left facial paralysis. He had three episodes of spontaneously resolving left facial paralysis in the past. The patient's mother had observed transient facial prior to this admission.

Physical examination revealed left facial paralysis and mild upper facial edema. Audiogram, CT scan of the temporal bones, and metabolic workup were all within normal limits. Nerve excitability testing revealed a 7 mA threshold difference between the normal and paralyzed sides. Because of the multiple episodes of previous left facial paralysis and the nerve excitability test findings, a transmastoid decompression of the facial nerve from the stylomastoid foramen to the geniculate ganglion was performed. Significant edema was noted in the horizontal portion of the nerve. Facial function returned to normal within 3 months.

S. F. Mucci and A. Sismanis (✉)
Department of Otolaryngology – Head and Neck Surgery,
Medical College of Virginia, Virginia Commonwealth University,
Richmond, Virginia, USA

Subsequently, the child had two more bouts of spontaneously resolving right-sided facial paralysis and was lost to follow-up for 9 years before presenting again to the emergency room in April 1990 at age 12 with another episode of complete right-sided facial paralysis and mild edema (Fig. 1). Audiogram, gadolinium-enhanced magnetic resonance imaging (Gad-MRI) of the head, and metabolic workup were all within normal limits. Electroneurography (ENOG) revealed 100% degeneration of the right facial nerve. Transmastoid decompression of the right facial nerve from the stylomastoid foramen to the geniculate ganglion was then performed. Again, severe edema was noted in the horizontal portion of the nerve. Full recovery of facial nerve function occurred within 3 months (Fig. 2). There has been no recurrence of facial paralysis since.

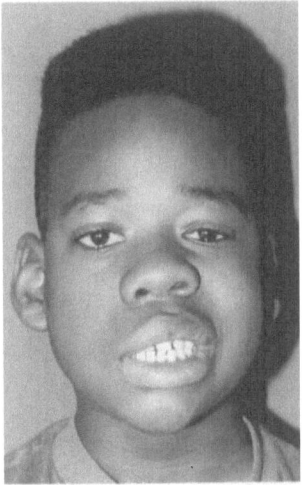

Fig. 1 Right facial paralysis and edema in a 12-year-old boy

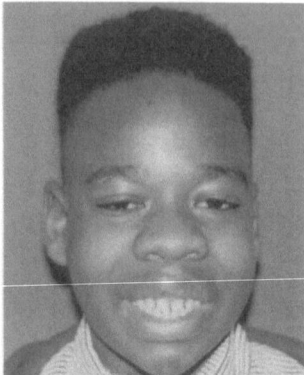

Fig. 2 Same patient as in Fig. 1. Resolution of paralysis 3 months postoperatively

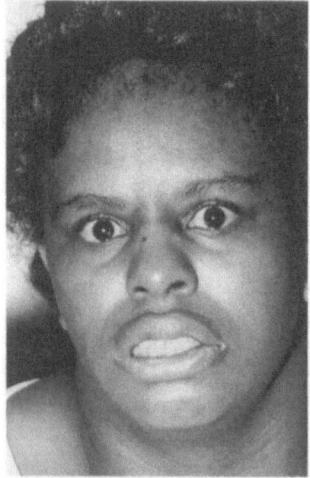

Fig. 3 Bilateral facial weakness and edema of the upper lip

Case 2

A 36-year-old black female was seen in our clinic in September 1990 with the chief complaint of bilateral progressive facial weakness of 6 months' duration.

Physical examination showed paresis of both sides of the face, the left greater than the right, and near complete paralysis of the upper face (Fig. 3). The tongue was deeply fissured, and there was edema of the upper lip (Fig. 4). The remainder of the head and neck was normal.

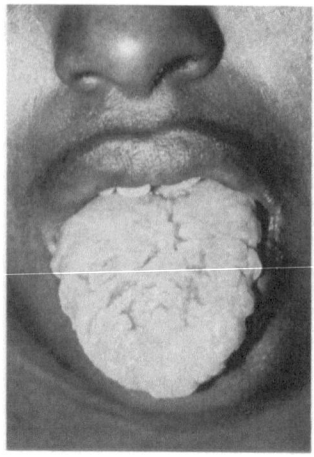

Fig. 4 Same patient as in Fig. 3. Deeply fissured tongue (lingua plicate)

Audiogram, Gad-MRI of the head and neck, and metabolic work up were all normal. ENOG showed 54% degeneration of the left facial nerve relative to the right. A diagnosis of MRS was made. At follow-up 3 months later, the patient was noted to have improving bilateral facial weakness.

Discussion

In 1928, Melkersson described a relationship between paralysis and swelling of the face. In 1931, Rosenthal added lingua plicata to the list of clinical manifestations; hence the modern name for the syndrome [11].

Clinical Features

Recurrent edeme of the lips and/or adjacent of the face is the most consistent feature of MRS. The tongue, hands, chest, and buttocks may also be involved [3].

Facial nerve involvement has been reported in 30%–90% of MRS cases throughout the literature [8]. Bouts may be unilateral or bilateral, and may involve all or part of the nerve. Associated cranial neuropathies have been described [7]. The least consistent component of the classic triad is lingua plicata [8].

Oligosymptomatic forms of MRS with only two of the three features of the classical triad have been reported [4]. Moreover, several reports describe variants of MRS in which only one symptom is present [11].

Etiology

The etiology of MRS remains unknown. Infectious, allergic, immunologic, and hereditary theories have all been postulated [1, 11].

MRS may have a hereditary predisposition. Several cases have been reported in which the disease appeared in four consecutive generations [6]. Others believe that MRS is an incomplete autosomal dominant trait with variable penetration [1].

Diagnosis

Clinic impression remains the mainstay of diagnosis. This can be confirmed by pathologic study of a punch biopsy from an involved area of mucosa [7]. Recently, serial acute and convalescent titers of angiotensin-converting enzyme have been recommended [8].

Treatment

Data on the efficacy of systemic steroids is conflicting [12]. For recurrent facial paralysis, decompression should be considered. Graham and Kemink reported good results with total facial nerve decompression in two patients [2]. For chronic lip edema, injections of triamcinolone acetonide seem to be effective [5].

Conclusions

In summary, MRS is rare condition classically presenting with a triad of facial and/or lip edema, fissured tongue, and relapsing facial palsy. We have presented two representative patients. Due to the rarity of this syndrome and its oligosymptomatic presentation, the disease is probably underdiagnosed. Treatment of this syndrome remains controversial, and the otolaryngologist should therefore be familiar with it.

References

1. Carr RD (1965) Is the Melkersson-Rosenthal Syndrome hereditary? Arch Dermatol 93 : 426–427
2. Graham MD, Kemink JL (1986) Total facial nerve decompression in recurrent facial paralysis and the Melkersson-Rosenthal Syndrome: a preliminary report. Am J Otol 7 : 34–37
3. Hornstein OP (1970) Melkersson-Rosenthal syndrome. In: Viken PJ, Bruyn GW (eds) Handbook of clinical neurology. American Elsevier, New York, pp 205–240
4. Klaus SN, Brunsting LA (19959) Melkersson-Rosenthal syndrome – Report of a case. Proc Mayo Clin 34 : 365–366
5. Krutchkoff D, James R (1978) Cheilitis granulomatosa: successful treatment with combined local triamcinolone injections and surgery. Arch Dermatol 114 : 1203–1206
6. Lygidakis C, Tsakanikas C, Ilias A, Vassilopoulos D (1979) Melkersson-Rosenthal syndrome in four generations. Clin Genet 15 : 189–192
7. Minor MW, Fox RW, Bukantz SC, Lockey RF (1987) Melkersson-Rosenthal syndrome. J Allergy Clin Immunol 80 : 64–67
8. Orlando MR, Atkins JS (1990) Melkersson-Rosenthal syndrome. Arch Otolaryngol Head and Neck Surg 116 : 728–729
9. Roseman B, Mulrihill JJ (1978) Melkersson-Rosenthal syndrome in a 7-year-old girl. Pediatrics 61 : 490–491
10. Streeto JM, Watters FB (1964) Melkersson's syndrome; multiple recurrences of Bell's palsy and episodic facial edema. N Engl J Med 271 : 308–309
11. Wadlington WB, Riley HD Jr, Lowbeer K (1984) The Melkersson-Rosenthal sydrome. Pediatrics 73 : 502–506
12. Wolk SM, Wagner JH, Davidson S et al. (1978) Treatment of Bell's palsy with prednisone: a prospective, randomized study. Neurology 2B : 158–161

Eur Arch Otorhinolaryngology (1994) [Suppl]: S 168 – S 170

INVITED LECTURES

H. L. J. Tanghe, K. H. Pauw, and A. Kasteel-van Linge

Course of the Facial Nerve in Congenital Dysplasia of the External Auditory Canal: A High-Resolution Computerized Tomography Study

Introduction

Congenital dysplasia of the external auditory canal (EAC) appars with a frequency of 1:10000 to 1:20000 births [4]. Surgical correction of congenital dysplasia of the EAC is difficult. The facial nerve almost always has an abnormal course and can be injured easily during operation [5]. Radiological identification of the facial nerve canal, however, is no guarantee that the facial nerve is enclosed. The purpose of this study was to provide a detailed analysis of the course of the facial nerve in congenital dysplasia of the EAC.

Material and Methods

The CT scan of 32 patients with congenital dysplasia of the EAC were reviewed. Contiguous CT sections of 1- or 1.5-mm thickness were obtained in the axial plane at 30° and in the coronal plane at 105° in relation of the antropologic baseline 0° [3]. Congenital dysplasia of the EAC was divided into bony or membranous atresia and stenotic EAC.

H. L. J. Tanghe (✉)
Departments of Radiology , University Hospital Rotterdam-Dijkzigt, Dr. Molewaterplein 40, 3015 GD Rotterdam, The Netherlands

K. H. Pauw
Departments of Radiology – Section of Neuroradiology, University Hospital Rotterdam-Dijkzigt, Dr. Molewaterplein 40, 3015 GD Rotterdam, The Netherlands

A. Kasteel-van Linge
Departments of Radiology – Section of Otorhinolaryngology, University Hospital Rotterdam-Dijkzigt, Dr. Molewaterplein 40, 3015 GD Rotterdam, The Netherlands

Results

This study included 32 patients (41 ears) with a unilateral ($n = 23$) or bilateral ($n = 9$) dysplasia of the EAC. The malformation was part of a syndrome in six cases: Goldenhar syndrome ($n = 2$), Treacher Collins syndrome ($n = 1$), Klinefelter syndrome ($n = 1$), cheilo-gnato-palatoschisis ($n = 1$), and congenital clavicular hypoplasia-agenesia (CCHA) syndrome ($n = 1$).

Bony atresias with a bony overgrowth of the deformed tympanic bone, referred to as the atresia plate, were found

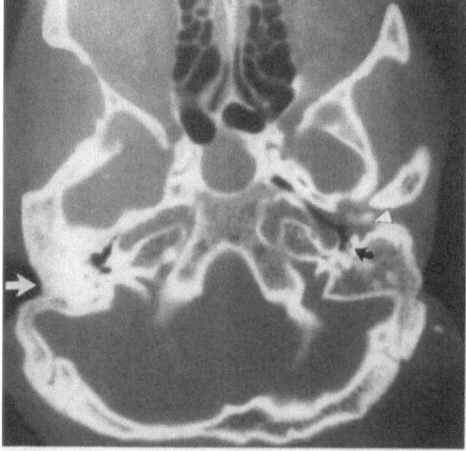

Fig. 1 Thick bony atresia plate on the right (*large white arrow*) and stenotic external auditory canal (EAC) on the left (*white arrow head*). Associated anomalies are on the *right* a small middle ear cavity and on the *left* side a displaced mandibular condyle, an anteriorly located mastoid segment (*curved black arrow*) of the facial nerve, and a small middle ear cavity

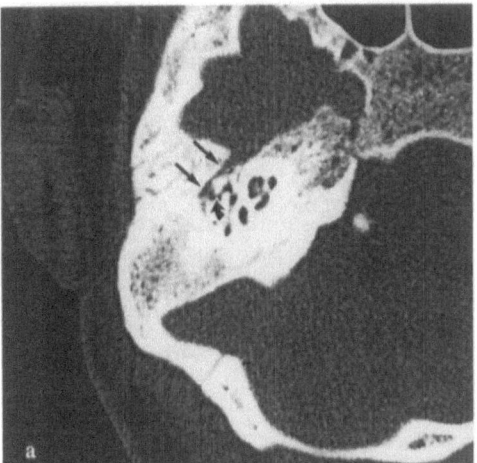

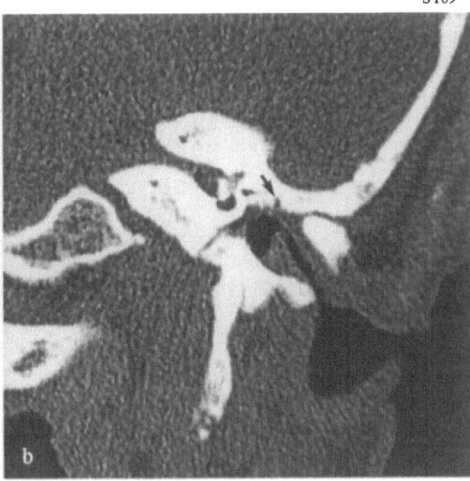

Fig. 2a Axial CT scan. Laterally displaced tympanic segment (*small arrows*); associated anomalies: the small middle ear cavity and fused ossicles (*curved arrow*). **b** Coronal CT scan. The laterally displaced tympanic segment in the roof of the middle ear cavity (*arrow*) in case of a stenotic external auditory canal (EAC)

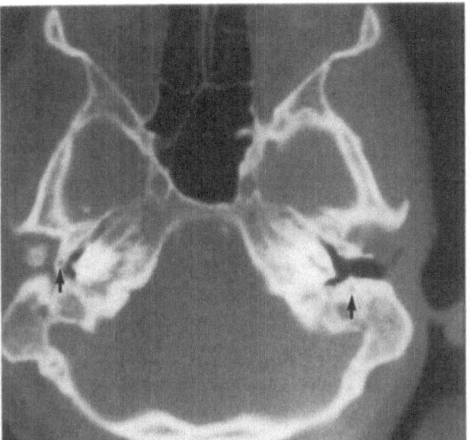

Fig. 3 Bony atresia on the *right* with an anteriorly displaced mastoid segment (*arrow*) in a thin atresia plate, constituting the medial wall of an abnormal temporomandibular joint. Small middle ear cavity. Compare with normal position of *left* mastoid segment (*arrow*)

in 25 and a normal bony EAC with a membranous atresia in three ears. Thirteen ears had a congenital stenosis of the EAC (Fig. 1).

The location of the labyrinthine segment of the facial nerve canal was always normal. The tympanic segment had an anomalous course in two ears: it was located laterally in the roof of the middle ear cleft (Fig. 2a, b) in one case with a stenotic EAC and in the lateral wall of the middle ear cleft in one case with bony atresia. In 15 (60%) ears with bony atresia and in three (23%) ears with a stenotic EAC (Fig. 3), the mastoid segment was found to be displaced anteriorly.

Discussion

Our findings concerning the mastoid segment concur with the results of Swartz et al. [7], who found a frequency of 55% with anterior displacement in a group of 13 ears with a bony and two with a membranous atresia and reported no anomalous course of the tympanic segment. In the presence of an anteriorly located mastoid segment, the facial nerve does not emerge from a stylomastoid foramen in a normal position, but from a position at the posterior or medial wall of an abnormal mandibular fossa (Fig. 3) or dehiscence within the jugular fossa.

There is a discrepancy between radiological and surgical findings concerning the frequency of variations of the facial nerve canal. Belluci [2] reported that the facial nerve was not covered by bone in 25 (35%) out of 71 patients with dysplasia of the EAC. It is known, however, that in the medial two thirds of the tympanic segment, the bony wall adjacent to the middle ear is often very thin or completely absent and cannot be resolved by high-resolution CT [6]. This congenital bony dehiscence in the facial canal is found in 55% of temporal bones and cannot therefore be regarded as an associated anomaly of dysplasia of the EAC [1]. The tympanic segment of the facial nerve was found in the lateral or superior wall of the middle ear cavity in two of our patients. To our knowledge, a facial nerve canal located in this position has not been reported before.

Conclusions

In bony atresia or stenotic EAC, most course anomalies of the facial nerve are present in the mastoid segment, consisting of an anterior displacement, and the tympanic segment of the facial nerve canal can be located in the lateral or superior wall of the middle ear cleft. No displacement of the facial nerve is found in membranous atresia of the EAC.

References

1. Baxter A (1971) Dehiscence of the fallopian canal: an anatomical study. J Laryngol Otol 85 : 587 – 594
2. Belluci RJ (1981) Congenital aural malformations: diagnosis and treatment. Otolaryngol Clin North Am 14 : 95 – 124
3. Chakeres DW, Spiegel PK (1983) A systematic technique for comprehensive evaluation of the temporal bone by computed tomography. Radiology 146 : 97 – 106
4. Jafek BW, Nager GT, Strife J, Gaylor RW (1975) Congenital aural atresia: an analysis of 311 cases. Ann Otol Rhinol Laryngol 80 : 588 – 595
5. Jahrsdoerfer RA, Yeakly JW, Aguilar EA, Cole RR, Gray LC (1992) Grading system for the selection of patients with congenital aural atresia. Am J Otolaryngol 13 : 6 – 12
6. Swartz JD (1984) The facial nerve canal: CT analysis of the protruding tympanic segment. Radiology 153 : 443 – 447
7. Swartz JD, Faerber EN (1985) Congenital malformations of the external and middle ear: high-resolution CT findings of surgical import. AJNR 6 : 71 – 76

Eur Arch Otorhinolaryngology (1994) [Suppl]:S171

ABSTRACTS

H.-J. Christen, F. Hanefeld, H. Eiffert, and R. Thomssen

Lyme Borreliosis – Main Cause of Acute Peripheral Facial Palsy in Childhood

The epidemiology and clinical features of acute peripheral facial palsy with respect to Lyme borreliosis were investigated in a prospective multicenter study. The study included seven pediatric departments serving a geographically well-defined region in Lower Saxony with a population of 350000 children. During a 3-year period (1987–1989), 76 consecutive cases with acute peripheral facial palsy were investigated. On the basis of their CSF findings 137 additional pediatric cases with facial palsy were included. They were examined by the same serological methods in our laboratory as the 76 cases but treated in other hospitals not participating in the multicenter study. Diagnosis of Lyme borreliosis was based on the detection of specific IgM antibodies against *Borrelia burgdorferi* in CSF, using an IgM capture assay. The demonstration of specific IgM and/or IgG antibodies in serum alone was not considered to be sufficient for the diagnosis of Lyme borreliosis.

The annual incidence of acute peripheral facial palsy was 6.6/100 000 children aged 0–14 years. Lyme borreliosis was the single most frequent verifiable cause of acute peripheral facial palsy and accounted for 32.9% of all cases. A further 18.4% of the children showed signs of para- or postinfectious geneses of facial palsy. Facial palsy due to Lyme borreliosis occurred only between May and November. In summer and autumn nearly every second case was due to Lyme borreliosis. Bilateral facial palsy was infrequent, but occurred exclusively in children with

Borrelia infections. In 58.1% of children with Lyme borreliosis a tick bite and/or erythema migrans were noticed, located in the head-neck region in the majority of cases. With only few exceptions, facial palsy manifested within 2 weeks and 3 months (median, 4 weeks) ipsilateral to the side of the tick bite. CSF findings were significantly different according to the cause of the facial palsy. All children with neuroborreliosis, except three, revealed an inflammatory CSF syndrome, consisting of lymphocytic pleocytosis and normal or elevated protein content. This was true in spite of the fact that three-fourths of these children showed no clinical signs of meningeal inflammation. All children with Lyme borreliosis were treated with intravenous penicillin. Independent of the etiology or the therapy administered, one-half of the children experienced improvement within the first 10 days after onset of illness.

Conclusion. Lyme borreliosis proved to be the main cause of acute peripheral facial palsy in children. Because of its high frequency, CSF examination including serological testing for antibodies against *Borrelia burgdorferi* should be performed in all cases. In patients with CSF pleocytosis, Lyme borreliosis has to be suspected unless proven otherwise. In view of the ipsilateral localization of the tick bite and the resulting nerve palsy, a direct invasion of the CNS via the affected nerve by *Borrelia burgdorferi* has to be assumed.

H.-J. Christen, F. Hanefeld, H. Eiffert, and R. Thomssen
Department of Pediatrics and Department of Medical Microbiology,
University Hospital, 37075 Göttingen

Eur Arch Otorhinolaryngology (1994) [Suppl]:S 172

ABSTRACTS

D. López-Aguado, M.E. Campos-Bañales, J. Alvarez, J. Rivero-Suarez, and B. Perez-Piñero

Dehiscences in the Fallopian Canal

Fifty human temporal bones from necropsies were studied, focussing basically on the presence of dehiscences in the fallopian canal and vascular comunications between the facial nerve and the surrounding bone. In our presentation we report the high incidence of dehiscences at the oval window (60%) and in the pyramidal segment (54%). The presence of dehiscences in the fallopian canal at different levels in the same temporal bone was a common finding.

D. López-Aguado, M.E. Campos-Bañales, J. Alvarez,
J. Rivero-Suarez, and B. Perez-Piñero
Hospital Universitario de Canarias, La Laguna, Spain

Eur Arch Otorhinolaryngology (1994) [Suppl]: S 173

ABSTRACTS

H. Nakatani, T. Haji, H. Saito, and T. Takeda

Macrodissection Study on Peripheral Facial Nerve Branches to Stensen's Duct

Electrical resistance of the skin and subcutaneous tissue is one of the major problems of neurophysiological facial nerve testing. The tests are sometimes abandoned due to the pain and stimulating initial artifacts. To overcome this disadvantage, the authors have found that the facial nerve can be stimulated with far less current through Stensen's duct.

Macrodissection of seven sides of the face from five cadavers fixed in a solution of 10% formalin and 5% alcohol were performed under a dissecting microscope. Structures over the facial nerve and Stensen's duct were dissected away, and the distance between the two structures was noted.

The duct was situated deeper than the facial nerve at the level of the orifice. It ran parallel to the facial nerve at a depth of 1.5 – 2.0 cm from the orifice. The closest site was at a depth of 6 – 7 cm from the orifice, where the duct occasionally crossed one of the branches of the nerve. The duct reached to the facial nerve trunk at a depth of 8.0 – 8.5 cm from the orifice. We conclude that Stensen's duct is a favorable site for stimulation of the peripheral branches of the facial nerve.

H. Nakatani, T. Haji, H. Saito, and T. Takeda
Department of Otolaryngology, Kochi Medical School, Nankoku, Kochi, Japan 783

Grading of Facial Palsies

Eur Arch Otorhinolaryngology (1994) [Suppl]: S 177 – S 179

S. A. Burres

The Quantification of Synkinesis and Facial Paralysis

Introduction

Any effective system of grading the paralyzed face must account for the disturbances in both the quantity and quality of motor function. Since adequate force is required for visible animation, the quantity of muscle contraction is the more critical of these two parameters in the face or in any other motor system. The total quantity of force in the facial muscles can be estimated objectively with the linear measurement index (LMI), a conglomerate of point measurements taken from key landmarks during different mimetic expressions [1]. This system of facial grading has been adapted to clinical situations and compares favorably with subjective schemes of facial grading [2, 3].

The reduction in the quality of muscle action is manifested by a loss of peripheral control over localized contraction, an impediment entitled synkinesis. Synkinesis is a more elusive disorder to measure than maximum function since it involves abnormalities in the co-contraction of muscles on the same half-face and also because these motions are purposeful, although not desirable. An index was derived in normal subjects to express the relationship between the integrated EMG (iEMG) activity and the changes in skin distances on the same half-face at maximum effort [1]. This relationship is called the peak electromechanical ratio (PEMR). An increase in the PEMR, indicating the pathologic spread of electrical activity in the face, constitutes a physiologic correlate of synkinesis.

Methods

A random group of 30 facial paralysis patients aged between 17 and 73 years (13 male, 17 female) was accumu-

S. A. Burres
Clinical assistant, Division of Otolaryngology/Head and Neck Surgery, University of California, Los Angeles, 100 UCLA Medical Plaza, Westwood, CA 90024, USA

lated. Acoustic neuroma patients were at least 18 months postoperative status and known to have synkinesis. Bell's palsy cases were studied at any stage of the disorder. Other patients had a wide variety of disorders such as temporal bone fractures, parotid tumors, etc. The facial biomechanical measurements used in this investigation have been detailed in previous publications [1, 2].

With the formula PEMR = log (iEMG)/fractional displacement, the resultant PEMR value has a linear relationship to facial nerve efficiency, i.e., the greater the PEMR, the more effective are the nerve fibers.

Results

In four subjects, the PEMR could not be calculated because the motion and electrical output were too small (Fig. 1). In 26 of the 30 subjects, the abnormally elevated PEMR provided evidene of disturbed facial nerve performance. After an injury to the facial nerve, there is a

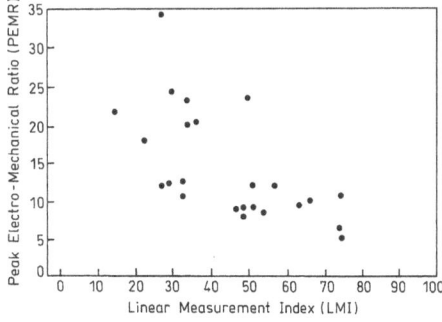

Fig. 1 Peak electromechanical ratio (*PEMR*) versus linear measurement index (*LMI*) for 26 paralysis patients

reduction in the number of fibers passing through the injured segment and a reduction in those reaching the intended muscles. More muscle fibers will be stimulated to produce a specific motion than normally required, because the aberrant branches are unavoidably triggered. In conjunction with the abnormal spread of tension to neighboring muscle groups that occurs in these synkinetic faces, there is a representative increase in EMG output and an elevated PEMR.

Early in recovery, when the LMI is less than 15%, axons begin to reinnervate muscle. During this phase, the PEMR is less than 12 and facial nerve function is fairly efficient. Most of the fibers are contributing to function, and there is little evidence of electromechanical mismatch. Selective control of muscle motion is developed at this point, indicating that if the peripheral pattern of the innervation is favorable, the central organization can adapt to control it.

As motor function improves (15% < LMI < 35%), a mild abnormality is still detected in some cases (PEMR less than 12), e.g., Bell's palsy patients, which may not represents clinically obvious synkinesis. If the abnormal spread of electrical activity is severe enough (PEMR greater than 12), synkinetic facial displays were frequent in the subjects expressions. At some point, the loss of the misdirected fibers has diminished the ultimate potential for normal recovery and limited the maximum tension that can be delivered by any single facial region. If the PEMR is significantly greater than 12, the maximum motor capacity rarely recovers more than 35% of the normal size, whereas if the PEMR remains within two to three times of normal and enough axons traverse the injured segment, the potential full recovery of motor function is greater.

As the LMI scores increased past 35%, the PEMR scores continually declined toward normal. Likewise, the physical recovery has been steadily more acceptable in these subjects. Pathologic levels of synkinesis are rarely detectable in cases with more than 80% symmetry of maximum effort.

Case Examples

The following cases are analyzed in detail and illustrate the nature of the information that was obtained with integrated EMG and the LMI.

Case 1

The patient in case 1 was a 76-year-old man with an incomplete Bell's Palsy of 2 weeks' duration. The LMI was 33% and the PEMR 10.2 (PEMR eye only, 7.0); iEMG on the paralyzed side was 14.3 μV; and on the normal side 35.2 μV (see Fig. 2). As far as the presumed status of the

facial nerve was concerned, 1030 fibers (15%) were intact and functional, 1840 (25%) were intact and misfunctional, and 4130 (59%) were nonfunctional.

The iEMG score on the paralyzed side (14.3 μV) was approximately 41% of that on the normal side, indicating that 41% of the motor units on the paralyzed side had been reinnervated or 41% of the fibers of the facial nerve were intact to innervate the muscle fibers producing the iEMG. Since there is a logarithmic relationship between iEMG and force in the normal face, 41% of the iEMG would be able to generate approximately 79% of the maximum motion if the facial nerve was connected at normal efficiency, yet the LMI indicates that only 33% of the maximum motion was actually being achieved. In fact, the logarithmic relationship predicts that 50% of the facial nerve could be destroyed and if the remaining 50% functions perfectly normally, it could generate about 90% of the maximum facial motion and the loss would be subclinical.

In this patient, a large percentage of the motor units that generate electrical activity were misfunctional, i.e., triggered muscles fibers that either do not contract in a visibly noticeable manner or contracted in a distant area of the face that was not being measured. The PEMR indicates the degree of inefficiency in their distribution. The normal mean value of the PEMR is 3.8, so that this patient's PEMR was approximately 2.7 times normal. For every normally functioning facial motor unit, 1.7 motor units were misfunctional.

Let us suppose there were 7000 fibers in this patient's facial nerve. If 41% of the facial motor units can fire, then presumably 41% of the nerve or 2870 fibers are intact and 4130 fibers have not yet recovered. Based on the PEMR, approximately 1030 of the 2870 are functioning normally and the remaining 1740 are connected to muscle fibers that can be stimulated by voluntary effort and contribute to the iEMG, but do not add to appropriate facial motion.

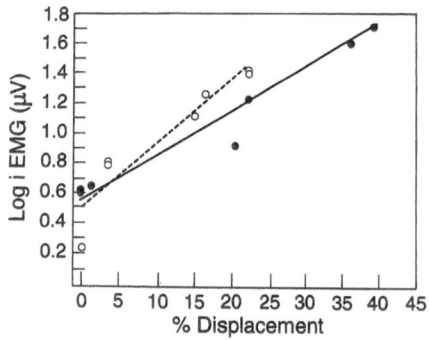

Fig. 2 Case 1. Percentage displacement versus log integrated EMG (iEMG) for eyes closed tightly. ●, normal side; ○, paralyzed side

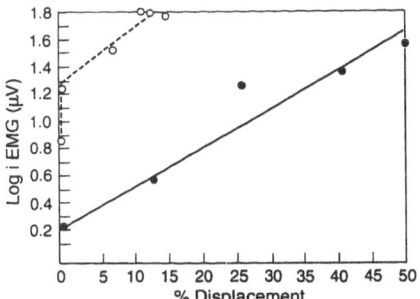

Fig. 3 Patient #2-percent Displacement versus log iEMG for Nose Wrinkle. ●-Normal side ○-paralyzed side

Case 2

The patient in case 2 was a 53-year-old man who was 2 years status post removal of an acoustic neuroma.

The LMI was 36% and the PEMR 18.3 (PEMR eye only 23.8); iEMG on the paralyzed side was 38.3 μV and on the normal side 18.3 μV (see Fig. 3). As far as the presumed status of facial nerve was concerned, 1400 fibers (20%) were intact and functional and 5600 (80%) were intact and misfunctional; there were no nonfunctional fibers.

This phase portrays a physiologic endstage in recovery after facial paralysis. The motor units and the reinnervation process is probably close to 100%, although the LMI shows that only 36% of the face is functional. A large proportion of the detectable electrical activity is not accompanied by purposeful motion in a desired area and, consequently, the PEMR is very high and facial motor efficiency very low. The quantity of motion in the other facial regions on the paralyzed half-face, besides the eye, is invariably less than on the normal side.

Although the number of intact facial nerve fibers on the tumor side may be less than on the normal side, enough had survived the surgery to totally reinnervate the face and so 7000 were presumed to be present.

The iEMG values for the two half-faces seem to be reversed, but they are not. The paralyzed side produces a normal level of maximum iEMG activity (normal means 46.9 μV ± 15.0 μV), again indicating that the face has been totally reinnervated. The output from the patient's normal half-face is subnormal because its effort is not truly maximal, an obstacle in dealing with voluntarily produced electrical activity rather than evoked responses. By habituation, he has learned to limit the motion on his normal side through a subconscious attempt to achieve symmetry

in his expressions. He is unable to voluntarily, without training, fully contract his normal side.

Discussion

Synkinesis and maximum motor function can be estimated objectively after facial nerve paralysis with clinically applicable techniques. Out data substantiates the assertion that maximum motor function is the most important feature to quantify because even when synkinesis is pathologic, there will be a ceiling on the force in any facial region, paralleled by a reduction in the LMI. The LMI also directly quantifies synkinesis by measuring paradoxical motion during several expressions. The percent of normal, misfunctional, and nonfunctional motor units can be estimated independently in all of the major regions of the face.

Synkinesis is a normal phenomenon. The normal human face resorts to synkinesis in order to mount a maximum contraction, e. g., vigorous eye closure is achieved in conjunction with contraction of labial levator and zygomaticus muscles. As more neurons fire to increase force, motor units from sites distance to the center of effort amplify the response, perhaps through anastomotic branches of the facial nerve.

In normal or pathologic faces, synkinesis begins at some threshold point. If the injury has been severe enough to allow the crossover of nerve axons into new myelin columns or fascicles, that threshold may be reset, far below the range that produced the maximum effort demonstrated in normal faces and may then cause a wide spread of electrical activity. In this case, synkinesis will occur every time the patient performs an expression with an intensity over their new threshold and this will be unique for each subject, as their PEMR.

From a biomechanical viewpoint, synkinesis is the result of the subject trying to achieve symmetry between a normal half-face and an abnormal half face. Since the force on the paralyzed half-face cannot match the force on the normal half face by using only the matching contralateral muscles, additional facial muscles are recruited in the effort, although the desired facial display is still not ultimately achieved.

References

1. Burres SA (1985) Facial biomechanics. The standards of normal. Laryngoscope 95 : 708 – 714
2. Burres SA (1986) Objective grading of facial paralysis. ORL 95 : 238 – 241
3. Burres SA (1986) The comparison of facial grading systems. 112 : 755 – 758

Eur Arch Otorhinolaryngology (1994) [Suppl]: S 180 – S 181

FREE PAPERS AND POSTERS

B. R. Ross, G. Fradet, and J. M. Nedzelski

Development of a Sensitive Clinical Facial Grading System

Abstract

Clinicians require a reliable and valid method of evaluating facial function following facial nerve injury. This tool should be clinically relevant, easy to administer, provide a quantitative score for reporting purposes, and be sensitive enough to detect clinically important change over time or with treatment. The objectives of this study were to develop and validate a well-defined grading system that would address the above mentioned points. All essential information, including precise definitions for each item, is presented on one page (Fig. 1, see next page). The facial grading system (FGS) is based on the evaluation of resting symmetry, degree of excursion of facial muscles and degree of synkinesis associated with each voluntary movement. Different regions of the face are examined separately using five standard expressions. All items are graded on point scales and a cumulative composite score, tabulated.

Construct validity was addressed by comparing the proposed FGS to pre- and post-rehabilitation treatment scores of 19 patients that had documented change in a controlled
study of facial feedback training [1]. It succeeds in reporting results in a more continuous manner with a wider response range than the gross House-Brackmann grades [2]. Tests of internal consistency confirmed that each component of the grading system is sensitive to change and individually contributes to a change in the composite score [3].

The proposed FGS, as an evaluative measure requires little time or specialized equipment, and is responsive to clinically important change. Test of intra-rater and inter-rater reliability are currently ongoing.

References

1. Ross BG, Nedzelski JM, McLean JA (1991) Efficacy of feedback training in long-standing facial nerve paresis. Laryngoscope 101: No 7, 744 – 750
2. Burres S, Fisch U (1986) The comparison of facial grading systems. Arch Otolaryngol Head Neck Surg 112: 755 – 758
3. Feinstein AR (1987) Clinimetrics. Yale University Press, New Haven and London, 179 – 181

B. R. Ross, G. Fradet, and J. M. Nedzelski
Department of Otolaryngology,
Sunnybrook Medical Centre, 2075 Bayview Av.,
North York, Ontario, Canada M4N 3M5

Facial Grading System

Resting Symmetry

Compared to normal side

Eye (choose one only)
- normal — 0
- narrow — 1
- wide — 1
- eyelid surgery — 1

Cheek (naso-labial fold)
- normal — 0
- absent — 2
- less pronounced — 1
- more pronounced — 1

Mouth
- normal — 0
- corner drooped — 1
- corner pulled up/out — 1

Total ☐

Resting symmetry score — Total × 5 ☐

Patient's name

Dx

Date

Symmetry of Voluntary Movement

Degree of muscle EXCURSION compared to normal side

Standard Expressions — columns: Unable to initiate movement/no movement; Initiates slight movement; Initiates movement with mid excursion; Movement almost complete; Movement complete

Standard Expressions	1	2	3	4	5	
Forehead Wrinkle (FRO)	1	2	3	4	5	☐
Gentle eye closure (OCS)	1	2	3	4	5	☐
Open mouth Smile (ZYG/RIS)	1	2	3	4	5	☐
Snarl (LLA/LLS)	1	2	3	4	5	☐
Lip Pucker (OOS/OOI)	1	2	3	4	5	☐

Gross Asymmetry / Severe Asymmetry / Moderate Asymmetry / Mild Asymmetry / Normal symmetry — Total ☐

Voluntary movement score: Total × 4 ☐

Synkinesis

Rate the degree of INVOLUNTARY MUSCLE CONTRACTION associated with each expression

NONE: No synkinesis or mass movement; MILD: Slight synkinesis; MODERATE: Obvious but not disfiguring synkinesis; SEVERE: Disfiguring synkinesis/Gross mass movement of several muscles

	0	1	2	3	
Forehead Wrinkle (FRO)	0	1	2	3	☐
Gentle eye closure (OCS)	0	1	2	3	☐
Open mouth Smile (ZYG/RIS)	0	1	2	3	☐
Snarl (LLA/LLS)	0	1	2	3	☐
Lip Pucker (OOS/OOI)	0	1	2	3	☐

Synkinesis score: Total ☐

Vol mov't score ☐ − Resting symmetry score ☐ − Synk score ☐ = Composite score ☐

Ross, Fradet, Nedzelski 1992

Fig. 1 Facial grading system

Eur Arch Otorhinolaryngology (1994) [Suppl]: S 182 – S 184

FREE PAPERS AND POSTERS

M. Frey, A. Jenny, E. Stüssi, S. Handschin, and R. Manktelow

Development of a New Paresis Scoring System for Pre- and Postoperative Evaluation of Facial Paresis

Introduction

Five years' experience with the International Muscle Transplant Registry [1, 2] showed that the Stennert's Scheme [3] and all the other paresis scoring systems are not able to represent the static and dynamic details of the face which are affected by facial paralysis or by surgical procedures for functional reconstruction. At that time, the International Muscle Transplant Registry included patients with facial paresis who were treated with free muscle transplantation. Analyzing 137 patients from six different countries, the description of the functional results by the improvement of the paresis scores was far too imprecise. The functional details of the different regions of the face treated by muscle transplantation were not sufficiently represented. Reorganizing the International Registry, we included three-dimensional measurements of facial movements for functional assessment.

Material and Methods

After some positive experiences with three-dimensional, computer-assisted measurements in patients with unilateral facial paresis, normal facial movements in 16 young sport students were studied. A VICON system together with four cameras was used for three-dimensional motion analysis [4].

M. Frey (✉) and A. Jenny
Klinik für Hand-, Plastische und Wiederherstellungschirurgie,
Department Chirurgie, Universitätspital, Rämistrasse 100,
8091 Zürich, Switzerland

E. Stüssi, S. Handschin
Laboratorium für Biomechanik der ETH Zürich, Switzerland

R. Manktelow
Department of Hand- and Reconstructive Microsurgery,
General Hospital, Toronto, Canada

Based on the measurements of the facial movements, a map of static and dynamic points in the face was designed. The consistency and importance of the different points were tested in ten different exercises, seven of them as bilateral exercises such as maximal lifting of eyebrows, closure of eyelids, screwing up the nose, maximal showing of the teeth, maximal pull of the corners of the mouth downwards, pursing of the lips, and biting the teeth. Two unilateral exercises included separate maximal pull of the corner of the mouth up and backwards on the right and on the left side. The tenth exercise was a complex smile. Every exercise was repeated three times in each tested individual and sufficient time was given for relaxation between the exercises. The stored data were analyzed later in terms of the following questions:

1. Do the static points really stay static during all the exercises?
2. Which of the dynamic points are most representative for the movements in the different regions of the face?
3. Which of the relations between the different dynamic and static points in the face best reflect regional function?

Results

Static Points

A minimum of three static points are necessary to define a three-dimensional space. In previous reports on functional results, the tragus point was frequently used as a static point, and Manktelow proposed the central chin point (CC). Because we had some doubts about the CC, we were looking for a third static point besides the two tragus points on the right and left side. We decided on the central nose point (CN), a small, constantly calm area in the dorsum of the nose. Motion analyses showed that only the two tragus points and the CN are real static points with an excursion of about 1% of the maximal distance or, in millimeters, less than 1 mm, whereas the CC was moved similarly to a dynamic point (e.g., excursion CC – CN = 4.21% of maximum distance, SD = 3.25, $n = 250$).

Dynamic Points

For clinical application, the number of points and the distances measured between the points have to be limited to a minimum which is both practicable and which gives a complete functional status of the face. The brow point at the crossing of the upper border of the eyebrow and the pupillar line were selected for the frontal region. Closing of the eyes is best represented by the upper and lower eyelid points at the crossing of the border of the eyelids with the pupillar line. The complex movements of the naso-oral region is described by the corner of the mouth point, the midlateral point of the upper lip in the middle between the philtrum point and the corner of the mouth at the vermillion border, the midlateral point of the lower lip, the philtrum point in the middle of the philtrum at the vermillion border, and the alar of the nose point at the lowest point of the alar in the crease to the upper lip.

Distances Relevant for Measurements

The functional assessment of the frontal region is restricted to one distance, i.e., the minimum and maximum distance between the CN and the brow point is measured on both sides during the exercise of maximal lifting of the eyebrows. The excursion was optimal for this distance and for this exercise.

For the function of eye closure, too, only one representative distance is measured during one exercise. The distance between the upper and the lower eyelid point is documented during closure of eyelids as in sleep.

Because the nose–mouth complex showed the need for more details to be described, four distances are used in clinical application. The changes in the distance between the tragus point and the mouth corner point mainly describe the lateral component of the movement of the mouth; those in the distance between the CN and the midlateral point of the upper lip describe more the upward component. The distance between the CN and the midlateral point of the lower lip is used to detect asymmetric disfigurement of the paralyzed lower lip. Although nose and mouth are mostly moved together in mimic activity, the distance between CN and the alar of the nose point gives important information on the symmetry of the nose and distorsion during movements. Shifting of the philtrum is best documented by the distance between the tragus point and the philtrum point. These distances are measured during four exercises: maximal showing of the teeth, smiling with lips losed, smiling with showing teeth, and pursing of the lips. All

selected points showed high reproducibility. The fixation of the luminescent half-spheres could be performed at the same defined place. Repeated fixation involving different investigators never produced a mistake of more than 1 mm.

Discussion

Using a VICON system for three-dimensional analyses of facial movements, a map of significant static and dynamic points in the face was successfully designed. Many of the relations of the different points were tested by distance measurements during ten different mimic exercises. The distances most representative for the regional functions in the face were selected, as well as the most important exercises. Measuring the minimum and the maximum values for the different distances, the excursions of the dynamic points can form a detailed, quantitative functional status of the face. This kind of functional assessment is the only one sensitive enough to detect and to describe partial or incomplete facial palsies and to describe functional recovery after surgical reconstructions. Measurements on both sides of the face give an exact description of symmetry of the face during rest and during mimic activation.

However, it is not enough to document facial function in millimeters. Therefore, in addition to integrating these movement measurements into the forms for "Paralysis Assessment" in the International Registry for Neuromuscular Reconstruction in the Face, we also used a questionnaire on the quality of facial function. Part of this involves asking about or investigating associated physiologic abnormalities, and we differenciate between complete and incomplete, and between total and partial, facial paresis. We judge exact preoperative documentation of the function that is expected to be improved by the procedure to be as important as the function that has recovered postoperatively. A description of the specific local function of the most important facial muscles is of high value in describing partial lesions or when reinnervation takes place in facial muscles.

Because of the extremely complex nature of facial palsy and its treatment, a complex documentation such as that of the International Registry for Neuromuscular Reconstruction in the Face is necessary. Attempting to make quantitative measurements of facial movements realistic for daily clinical application, we developed a simple instrument for distance measurements in the face. After documentation of a sufficient number of patients with facial palsy, it will be possible to correlate scoring to the stored data; studies on details of facial palsy and its treatment should be only performed on pooled, detailed data.

References

1. Frey M, Sing D, Harii K, Hakelius L, Stevenson T, Freilinger G, Nicolai J-P A, Sing C (1991) Free muscle transplantation for treatment of facial palsy – first experiences with the International Muscle Transplant Registry. Eur J Plast Surg 14:212–218
2. Plummer EA, Sing DB, Faulkner JA, Sing CF (1985) Software for a muscle transplant registry. In: Frey M, Freilinger G (eds) 2nd Vienna Muscle Symposium – proceedings. Facultas, Vienna, pp 371–375
3. Stennert E, Limberg CM, Fentrup KP (1979) Paralysis and secondary defect score. In. Miehlke A, Stennert E, Hilla R (eds) New aspects in facial surgery. Clin Plast Surg 6:458
4. Stüssi E, Handschin S, Frey M (1992) Quantifizierung von Gesichtsasymmetrien – eine Methode zur Objektivierung von Beeinträchtigungen der Gesichtsmotorik; eine Pilotstudie. Biomed Tech (Berlin) 37:14–19

Eur Arch Otorhinolaryngology (1994) [Suppl]:S185–S186

T. Minatogawa, Y. Nishimura, and T. Kumoi

Prediction of Prognosis in Facial Nerve Palsy using Constellation Diagram

Introduction

Prediction of the prognosis of facial nerve palsy has been attempted using values obtained by neurophysiological examinations. However, the values obtained by these methods are only a cross-section of the entire course of the palsy. In order to assess more simply and concisely the prognosis of the disease during the early stage, we applied the constellation diagram method to depict the course of mimetic movement diagrammatically.

Materials and Methods

The subjects were 31 patients with Bell's palsy and 18 with Hunt's syndrome in whom mimetic movement had been recorded (every fifth day for the former and every tenth day for the latter) from the onset of palsy. To evaluate mimetic movement, we adopted a scoring system of $0-100$ points [1, 2] in which mimetic movement is divided into ten items.

Values obtained every 5 days for 25 days in Bell's palsy and every 10 days for 40 days in Hunt's syndrome were analyzed with two-way layout ANOVA (analysis of variance) to determine the significance of differences and the variance patterns of the progress between groups with complete and incomplete recovery.

Results

Bell's Palsy

Calculation of the values with a stepwise discriminant analysis of multivariate analysis was performed using the scores of A (fifth day), B (tenth day), C (15th day), D (20th day) and E (25th day). The rate of accuracy in forecasting the outcome of recovery with scores A and B was 74.7% (probability of error rate, 1%), with A, B and C, 75.8% (probability of error rate, 0.7%), with A, B, C and D, 85.5% (probability of error rate, 0.1%) and with A, B, C, D and E, 90% (probability of error rate, 0.02%). Figure 1 shows an example of a scatter diagram of discriminant analysis plotting the scores of A (5th day) on the abscissa, and those of B (10th day) on the ordinate, and the linear discriminant line is drawn using the linear discriminant junction

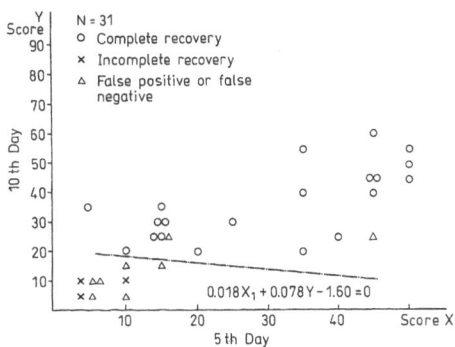

Fig. 1 Scatter diagram of patients with Bell's palsy. The line of linear discriminant function ($0.018X + 0.078Y - 1.60 = 0$) is drawn. *Abscissa*, score of mimetic movement on fifth day after onset of paralysis. *Ordinate*, score of mimetic movement on tenth day after onset of paralysis

H. Minatogawa (✉), Y. Nishimura, and T. Kumoi
Department of Otolaryngology, Hyogo College of Medicine,
1-1, Mukogawa-cho, Nishinomiya, 663 Japan

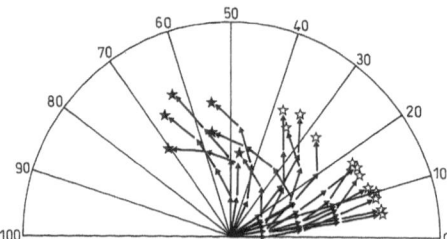

Fig. 2 Constellation diagram of 18 patients with Hunt's syndrome. Cases of complete recovery are represented by *black stars* and cases of incomplete recovery are represented by *white stars*

day, with a score of 16.7 ± 16.5 in the complete recovery group and 7.5 ± 5 in the incomplete recovery group. In cases of Hunt's syndrome with scores of mimetic movement above 15 at 10 days after onset, complete cure ensued, whereas those with a score below 10 resulted in only incomplete cure ($p < 0.01$, Fisher's exact probability test).

The variance patterns of the complete and incomplete recovery groups obtained from three classes (A, B and C) were significantly different ($p < 0.01$). The constellation diagram drawn from 18 cases is shown in Fig. 2. The vector of most of the complete recovery patients shows anticlockwise rotation at the P3 points, suggesting a favourable recovery process.

(Z) of $0.018X + 0.078Y - 1.60 = 0$. When a dot of one patient's score of A and B comes above the line, then complete recovery is expected with a probability of 74.7%. Triangles indicate false positive or false negative cases which did not meet the prediction from the data of A and B.

The data of the present series of Bell's palsy were also analyzed by two-way ANOVA using two groups (complete and incomplete recovery) and five classes, A, B, C, D and E. The variance pattern obtained from A, B, C and D showed a significant difference between the two groups ($p < 0.01$).

Hunt's Syndrome

The same method of analysis as for Bell's palsy was performed on 18 cases of Hunt's syndrome, with two groups of recovery (complete and incomplete) and four classes: A (10 days), B (20 days), C (30 days) and D (40 days).

The discriminant analysis of scores of mimetic movement showed a significant difference as early as the tenth

Discussion

This study demonstrated that the constellation diagram, which does not involve complex mathematical calculations, is very useful in the follow-up of facial nerve palsy. This method may also be of use in the follow-up of numerical data in other fields of clinical investigation.

Although the number of cases in the present series is quite limited, if a large number of patients could be obtained through a co-operative field study, a more exact linear discriminant function equation would be expected, and thus within 5, 10 or 15 days after the onset of facial nerve palsy we could predict the patient's outcome and select the optimal treatment modality for that patient.

References

1. Kinishi M et al. (1983) Evaluation method for the degree of facial palsy. Facial N Res Jpn 3 : 1–3
2. May M (1970) Facial paralysis, peripheral type: a proposed method of reporting. Laryngoscope 80 : 331–390

Eur Arch Otorhinolaryngology (1994) [Suppl]: S 187–188

FREE PAPERS AND POSTERS

V. Gallati and H. Scriba

Computer-Assisted Grading of Facial Function

Introduction

A standardized method has been developed to measure objectively the degree of facial nerve palsy of a patient. This problem has not yet been solved [1–6]. Such an objective method would enable a comparison of results between different researchers. Facial function can be measured optically by observing structural movement and the creation of new creases in the face on change of expression. These optical observations can be evaluated using a computer-aided image-processing system.

Materials and Methods

An IBM-compatible 386 PC was used with the image-processing program Optimas running under Microsoft Windows. For evaluation we used the built-in macro-language in connection with compiled C modules. The images were taken with a black-and-white high-resolution video camera fitted with a lens of fixed focal length. This camera was adjusted to a fixed position and was directly connected to the computer system. In order to make picture subtractions, the position of the head should not change while being photographed. This problem was solved by means of a head fixation system (cephalostat), which is a modified version of an instrument used for X-ray tomography at the Department of Maxillofacial Surgery at the University of Zurich. By this method, all necessary pictures can be taken in less than 5 min.

V. Gallati (✉)
ORL Klinik, Universitätsspital Zürich, Rämistrasse 100, 8091 Zürich, Switzerland

H. Scriba
Department of Dentofacial Orthopedics, Universität of Zurich, Director Prof. P. W. Stöckli, Switzerland

The starting point for a subtraction is the picture of the face at rest. From this, a picture of the face in motion is subtracted, in our example a person smiling. The difference in the corresponding gray-scale values at each point in the pictures is displayed: This subtracted picture is binarized using a fixed threshold. The luminance values above the threshold are counted in the corresponding areas (Fig. 1). In the case of a complete paralysis, there is a further difficulty. Owing to the strictly one-sided movement, the paralyzed side is drawn towards the healthy side. This "pseudomovement" must be eliminated, which was achieved by pixelwise subtraction accompanied by the elimination of negative values.

Results

In subjects with normal facial function, an asymmetry of up to 13% was found. In patients with paresis, we obtained

Table 1 First results of the computer-assisted grading system compared with the grading system of House and Fisch

	Grading system		
	House (class)	Fisch (%)	Computer-assisted (%)
Normal			
Patient 1	I	100	94
Patient 2	I	100	90
Patient 3	I	100	87
Paresis			
Patient 4	II	79	74
Patient 5	IV	38	34
Patient 6	III	66	60
Paralysis			
Patient 7	VI	0	7
Patient 8	VI	0	10
Patient 9	VI	0	11

Fig. 1 **a** Face at rest. **b** Face in motion. **c** Subtraction of **a** and **b**. **d** Binarized picture of **c**

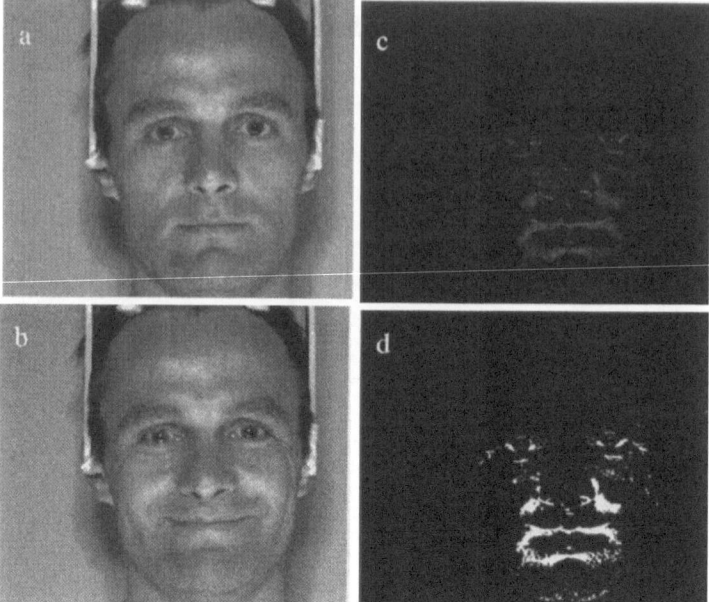

results similar to the grading systems of Fisch and House (Table 1). Even with patients suffering from facial paresis together with synkinesis, both the paresis and the synkinesis can be clearly recognized and assessed.

There are preliminary results. At present the method is in clinical use to obtain results with a large number of patients with different types of facial palsy.

References

1. Burres S (1985) Facial biomechanics: the standards of normal. Laryngoscope 95 : 708 – 714
2. Burres S (1986) The comparisons of facial grading systems. Arch Otolaryngol Head Neck Surg 112 : 7
3. Damenz W (1990) FANDOS – eine standardisierte computergestützte Dokumentation und Auswertung von Erkrankungen des Nervus facialis. HNO 38 : 116 – 118
4. Fisch U (1981) Surgery of bells palsy. Arch Otolaryngol 90 : 1 – 11
5. House JW (1985) Facial nerve grading system. Otolaryngol Head Neck Surg 93 : 146
6. Stennert E (1990) Objective clinical measurement and scoring of facial nerve function and paresis. Facial nerve. Kugler and Ghedini, Amsterdam, pp 563 – 566

Eur Arch Otorhinolaryngology (1994) [Suppl]: S 189

ABSTRACTS

C. Jaquenod and A. Boehmer

Subjective Evaluation of Facial Function by the Patient

Forty-seven patients with a history of clinical complete facial nerve palsy were enrolled in a case control study to determine the accuracy of the results of a questionnaire including a subjective global self-estimation by the patients (SGE), a section of 12 questions, and a card to measure voluntary facial movements by the patients themselves.

All patients underwent clinical examination after having returned completed questionnaires. Their facial function was recorded by the video. The recordings were then judged by a board of five experts in facial-function estimation. The median of their objective global estimations (OGE) was regarded as the standard of facial function for each patient. Comparing the results of the questionnaire with the OGE of the experts established a good correlation between the self-measurement by the patients and the OGE and revealed a good predetermination of a possible range of estimation of the remaining facial functions through answering the 12-question section of the questionnaire.

In conclusion the questionnaire and the self-measurement of facial movements by the patient have to be considered a good tool for the predetermination and estimation of remaining facial function as a subjective method of evaluation of facial function by the patient.

C. Jaquenod and A. Boehmer
Clinic and Policlinic of Otorhinolaryngologia, Head-Necksurgery,
University-Hospital of Zürich, 8091 Zürich, Switzerland

Eur Arch Otorhinolaryngology (1994) [Suppl]: S 190

ABSTRACTS

J. Rickenmann, C. Jaquenod, and U. Fisch

Comparative Value of Facial Nerve Grading Systems

The Fisch grading system (Fisch 1981) and the House-Brackmann grading systems were compared by statistical examination for their reliability and interobserver variability. Furthermore their correlation and their agreement with a standard global evaluation were compared. Forty-seven patients with facial palsies of different etiology were evaluated with the two systems and with a global overall evaluation performed by five ENT surgeons familiar with facial palsy. The Fisch grading system showed a high reliability of 0.93 compared to a reliability of 0.77 with the House grading system (the international standard requires a reliability of at least 0.8). The mean interobserver variability was 5.24% (SD = 3.2) for the Fisch grading system and 9.26% (SD = 5.0) for the House-Brackmann grading system. With a confidence limit of 95% the interobserver variability is not more than 11.6% for the Fisch grading system and 19.26% for the House grading system. The correlation of both gradings with the global evaluation was high with $r = 0.98$ and $r = 0.97$, respectively. The Fisch grading system showed excellent agreement (difference to the global evaluation less than 10%) with the global overall evaluation in 41 of 47 cases (87%) and the House grading system in 32 of 47 cases (66%). These results demonstrate that the Fisch grading system is a highly reliable and valid method of facial nerve evaluation. Due to the low interobserver variability it allowed evaluation in 10% steps, in contrast to the House grading system, which allowed steps of only 20%.

Reference

Fisch U (1981) Surgery for Bell's palsy. Arch Otolaryngol 107:1

J. Rickenmann, C. Jaquenod, and U. Fisch
Department of Otorhinolaryngology, Head and Neck Surgery,
University Hospital, 8091 Zürich, Switzerland

Botulinum Toxin

Eur Arch Otorhinolaryngology (1994) [Suppl]: S 193 – S 194

T. Kobayashi, K. Sugasawa, K. Ishii, and N. Takeuchi

Treatment of Hemifacial Spasm with Botulinum Toxin

Introduction

In our otolaryngology clinic, following dystonias in the head and neck, hemifacial spasm, blepharospasm, Meige syndrome, facial synkinesis, and spastic dysphonia have been observed. Hemifacial spasm is the most frequently seen. A vascular compression of the facial nerve root in the cerebellopontine angle can be demonstrated in most cases. Although microvascular decompression surgery (Jannetta) at the facial nerve root exit has been widely introduced, the success rate is not 100%. Some patients are reluctant to undergo such a procedure beause of the treatment failure and the risk of facial paralysis, hearing loss, and other complications. Selective resection or blocking of the facial nerve branch is not so popular these days, because of the high recurrence rate. Since 1988, we have been using botulinum toxin to control various conditions of dystonia in the head and neck area.

Patients

A total of 65 patients had hemifacial spasm, all of which had failed to respond to medication and/or nerve blocking. Five patients had recurrences after Jannetta surgery. The severity of spasm was classified as follows: grade 0, normal; grade 1, mild; grade 2, moderate; grade 3, severe; and grade 4, extreme. Pretreatment grades of our patients were from 1 to 4.

T. Kobayashi (✉)
Department of Otolaryngology, Teikyo University Hospital, Anesaki 3426, Ichihara City, Chiba 299, Japan, and Department of Otolaryngology, Japan Railway Tokyo General Hospital, Yoyogi 2-1-3, Tokyo 151, Japan

K. Sugasawa, K. Ishii, and N. Takeuchi
Department of Otolaryngology, Faculty of Medicine University of Tokyo, Hongo 7-3-1, Tokyo 113, Japan

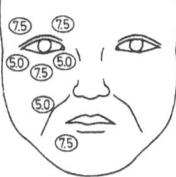

Fig. 1. Treatment plan of hemifacial spasm (grade 3) in a 59-year-old woman, (*numbers* indicate units of drug injected)

Four further patients had blepharospasm and four had synkinesis of the facial muscles as sequelae of palsy (three post-Bell's palsy and one post-traumatic palsy). Another two patients had Meige syndrome.

Drug and Method

We used botulinum toxin (type A), which was prepared by the Chiba Serum Institute of Japan. The freeze-dried toxin was used. A solution with a concentration of 5 units/0.1 ml was freshly prepared just before injection. A 1-ml syringe with a minute scale of 0.05 ml was used. The 23-gauge injection needle was completely coated except for its tip; this was used as an electrode for EMG monitoring. In hemifacial spasm, the most frequently involved area is the orbicularis muscle. Figure 1 shows the treatment plan for injection in one specific case.

Results

In hemifacial spasm, all patients showed improvement. The patients with higher grades (grades 3 and 4) of severity were found to have a higher success rate, both subjectively and objectively. However, none of our series showed grade 0 after injection. Neither history of previous treatments (nerve blocking and Jannetta surgery) nor duration of symptoms influenced the results.

Relief of spasm began the day after injection. The maximum effect was obtained on the third or fourth day after the injection. The beneficial effect showed gradual decrease between 8 and 16 weeks (12 weeks on average).

In blepharospasm, synkinesis, and Meige syndrome, the results were poorer than in hemifacial spasm. In one patient with blepharospasm (a 77-year-old man), accompanying pain was relieved each time after the botulinum toxin treatments.

Complications were upper eye lid ptosis, disappearance of the nasolabial fold, and mouth droop. During this study, two patients with hemifacial spasm asked to proceed to Jannetta surgery, because of the inconvenience of frequent treatments. These patients had two and four treatments of botulinum toxin, respectively, before surgeries were subsequently and successfully performed.

Comments

Site of Injection

In hemifacial spasm and blepharospasm, we injected directly into the oribicularis oculi muscle. In the upper periorbital area, injections were placed at the extreme medial and lateral portion of the orbicularis oculi muscle. Injection at the center of the upper eye lid must be avoided, because of ptosis following injection. In some cases, further injections were given to the zygomaticus, the levator labii superioris, and the mentalis muscles for control of the lower face (Fig. 1).

Doses of Toxin and Duration of Therapeutic Effect

The doses of the toxin at one treatment in hemifacial spasm should be less than 50 units. Doses of more than 50 units around the periorbital area may produce ptosis and incomplete closure of the eye. The duration of effect lasted for 8–16 weeks. Even within a given case and dose, the duration of the effect varied with sequential injections.

Complications

Complications were related to the injection site and the amount of toxin injected. No systemic effects were observed in our study. So far, there has been no evidence of antibody formation against botulinum toxin in patients' serum in our Japanese group study. An animal experiment in which large doses were given showed rapid induction of antibody with in 10–14 days after injection of the toxin. Therefore, an injection interval of at least 2 months is recommended [1]. Injections with an interval of 6 months produce practically no antibody at all, because doses are so small.

Indications

Patients with hemifacial spasm experienced better control than other dystonic conditions such as blepharospasm, synkinesis, or Meige syndrome. Swift muscular movements, as seen in hemifacial spasm, were more easily controlled than somewhat sluggish movements, as seen in blepharospasm and Meige syndrome. The pathomechanism of involuntary muscle movements appears to differ in these conditions. Another principle we studied is that the more specific and well-localized the muscles involved, the more easily the disorders are controlled.

In hemifacial spasm, we inject botulinum toxin in following cases:

1. Patients who do not want Jannetta surgery
2. Patients whose physical condition does not permit surgery
3. Patients with recurrence after surgery
4. Patients who have hearing only in the spastic side
5. Patients whose occupation does not permit even temporary facial palsy (actors, singers, and other public figures)

International Agreement

Grading of hemifacial spasm and unification of drug units must be considered in the near future.

Reference

1. Chiba Serum Institute (1992) Botulinum toxin note, no 3

Eur Arch Otorhinolaryngology (1994) [Suppl]: S 195 – S 199

R. Laskawi, W. Damenz, P. Roggenkämper, and A. Baetz

Botulinum Toxin Treatment in Patients with Facial Synkinesis

Introduction

Botulinum toxin therapy (BTT), originally applied to treat strabism (for review see [8]), is now established as a minimally invasive, successful therapy in a number of diseases. The treatment of mass movements (synkinesis) following paralysis of the facial nerve, which may have various etiologies, has recently been reported as another indication. First experiences with BTT, applied to several patients with such synkinesis, were published by Roggenkämper et al. [7]. This indication was also confirmed by case reports by other authors [2, 6]. According to Roggenkämper et al. [7] this treatment is effective for an average of 11 weeks after the first injection, according to patients' personal assessment.

In this paper we describe our extended experience, the technique of botulinum toxin injection, the choice of an appropriate dose, experience concerning the length of the effective period, control of the therapeutic effect, and possible side effects.

Patients and Methods

Altogether 23 patients (six men, 17 women) with synkinesis after facial nerve paralysis of various etiologies – 14 Bell's palsy (61%), six after hypoglossal-facial nerve anastomosis (26%), three zoster oticus (13%) – were treated at the ENT Department of the University of Göttingen. The patients' ages ranged from 25 to 87 years ($\bar{x}$, 53.7 years).

R. Laskawi, W. Damenz, and A. Baetz
ENT-Department, University of Göttingen, Robert-Koch-Str. 40, 37075 Göttingen, Germany

P. Roggenkämper
Department of Ophtalmology, University of Bonn

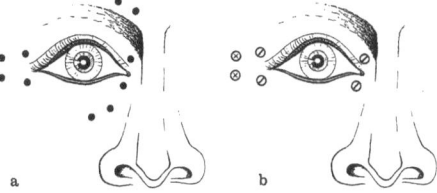

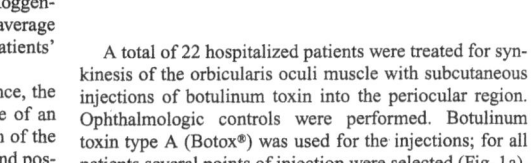

Fig. 1 a Possible periocular injection points. b Example of a upright *first* total dose with injection points and single-point doses. ⊘ 1.25 U; ⊗ 2.5 U

A total of 22 hospitalized patients were treated for synkinesis of the orbicularis oculi muscle with subcutaneous injections of botulinum toxin into the periocular region. Ophthalmologic controls were performed. Botulinum toxin type A (Botox®) was used for the injections; for all patients several points of injection were selected (Fig. 1a). The total number of treatments was 59.

For an exact assessment of different degrees of BTT efficacy, the width of the palpebral fissure (PFW; maximum distance in millimeters between directly opposed points on the lower and upper lid) was measured with sliding callipers during various facial movements not involving the eye itself (e.g., frowning or exposing teeth).

In principle, mass movements after defective healing of facial paralysis can manifest themselves in a variety of ways (Fig. 2), e.g., after only one or more movements of various facial regions that normally are not accompanied by eye movements. These movements will be referred to below as "non-eye movements" (NEM). We always tested five standard movements before and after therapy: frowning, closing eyes, exposing teeth, turning up nose, and pouting. The reason for also checking eye closure was to estimate its possible influence on mass movements in other facial areas such as the perioral region. Knowledge about therapy of such synkinesis is scant. We only treated two of our patients in the perioral region. Documentation of the

Fig. 2 Variations of m. orbicularis oculi mass movements. *top (Ia, b)*, various "non-eye movements" cause eyelid closure on the affected ide. *Middle (IIa, b)*, palpebral fissure width on the right side during smiling and frowning is identical, but esthetically less satisfactory during frowning since the difference in PFW is greater. *Bottom (IIIa, b)*, eyelid closure only during pouting

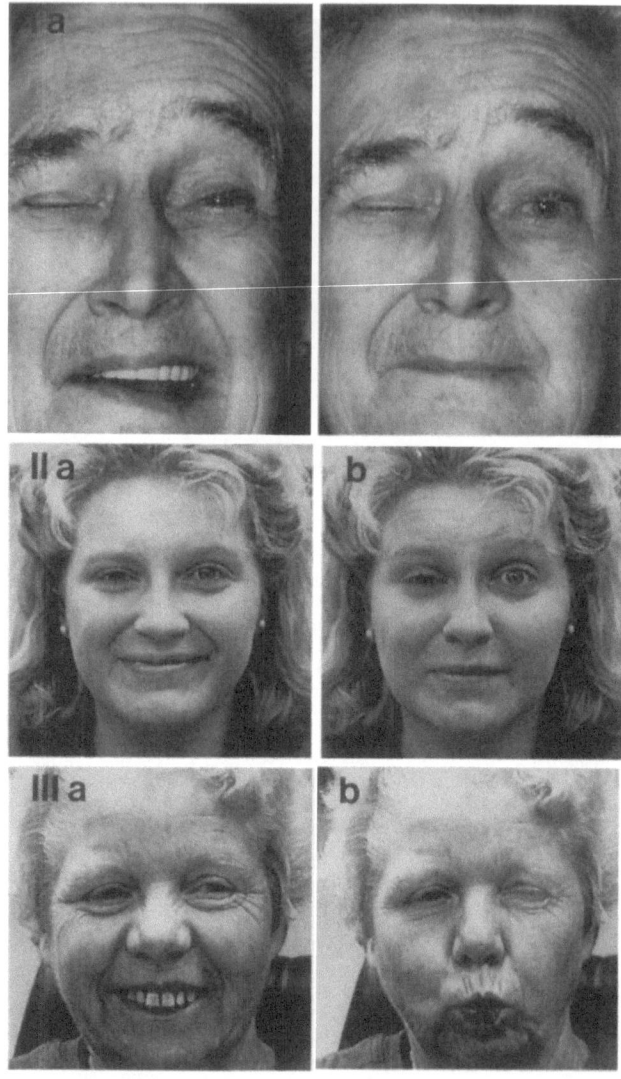

therapeutic result was done by referring to the standard movement (looking straight ahead) which produced the greatest difference in PFW between the affected and the healthy eye before therapy.

If, however, an NEM caused a greater difference of PFW after therapy than any of the NEM before, then this post-therapeutic NEM served as the basis of comparison. This occurred, however, in only two cases. Values of the affected side were expressed as percentages of PFW of the healthy side before and after therapy.

Control measurements, performed at two different times in seven healthy adult volunteers (five men, two women), revealed that the absolute values of PFW produced by identical NEM in different subjects (Fig. 3) varied considerably (from 3 to 13 mm). The increase in PFW alone was therefore not taken as the basis for evaluat-

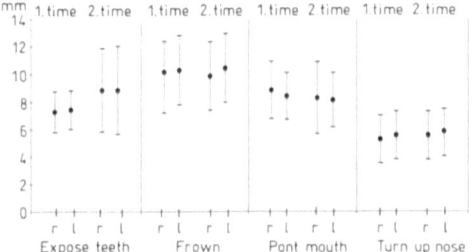

mm 1.time 2.time 1.time 2.time 1.time 2.time 1.time 2.time
14
12
10
8
6
4
2
0
    r l   r l   r l   r l   r l   r l   r l   r l
     Expose teeth   Frown   Pont mouth   Turn up nose

Fig. 3 Normal values (± SD; $n = 7$) for palpebral fissure width (PFW) during various movements not involving the eye

ing therapeutic success; to make an assessment of the degree of convergence of the two sides, its relation to the healthy side was used instead. Side differences (between right and left eye) did not exceed 1 mm in healthy subjects. Patients were questioned as to the persistence of the therapeutic effect and the possible presence of side effects.

Results

All synkinesis of the orbicularis oculi muscle improved or was at last arrested, resulting in an approximation of PFW

to the healthy side during various facial movements. A number of patients reported an improved motility of the forehead. This can be explained by weakened orbicularis oculi muscles [12].

It is interesting to note that our patients (see Fig. 4a, b) usually had no complete paralysis of the treated muscles, but rather showed a change which can be characterized as a "weakening" or incomplete paralysis. In those patients in whom we performed an electromyogram (EMG) of the orbicularis oculi muscle, we found voluntary innervation pattern, indicating that muscle innervation was still possible (Fig. 1, d).

The number of single points of injection (eye region) varied between three and ten. Figure 1a shows the location of points being used. The total dose per patient (eye region) varied from 3.75 units Botox® (U) to 23.75 U. On average, 10.9 U ± 5.67 was administered. Single doses per injection point varied from 1.25 to 2.5 U.

Our measurements showed that an effect could be observed in all patients as early as 3 days after the initial or the follow-up treatment. The subjective assessment of the full effect of the first injection by patients who had at least two injections was on average, 8.6 weeks. Figure 5a shows, in percentages, the maximum approximation of PFW of all patients following the first treatment for the various doses selected and for a time interval sufficient to safely assume an effect of BTT having set in. As can be seen, higher doses

Fig. 4a, b Patient after hypoglossal-facial nerve anastomosis following excision of an acoustic neurinoma. **b** Palpebral fissure width (PFW) after botulinum toxin therapy (BTT). **a** By associated movement of the orbicularis oculi muscle, PFW is distinctly narrower on the operated side when the patient exposes her teeth. **c, d** EMG 2 weeks after BTT (distinct voluntary innervation pattern, arrow in **d** marks begin of innervation)

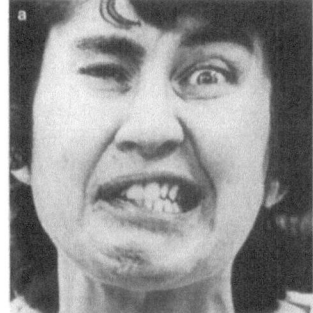
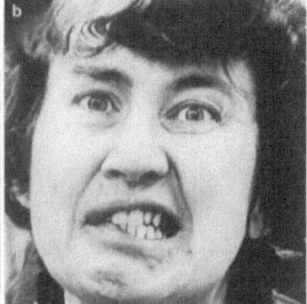
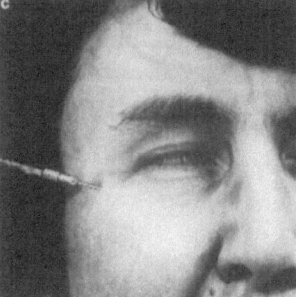
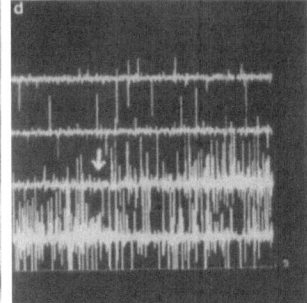

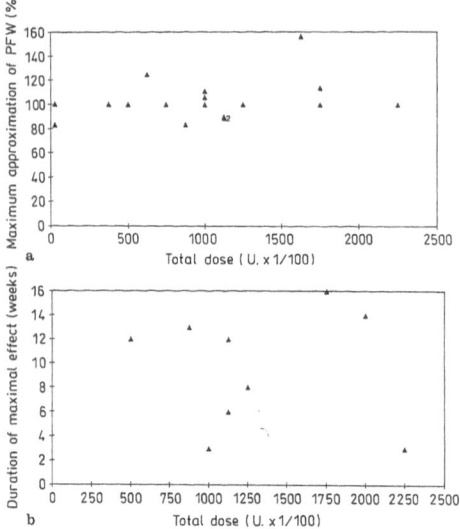

Fig. 5a, b First botulinum toxin treatment for synkinesis. **a** Maximum approximation of the palpebral fissure width (*PFW*) measured (%) for various doses (days 3–40). **b** Subjective assessment of length of effective period for different doses selected

do not result in wider PFW. Figure 5b shows, for the different doses applied, the length of time following the first injection during which the patients subjectively felt the full effect of treatment. The average time ($\bar{x}$) stated was 8.6 ± 4.07 weeks.

Figure 6 depicts the time course of PFW measurements in all patients after the first treatment. The total dose given to those patients who attained an approximation between

90% and 110% after the first injection for several measurements varied from 3.75 U to 22.5 U, with an average of $10.7 U \pm 5.38$. In choosing the starting dose (see Fig. 1b), one should be led by the clinical grade of severity of synkinesis. In patients having, for instance, a complete eye closure, a higher dose should be given rather than a lower. Since the response seems to differ individually, the dose will have to be modified (lower or higher) for the next injection, depending on the patient's reaction.

In eight patients in whom measurements were performed before the first and second treatment, we found that at an average time ($\bar{x}$) of the second injection of 16.6 ± 3.05 weeks after the first, the mean value (%) of the approximation to the healthy side before the second injection ($\bar{x}$, 48.76%) was even higher than before the first injection ($\bar{x}$ before first injection, 36.87%). This makes a slow but steady loss of efficacy likely.

Passing side effects of all treatments were hematoma (5%), tearing (7.7%), and foreign body sensation (3.3%).

Discussion

A number of authors have studied the topic of synkinesis after defective healing following paralysis of the facial nerve and its causes. In 1905, Lamy [5] gave an exact description of the special role played by the frontal region in defective healing after facial nerve paralysis. In 1939, Fowler [4] tried, in experiments with monkeys, to demonstrate the peripheral genesis of mass movements. Sunderland [13] gave an overview of important factors that may influence the clinical picture of synkinesis.

Stennert [10–12] studied the problem of defective healing after facial nerve paralysis. He explained their "mechanics" by demonstrating the autoparalytic syndrome and by proving through EMG studies that for example, in most cases the clinically "missing" innervation of the forehead has its true origin in a muscular system of trac-

Fig. 6 Palpebral fissure width (*PFW*; affected side as percentage of healthy side) at various times after therapy (*n* = 61; all measurements after first treatment for synkinesis)

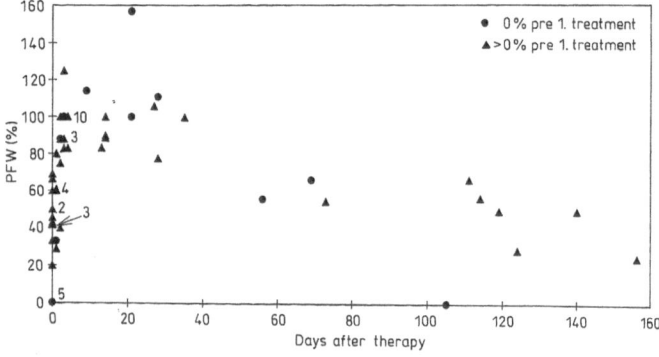

tion/countertraction, and not in an actually defective (absent) innervation in this area. This supposition explains our observation that some patients had improved motility in their frontal region after BTT because their "countertraction system," the orbicularis oculi muscle, was weakened.

The problem of mass movements and their therapy, however, is far from being solved. Fisch [3] presented a surgical model of selective neurectomy of certain facial nerve branches and stated: "Because a reduction in associated movements could only be achieved at the expense of increased periorbital paresis, in all cases there was a tendency to a narrower eyelid opening on the operated side two to three years after surgery."

This justifies BTT was a possible supplementary measure to surgical procedures and its repeated application in caes in which PFW tends to decrease again after surgery. Mass movements are responsible for patients' facial expression – normally the"mirror of emotions" – becoming uncoordinted on the involved side. Synkinesis in the ocular region is caused by involuntary activation of the orbicularis oculi muscle during other movements normally not involving the eye. According to our results, which are based on observation of patients' degree of reduction of PFW differences associated with certain facial movements over a certain period of time, BTT offers a minimally invasive, effective possibility to improve these associated movements.

The results obtained so far also show that the differences between length of the effective period and maximum PFW can obviously vary considerably among individuals, excluding a simple dose-response relationship. Compared with other indications (blepharospasm, hemifacial spasm, spasmodic torticollis), a lower dose of botulinum toxin is sufficient for the synkinesis dealt with here. This may be one reason for the low incidence of side effects. Another reason is the appropriate choice of the injection points.

The time of our measurements shows that for a period ob about 40 days nearly 100% approximation of the PFW of the affected to the healthy side, as well as a diminished muscular activity, can be achieved without complete paralysis of the orbicularis oculi muscle. This was demonstrated by EMG.

A slight effect persisted in the treated patients before the second injection, as evidenced by the higher average PFW values compared with the status before the first injection. Still later, the pretherapeutic status was reached again [7]. Roggenkämper et al [7] observed a longer period (20.4 weeks) between first and second injection and found that the force of eyelid closure on the affected side approached the situation before therapy.

Recent results after various training methods [1, 9] have raised hopes for achieving even better results in the neces-sary suppression of synkinesis by a combination of these methods.

Finally, it can be stated that BTT is an effective therapeutic method to improve mass movements following defective healing. Its advantages include the low degree of invasiveness, the possibility of approaching the neuromuscular junction, the most peripheral connection between muscle and nerve, the possible combination with surgical procedures, the reversibility of side effects, the technical simplicity, the possibility of modifying follow-up injections, and the low dose necessary for treatment.

Patients presenting with mass movements should be informed about this therapeutic option so that, depending on the severity of their defects, they can take advantage of BTT.

References

1. Brudny J, Hammerschlag PE, Cohen NL, Ransohof J (1988) Electromyographic rehabilitation of facial function and introduction of a facial paralysis grading scale for hypoglossal-facial nerve anastomosis. Laryngoscope 98 : 405–410
2. Dressler D, Schönle PW (1990) Botulinum toxin to suppress hyperkinesias after hypoglossal-facial nerve anastomosis. Eur Arch Otorhinolaryngol 247 : 391–392
3. Fisch U (1986) Extracranial surgery for facial hyperkinesis. In: May M (ed) The facial nerve. Thieme, Stuttgart, chapter 27, pp 509–523
4. Fowler EP (1939) Abnormal movements following injury to the facial nerve. J AMA 1003–1008
5. Lamy H (1905) Note sur les contractions "synergiques para-doxales" observé á suite de la paralysie faciale périphériques. Nouv Iconogr Salpetr 18 : 424–425
6. Putterman AM (1990) Botulinum toxin injections in the treatment of seventh nerve misdirection. Am J Opthalmol 205–206
7. Roggenkämper P, Laskawi R, Damenz W, Schröder M, Nüßgens Z (1990) Botulinus-Toxin-Behandlung bei Synkinesien nach Fazialisparese. HNO 38 : 295–297
8. Scott AB (1989) Botulinum-toxin therapy of eye muscle disorders. Safety and effectiveness (ophthalmic procedures assessment, American Academy of Ophthalmology). Ophthalmology, instrument and book issue
9. Shimono T, Hattori N, Yamamoto T, Takimoto I (1989) EMG-biofeedback therapy for reduction of synkinesis. Facial N Res Jpn 9 : 189–192
10. Stennert E, Limberg CH, Frentrup KL (1977) Parese und Defekt-heilungsinder – ein leicht anwendbares Schema zur Objektivierung und Bewertung von Therapieerfolgen bei Fazialisparesen. HNO 25 : 238–245
11. Stennert E (1981) Komplikationen und Rückstände nach operativen Eingriffen am Nervus facialis. In: Miehlke A, Stennert E, Arold R (eds) Motorische Nerven. Arch Ohren Nasen Kehlkopf-heilkd, 231, (1 T A)
12. Stennert E (1982) Das autoparalytische Syndrom – ein Leit-symptom der postparetischen Fazialisfunktion. Arch Otorhino-laryngol 236 : 97–114
13. Sunderland S (1977) Mass movement after facial nerve injury. In: Fisch M (ed) Facial nerve surgery. Kugler, Amstelveen, pp 285–289

Eur Arch Otorhinolaryngology (1994) [Suppl]: S200 – S202

P. Hambleton

Botulinum Toxin: Structure and Pharmacology

Botulism

Strains of Clostridium botulinum produce seven antigenically distinct neurotoxic proteins (neurotoxins types A – G) that act primarily at peripheral cholinergic synapses blocking release of the neurotransmitter substance acetylcholine. This gives rise to Botulism, a rare but often fatal disease of man and other animals. The symptoms of the disease are a symmetrical, descending paralysis with impaired vision, dysphagia, widespread muscular weakness and, ultimately, death from respiratory failure. In humans, the most common cause of the disease is the ingestion of food containing pre-formed toxin produced as a result of the germination of contaminating C. botulinum spores and subsequent primarily with types A, B and E toxins, with type F responsible for a minority of outbreaks only.

Infection with C. botulinum can give rise to other forms of human botulism. Wound botulism is a rare form of the disease that results from the organisms contaminating deep wounds. Where wounds become necrotic or where there is growth of other bacteria, the tissues associated with the wound may become anaerobic, allowing the C. botulinum spores to germinate, grow and produce toxin in a manner analogous to tetanus. Infant botulism, so called because only children of up to 35 weeks appear to be susceptible, results from colonisation of the intestinal tract by C. botulinum. In the USA, this is now the most prevalent form of botulism.

There is no known cure for the toxic paralysis of botulism. Although preparations of antitoxins are available and may form part of the clinical treatment, by the time clinical symptoms present, the toxin has been irreversibly bound and the blockade of acetylcholine release cannot be overcome. With infant botulism, antitoxin therapy forms a useful adjunct to the antibiotic therapy used to eliminate the intestinal colonisation. Prophylaxis with toxoid vaccines is the only effective means of preventing the neuroparalytic effects of the toxins.

Toxin Structure

Complexed Toxins

The botulinum toxins are proteins, often found in association with other, non-toxin, proteins in both naturally and in vitro grown cultures. Toxin complexes from types C, E and F and haemagglutinin-negative strains generally consist of the neurotoxin moiety (M_r, ~ 150 kDa) in association with one or more non-toxin proteins of similar molecular weight. These so-called M complexes vary in molecular mass between 230 – 350 kDa, depending on the toxin type. Toxin complexes from types A, B and haemagglutinin-positive strains of type D may be larger and contain a third protein having haemagglutinin activity. Therapeutic type A toxin contains complexes of this latter type. The proteins of the various complexes dissociate at high pH values (about pH 8), but reassociate spontaneously when the pH is lowered. The current therapeutic toxin formulations are based on toxin complexes of the M type.

Neurotoxins

All the botulinum neurotoxins have similar molecular structures and molecular masses (M_r, 140 – 170 kDa). They are probably all synthesised as single polypeptide chains which are cleaved by proteolytic enzymes during secretion from the organism to give a dichain comprising two asymmetric subunits: a heavy (H) chain (M_r, 85 – 105 kDa) and a light (L) chain (M_r, 50 – 50 kDa) linked together by at least one disulphide bond (Fig. 1).

P. Hambleton
Division of Biologics, PHLS CAMR, Porton Down, Salisbury, Wiltshire SP4 0JG, U. K.

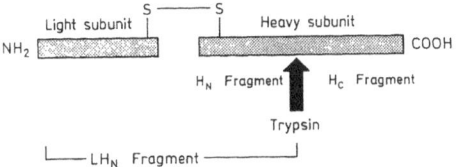

Fig. 1 Dichain structure of the botulinum neurotoxins

Modern techniques of biochemical separation and genetic engineering are being used to further elucidate the molecular structure of the toxins. In the presence of reducing and chaotropic agents, the H and L subunits dissociate and can be separated by chromatographic or electrophoretic means and obtained with high purity. Toxins are susceptible to proteolytic enzymes and further fragments of toxins can be purified. For example, trypsinisation of type A toxin first yields a modified toxin lacking a small region near the carboxyl-terminal of the H chain and which is incapable of binding to acceptor sites on the nerve ending. Subsequently, a larger portion of the H chain (the H_C fragment) is cleaved off, leaving the $H_N L$ fragment (M_r, ~100 kDa) comprising the L chain and the amino-terminal half of the L chain. The biological activities of these various toxin fragments have been investigated using a variety of experimental systems and a fuller understanding of how the toxins act is now being obtained.

Fragments of botulinum toxin genes have been cloned into Escherichia coli in order to sequence the toxin genes. Using this approach, the complete amino acid sequence of toxins A-F have now been deduced. For type A toxin the predicted amino acid sequence corresponds to a polypeptide of 149580 Da. Analysis of the sequences has shown some regions of homology conserved in the different toxin genes which may prove to be associated with common biological activities. Sites of proteolytic cleavage, including that which produces active toxin from protoxin, have been tentatively identified. Regions of high hydrophobicity having the potential to span mammalian cell membranes have been identified that may be associated with the observed in vitro channel-forming activity. The sequences will allow predictions to be made of the likely secondary structures of the toxin molecules. Perhaps the most exciting recent observation is that a conserved region of the L_c subunit of botulinum and tetanus toxins containing three histidine residues closely resembles similar domains present in some 42 zinc metalloproteases, suggesting a possible enzymatic character for the neurotoxins.

Mode of Action

The botulinum neurotoxins are extremely potent agents having specific toxicities ranging from 4×10^7 to 2×10^8

mouse median lethal doses per milligram of protein. They act presynaptically by blocking the release of the neurotransmitter acetylcholine at the neuromuscular junction. Three stages may be involved in inhibition: a primary step involving rapid and irreversible binding to acceptors on the presynaptic nerve surface; an internalisation phase in which toxin crosses the cell membrane and enters the nerve terminus; toxic activity involving one or more steps giving rise to disabling of the acetylcholine release mechanism.

Binding

The acceptor molecules to which the botulinum toxins bind on the presynaptic nerve surface have not been characterised. Studies are complicated by the fact that the toxins do not all appear to bind to the same acceptors. For example, types A and B neurotoxins do not compete for acceptors on the surface of rat brain synaptosomes. In contrast, types A and E appear to recognise the same acceptors as do types C and D neurotoxins. Furthermore, the neurotoxins seem to bind to more than one type of acceptor on the synaptosomes. Binding to a small pool of high-affinity acceptors is such that the toxin is effectively irreversibly bound. Treatment of synaptosomes with proteases or neuraminidase reduces toxin binding, suggesting that protein and sialic acid residues may be components of the acceptors. It is not known whether the acceptors on the brain synaptosomes bear any resemblance to those on the peripheral nerve terminal. It is, however, now recognised that the neurotoxins probably bind to these acceptors by an active (binding) site region located on the carboxyl-terminal half of the H subunit (H_c fragment; Fig. 1).

Internalisation

Once bound to the acceptor(s) on the presynaptic nerve surface, the neurotoxin is internalised into the nerve terminal by an energy-dependent process, probably resembling that of receptor-mediated endocytosis, in which the toxin-acceptor complex becomes encapsulated in clathrin-coated endosomes. The H chain of the neurotoxin is capable of forming channels in lipid membranes at low pH, which may be relevant to the internalisation process. It is not known whether the toxin remains within a membrane or whether whole toxin or a fragment is released into the cytosol.

Toxic Activity

It is now clear that the toxic activity of the neurotoxins is a function of the L chain, the H chain being associated with binding and internalisation. Studies involving direct injection into nerves and permeabilised cultured cell systems have shown that the action of the L_c subunit is not specifically to block acetylcholine release, since it is capable of blocking calcium-mediated exocytosis of other neurotransmitter substances. The non-specificity of the intracellular toxicity indicates clearly that the characteristic specificity of the botulinum neurotoxins is a function of their binding, rather than of inhibitory activity.

The nature of the inhibitory action of the toxins is not understood. In normal conditions, an action potential reaching the nerve ending triggers an influx of calcium ions that in turn stimulates exocytosis of acetylcholine-containing vesicles from active zones on the plasma-lemma. The toxins do not affect the evoked influx of calcium, rather they seem to affect some subsequent stage.

Various mechanisms for inhibition have been proposed. The toxins may act directly on components of the exocytosis mechanism, perhaps a vesicle protein, elements of the cytoskeleton or a component of the vesicle trafficking system. Alternatively, the toxins may stimulate calcium disposal so that, despite the rapid influx to the nerve terminal, the concentration necessary for neurotransmitter release is not achieved. Another possibility is that neurotransmitter release may require entry of calcium to some internal milieu, a process that may be blocked by the toxins. There are insufficient data to favour any one of the above. There is evidence that not all the botulinum neurotoxins block neurotransmitter release by the same mechanism and they may affect different components of the exocytosis system.

Because of their highly specific toxicity and the longevity of their inhibitory effect, it has been considered that the botulinum neurotoxins exert their biological effect by enzymic activity. Hitherto, no such enzymic activity has been demonstrated. However, as mentioned above, the recognition of a sequence in the L_c portion that closely resembles sequences in zinc-containing proteases suggest that the toxins may ultimately prove to also be zinc metalloproteases. What remains unclear is the nature of the substrate for such enzymic activity; one would predict this to be a key protein component of the neurotransmitter exocytosis mechanism.

Botulinum Toxin as a Therapeutic Agent

The very characteristics that make botulinum toxin such a potent cause of neuroparalytic disease also exquisitely fit the toxin for use as a therapeutic drug. It was knowledge of the potency and specificity of the toxin that prompted A.B.Scott to introduce the technique of injecting small quantities of the type A toxin into extraocular muscles to deliberately induce muscle weakness in the treatment of strabismus. This novel therapy has now been extended to other conditions associated with involuntary spasmodic contraction of muscles, specifically focal dystonias. Botulinum toxin therapy has become established as the treatment of choice for benign essential blepharospasm in preference over the surgical alternatives of stripping of the orbicularis oculi or bilateral avulsion of the facial nerve. The treatment is not a cure, as motor fusion may become re-established, but repeat injections usually serve to maintain effective control of the condition. Symptoms of hemifacial spasm, Meige syndrome, facial synkinesis, spasmodic dysphonia and spasmodic torticollis may all respond well to toxin therapy.

Generally, side-effects from neurotoxin therapy are minor, self-limited and localised and can be minimised by careful selection of dose and placement of injections. The long-term effects of continued treatment, as well as the maximum dose, have not been determined, but there have not been reports of adverse systemic side-effects in patients who have received long-term multiple treatments.

Some concern has been voiced about the possible chronic stimulation of the immune system by repeated injections, since the presence of circulating antibody would neutralise the efficacy of the treatment. This appears not to be a general problem, except for a very few patients with conditions that require the administration of higher doses. A study in our laboratory showed that in a group of ten torticollis patients who had either stopped responding or had a diminished response to toxin treatment, seven had clearly developed toxin-neutralising antibodies. Patients in a matched group who continued to respond had no toxin antibodies. There is, as yet, no indication of the dose and/or duration of treatment that might predispose to induction of antitoxin, and it is clear that only a small minority of patients develop such a response. Approaches that might contribute to preventing antibody formation might include the use of low doses and perhaps the use of more highly purified neurotoxin, since the latter could represent a lower challenge of clostridial protein. Where patients develop antitoxin, there is presently no alternative to ceasing the treatment. However, since the various toxin serotypes do not cross-react with each other, the possibility of resuming treatment with alternative toxin serotypes exists. Although the practicality of this has been recently demonstrated, the clinical efficacy of other toxin types remains to be fully evaluated and no alternative therapeutic formulations are presently available.

**Diagnostic Procedures:
Electrophysiology**

Eur Arch Otorhinolaryngology (1994) [Suppl]: S205–S207

FREE PAPERS AND POSTERS

K. Date, Y. Nishimura, T. Minatogawa, H. Iritani, F. Satomi, and T. Kumoi

The Utility of Single-Fiber Electromyography in Facial Nerve Paralysis

Introduction

Many studies on the etiology, diagnosis, treatment, and other aspects of facial nerve paralysis have been performed; however, the precise pathophysiology of facial nerve paralysis has not yet been resolved.

Single-fiber electromyography (SFEMG) is a recently developed method of evaluating the characteristics of neurologic and neuromuscular disease employing a specifically designed fine-needle electrode; it is based on the principle that a pair of action potentials recorded from two muscle fibers, both of which are innervated by a single motoneuron fiber, can be obtaiend simultaneously. The SFEMG technique has been described in detail by Stålberg and Trontelj [4]. In cases of disturbed neuromuscular transmission, for example during the early stages of reinnervation, different findings can be obtained with this technique.

In the present study, we investigated the severity of facial nerve damage during the recovery process in patients with facial nerve paralysis and in a cat model of ischemic facial nerve paralysis using the SFEMG method and compared the values with those of normal controls.

Materials and Methods

SFEMG on the orbicularis oris muscle, as the representative of the facial mimetic muscles, were obtained in ten normal human subjects and nine patients with peripheral

K. Date (✉), Y. Nishimura, T. Minatogawa, H. Iritani, F. Satomi, and T. Kumoi
Department of Otolaryngology, Hyogo College of Medicine, 1-1, Mukogawa-cho, Nichinomiya, 663 Japan

facial nerve paralysis during different stages of recovery from complete paralysis in normal facial movement.

In the human study, the group with peripheral-type facial nerve palsy comprised five patients with Bell's palsy and three patients with Ramsay Hunt syndrome. In an animal model of facial nerve paralysis, six healthy adult cats were used; right ischemic facial nerve paralysis was established according to our previously reported method [1, 2]. Three experimental animals underwent surgery to chronically implant stimulating bipolar electrodes over the left motor cortex for orthodromic activation of the right facial mimetic muscles.

SFEMG were obtained using a specifically designed concentric fine needle electrode with a small hole of 500-μm diameter near the tip and a fine wire of 25-μm diameter was threaded through the hole in order to record the muscle action potentials within the area.

The recording system of SFEMG is a computerized myography instrument (Medelec, MS-20, Vickers Healthcare, England). When the needle electrode is brought to a position from where it is possible to record the action potentials of muscle fibers innervated by the same motoneuron fiber, the preceding spike component is taken as the triggering potential and the interval between the two spike components is measured.

When a nerve fiber is activated during weak voluntary movement and responses are recorded from a single muscle fiber, a latency variability in the order of tens of milliseconds, the jitter phenomenon, is obtained. The interval (in milliseconds) between the two potentials (interpotential interval, IPI) expresses the difference between the conduction times along the two paths and thus reflects the differing conduction velocities in nerve branches and muscle fibers. The IPI mean consecutive difference (MCD) is also designated as a value of SFEMG jitter. MCD (in microseconds) is defined by the following formula:

$$MCD = \sum \mid IPI_n - IPI_{n+1} \mid /n$$

where n is 1, 2, 3, ...100.

Results

Normal Values of Single-Fiber Electromyography
in Humans and in an Animal Model

In this study, a total of 35 montoneurons innervating the orbicularis oris muscle were studied in humans and 22 montoneurons in the animal model. The mean IPI and MCD of the orbicularis oris muscle obtained in humans are 0.50 ms (SD, 0.32) and 29.9 μs (SD, 8.9) and in the animal model 0.56 ms (SD, 0.19) and 32.6 μs (SD, 10.4), respectively. The statistical rejection ellipses ($p = 0.05$) plotted

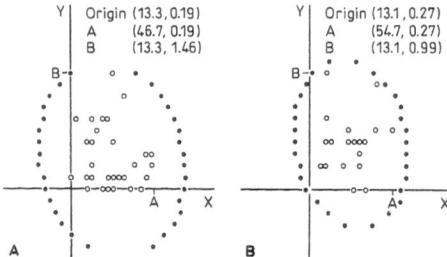

Fig. 1 **A** Statistical rejection ellipse of mean consecutive difference (MCD) and interpotential interval (IPI) calculated from 35 normal single motoneuron fibers to the orbicularis oris muscle in humans. **B** Statistical rejection ellipse of MCD and IPI calculated from 22 normal single motoneuron fibers to the orbicularis oris muscle in cats. *Abscissa*, MCD values of jitter (μs). *Ordinate*, IPI values of jitter (ms)

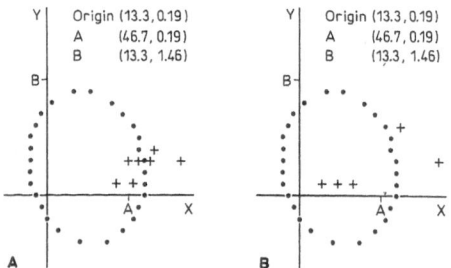

Fig. 2 A, B Single-fiber electromyography (SFEMG) values obtained from one patient with Bell's palsy plotted on the diagram of SFEMG jitter. **A** 5 days after onset of facial nerve palsy (score of mimetic movement was 40/100). Note that three of seven values (*crosses*) deviate outside the normal rejection ellipse. **B** 43 days after onset of facial nerve palsy (mimetic movement was fully recovered, 95/100). Two of five values (*crosses*) of mean consecutive difference (MCD) and interpotential interval (IPI) are still deviated outside the normal rejection ellipse

for normal humans and for the animal model using coordinates of IPI and MCD were very similar and are given in Fig. 1.

Single-Fiber Electromyography During the Recovery
Phase of Facial Nerve Paralysis

Abnormal jitter values were obtained during the recovery phase of facial nerve paralysis in both humans and the cat model. The more severe the facial nerve damage, the greater the deviation from the normal rejection ellipse range in humans (Fig. 2). Findings obtained from the animal model are very similar to those obtained from humans. Furthermore, as recovery proceeded, the coordinates of IPI and MCD gradually approached and finally came into the normal ellipse range.

Discussion

Following the loss of conduction of facial nerve fibers or denervation, whatever the cause, the reinnervation process occurs to restore their function. In most cases of Bell's palsy, complete functional recovery can be expected, but in a few cases recovery does not occur. Thus, it is desirable to have an accurate method to predict the chance of full recovery of patients with facial nerve paralysis. Many methods, such as nerve excitability test and electroneuronography, have been proposed, and among them, SFEMG is a recently developed method of evaluating the characteristics of neurologic and neuromuscular disease. The principle of this technique is based on the recording of a pair of muscle action potentials from a few muscle fibers, each of which is innervated by a single motoneuron fiber. It has been reported that one facial motoneuron fiber to the major zygomatic muscle in humans innervates eight more muscle fibers [3].

When motor units are voluntarily activated, jitter results from variation in the conduction times taken by impulses: (a) from the nerve-branching point to the motor end plates, (b) at the motor end plates, and (c) from the motor end plates to the recording electrode. In normal muscle at a regular innervation frequency, the jitter in SFEMG arises mainly at the motor end plate [4] and is related to a physiologic property or safety factor of the motor end plate.

In the present series conducted in humans and in a cat model, the utility of SFEMG technique was evaluated. First, jitter values recorded and calculated from 35 normal motoneuron fibers of the orbicularis oris muscle in humans and those from 22 fibers in an animal model were similar; in addition, their statistical rejection ellipses showed almost identical patterns.

Second, with the recovery process of facial nerve paralysis, the plots of IPI and MCD, which initially deviated outside the normal rejection ellipse range, come to be within the normal range.

These results indicate that the follow-up study of jitter values in patients with facial nerve paralysis can offer valuable information for determining their treatment.

References

1. Iritani H, Nishimura Y, Minatogawa T (1991) Neurophysiology of ischemic facial nerve paralysis in an animal model. Acta Otolaryngol (Stockh) 111 : 934 – 942
2. Iritani H, Nishimura Y, Minatogawa T, Kumoi T (1989) An animal model for ischemic facial nerve paralysis with a selective embolization. Ear Res Jpn 20 : 195 – 196
3. Hamilton SGL, Terzis JK, Carraway JT (1987) Surgical anatomy of the facial musculature and muscle transplantation. In: Terzis JK (ed) Microreconstruction of nerve injuries. Saunders, Philadelphia, pp 571 – 586
4. Stålberg E, Trontelj JT (1979) Single fiber electromyography. Mirvalle, Old Woking, Surrey, UK

Eur Arch Otorhinolaryngology (1994) [Suppl]: S 208 – S 211

FREE PAPERS AND POSTERS

C. Pototschnig, J. Gubitz, and W. F. Thumfart

Computer-Aided Neuromyography with Repetitive Stimuli for Diagnosis of Facial Nerve Disorders

Introduction

Different diagnostic methods were used to classify lesions of peripheral nerves, especially the facial nerve in ENT patients. In addition to clinical aspects and anamnesis, two further diagnostic steps should be pointed out: examination of tear secretion, stapedial reflex, and gustatory sensation for topodiagnostic questions as well as neurophysiological tests such as nerve excitability test (NET), maximal stimulation test (MST), electromyography (EMG), and neuromyography (NMG) to differentiate neurapraxia, axonotmesis, and neurotmesis.

Magnetic stimulation, developed by Barker in 1985 [2], allowed us to examine the whole course of the facial nerve from its origin in the motor cortex, to the cerebellopontine angle, and the peripheral areas. Muscle answer potentials were measured after electric or magnetic stimulation, depending upon nerve conduction. Investigation of neuromuscular transmission in the synaptic area of the motoric end plates was not included in daily routine diagnosis of facial palsies.

Degenerative lesions such as axonotmesis and neurotmesis induce Wallerian degeneration by destroying the axon as well as the enveloping structures. Much earlier changes can be seen in the motoric endplates with dissociation of acetylcholine receptors over the whole muscle cell. Significant decrease of muscle answer potentials can be seen in NMG after a few days, while in EMG spontaneous activities appear after 2 weeks in cases of degeneration.

Up to now all neurophysiologic tests were practiced with a stimulus frequency not reaching the refractory period. Therefore, injured neuromuscular systems were able to compensate and show a normal pattern. In contrast, normal activity means a nearly tetanic frequency of nerval impulses.

Material and Method

A diagnostic method is needed that stimulates with repetitive stimuli similarly to normal function. Standard parameters of NMG were used with supramaximal stimulation at the stylomastoid foramina (SMF) and recording at the nasolabial fold. A four-channel electromyography with external stimulation and recording was used. The external stimulator was our own design, offering multiple kinds of stimulus characteristics and adjustable frequencies (Fig. 1). After analog-digital transformation, computer-aided evaluation was performed. Three types of stimulation were used: (1) 15 repetitive stimuli supramaximal at 10 Hz, 20 Hz, and 50 Hz; (2) double stimuli were approached between 10 and 1.5 ms; and (3) 15 repetitive stimuli supramaximal at 10 Hz, 20 Hz, and 50 Hz were followed by double stimuli between 10 and 1.5 ms. Latency, amplitude, and integral on the muscular answer potential were evaluated.

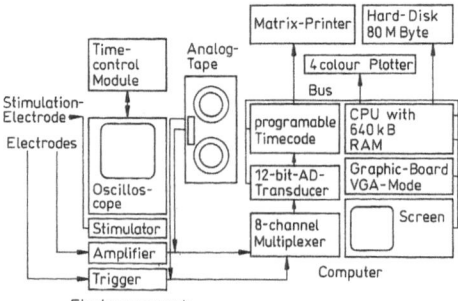

Fig. 1 Stimulation unit (flow chart): repetitive stimuli in the diagnosis of facial nerve disorders

Fig. 2 20-Hz train in a healthy subject

Train: 20 Hz
15 stimuli

Healthy person

Parameter :
Bandpass [20 Hz-10 kHz]
Sens / U 200 μV
Time-Window 800 ms

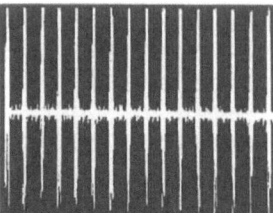

Fig. 3 Progress of amplitude
and latency in a healthy subject

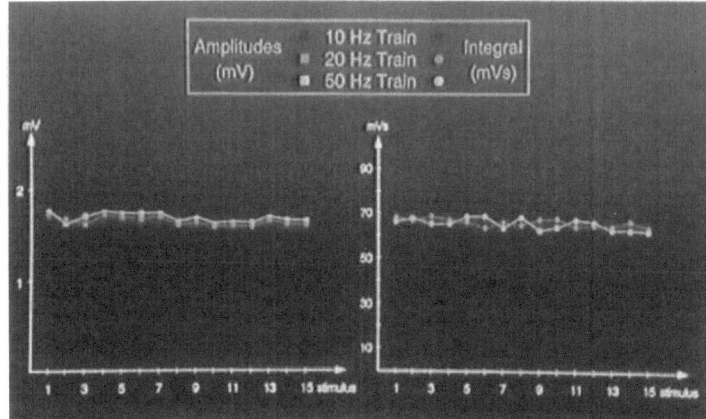

Fig. 4 Course of muscle answer potentials in 10-Hz train
(second day of axonotmesis)

Train : 10 Hz
15 stimuli

Axonotmesis
2nd day

Parameter :
Bandpass [20 Hz-10 kHz]
Sens / U 200 μV
Time-Window 800 ms

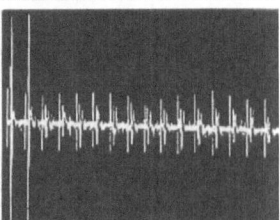

Fig. 5 Progress of amplitude
and integral on second day
of axonotmesis

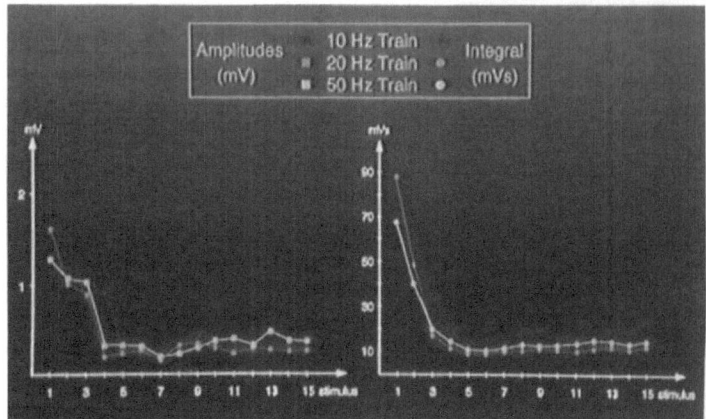

S210

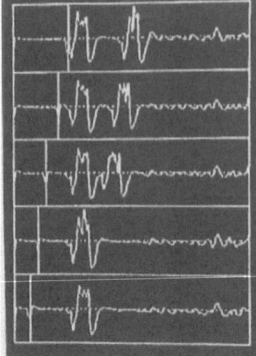

No Train
approached double stimulu:
Delay: 5,4,3, 2, 1.5 ms

Axonotmesis / Neurapraxia
loss of MAP Delay < 3 ms

Parameter :
Bandpass [20 Hz – 10 kHz]
Sens / U 200 μV
Time-Window 25 ms

Fig. 6 Double stimuli with an approach of the second muscle answer potential (*MAP*) up to 3 ms

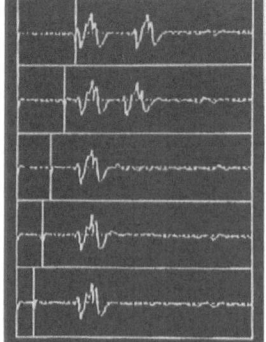

Train : 10 Hz
approached double stimulu:
Delay: 5,4,3,2, 1.5 ms

Axonotmesis / Neurapraxia
loss of MAP Delay < 4 ms

Parameter :
Bandpass [20 Hz – 10 kHz]
Sens / U 200 μV
Time-Window 25 ms

Fig. 7 Double stimuli after repetitive stimuli up to an approach of 4 ms with reduced shape

Results

In healthy patients, no severe changes in amplitude, latency, or integral were seen in 20-Hz stimulation (Fig. 2). The progress of amplitude and latency showed no change (Fig. 3). Axonotmesis with degeneration induced even at 10 Hz a significant decrease in the answer potentials at an early period of lesion (Figs. 4, 5). An early decrease in the answere potential with a nearly complete loss of amplitude and integral was seen in 10-Hz and 50-Hz stimulations after four pulses. The neuromuscular system showed a significant overstress after high-frequency stimulation of

the injured nerve, while the first muscle answer potentials were regular. In neurapractic lesions, only slight decreases in muscle answer potentials were seen in stimulation frequencies up to 20 Hz (Figs. 6, 7).

Conclusion

Up to now a lower frequency limit of 350 Hz was described for peripheral motor nerves, that means a refractory period of 2.9 ms. In our measurements significant decreases were found in healthy subjects at 50 Hz, and in injured nerves from 10 Hz on.

Measurement of the neuromuscular transmission, in contrast to exclusively neural to neural deduction, allows an earlier assessment of lesions. Neurapractic lesions show a higher vulnerability of the neuromuscular area with diminished muscle answer potentials after repetitive stimulation as a consequence of acute dysbolic changes. Axonotmesis and neurotmesis show an early decrease and almost complete disappearance of muscle answer potentials in the progress of repetitive stimulation.

In the regeneration phase, significant changes in muscle answer potentials can be seen after repetitive stimulation with clinically normal activity. Longterm damage of the neuromuscular area must be postulated.

In the differentiation of facial nerve lesions, no exact rating can yet be done, but further investigations based on repetitive stimulation will open up new possibilities in the diagnosis of facial nerve disorders.

References

1. Amoiridis G, Haan J (1990) Motorische Neurographie: Simultanableitung mittels Oberflächen- und Nadelelektroden. Z EEG EMG 21 : 51 – 55
2. Barker AT, Talinous R, Freeston IL (1985) Non-invasive magnetic stimulation of human motor cortex. Lancet i (8437): 1106 – 1107
3. Bergmanns J (1973) Physiological observations on single human nerve fibres. In: Desmedt (ed) New developments in electromyography and clinical neurophysiology, vol 2. Karger, Basel
4. Besser R, Dillmann U, Gutmann L, Hopf HC (1988) Das repetitive Muskelantwortpotential bei neuromuskulärer Übertragungsstörung durch Hemmung der Azetylcholinesterase. Z EEG EMG 19 : 85 – 91
5. Crespi V, Passerini D, Bassi S, Albizzati MG (1976) Repetitive stimulation of the facial nerve in myasthenic and normal subjects. Electromyogr Clin Neurophysiol 16 : 433 – 448
6. Esslen E (1973) Electrodiagnosis of facial palsy. In: Miehlke A (ed) Surgery of the facial nerve. Urban and Schwarzenberg, Munich, pp 45 – 51
7. Esslen E (1977) Electromyography and electroneuronography. In: Fisch U (ed) Facial nerve surgery. Kugler, Amstelveen, pp 93 – 100
8. Hopf HC (1962) Untersuchungen über die Unterschiede in der Leitgeschwindigkeit motorischer Nervenfasern beim Menschen. Dtsch Z Nervenheilkd 183 : 579 – 588
9. Jacobi HM, Struppler A (1968) How to evaluate variations in muscle action potentials following repeated nerve stimulation. EEG Clin Neurophysiol 25 : 402

10. Lehmann HJ, Tackmann W (1974) Neurographic analysis of trains of frequent electric stimuli in the diagnosis of peripheral nerve diseases. Eur Neurol 12 : 293 – 308

11. Pototschnig C, Stennert E (1990) Magnetic stimulation: new possibilities in the assessment of facial nerve dysfunction. In: Castro D (ed) The facial nerve. 6th international symposium on the facial nerve, 1988, Rio de Janeiro, Brasil. Kugler and Ghedini, Amstelveen, pp 183 – 190

12. Thumfart WF, Daun H, Berg M (1985) Computerized electromyography versus electroneurography in the diagnosis of facial nerve paralysis. In: Portman M (ed) The facial nerve. Masson, Bordeaux

Eur Arch Otorhinolaryngology (1994) [Suppl]: S212–S213

K. Tashima, T. Takeda, and H. Saito

Antidromically Evoked Facial Nerve Response in Guinea Pigs with Partial Nerve Injury

Introduction

Since the most common site of lesion in facial palsy is in the intratemporal course, we need a test to evaluate facial nerve function in the temporal course. Antidromically evoked facial nerve response (AFR) allows real time evaluation of the functional alterations of the facial nerve. Some papers state that the prolongation of latency was demonstrated on the damaged facial nerve [2, 3, 5]. However, there is no chronological study on the prolongation of latency in the damaged facial nerve. The purpose of this study is to show the chronological changes in latencies of this response after nerve damage in guinea pigs.

Materials and Methods

Fifty-eight guinea pigs, weighing 220–710 g, were used in this study. The experimental animals were divided into two groups. The first group, comprising 24 animals weighing 220–710 g, served as controls. The second group, comprising 34 animals weighing 230–600 g, was used to examine the chronological changes in the action potential after partial nerve transection.

Facial nerve transections were performed at the geniculate ganglion. The tympanic bulla was opened via the superior approach under general anesthesia with an intraperitoneal injection of pentobarbital sodium (25 mg/kg). The facial nerve was exposed at the geniculate ganglion and half of the nerve was transected.

K. Tashima (✉)
Department of Otolaryngology, Kochi Municipal Hospital, 1-7-45, Marunouchi, Kochi, 780, Japan

T. Takeda and H. Saito
Department of Otolaryngology, Kochi Medical School, Nankoku, Kochi, 783, Japan

In the recordings of AFR, the animals received a tracheotomy and were artificially respirated. A muscle relaxant (pancuronium bromide, 0.4 mg) was used. An active electrode was placed on the fenestrated facial canal between the geniculate ganglion and the stylomastoid foramen, and a reference electrode was placed on the scalp. The facial nerve was stimulated on the nerve trunk near the stylomastoid foramen. In all the animals (expect for two cases in which no response was recorded), triphasic AFR recorded, and the latencies of the responses were measured. The latency of the action potential was defined to be an interval from the onset of the stimulation to the peak of the negative wave [5].

In the first group, AFR were recorded without any nerve damage. In the second group, they were recorded immediately after the transection in two guinea pigs, on the first, second, fifth, and 14th day in five guinea pigs each, and on the third and seventh day in six animals each.

Results

In the first group, triphasic action potential was recorded in all animals. The mean value of the latencies was 0.43 ms and the standard deviation was 0.15 ms. These data were used as controls (Fig. 1).

In the second group, triphasic action potential was recorded in 30 out of 32 cases. In the remaining two cases, no responses were identified, i.e. in those recorded on the third and the seventh day. Immediately after the partial transection, the amplitude of the potential decreased, but the latency had not changed. Figure 1 shows the chronological changes in the latencies of the recorded triphasic waves. On the first and second day, the mean latencies were already prolonged compared with the controls, but the differences were not significant. The prolongation of the latencies became significant after the third day ($p < 0.01$). On the 14th day, the mean latency became shorter compared with the seventh day, but the latencies were still significantly prolonged ($p < 0.05$).

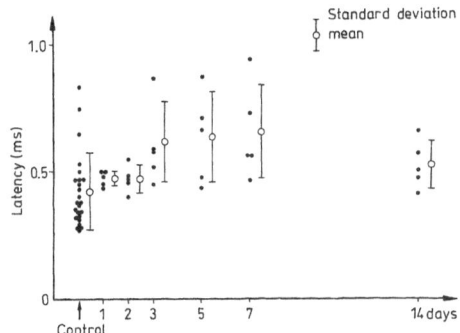

Fig. 1 Chronological changes in the latencies of the recorded triphasic waves after partial transection

In this experiment, the prolongation of the latencies was not significant within 2 days after the transection, but there were three abnormally long latencies in the controls. These three could be rejected by Smirnov's rejection test. If the remaining 21 data were used as controls, the latencies of the first and second day were already significantly prolonged compared with the controls.

Discussion

In 1974, Bumm first described the AFR and suggested that this test provided cross- lesion testing in the temporal bone [1]. It should be the best method for early diagnosis of facial palsy. Some papers state that the prolongation of latency is demonstrated on the damaged facial nerve [2, 3, 5]. This means that the latency of this response is a good indicator of facial nerve damage.

In this experiment the latencies were prolonged compared with controls on the first and the second day. After the third day the latencies significantly prolonged and then shortened by the 14th day. Nakatani et al. reported the chronological changes of the facial nerve swelling after nerve damage [4]. They reported that the diameter of the half-sectioned nerve had reached maximum value on the fifth postoperative day and the nerve returned to its original size by the 14th day. Our own results correlated well with Nakatani's report of facial nerve swelling after nerve damage. We can estimate the real time degree of the nerve damage by the latency changes of the action potential. On the basis of this study, we assume that we can diagnose the degree and the progression of nerve damage in the temporal bone at an early stage.

References

1. Bumm P, Finkenzeller P, Kallert S (1974) Ableitung von intratemporalen des N. facialis im äußeren Gehörgang. Arch Otorhinolaryngol 207 : 484 – 486
2. Herzon GD, Zealear DL (1988) Facial nerve antidromic recordngs in patients with Bell's palsy. Otolaryngol Head Neck Surg 99 : 584 – 589
3. Kitani S, Yanagihara N (1988) Experiments on antidromic evoked potentials of the facial nerve. A possible electroneurodiagnostic examination of intratemporal facial nerve paralysis. Acta Otolaryngol Suppl (Stockh) 446 : 119 – 125
4. Nakatani H, Saito H (1986) Facial nerve swelling after damage. An experimental study. Facial N Res Jpn 6 : 45 – 48
5. Tashima K, Takeda T, Saito H (1989) Antidromically evoked facial nerve response in guinea pigs. In: Sacritistan T et al. (eds) Otorhinolaryngology, head and neck surgery. Kuguler and Ghedini, Amsterdam, pp 691 – 694

Eur Arch Otorhinolaryngology (1994) [Suppl]: S214–S215

H. Nakatani, T.Takeda, H. Saito, and T. Haji

Antidromically Evoked Facial Nerve Responses in Human Subjects: Modification of Recording Techniques

Introduction

Antidromically evoked facial nerve response was first introduced by Bumm and his coworkers in 1974 [1] as the only method to evaluate function of the facial nerve in the temporal bone. This response allow us to diagnose the degenerating process of the facial nerve earlier than the neurophysiological tests wich are currently in use, such as electroneurography [2, 3]. However, this small response with short latency is easily interfered with by initial stimulus artifacts and compound muscle action potentials in clinical cases. In this study, we tried various kinds of recording techniques and we show our method of recording the nerve response in human subjects.

Materials and Methods

Normal human subjects who did not have any history of facial nerve disorders were used in this study.

Stimuli used were a square-wave pulse of 0.1-ms duration at a frequency of 10/s. Responses were amplified with filter settings of 50–3000 Hz, and 100 series of responses were averaged by a signal processor (Nihon Koden MEB-5304 or 7102). The following experiments were performed to record a clear response.

Experiment 1. We compared responses evoked by pulses with either positive or negative only, or both polarity alternately for stimulation.

Experiment 2. The facial nerve was stimulated with a bipolar catheter electrode of 0.8-mm diameter (Unique

H. Nakatani (✉), T. Takeda, H. Saito, and T. Haji
Department of Otolaryngology, Kochi Medical School, Okocho, Nankoku, Kochi, 783, Japan

Medical, UKG100-2PM) via the parotid duct, conventional transcutaneous stimulation was also carried out to compare the responses with the periductally stimulated responses.

Experiment 3. A silver-ball electrode and a monopolar needle electrode were compared as active electrodes.

Experiment 4. We recorded responses at the entrance of external auditory canal, at the posterior wall near the eardrum, and on the promontorium through the eardrum.

Experiment 5. We eliminated muscle action potentials by subtracting the response recorded at a lateral site from that at a more medial site.

Results

Experiment 1. When only positive and negative pulses were summed for stimulation, the nerve responses were interfered with by initial stimulus artifacts. On the other hand, the responses evoked with pulses changing polarity alternately were almost free from stimulus artifacts.

Experiment 2. Transcutaneous stimulation produced large stimulus artifacts, and clear nerve responses were not obtained in most cases. However, transductal stimulation elicited a clear nerve response without the interference of stimulus artifacts.

Experiment 3. The nerve response reporded with a silver-ball electrode was very small and was easily disturbed by artifacts originating from stimuli and muscular contraction. The response recorded with a needle electrode, however, had enough amplitude to be identified.

Experiment 4. Amplitude of the nerve response increased when an active electrode was placed at a more medial site. On the other hand, compound muscle action potentials showed almost similar configurations at every place.

Experiment 5. Subtraction of the response recorded at a lateral site from that a more medial site eliminated compound muscle action potentials and made it easier to analyze waveform of the nerve response.

Discussion and Conclusion

After Bumm's report [1], antidromically evoked facial nerve response has been considered by otologists to be an indicator of nerve damage within the temporal bone at the earliest stage of facial palsy. However, it is not as easy to obtain the responses in human subjects as in animals, because we cannot approach the facial nerve directly for stimulation and recording or use a muscle relaxant. Therefore, the responses recorded in human subjects are very small and are easily interfered with by various kinds of artifacts. In this study, we were able to obtain a clear response by modifying some of the recording techniques. We suggest that stimulation with alternative polarities, transductal stimulation, recording with a needle electrode, intratympanic recording, and subtraction of the responses recorded at two different sites are necessary to obtain a clear and analyzable response.

Acknowledgement This research was supported by a grant from the Ministry of Education (grand no. 1480407).

References

1. Bumm P, Finkenzeller D, Kallert S (1974) Ableitung von intratemporalen Aktionspotentialen des N. Facialis im äußeren Gehörgang. Arch Otorhinolaryngol 207:484–486
2. Herzon DL, Zealear DL (1988) Facial nerve antidromic recordings in patients with Bell's palsy. Otolaryngol Head Neck Surg 99:584–589
3. Kitani S, Yanagihara N (1988) Experiments on antidromic evoked potentials of the facial nerve. Acta Otolaryngol Suppl 446:119–125

Eur Arch Otorhinolaryngology (1994) [Suppl]: S216–S217

S. Poignonec, M. Vidailhet, G. Lamas, I. Fligny, J. Soudant, P. Jedynak, and J.-C. Willer

Electrophysiological Evidence for Central Hyperexcitability of Facial Motoneurons in Hemifacial Spasm

With the use of qualitative and quantitative electrophysiological methods, the aim of the present study was to substantiate the idea that a central hyperexcitability exists in the facial motoneurons in hemifacial spasm (HFS). The study was carried out on eight patients (six men, two women, 40–65 years) affected with HFS from both idiopathic ($n = 6$) and postparalytic ($n = 2$) origin. In a first set of experiments, we studied trigeminofacial reflexes elicited by electrical stimulation of supraorbital nerves on both the normal and affected side of HFS patients and in four control subjects using classical conventional techniques as described previously [1, 3, 5]

On the patients' normal side as well as in control subjects, supraorbital nerve stimulation elicited the well-known double-component (R1-R2) blink reflex response in the ipsilateral orbicularis oculi muscles, while no reflex was ever observed in the other ipsilateral facial muscles, i. e., orbicularis oris and chin muscles. In patients, such a stimulus also elicited a double-component (R1-R2) blink response in the contralateral orbicularis oculi muscles (HFS side), while in control subjects only the R2 component was usually recorded. This crossed R1 blink response was observed in all patients, whatever the cause of HFS. Furthermore, supraorbital nerve stimulation on the affected side elicited ipsilaterally the R1-R2 blink reflex responses of the blink-type (R1 and R2) in the other facial muscles, i. e., orbicularis oris and chin muscles. Such blink-type reflex responses were not observed in homologous muscles of patients' normal side and in control subjects, at least during this specific experimental procedure, in which subjects were required to relax as much as possible. These first data clearly show a qualitative aspect of a hyperexcitability of the facial motoneurons involved in the blink reflex and a wide spread of the hyperexcitability to the whole facial motoneuronal pool.

Since the central pathway of the R1 response is known to be oligosynaptic (two or three synapses) [2], we decided to explore the facial motoneuronal excitability for this R1 reflex response in order to quantify the hyperexcitability of the facial nucleus in a second set of experiments. For this purpose, we used a classical double-shock technique described elsewhere [6]. Briefly, the test stimulus (ipsilateral supraorbital nerve) was adjusted to elicit stable R1 and R2 reflex responses, while the conditioning stimulus (contralateral supraorbital nerve) was adjusted so as to be just infraliminal to any reflex response. Numerical values of the R1 response were then converted into percentages in order to allow intra- and interindividual comparison. For each muscle, the 100% value represented the mean of 40 responses obtained during the control period preceding each conditioning procedure.

In all patients and only on the affected side, the infraliminal conditioning stimulus induced an important facilitation on the R1 reflex response elicited by the test stimulus in all facial muscles reflexly tested. In the orbicularis oculi muscles, the onset of the facilitatory effect occurred for a shorter interstimulus interval (Δt, 0 ms) than that was observed on the patients' normal side and in controls (Δt, 30 ms). The maximum facilitatory effect was significantly higher (+330%) than for the normal side (+220%) and remained significantly higher for a longer interstimulus interval (+50% for $\Delta t = 100$ ms) than for the normal side (+2% for $\Delta t = 100$ ms). In orbicularis oris and chin muscles, a similar pattern of the R1 excitability curve was observed on the affected side, while, as already mentioned above, no reflex response was elicited in homologous muscles from the normal side or in control subjects. Furthermore, in these latter cases, the conditioning stimuli were ineffective in the production of any reflex activity.

S. Poignonec, G. Lamas, I. Fligny, and J. Soudant
Department E.N.T., Faculté de Médecine Pitié-Salpêtrière 91, Bd. de l'Hôpital, 75634 Paris Cédex 13, France

M. Vidailhet and P. Jedynak
Department Neurology, Faculté de Médecine Pitié-Salpêtrière 91, Bd. de l'Hôpital, 75634 Paris Cédex 13, France

J.-C. Willer (✉)
Lab. Neurophysiology, Faculté de Médecine Pitié-Salpêtrière 91, Bd. de l'Hôpital, 75634 Paris Cédex 13, France

This second set of data clearly shows that the central hyper-excitability of facial motoneurons observed in HFS can be quantified accurately with paired stimuli. Futhermore, since the onset of facilitation observed in the R1 reflex response occurred early in the excitability curve, i.e., when both conditioning and test stimuli were delivered simultaneously (Δt, 0 ms), one can suggest that those facial motoneurons involved in the R1 reflex response receive convergent afferent messages with a similar oligosynaptic pathway from both conditioning (contralateral) and test (ipsilateral) stimuli. This idea is supported by the fact that a crossed R1 response was recorded in the orbicularis oculi muscle of the affected side when the contralateral supraorbital nerve was excited, showing the existence of a crossed di- or trisynaptic afferent pathway projecting to the same motoneuronal pool as the ipsilateral one.

Although direct anatomical connections between the trigeminal sensory nucleus and the contralateral facial nucleus have been described [4], most authors agree on the strictly ipsilateral distribution of the R1 component. Consequently, our present data raise the question as to whether these crossed oligosynaptic excitatory effects and the ectopic R1 responses are produced by abnormal synaptic connections or by existing synapses that are normally irresponsive to contralateral supraorbital nerve stimulation.

Acknowledgements This work was supported by INSERM (CRE), AP-HP (CRC 92–93), and by the Fondation pour la Recherche Médicale.

References

1. Anger RG (1979) Hemifacial spasm: clinical and electro-physiological observations. Neurology (Minneap) 29:1261–1272
2. Holstege G (1990) Neuronal organization of the blink reflex. In: Paxinos G (ed) The human nervous system. Academic, New York, pp 287–296
3. Kugelberg E (1952) Facial reflexes. Brain 75:385–396
4. Ramon y Cajal SR (1909) Histologie du système nerveux de l'homme et des vertébrés. Maloine, Paris, pp 859–888
5. Willer JC, Lamour Y (1977) Electrophysiological evidence for a facio-facial reflex in the facial muscles in man. Brain Res 119:459–464
6. Willer JC, Roby A, Boulu P, Boureau F (1982) Comparative effects of electroacupuncture and transcutaneous nerve stimulation on the human blink reflex. Pain 14:267–278

Eur Arch Otorhinolaryngology (1994) [Suppl]: S218 – S219

K. Nakamura and Y. Koike

Prognostic Diagnosis of Peripheral Facial Palsy by an Impedance Method

Introduction

A satisfactory prognostic test for peripheral facial paralysis has not yet been established. Electroneurography (ENoG) is useful, but alone it is not effective enough for an accurate prognostic diagnosis. Therfore, a new method is required for accurate diagnosis. As an impedance meter is often used clinically for purposes such as impedance plethysmography [5] and impedance cardiography [2], we examined the possibility of using it for accurate prognostic diagnosis of facial palsy.

Materials, Methods, and Subjects

Figure 1 is a block diagram of the impedance method. Change in the impedance between a pickup electrode and a reference electrode is measured with an impedance meter. The impedance meter has four electrodes. The pickup electrode is placed on the center of the upper lip and the reference electrode on the dorsum of the nose. The two exciter electrodes are placed bilaterally on the cheeks. The stimulating surface electrode is placed over the stylomastoid foramen of the normal side. First, the stimulation voltage is slowly increased from zero until a movement of the upper lip is observed, and the waveform of change in the impedance is recorded with a pen oscillograph. The stimulation voltage is then gradually increased, resulting in gradual increase in amplitude of the waveform (Fig. 2). The deviation of the upper lip correlates well with the change in the impedance. We define the amount of change in the impedance at supramaximal stimulation as ΔZ. This procedure is then repeated on the affected side. We ex-

pressed the ratio of ΔZ on the affected side to that on the healthy side as $\Delta Z\%$ and used this ratio as an index to determine the prognosis.

The subjects examined were 61 patients with Bell's palsy or Hunt's syndrome. All patients were seen within 7 days after the onset of disease and received conservative treatment. We repeatedly applied the impedance method together with ENoG during the acute phase of facial paralysis and recorded only the lowest values of ENoG (ENoG%) and $\Delta Z\%$ measured at the same time.

The degree of paralysis was evaluated by the 100-point facial movement assessment procedure [3]. Patients were assigned to the complete recovery group when their score was 90 or more points with no sequelae and to the incomplete recovery group when their score was 85 or less points or they had sequelae after 6 months from the onset of the disease.

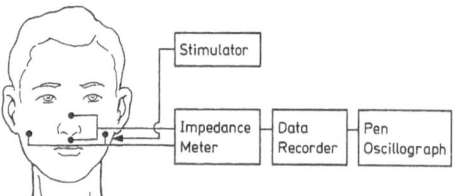

Fig. 1 Block diagram of the impedance method

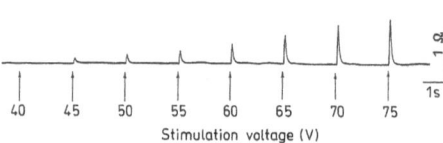

Fig. 2 Waveforms obtained by the impedance method. The amplitude of the waves gradually increased with increase in the stimulation voltage

K. Nakamura (✉) and Y. Koike
Department of Otolaryngology, The University of Tokushima School of Medicine, 3 Kuramoto, Tokushima, 770, Japan

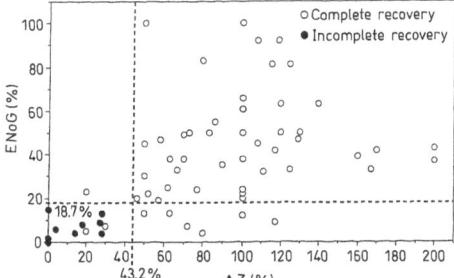

Fig. 3 Relationship between lowest values of electroneurography (*ENoG%*) and the ratio of ΔZ on the affected side to that on the healthy side ($\Delta Z\%$, where ΔZ is the amount of change in the impedance at supramaximal stimulation) of 61 patients with Bell's palsy or Hunt syndrome and their prognosis. The accuracy of assessing a poor prognosis by ENoG alone and in combination with the impedance method as 56% and 82%, respectively

Results

Figure 3 shows the relationship between the ENoG% and $\Delta Z\%$ of the 61 patients and shows their prognosis. Fifty-two patients recovered completely and nine patients showed incomplete recovery. An unfavorable prognosis was associated with an ENoG% of less than 18.7% and a $\Delta Z\%$ of less than 43.2%. These values were calculated statistically as the 5% critical limits of our group with an unfavorable prognosis.

First, we predicted the prognosis by ENoG alone. Patients with an ENoG% of 18.7% or more were defined as having a good prognosis, and those with an ENoG% less than 18.7% as having a poor prognosis. Based on this criteria, 44 patients were determined to belong to the good prognosis group, and in fact all these patients recovered completely. Seventeen patients were determined as belonging to the poor prognosis group, but eight of these patients revovered completely. Thus, the accuracy of predicting a poor prognosis by means of ENoG alone was only 56%.

Then, prognostic diagnosis by a combination of EnoG and the impedance method was examined. Patients with an ENoG% of 18.7% or more or those with a $\Delta Z\%$ of 43.2%

or more were defined as having a good prognosis, whereas those with an ENoG% of less than 18.7% and those with a $\Delta Z\%$ of less than 43.2% were defined as having a poor prognosis. Based on these criteria, 50 patients were determined as belonging to the good prognosis group, and all of these patients recovered completely. Of the 11 patients determined as belonging to the poor prognosis group, only two patients recovered completely. Thus the accuracy of predicting a poor prognosis by a combination of ENoG and the impedance method was 82%.

Discussion

We have found that some patients who were determined to have a poor prognosis for facial palsy by ENoG showed good facial movements at the supramaximal stimulation on visual examination (maximum stimulation test) [4], and many of these patients recovered completely. Thus, we thought that objective quantification of facial movements should be useful in assessing the prognosis. We developed the impedance method described her for quantitative comparison of the facial movement (upper lip movement) on the affected side and healthy side. Our results showed that the impedance method alone was fairly effective for prognostic diagnosis, but it is more accurate to determine the prognosis by a combination of ENoG and the impedance method. It was concluded that a combination of ENoG and the impedance method was more effective than ENoG alone for prognostic diagnosis of peripheral facial palsy.

References

1. Esslen E (1977) Electromyography and electroneurography in facial nerve surgery. Kugler Medical, Amstelveen
2. Kubicek WG, Kottke FJ, Ramos MU, Patterson RP, Witsoe DA, Labree JW, Layman TE, Schoening H, Garamela JT (1974) The Minnesota impedance cardiograph, theory and applications. Biomed Eng 9:410–416
3. May M (1970) Facial paralysis, peripheral type: a proposed method of reporting. Laryngoscope 80:331–390
4. May M, Harvey JE, Marovitz WF, Stroud M (1971) The prognostic accuracy of the maximal stimulation test compared with that of the nerve excitability test in Bell's palsy. Laryngoscope 81: 931–938
5. Nyboer J (1950) Electrical impedance plethysmography. Circulation 2:811–821

Eur Arch Otorhinolaryngology (1994) [Suppl]:S220

ABSTRACTS

S. R. Whitaker, H. R. Blanks, and P. Laue

Facial Nerve Antidromic Evoked Potentials

Recording facial nerve potentials generally involves peripheral stimulation of the extratemporal facial nerve and recording a combined electrical potential representing: (1) the peripheral facial muscular response (EMG) and (2) a small proximal antidromic response. In most cases, the very small antidromic facial nerve potential cannot be differentiated from the much larger EMG muscular response. The antidromic response occurs from a progressive depolarization along the intratemporal portion of the nerve into the facial motor nucleus. The spatial orientation of the motor cells within the facial nerve nucleus may account for some of the difficulty in recording this potential. Antidromic responses of the facial nerve are affected by pathologic injury to the facial nerve, i.e., nerve compression. Experimental results in animals with recording of the antidromic evoked potential along the facial nerve and within the facial nerve nucleus are presented. Suggestions for improved recordings in humans are discussed.

S. R. Whitaker, H. R. Blanks, and P. Laue
University California Irvine, Department of Otolaryngology,
Build 25, RT 81, 101 The City Drive South, Irvine, USA

Eur Arch Otorhinolaryngology (1994) [Suppl]:S221

ABSTRACTS

P. J. Catalano, D. M. Simpson, and A. R. Eden

Infraorbital (V₂) and Mental (V₃) Nerve Stimulations Produce Correspondingly Specific Facial Nerve Reflexes Analogous to the Blink Reflex

This study investigated reflex arcs between the second (V_2) and third (V_3) divisions of the trigeminal nerve and their corresponding branches of the facial nerve. Although electromyographic presence of the traditional (V_1) blink reflex is an important clinical prognostic of facial nerve function, it tests only one of the five major branches of the facial nerve, or about 20% of facial nerve function. Studies were performed in adult humans with facial palsy. The infraorbital and mental nerves were stimulated, and the resultant electromyographic activity measured bilaterally in the nasalis and mentalis muscles, respectively. Results demonstrated the presence of reflex arcs between all divisions of the trigeminal nerve and their corresponding branches of the facial nerve.

P. J. Catalano, D. M. Simpson, and R. Eden
Mount Sinai School of Medicine, Departments of Otolaryngology
and Clinical Neurophysiology,
Box 1191, Fifth Avenue and 100th Street,
New York, NY 10029-6574, USA

Eur Arch Otorhinolaryngology (1994) [Suppl]:S222

ABSTRACTS

S.A. Burres

Electrophysiologic Evaluation of Facial Nerve.
Function After Paralysis

Usually, the clinical evaluation of facial paralysis is limited to a perfunctory appraisal of facial motion based on meager clinical guidelines. We have shown that using linear measurement and integrated electromyography it is possible to obtain meaningful, accurate data about the function of the facial nerve in various regions. By applying these techniques to facial paralysis patients it is possible to estimate the force of the facial muscles and the number of intact fibers in the facial nerve in different regions during maximum motion. Of even greater significance, it is possible to analyze the activity of the facial motor units during grades contractions. In 30 patients with facial paralysis of different etiologies, the number of nonfunctioning, partially functioning, and normally functioning motor units in several regions of the face was determined and motion vs. force graphs were derived.

S.A. Burres
100 UCLA Medical Plaza, Suite 522, Los Angeles, California, USA

Eur Arch Otorhinolaryngology (1994) [Suppl]:S223

ABSTRACTS

N. Yanagihara, T. Kozawa, Y. Miyamoto, and S. Murakami

Clinical Value of a Battery Electrodiagnostic Test

For the last 20 years we have used the standardized electrodiagnostic tests to assess grade of nerve injury and prognosis of facial palsy. The tests involve (1) conventional nerve excitability test, (2) strength-duration curve testing at the orbicularis oris, orbicularis oculi, and frontalis muscle and (3) evoked compound muscle action potential of the orbicularis oris and oculi muscle. The test battery was applied to more than 2000 patients with conditions including Bell's palsy, Hunt's syndrome, traumatic facial palsy, facial palsy due to otitis media, and other intratemporal facial palsies. Reliability, advantages, and disadvantages of each test are described. We emphasize the importance of a battery test for evaluation of prognosis of facial palsy due to different etiologies.

N. Yanagihara, T. Kozawa, Y. Miyamoto, and S. Murakami
Department of Otolaryngology, Ehime University,
School of Medicine, Ehime, Japan

**Diagnostic Procedures:
Electroneurography**

Eur Arch Otorhinolaryngology (1994) [Suppl]: S 227 – S 229

D. Hoehmann, C. DeMeester, and L. G. Duckert

Electrical Evaluation of the Facial Nerve in Acoustic Neuroma Patients Comparing Transcranial Magnetic Stimulation and Electroneurography

Introduction

Electroneurography is the standard in electrodiagnostic tests to evaluate facial nerve function [3 – 7]. The test measures the integrity of the extratemporal facial nerve and does not assess the proximal portion within the internal auditory canal until the neural degeneration has progressed towards the periphery.

As an alternative means of facial nerve stimulation, the transcutaneous magnetic technique may provide a non-invasive and painless stimulation of the intratemporal and proximal portion of the nerve [8, 12, 14].

Pulsed magnetic fields induce electrical current in neural tissue, resulting in depolarization and generation of action potentials. The amplitude of the action potential compares favorably with those induced by electroneurography ENOG. The exact location of stimulation of the seventh nerve is still under investigation and suspected to be in the labyrinthine segment [12], the proximal intratemporal segment [8], and the intracisternal segment [10]. Recent data identified the "route exit zone" segment of the nerve as the stimulus site [9, 13]. Based on this experience, it is most likely that the nerve is depolarized by the magnetic field along its intracisternal course. In patients with known acoustic neuromas, magnetic field stimulation might show evidence of earlier or more complete conduction aberrations in comparison to ENOG. It could be expected that responses are more likely to be altered if the nerve could be tested proximal to or at the side of the lesion.

To confirm this theory a series of patients with known acoustic neuromas were examined using ENOG and magnetic coil stimulation (MCS) just prior to surgery and 1 week postoperatively. Responses to both stimuli were compared with the size of the tumor and the pre- and postoperative facial nerve function using the Stennert grading system.

Methods

A pulsed magnetic field is generated by a circular coil through which a large current flow transiently to induce a peak magnetic field of approximately 2 T. The position of the coil over the patient's skull determines whether the face-associated motor cortex or the cranial nerve itself is stimulated. For cortical stimulation, the direction of the current within the coil determines which hemisphere is excited preferentially. Short-latency responses with latencies up to 6 ms were induced with the center of the stimulating coil 6 cm lateral to the vertex in the intra-aural line [2]. Long-latency responses were induced by activation of either the ipsilateral or contralateral facial motor cortex if the stimulating coil was placed 2 cm medial to the vertex.

Stimulation thresholds for nerve action potentials as well as suprathreshold and supramaximal stimulation measurements of latency and amplitude for both the unaffected ear and the neuroma ear were obtained preoperatively and 1 week postoperatively with ENOG, which was performed with a Nicolet pathfinder signal processor and magnetic stimulation was performed using a Magstim 200. Electromyograms were taken both ipsilaterally and contralaterally from the orbicularis occuli and orbicularis oris musculature. For calculation of amplitude and latencies of the muscle action potentials generated by the magnetic stimulation, five consecutive responses were averaged and analyzed.

Twenty patients were initially enrolled in the study. Three patients failed to complete the test battery and were eliminated from the study.

D. Hoehmann (✉), C. DeMeester, and L. G. Duckert
Dept. Otolaryngology Universität Würzburg,
Josef-Schneider-Str. 11, 97080 Würzburg, Germany

Table 1 Pre- and postoperative results of studied patients

Patient	Tumor size (cm)	Preop. ENOG threshold elevation (%)	Preop. MCS threshold elevation (%)	ENOG amplitude reduction (%)		MCS amplitude reduction (%)		Postop. facial function (score)
				Preop.	Postop.	Preop.	Postop.	
1	1.5	0	0	0	90	65	35	0
2	> 2.5	50	0	19	–	36	74	9
3	2	0	0	0	0	40	0	2
4	1	0	0	65	64	59	57	2
5	0.5	0	0	0	0	49	0	0
6	1.5	40	0	41	37	15	89	0
7	1.5	0	0	76	99	20	98	6
8	> 2.5	0	25	52	52	55	74	2
9	> 2.5	0	33	0	–	58	27	7
10	> 2.5	50	0	0	–	0	58	10
11	1	0	0	29	0	0	33	0
12	2.5	0	0	15	90	0	0	1
13	1.5	0	0	42	95	0	0	10
14	2.5	0	28	72	–	58	0	10
15	1.5	0	33	0	88	0	86	2
16	1	0	42	17	–	29	0	6
17	2	0	37	67	92	80	79	0

ENOG, electroneurography; MCS, magnetic coil stimulation.

Results

None of the 17 patients demonstrated clinical evidence of facial weakness preoperatively. Results are summarized in Table 1. Postoperatively 12 patients demonstrated worsening of their facial nerve function. Seven patients had moderate to severe facial nerve dysfunction documented by Stennert scores in excess of 5. In four of these patients, the tumor was in excess of 2.5 cm in diameter. A comparison of preoperative interside threshold differences revealed significant threshold differences in three patients using ENOG and in six patients using MCS. These threshold shifts were observed in six of eight patients who were found to have tumors of 2 cm or more intraoperatively ($p < 0.04$, Fisher exact probability test).

For comparison of interside amplitude differences, values in excess of 10% or more between normal and abnormal were reported. Eleven out of 17 patients (65%) demonstrated amplitude reduction using ENOG. Twelve patients (70%) demonstrated amplitude reduction of ipsilateral short-latency responses following MCS. Collectively, the ENOG and MCS interside amplitudes were preoperatively reduced in 15 patients (88%). There was no statistically significant correlation between tumor size and postoperative outcome. While there was a tendency to interside latency interval prolongation with larger tumors, in general this could not be confirmed by statistical analysis.

A comparison of pre- and postoperative action potential amplitudes using ENOG revealed significant amplitude reduction in 14 of 17 patients (82%). In five of these pa-

tients, the postoperative ENOG was unobtainable. In each case, the postoperative facial nerve function was significantly altered. Using MCS, a postoperative amplitude shift greater than 10% was documented in 11 of 17 patients. There was no correlation between the amount of amplitude reduction and postoperative facial function. Postoperative nerve action potentials were obtained with MCS in each of the five patients who had ablation of ENOG responses.

Discussion

The value of electrocochleography and MCS used to assess the presence and degree of neural blockade in patients with Bell's palsy and acoustic tumors has been documented [5, 6, 8, 10].

The theory that magnetic stimulation would allow us to assess conduction abnormalities in a greater percentage of patients with acoustic neuromas pre- and postoperatively than ENOG remains subject to further review. It is valid to conclude, based on statistical analysis, that ENOG and MCS are more likely to demonstrate threshold differences in patients with neuromas in excess of 2 cm. Interside amplitude reduction was present in a high percentage of patients using both ENOG and MCS. Similar rates of preoperative ENOG reduction were reported by Kartush [5, 6], who indicated that the degree of ENOG reduction could not consistently predict early postoperative facial function. The data of the present study are similar in that there was no apparent correlation between tumor size, postoperative function, and the degree of amplitude reduction measured by either ENOG or MCS. With regard to a comparison of pre- and postoperative facial nerve action potential amplitudes, ENOG and MCS are both sensitive to the trauma of surgical manipulation. It is of interest that the nerve remained excitable using MCS in each case, where as sensitivity to stimuli was lost postoperatively using ENOG. It may be that MCS is a more sensitive indicator of facial nerve integrity along the whole of its course, including the corticonuclear projections and primary genu, regardless of its electrical activity at the stylomastoid foramen.

Longer follow-up, will be needed to assess facial nerve recovery at 6 months to 1 year before and further conclusions can be drawn regarding the predictive value of ENOG, or MCS facial nerve action potential amplitude reduction seen at 1 week. It appears that neither ENOG or MCS offers a greater advantage in predicting facial nerve function in the immediate postoperative recovery period. MCS may ultimately offer an alternative to ENOG to assess patients with acoustic neuromas pre- and postoperatively.

References

1. Beck DL, Benecke R (1990) Intraoperative facial nerve monitoring. Technical aspects. Otolaryngol Head Neck Surg 102: 270–272
2. Benecke R, Meyer BU, Schoenle P, Conrad B (1988) Beurteilung motorischer Hirnnervenfunctionen mit Hilfe der transkraniellen magnetischen Stimulation. EEG EMG 19: 228–233
3. Esslen E (1973) Electrodiagnosis of facial palsy. In: Miehlke A (ed) Surgery of the facial nerve. Urban and Schwarzenberg, Munich, Saunders, Philadelphia
4. Kartush JM, Lilly DJ, Kemink JL (1985) Facial electroneurography: clinical and experimental investigations. Otolaryngol Head Neck Surg 93: 516–523
5. Kartush JM, Graham MD, Kemink JL (1986) Electroneurography: preoperative facial nerve assessment in acoustic neuroma surgery: a preliminary study. Am J Otol 7: 322–325
6. Kartush JM, Niparko JR, Graham MD, Kemink JL (1987) Electroneurography preoperative facial nerve assessment for tumors of the temporal bone. Otolaryngol Head Neck Surg 97: 257–261
7. Kartush JM (1989) Electroneurography and intraoperative facial monitoring in contemporay neurotology. Otolaryngol Head Neck Surg 101: 496–503
8. Kartush JM, Bouchard KR, Graham MD, Linstrom CL (1989) Magnetic stimulation of the facial nerve. Am J Otol 10: 14–19
9. Metson R, Rebeiz E, West C, Thornton A (1991) Magnetic stimulation of the facial nerve. Laryngoscope 101: 25–30
10. Meyer BU, Britton TC, Benecke R (1989) Investigations of unilateral facial weakness: magnetic stimulation of the proximal facial nerve and the face-associated motor cortex. J Neurol 236: 102–107
11. Meyer BU, Kloten H, Britton TC, Benecke R (1990) Technical approaches to hemisphere-selective transcranial magnetic brain stimulation. Electromyogr Clin Neurophysiol 30: 311–318
12. Schriefer TN, Mills KR, Murray NM, Hess CW (1988) Evaluation of proximal facial nerve conduction by transcranial magnetic stimulation. J Neurol Neurosurg Psychiatry 51: 60–66
13. Seki Y, Krain L, Yamada T, Kimura J (1990) Transcranial magnetic stimulation of the facial nerve: recording technique and estimation of the stimulated side. Neurosurgery 26: 286–290
14. Windmill IM, Martinez SA, Shields CB, Paloheimo M (1989) Magnetically evoked facial nerve potential. Otolaryngol Head Neck Surg 100: 345–347

Eur Arch Otorhinolaryngology (1994) [Suppl]: S 230 – S 232

I. M. Smith, J. A. M. Murray, and R. Mountain

The Prognostic Value of Electroneurography in Bell's Palsy

Facial electroneurography (ENoG), introduced by Esslen in 1977 [2], is now established as a recognised investigation of facial nerve function. It offers the major advantage over other electrical tests of providing an objective, quantitative assessment of facial nerve degeneration. Using the healthy side as a reference, the reduction in amplitude of the action potential on the affected side is thought to represent the percentage of nerve fibres which have degenerated.

In 1981 Fisch [3] suggested that all patients with idiopathic facial palsy who have less than 90% degeneration 3 weeks after onset would regain normal facial movements spontaneously. These findings have been disputed, however; in 1983 May [6] found that patients whose involved side had a response of less than 25% tended to have an incomplete return of facial function. Our own initial results [4] using this test also failed to agree with those of Fisch.

We used ENoG to investigate 49 patients with Bell's palsy presenting within 10 days of the onset of symptoms. Their clinical outcome was graded into three groups: complete recovery within 6 weeks (group A), delayed recovery, reasonable function at 3 months (group B) and severe palsy at 3 months (group C).

The compound action potentials (CAP) in millivolts and latency times in milliseconds were measured for the normal and affected sides at the time of onset (Table 1).

The initial amplitude of the CAP on the affected side failed to show any correlation with the final outcome. Similarly, the latency time provided no indication of final recovery, there being no significant difference between the three groups.

These results made us question the claimed sensitivity of ENoG in predicting prognosis for these patients. As a result, the technique was scrutinised and by experimenta-

I. M. Smith (✉)
ENT Department, Bristol Royal Infirmary, Bristol, U. K.

J. A. M. Murray and R. Mountain
ENT Department, Royal Infirmary Edinburgh

Table 1 The mean ± 1 s.d of the latency (ms) and amplitude (mv) of the response of orbicularis oculi in the three groups, A, B and C

	A[a] (n = 33)	B[b] (n = 9)	C[c] (n = 7)
Normal side			
Latency	2.5 ± 0.3	2.5 ± 0.3	2.5 ± 0.3
Amplitude	1.6 ± 0.7	1.6 ± 0.9	1.8 ± 1.1
Affected side			
Latency	2.6 ± 0.6	3.0 ± 0.8	2.6 ± 0.3
Amplitude	1.2 ± 0.8	0.6 ± 0.7	1.0 ± 1.0

[a] Complete recovery within 6 weeks.
[b] Delayed recovery, reasonable function at 3 months.
[c] Severe palsy at 3 months.

tion a standardised optimum method was derived in the hope of achieving greater consistency and reliability.

Twelve healthy volunteers were used to measure the action potential amplitude and latency times using 11 different standard positions of the recording and stimulating electrodes [7]. The different positions of the electrodes ensured a change not only in position, but also in the intercentre distance. Great care was taken in positioning electrodes, ensuring a low interelectrode resistance and using supramaximal stimulation when possible.

The optimum electrode position was determined by those sites which gave consistantly high CAP amplitudes. There was no single position clearly superior for the stimulating electrode. Instead, there appeared to be a fairly large suitable area which still enabled a maximum stimulus to be delivered to the nerve trunk (Fig. 1). The optimum intercentre distance appeared to be 2 or 2.5 cms, 1.5 cm being too small.

The results for the recording electrodes confirmed the findings of Esslen that if the electrodes are moved away from the alar margin, the resulting waveform is unsuitable for use (Fig. 2); again, the optimum intercentre distance appeared to be 2 cm.

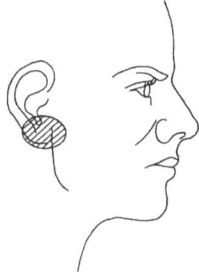

Fig. 1 Optimum area for stimulating electrodes

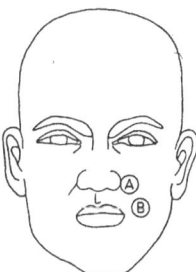

Fig. 2 Optimum position for recording electrodes. *B* Cathode; *A* Anode

The latency time in the majority of positions showed little variation, but showed a significant negative correlation with the CAP amplitude, i.e. as the latency time increased, the CAP amplitude decreased. Latency time is known to increase with submaximal voltage stimulation; a change in the position of the stimulating electrodes probably resulted in a reduced voltage to the nerve trunk in some positions, thus explaining the change in latency times found.

This standardised technique was then used in the investigation of a further group of patients with Bell's palsy; 26 patients with a unilateral palsy, 21 of whom had a total paralysis were studied. The majority of patients were again tested electrophysiologically within 10 days of onset.

Patients were analysed retrospectively according to their clinical recovery and the results of the ENoG investigation. They were divided into two groups, A and B. Patients in group A achieved a complete return of function, whereas those in group B had a delayed and incomplete recovery, some individuals being left with a significant residual defect. On the basis of the ENoG results, they were also divided into those with more or less than 90% degeneration.

Table 2 Results of electroneurography (ENoG) expressed as the mean amplitude ±1 s. d for the muscle action potential (mv)

	A[a] ($n = 18$)	B[b] ($n = 8$)
Normal side		
Number of responses	18	8
Absent responses	0	0
Amplitude (mv)	2.32 ± 1.47	2.42 ± 0.6
Affected side		
Number of responses	16	4
Absent responses	2	4
Amplitude (mv)	1.32 ± 1.08	0.06 ± 0.09
Recovery time (months)	2.8 ± 1.9	11.2 ± 6.9

[a] Patients in group A achieved complete return of function.
[b] Patients in group B had delayed and incomplete recovery.

Group A comprised 18 patients (69.2%) and group B, eight patients (30.7%). The mean age in group A was 47.7 years, which did not differ significantly from that in group B (49.6 years). There were 19 women and seven men.

The mean values for the muscle CAP are given in Table 2. There is a significant difference in the values for patients in group A compared to those in group B ($p = 0.01$, Student's t test). In line with this, the time for recovery was significantly shorter in group A (2.8 ± 1.9 months) compared to the mean for group B (11.2 ± 6.9 months; $p = 0.05$, Student's t test).

The patients were also divided into those who had more or less than 90% degeneration as determined by ENoG. All but one of those whose degeneration was *less* than 90% made a complete recovery. In contrast, only two of those with *more* than 90% degeneration achieved a complete recovery of function.

Bell's palsy probably represents a spectrum of nerve injury, with the chances of recovery being directly proportional to the number of fibres which have degenerated. This concept is supported by the work of Esslen [2], who has shown, using ENoG, that in 145 cases of idiopathic facial palsy, 2.75% showed no sign of degeneration, whilst 6.2% had degeneration of all motor fibres.

The persistence of some voluntary movement of the face implies that significant degeneration has not occurred and the prognosis for a complete return of function is therefore excellent. Difficulties arise in those patients who present with a total paralysis where there are no clinical signs to indicate the degree of injury. The results of our last study have given us confidence in using this investigation in that, providing a careful and standardised technique is used, it is capable of providing an accurate prediction of prognosis.

The controversy over definitive treatment for Bell's palsy continues. By predicting the natural prognosis of the disease, this investigation facilitates the evaluation of any therapy which may be considered. Until an effective treatment is available a method of accurately predicting prognosis at an early stage is essential. Only then can patients either be reassured or start active therapy at the earliest possible moment in the disease process. ENoG appears to offer an early and reliable prognostic indicator which hopefully will be of benefit to many patients.

References

1. Adou KK, Sheldon MI, Kahn AM (1977) Comparative prognostic value of maximal nerve excitability testing (NET) versus neuromyography (NMG) in patients with facial paralysis. Trans Pac Coast Otoophthalmol Soc 58 : 29–42

2. Esslen E (1977) Electromyography and electroneurography. In: Fisch U (ed) Facial nerve surgery. Aesculapious, Birmingham, pp 93–100

3. Fisch U (1981) Surgery for Bell's palsy. Arch Otolaryngol 107 : 1–11

4. Heath JP, Cull RE, Smith IM, Murray JAM (1988) The neurophysiological investigation of Bell's palsy and the predictive value of the blink reflex. Clin Otolaryngol 13 : 85–92

5. House JW, Brackman DE (1985) Facial nerve grading systems. Otolaryngol Head Neck Surg 93 : 146– 147

6. May M, Blumenthal F, Klein SR (1983) Acute Bell's palsy, prognostic value of evoked electromyography, maximal stimulation, and other electrical tests. Am J Otol 5 : 1–7

7. Smith IM, Murray JAM, Prescott RJ, Barr-Hamilton R (1988) Facial electroneurography – standarisation of electrode position. Arch Otolaryngol Head Neck Surg 114 : 322–325

Eur Arch Otorhinolaryngology (1994) [Suppl]:S233

POSTERS

M. Asai, S. Kitani, S. Murakami, and N. Yanagihara

Innervation Pattern of the Extratemporal Ramification of the Facial Nerve; Intraoperative Evoked Electromyographic Study: Second Report

We reported the innervation pattern of the extratemporal ramification of the facial nerve in man at the VI International Symposium in the Facial Nerve. By further investigation, we obtained additional information on the innervation pattern.

The investigation was performed during parotid tumor surgery or partial selective neurectomy for hemifacial spasm. An electrical stimulation was given first to the facial nerve trunk and then to each discrete branch. Using bipolar needle electrodes, the evoked electromyography was recorded from the frontalis, orbicularis oculi, orbicularis oris, and depressor labii inferioris muscles, respectively.

In all 11 patients with the parotid tumor and 9 out of 11 patients with the hemifacial spasm, innervation pattern of the extratemporal facial nerve was the same as in the previous report; the nerve fiber innervating the frontalis muscle existed only in the upper major branch, and the nerve fiber innervating the depressor labii inferioris muscle only in the lower major branch. But in two cases with hemifacial spasm the nerve fiber innervating the frontalis muscle existed not only in the upper but also in the lower major branch. In one case with hemifacial spasm the nerve fiber innervating the depressor labii muscle existed in both the upper and lower branches. These results suggest a very complex peripheral innervation pattern with intricate anastomosis in the facial nerve fibers.

M. Asai (✉), S. Kitani, S. Murakami, and N. Yanagihara
Department of Otolaryngology, Ehime University, Shigenobu-cho,
Onsen-gun, Ehime, 791-02, Japan

Eur Arch Otorhinolaryngology (1994) [Suppl]: S234–S235

L. Parisi, G. Valente, G. Ralli, M. Terracciano, and E. Calandriello

Bell's Palsy and Magnetic Stimulation: Longitudinal Study

Introduction

Neurophysiological investigation of unilateral facial palsy is routinely based upon studies of the excitability and conduction velocity of the facial nerve in its intracranial course. For lesions of the facial nerve lying proximally, electrical stimulation of the nerve at the stylomastoid foramen can only reveal effects caused by anterograde degeneration of the nerve fibres [2–3]. Transcranial magnetic stimulation of the motor cortex or of peripheral nerves has been used to evoke responses in limb muscles. Recently, this technique has also been applied to stimulate the intracranial portion of the facial nerve. Brief magnetic pulses generated by a coil held over the ipsilateral scalp elicit a cortical magnetic action potential (cMAP) of similar morphology to that obtained with routine electroneurography (ENoG) [1, 6–8]. The aim of this study was to investigate whether the technique of magnetic stimulation could be helpful in the neurophysiological assessment of facial palsy and of prognosis for recovery of facial nerve function.

Patients and Methods

Twenty-eight patients with unilateral Bell's palsy (16 men and 12 women; age range, 16–66 years, with a mean of 30.1 years) were studied with transcranial magnetic stimulation (SMT). The severity of the facial paralysis was objectively graded. The onset of facial weakness occurred from 1 day to 2 weeks prior to testing.

Furthermore, the patients were investigated at 15, 30 and 60 days and 1 year after onset of idiopathic facial palsy. Electromyographic recordings were taken from both superior orbicularis oris muscle using surface electrodes.

L. Parisi, G. Valente, G. Ralli, M. Terracciano, and E. Calandriello
Istituto II Clinica Neurologica, Università "La sapienza",
Viale Università 30, 00185 Roma, Italy

For transcranial peripheral nerve stimulation, a Cadwell MES 10 stimulator generated a brief magnetic field at the center of the coil. The coil was placed tangentially on the parieto-occipital surface of the scalp. In order to minimise the baseline irregularities from continuing activity and render latency measurements more reliable, eight responses were averaged. A supramaximal response was usually obtained with the magnetic field at only 35% of its maximal strength.

Results

In all patients no response to magnetic stimulation could be recorded from the affected side, even in those who

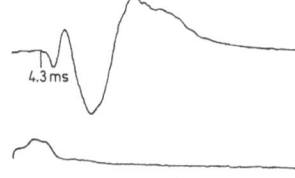

Fig. 1 Compound muscle action potentials recorded over orbicularis oris in a 21-year-old patient affected by right Bell's palsy in response to magnetic stimulation of the facial nerve at 1 day after onset of facial palsy

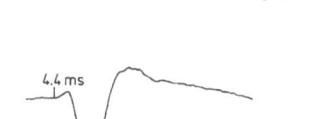

Fig. 2 Compound muscle action potentials recorded over orbicularis oris in the same patient as in Fig. 1 at 60 days onset of facial palsy

S235

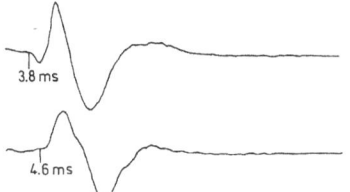

Fig. 3 Compound muscle action potentials recorded over orbicularis oris at 1 year after onset of Bell's palsy in the same patient as in Fig. 1

developed facial palsy 1 day prior to testing (Fig. 1). Repeated examinations 30 and 60 days later (Fig. 2) showed a persisting lack of response of the facial nerve to transcranial stimulation even after an appreciable recovery from the palsy in 15 out of the 28 patients. On repeated examination 1 year later in all patients, the facial weakness had completely resolved and normal responses to magnetic stimulation were obtained (Fig. 3).

Discussion

Since the first report by Murray et al. in 1987 [5] on magnetic facial nerve stimulation, it has been possible to stimulate this nerve non-invasively and intracranially and to assess conduction in its proximal segment. Schriefer et al. [7] and Rosler et al. [6] speculated that magnetic stimulation excites the facial nerve within the labyrinthine segment of the facial canal. Macabee et al. [4] calculated the site of stimulation to be close to the exit of the facial nerve from the brainstem to its entrance in the internal auditory meatus. However, the excitation occurs within the proximal segment of the facial nerve where the lesions is known

to reside in Bell's palsy. This explains the absence of a response to magnetic stimulation in acute Bell's palsy. Facial nerve remains inexcitable, however, to transcranial magnetic stimulation despite considerable clinical improvement. A still demyelinated area of nerve injured portion would give rise to such a persisting absence of response.

One year later the facial palsy had completely recovered and normal responses to magnetic stimulation were obtained. Therefore, the absence of a response to facial nerve magnetic stimulation in Bell's palsy patients can be due to the proximity of the stimulation to the injured proximal segment of the nerve, yet this does not necessarily predict a bad prognosis. Thus magnetic stimulation does not reliably prove useful in the assessment of prognosis for recovery of facial nerve function in Bell's palsy.

References

1. Benecke R, Meyer BU, Schonle P, Conrad B (1988) Transcranial magnetic stimulation of the human brain: responses in muscle supplied by cranial nerves. Exp Brain Res 71 : 623–632
2. Essler E (1977) The acute facial palsy. Springer, Berlin Heidelberg New York
3. Fisch U (1984) Prognostic value of electrical tests in acute facial paralysis. Am J Otol 5/6 : 494–498
4. Maccabee PJ, Amassian VE, Cracco JB (1984) Intracranial stimulation of facial nerve in humans with magnetic coil. Electroencephalogr Clin Neurophysiol 70 : 350–354
5. Murray NMF, Hess CW, Mills KR, Schriefer TN, Smith SFM (1987) Proximal facial nerve conduction using magnetic stimulation. Electroencephalogr Clin Neurophysiol 66 : S71
6. Rosler KM, Hess CW, Schmid UD (1989) Investigation of facial motor pathways by electrical and magnetic stimulation: sites and mechanisms of excitation. J Neurol Neurosurg Psychiatry 52 : 1149–1156
7. Schriefer TN, Mills KM, Hess CW (1988) Evaluation of proximal facial nerve conduction by transcranial magnetic stimulation. J Neurol Neurosurg Psychiatry 51 : 60–66
8. Seki J, Krain L, Yamada T, Kimura J (1990) Transcranial magnetic stimulation of facial nerve: recording technique and estimation of the stimulated site. Neurosurgery 26/2 : 286–290

Eur Arch Otorhinolaryngology (1994) [Suppl]: S236–237

A. Pirodda, F. Calbucci, G. C. Modugno, F. Tognetti, and A. Rinaldi Ceroni

Electromyography of Evoked Activity of the Facial Nerve in Cerebellopontine Angle Surgery

Introduction

Intraoperative facial nerve monitoring is commonly used in cerebellopontine angle surgery; recording of evoked activity has proved to be the most sensitive method [1, 2] to detect potential injuries at an early stage.

Patterns of evoked activity can be generally correlated to a specific etiologic mechanism [1]. It seems sufficiently demonstrated [1] that nonrepetitively grouped discharges (bursts and pulses) are to be considered as an expression of probably noninjurious stimuli. They are especially helpful in verifying the location and course of the nerve [3] and its functional integrity after surgery. In contrast, repetitive discharges (trains) are observed after a potentially injurious stimulus [1]; thus they are attributed the function of detecting the possibility of even slight impairments due to excessive manipulation [3].

Materials and Methods

Electromyography (EMG) of evoked activity has been applied to 18 patients (ten men and eight women) who underwent cerebellopontine angle surgery between January 1991 and April 1992. Average age was 48 years (range, 34–68 years). Seventeen had a neuroma and the remaining one had a meningioma. The kind of surgical approach was selected essentially on the grounds of the degree of sensorineural hearing loss: the translabyrinthine approach was used in four cases and the suboccipital

A. Pirodda and G.C. Modugno
ENT Clinic, University of Bologna, Italy

F. Calbucci and F. Tognetti
Department of Neurosurgery, Bellaria Hospital, Bologna, Italy

A. Rinaldi Ceroni
ENT Clinic, University of Cagliari, Italy

approach was used in 14 cases. Tumor sizes ranged from 10 to 40 mm (average, 21 mm). In only one patient, who showed a complete paralysis of the seventh cranial nerve at first observation, did the preoperative electroneurographic study [4] demonstrate a degeneration degree of 80%. In all the patients an EMG intraoperative monitoring (online technique) was performed using a two-channel device: the recording was made using subdermal monopolar needle electrodes inserted into the nasolabial fold, the midline forehead, the orbicularis oculi, and the corner of the mouth.

The number and the total duration of the trains were evaluated. In 17 patients, anatomic integrity of the nerve was preserved. In the patient showing preoperative damage a neurorrhaphy was necessary. Preoperative functional evaluation was effected following House-Brackman grading [5]. In all the cases a control electroneurography was performed 1 week after surgery (and was subsequently repeated every month).

In order to work out some prognostic criteria, a logistic regression analysis was used: the age, the kind of approach, the size of the tumor, and the number and total duration of the train were considered as independent variables.

Results

The short-term results of intraoperative facial monitoring are shown in Table 1. In 11 patients out of 18 (61%), the postoperative function of the seventh cranial nerve was found to be satisfactory at electroneurographic control 1 week after surgery. In all these patients the size of the tumor ranged from 10 to 30 mm (average, 18 mm) and the intraoperative recordings showed nine trains or less, lasting no more than 10 min in total.

In six cases (33%), a class V fuctional impairment and in one case (6%) a class III functional impairment was observed: the size of tumor ranged from 15 to 40 mm

Table 1 Short-term results of intraoperative facial monitoring ($n = 18$)

	House grade	
	I–II	III–VI
No. of patients	11 (61%)	7 (39%)
Size of tumor (average mm)	18	27
Number of trains	< 9	> 5
Total duration of trains (min)	< 10	> 13
Suboccipital approach (n)	4	–
Translabyrinthine approach (n)	7	7

(average, 27 mm) and the total duration of trains always exceeded 13 min.

The logistic regression analysis showed that older age, suboccipital approach, big size of the tumor, and total duration of the trains are significantly related ($p < 0.01$) to immediately postoperative functional impairment of the seventh cranial nerve.

Three patients out of six had a complete recovery of the function of the facial nerve within 6 months. In the remaining three patients, the follow-up did not exceed 2 months.

Discussion

Our findings must be considered as preliminary observations because the number of cases does not allow us to draw definitive conclusions. The relationship between age of the patient, size of the tumor, surgical approach, and injury of the seventh cranial nerve is easy to understand; a more interesting observation concerns the close relationship between the duration of the trains and the functional impairment of the nerve.

In the cerebellopontine angle, a lack of perineural and epineural sheets makes the facial nerve particularly vulnerable to trauma [6]; if confirmed, the above findings could indicate another prognostic criterion, yielding a practical and easily employable technique to provide useful intraoperative information about the functional integrity of the nerve in this kind of surgery.

References

1. Prass RL, Kinney SE, Hardy RW, Hann JF, Luders H (1987) Acoustic (loudspeaker) facial EMG monitoring. II. Use of evoked EMG activity during acoustic neuroma resection. Otolaryngol Head Neck Surg 97:541–551
2. Dickins JRE, Graham SS (1991) A comparison of facial nerve monitoring system in cerebellopontine angle surgery. Am J Otol 12:1–6
3. Kileny PR, Niparko JK (1988) Intraoperative monitoring of auditory and facial function in neurotologic surgery. Adv Otolaryngol Head Neck Surg 2:55–88
4. Gantz BJ, Gmuer AA, Holliday M, Fisch U (1984) Electroneurographic evaluation of the facial nerve. Method and technical problems. Ann Otol Rhinol Laryngol 93:394–398
5. House JW, Breackmann DE (1985) Facial nerve grading system. Otolaryngol Head Neck Surg 93:146–147
6. Kartush JM, Niparko JK, Bledsoe SC, Graham MD, Kemink JL (1985) Intraoperative facial nerve monitoring: a comparison of stimulating electrodes. Laryngoscope 95:1536–1540

Eur Arch Otorhinolaryngology (1994) [Suppl]: S238

ABSTRACTS

J. M. Fernández, V. Baecker, O. Romero, N. Raguer, F. Crespo, and P. Quesada

Electroneurographic Evaluation of Facial Palsy.
Early and Late Results in 350 Patients

Electroneurography (ENoG) is a rapid and reliable technique in the early prognosis of Bell's palsy, but is less commonly used in the evaluation of the final outcome. Early and late results of 350 patients studied over the last 10 years (1981–1991) were prospectively assessed. ENoG examinations were performed on days 10–12 and 30 in all cases, and 150 patients were also examined on days 4–6. Patients with severe axonal degeneration (80%) were followed for a minimum of 2 years. Clinical recovery was evaluated following Zander Olsen criteria (1975). On days 10–12 compound muscle action potentials (CAMPs) of the parietic side of over 25% compared with the normal side were found to predict complete recovery within 1–6 months with very mild or no sequelae. Patients with CMAPs between 25% and 10% usually recovered with minor sequelae while those with CMAP amplitudes of 10% or less recovered slowly with moderate-to-severe sequelae. When CMAPs were less than 40% on days 4–6, the percentage on day 10–12 was less than 10%. Two years after onset, even patients with poor recovery (early CMAPs <10%) had CMAPs over 50%, a finding that suggests that the sequelae were due to aberrant rather than faulty reinnervation.

J. N. Fernández, V. Baecker, O. Romero, N. Raguer, F. Crespo, and P. Quesada
Department of Clinical Neurophysiology, Hospital Valle Hebrón, 08035 Barcelona, Spain

Eur Arch Otorhinolaryngology (1994) [Suppl]:S239

ABSTRACTS

M. Podvinec

Neuronography in Facial Palsy-Results of Long-term Observations

Three hundred ad twenty-six patients with idiopathic (Bell's) palsy and 21 patients with traumatic facial palsy were seen by the author between 1972 and 1983. The course of the palsy was followed by neuronography and rheobase-chronaxy measurements. Nineteen of 27 patients with sigs of denervation at the time of disease were re-evaluated clinically between 1989 and 1990; 8 were lost to control; 5/15 patients with idiopathic facial palsy had tympanomastoidal decompressive surgery and steroids; 10/15 had only steroid therapy. In both groups distribution of final results within the House grading system were comparable with each other and in general surprisingly satisfactory. Similar results were found in trauma cases, where 5/21 fulfilled denervation standards, and 4/21 were seen and tested. Of these 4, 3 had an indication of severe nerve damage, confirmed by surgery in 2 (subtemporal); in a further case there was only compression by bone particles. One was not operated on.

In conclusion, neuronography results are to be interpreted exclusively in the clinical context. Denervation signs in the first 10 days do not form a decisive indication for surgery, which we have abstained from in idiopathic cases since 1979. The degree of a traumatic intratemporal lesion is not to be identified by neuronography, whose value is, however, greater in trauma than in idiopathic cases. It seems possible that neuronography results are greatly influenced by neuropathologic processes in idio-pathic palsy, which may be reversible even in cases of temporary denervation signs during early testing.

M. Podvinec
Kantonsspital, 5001 Aarau, Switzerland

Magnetic Stimulation

Eur Arch Otorhinolaryngology (1994) [Suppl]: S 243 – S 246

T. Ohira, R. Shiobara, J. Kanzaki, and S. Toya

Identification of the Exact Stimulated Site in Transcranial Magnetic Stimulation of the Facial Nerve

Introduction

The exact stimulated site of the facial nerve in transcranial magnetic stimulation is unclear. Some authors reported that the stimulated site was the root exit zone of the facial nerve, from assumptions based on conduction velocity and extracranial electrical stimulation studies [1, 6]. However, other authors reported that the site was located at the more distal part of the facial nerve: the labyrinthine or intracanalicular portion [3 – 5]. One of the reasons why this ambiguity exists is that most of these authors did not compare responses of intracranial electrical stimulation (IES) and transcranial magnetic stimulation (TMS). In this study we performed IES and TMS simultaneously during operations and compared the onset latency of these responses.

Materials and Methods

Six patients with hemifacial spasm and three patients with acoustic neurinoma were studied. In our institution, intraoperative facial muscle EMG monitoring with IES is routinely performed to determine the effectiveness of decompression on the facial nerve in microvascular decompression operations for hemifacial spasm and to localize the position of the facial nerve in the tumor during acoustic neurinoma surgery. In this study, informed consent was received from the patients for performing TMS during surgery.

T. Ohira, R. Shiobara, and S. Toya
Department of Neurosurgery, Keio University, Shinanomachi 35, Shinjuku-ku, Tokyo 160, Japan

J. Kanzaki
Department of Otolaryngology, Keio University, Shinanomachi 35, Shinjuku-ku, Tokyo 160, Japan

Facial nerve-evoked EMG (eEMG) was recorded from the orbicularis oris muscle and orbicularis oculi muscle using needle electrodes. Another pair of needle electrodes was also placed near the stylomastoid foramen to stimulate the extracranial portion of the facial nerve.

The magnetic stimulator for TMS has a maximum strength of 1000 V. Two types of coils were used: a single coil of 90 mm in diameter and an 8-shaped double coil, each part 80 mm in diameter. IES was performed with bipolar coagulator forceps connected to the electrical pulse generator (0.2-ms duration). TMS was performed repeatedly during operations simultaneously with IES.

Results

Ipsilateral eEMG was produced by TMS with the single coil placed around the retroauricular area. Ipsilateral eEMG was also evoked by TMS with the 8-shaped double coil. In 8-shaped double coil TMS, the positioning of the coil was very precise and orientation of the coil was also important to evoke eEMG response. However, the morphology and onset latency were completely equal in these two types of TMS (Fig. 1). Morphology of eEMG by TMS was similar to that following extracranial electrical stimulation, although onset latency was longer in TMS than in extracranial electrical stimulation (Fig. 2).

In intraoperative monitoring, morphology and onset latency of eEMG by TMS was not affected at all during any stages of the surgical procedure, such as craniectomy, opening of dura mater, and suctioning cerebrospinal fluid. The onset latency of eEMG by TMS was shorter than that by IES at the root exit zone in a patient with hemifacial spasm (Fig. 3). The results of monitoring in six patients with hemifacial spasm are summarized in Table 1. The onset latency of eEMG by TMS was shorter than that by IES at the root exit zone in all of the six cases. The mean onset latency of eEMG by TMS and by IES at the root exit zone was 5.15 and 5.71 ms, respectively. The mean dif-

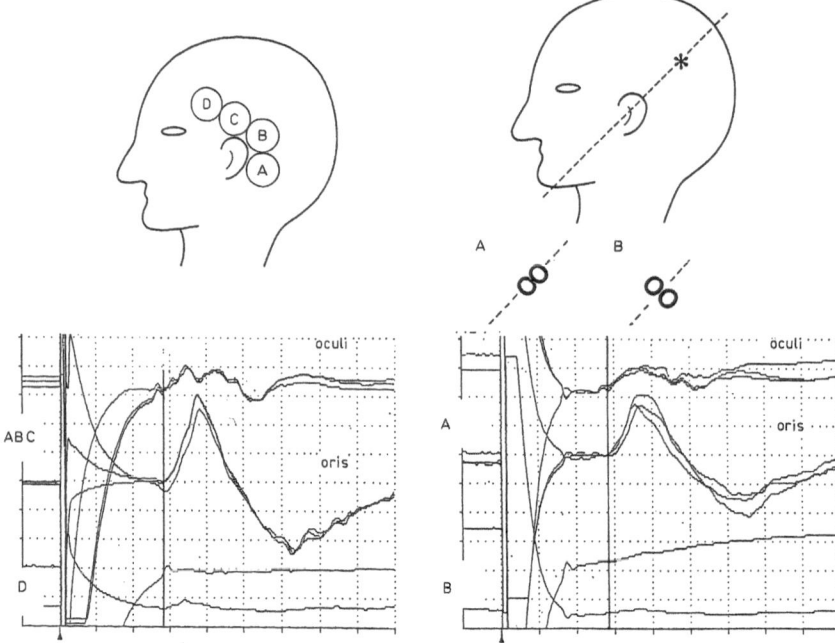

Fig. 1 Facial responses were evoked by magnetic stimulation with the single coil placed around retroauricular area (*left*). The 8-shaped double coil evoked a similar response, although the positioning of the coil was very precise (*) and orientation of the coil eas also important to evoke the facial nerve-evoked EMG (eEMG) response (*right*). Onset latency in both cases, 5.68 ms

Table 1 Intraoperative monitoring in six patients with hemifacial spasm

Patient	Magnetic stimulation (ms)	Electrical stimulation at root exit zone (ms)	Difference (ms)
1	4.76	5.24	−0.48
2	5.20	5.62	−0.44
3	6.12	6.88	−0.76
4	5.20	5.76	−0.56
5	4.32	4.80	−0.48
6	5.32	5.92	−0.60
Mean	5.15	5.71	−0.55
SD	0.55	0.64	0.11

Table 2 Intraoperative monitoring in three patients with acoustic neurinoma

Patient	Magnetic stimulation (ms)	IAC (ms)	Difference (ms)
7	6.48	6.48	0.00
8	5.44	6.00	−0.56
9	5.84	6.04	−0.20

IAC, electrical stimulation in the internal auditory canal.

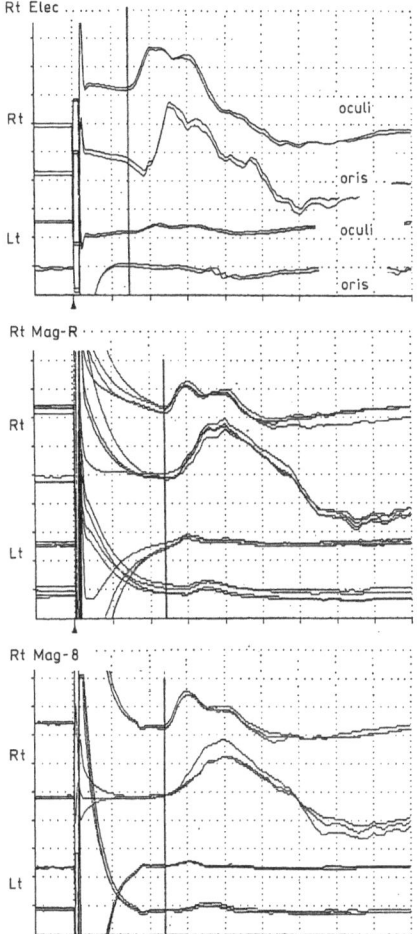

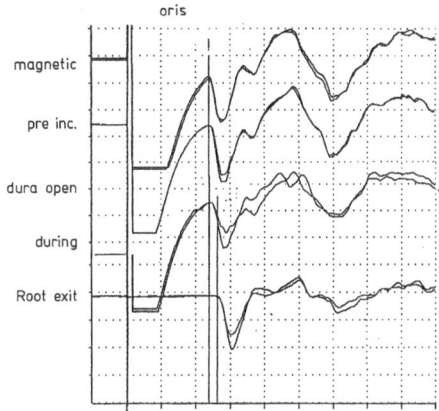

Fig. 3 Intraoperative monitoring in a patient with hemifacial spasm (patient 1; see Table 1). The morphology and onset latency of facial nerve-evoked EMG (eEMG) by magnetic stimulation (*Magnetic*) was not affected at all during stages of surgical procedure (*pre inc*, before incision; *during*, during surgical procedure). The onset latency of eEMG by magnetic stimulation was shorter than that by electrical stimulation at the root exit zone (*Root exit*): 4.76 versus 5.24 ms

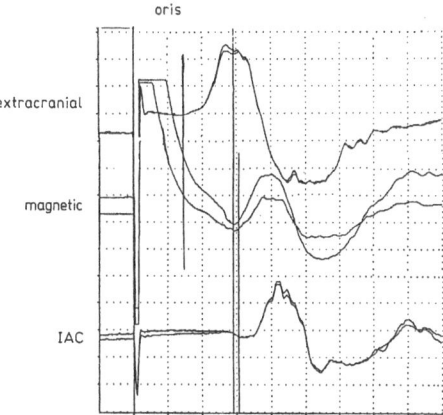

Fig. 2 The evoked EMG by magnetic stimulation with the single coil (*Mag-R; middle*) and the 8-shaped double coil (*Mag-8; bottom*) were ipsilateral and completely identical; onset latency, 4.8 ms. Their morphology was identical to that by extracranial electrical stimulation (*Elec; top*), although the onset latency was different (2.88 ms)

Fig. 4 Intraoperative monitoring in a patient with acoustic neurinoma (patient 9; see Table 2). The onset latency of facial-nerve-evoked EMG (eEMG) by magnetic stimulation (*Magnetic*) was even shorter than that by intracranial electrical stimulation in the internal auditory canal (*IAC*): 5.84 versus 6.04 ms

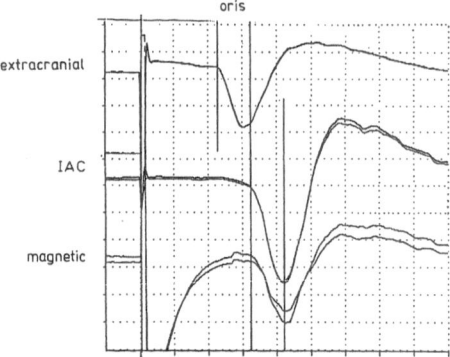

Fig. 5 Intraoperative monitoring in a patient with acoustic neurinoma (patient 7; see Table 2). The onset latency of facial-nerve evoked EMG (eEMG) by magnetic stimulation *(Magnetic)* was identical to that by electrical stimulation in the internal auditory canal *(IAC)* i.e., 6.48 ms

ference between these two kinds of eEMGs was 0.55 ms, ranging from 0.44 to 0.76 ms. Intraoperative monitoring in the patients with acoustic neurinoma showed that onset latency of eEMG by TMS was even shorter than that by IES in the internal auditory canal in two acoustic neurinomas (0.20 and 0.56 ms, respectively, Fig. 4) and identical in one (Fig. 5, Table 2).

Discussion

Our results suggest that TMS excites the same site of the intracranial facial nerve independent of the types of the magnetic coil. Our results also suggest that the stimulated site of the facial nerve in TMS is not the root exit zone, but in the more peripheral part of the nerve. The length of the facial nerve in the cerebellopontine angle and in the internal auditory canal is reported to be 15.8 mm (9–16 mm) and 12.7 mm (9.3–17.6 mm) respectively [2]. As conduction velocity of the facial nerve is approximately 50–60 m/s [7], a mean difference of onset latency between TMS and IES at the root exit zone of 0.55 ms means that the stimulated site is approximately 25–30 mm distal from the root exit zone, i.e., in the distal part of the intrameatal facial nerve. The results from the patients with acoustic neurinoma support this conclusion that the stimulated site is in the distal part of the internal auditory meatus.

References

1. Maccabee PJ, Amassian VE, Cracco RQ, Cracco JB, Anziska BJ (1988) Intracranial simulation of facial nerve in humans with the magnetic coil. Electroencephalogr Clin Neurophysiol 70: 350–354
2. Lang J (1981) Neuroanatomy of the optic, trigeminal, facial, glossopharyngeal, vagus, accessory, and hypoglossal nerves. Arch Otorhinolaryngol 231 : 1–69
3. Rosler KM, Schmid UD, Hess CW (1991) Transcranial magnetic stimulation of the facial nerve: where is the actual excitation site? Electroencephalogr Clin Neurophysiol Suppl 43 : 362–368
4. Schmid UD, Moller AR, Schmid J (1991) Transcranial magnetic stimulation excites the labyrinthine segment of the facial nerve; an intraoperative electrophysiological study in man. Neurosci Lett 124 : 273–276
5. Schriefer TN, Mills KR, Murray NMF, Hess CW (1988) Evaluation of proximal facial nerve conduction by transcranial magnetic stimulation. J Neurol Neurosurg Psychiatry 51 : 60–66
6. Seki Y, Krain L, Yamada T, Kimura J (1990) Transcranial magnetic stimulation of the facial nerve: recording technique and estimation of the stimulated site. Neurosurgery 26:286–290
7. Taverner D (1965) Electrodiagnosis in facial palsy. Arch Otolaryngol 81:470–477

Eur Arch Otorhinolaryngology (1994) [Suppl]:S247–S248

R. Quester, W. Thumfart, J. Menzel, and C. Pototschnig

Pre- and Postoperative Electrophysiological and Magnetic Stimulation Control of Facial Nerve Function in Hemifacial Spasm

Introduction

Facial spasm is one of the most distressing disorders of facial nerve function. It is characterized by paroxysmal and involuntary contractions of the mimic muscles. The spasms usually originate in the orbicularis oculi muscle, tending to extend to all the muscles innervated by the facial nerve. Intensity and frequency of spasms slowly progress.

While sedatives, relaxants, and antispasmodics are of little value in therapy, botulinum toxin has proved to be effective in many cases as temporary treatment. However, in cases of long-lasting and intensive spasms, surgical treatment is usually more effective. Microsurgical decompression of the facial nerve in the cerebellopontine angle, initiated by Jannetta, leads to the best results in comparison to the other surgical treatments such as partial nerve dissection.

This report is one of the rare studies concerning the long-term results of microsurgical vessel loop or, in one case, tumor decompression. The results of pre- and postoperative electrophysiological and magnetic stimulation testing are presented and discussed as well as postoperative auditory, vestibular, and facial nerve function.

Material and Methods

Thirteen patients with hemifacial spasms were treated by facial nerve decompression from 1983 to 1992. The age of the 11 females and two males ranged from 36 to 72 years, with an average age of 50 years. The duration of symptoms varied from 1.5 to 20 years, with a mean value of 6.5 years.

R. Quester (✉) and J. Menzel
Neurochirurgische Klinik, Krankenhaus Merheim,
Kliniken der Stadt Köln, Ostmheimer Str. 200,
51109 Köln, Germany

W. Thumfart and C. Pototschnig
ENT Department of the University of Cologne

Ten patients had spasms on the left side and three patients on the right side. One patient had been treated previously by partial peripheral nerve dissection.

The facial spasms were accompanied by a hypacusis in four cases, by a complete hearing loss in one case, and by vestibular symptoms in five patients. One case showed a temporary sensorial and motor hemisyndrome and another one a hypesthesia of one side of the face. Two patients suffered from tinnitus.

All patients had preoperative computerized tomography and in some cases magnetic resonance imaging. Clinical examination included pre- and postoperative otolaryngological testing with audiometry, caloric test, and brain stem evoked response audiometry (BERA). The facial nerve function was controlled by electromyography and neuromyography as well as magnetic stimulation. In this technique, a peak current flow through a coil consisting of 20 windings of up to 5000 Å was applied for a period of 300–500 μs, inducing a magnetic flow of up to 2 T for a period of 60–150 μs. The magnetic impulse induced an electric current in the surrounding tissue of up to 0.25 mA per cm². Depending on the coil position, the flow of current stimulated a nerve activity potential and led to muscular response. Nerve stimulation was performed from the contralateral cortex, the ipsilateral vertex, and the ipsilateral skull base area for cisternal stimulation.

A Tönnies TESY II two-channel electromyography was used for registration of muscle activity with bipolar hooked wire electrodes.

Surgery was done by a retromastoid craniectomy, and after moderate retraction of the cerebellum the entire intracranial facial nerve was inspected. The offending vessel was mobilized and a piece of Teflon interposed with fibrin glue sealing.

Results

Facial spasm completely disappeared after surgery in ten cases, in six of them directly and in the other cases within

S 248

3 – 12 months. Three patients showed a considerable reduction of intensity and frequency of spasms.

Three patients developed a temporary facial paresis, that completely disappeared within 6 months, while three other patients had a palsy that almost completely disappeared within a few years. In the postoperative course a permanent ipsilateral hearing loss occurred in five cases. Three patients had a complete, one patient a severe, and another one a mild hearing loss. A temporary hearing loss completely disappearing within a few weeks was observed in three other patients.

Two patients suffered from permanent vestibular disturbance on the operated side, while five had mild symptoms. During the long-term follow-up examinations, two patients showed severe spasms again after 6 and 18 months, respectively. Two other patients developed mild spasms after 4 and 5 years, respectively, remaining stable over the following years.

An offending vessel had been found in all cases intraoperatively, with exception of one patient with an epidermoid tumor. Vascular compression had been caused by the anterior inferior cerebellar artery (AICA) in seven cases and in the other cases by the basilar or vertebral artery.

EMG revealed the facial spasms in the registrations from the orbicularis oris and oculi muscles. Electroneuromyography showed normal latencies in nearly all cases (3 – 4 ms). EMG proved a discrete paresis of the orbicularis oculi muscle clinically not observable in the tumor patient. Intraoperatively, the nerve was compressed by tumor and the patient developed a complete facial paresis postoperatively. One patient showed discrete fibrillations in the innervated muscle of the ramus zygomaticofrontalis. Spontaneous activity and polyphasic potentials were found in the patient with peripheral nerve dissection before decompression surgery.

Postoperative EMG controls in cases of facial pareses normalized with restitution of nerve function.

Magnetic stimulation also proved to be effective in registration of facial spasms. Spasms were showed in ipsi- and contralateral cortical stimulation in the mimic muscles.

The latency was normal, with mean values of 5 ms in the ipsilateral and in the contralateral registration. Magnetic stimulation, near the stylomastoid foramen (SMF), and cisternal stimulation were also performed, with registrations of the orbicularis oris and oculi muscles. SMF stimulation revealed latencies of 3.80 – 4.45 ms in ipsilateral and 3.75 – 4.00 ms in contralateral registrations. Cisternal stimulation showed values of 5.10 ms in ipsilateral and 5.00 ms in contralateral registration. In all the examined cases, the latencies were normal.

A postoperative latency delay was observed in this case of facial paresis. This patient showed normal magnetic stimulation registrations and values of latencies before surgery. Latency delays after surgery nearly normalized within a year, correlating well with restitution of facial nerve function.

Discussion

The study has proved the effectiveness of facial nerve decompression, with disappearance or important diminishing of facial spasms in all cases. During the long-term follow-up, only two patients developed severe spasms again. Long-term results are described in studies by Goya and Jannetta [1, 2], reporting similar success rates of decompression surgery.

The major complication is a permanent sensorineural hearing loss on the operated side with an incidence of 61%, ranging from discrete to severe symptomatology. This can be explained by the fact that in many cases not only the facial, but also the vestibulocochlear nerve is irritated by the same vessel. This is also the reason for the high rate (more than 60%) of preoperative hearing or vestibular disturbancies. Similar results were reported by Moller [3].

In 46% of the patients, facial paresis was observed postoperatively with a high restitution rate.

Exact preoperative registrations of facial spasms were possible with electromyography. This method proved to be sensitive in detecting discrete signs of preoperative facial nerve irritation. Neuromyography showed normal latencies in the majority of cases.

Magnetic stimulation led to regular muscle action potentials. With this method a stimulation of the motor cortex as well as of the nuclear regions of the facial nerve was possible ipsi- and contralaterally. The preoperative latencies were normal with cortical stimulation (standard range, 9.5 – 12.0 ms). Quite normal results were obtained with cisternal stimulation (standard range, 4.0 – 6.6 ms) and SMF stimulation (standard range, 3.0 – 4.5 ms).

Postoperative latency delays were observed in the case of a facial paresis. They slowly normalized with restitution of facial nerve function.

With magnetic stimulation it was clearly possible to show that neural pathways were not affected in cases of facial spasm.

References

1. Goya T, Kinoshita K, Yamakawa Y, Morita Y, Ueda T, Nihara K, Fukui M (1983) Hemifacial spasm. Analysis of 40 cases of neurovascular decompression. Neurol Med Chir 23 : 651 – 658
2. Jannetta PJ (1987) Hemifacial spasm: etiology and treatment. In: English GM (ed) Otolaryngology. Harper and Row, Philadelphia
3. Moller MB, Moller AR (1985) Loss of auditory function in microvascular decompression for hemifacial spasm. J Neurosurg 63:17 – 20

Eur Arch Otorhinolaryngology (1994) [Suppl]: S249–S252

FREE PAPERS AND POSTERS

C. Pototschnig, I. Schneider, J. Gubitz, and M. Schneider

Influence of Different Electrodes on Electric and Magnetic Stimulation of the Facial Nerve

Introduction

Diagnoses of lower cranial nerve lesions, especially of the facial nerve, are based upon neurophysiological tests. Electromyography and a variety of stimulation tests are used. Because of the petrous bone, an approach to the most common area of lesions is difficult. Only distal parts of the nerve can be investigated.

Neuromyography, inaugurated by Esslen, shows good results using bipolar surface electrodes for stimulation at the stylomastoid foramina and deduction at the nasolabial fold. A highly significant correspondence in the number of injured nerve fibres to the altitude of the muscle answer potential was found.

Magnetic stimulation as a new technique, developed by Barker in 1985 [1] (Fig. 1), now allows a painless examination of the whole course of the nerve; beginning at its origin, the motor cortex, the cerebellopontine angle and the peripheral parts can be checked. Magnetic impulses induce a non-selective excitation of the surrounding tissue, meaning that by stimulation at the stylomastoid foramina, a direct excitation of the masseter muscle is induced; in transcranial stimulation, all other lower cranial nerves can be reached. A highly selective deduction of the appertaining musculature is necessary.

Two types of electrodes are used: (1) bipolar surface electrodes, producing good summation potentials and (2) concentric bipolar needle electrodes. These should be positioned very close to the muscular end plates. Using needle electrodes an exact determination of latency is possible, while no representative summation potentials can be deduced. In contrast, surface electrodes allow highly representative potentials, but a varying start of the muscle answer potential.

C. Pototschnig, I. Schneider, J. Gubitz, and M. Schneider
Klinik und Poliklinik für Hals-, Nasen- und Ohrenheilkunde
der Universität zu Köln, Joseph-Stelzmann-Strasse 9,
50924 Köln

In contrast to electric stimulation, we found significant differences in amplitudes and latencies when stimulating magnetically, with the small coil at the stylomastoid foramina and the large coil transcranially, using bipolar surface electrodes for deduction instead of using needle electrodes. A significant increase in the muscle answer potential can be seen in surface electrodes. The reason for this is the non-assessable influence of the magnetic impulse to the surrounding tissue (Figs. 2, 3).

Needle electrodes used for deduction did not show such a divergence, but unfortunately no representative potentials according to the type of lesion can be deducted (Figs. 4, 5). Therefore, no electrode to exactly determine the amplitudes was available.

Material and Methods

We designed and developed a deduction electrode producing representative potentials which was not susceptible to magnetic artefacts and was easy to apply:

A so-called double-needle electrode with a distance between the electric poles of 4 mm was used. Direct application to the muscle as well as a wide-ranged measure field were provided. Stimulation with electric and magnetic impulses at the stylomastoid foramina and magnetic impulses at the cerebellopontine angle was performed.

A total of 40 healthy subjects were examined, using all three types of deduction electrodes at the nasolabial fold. Intra- and interindividual differences in amplitudes and latencies depending on the deduction electrode and stimulation technique were assessed.

Results

Depending on the kind of stimulation, a mean increase in amplitudes from 2.44 mV to 4.47 mV was seen using bipolar surface electrodes. The increase ranged from 1.1 to 7.8 mV; the standard deviation was about 1.32.

Fig. 1 Area of stimulation

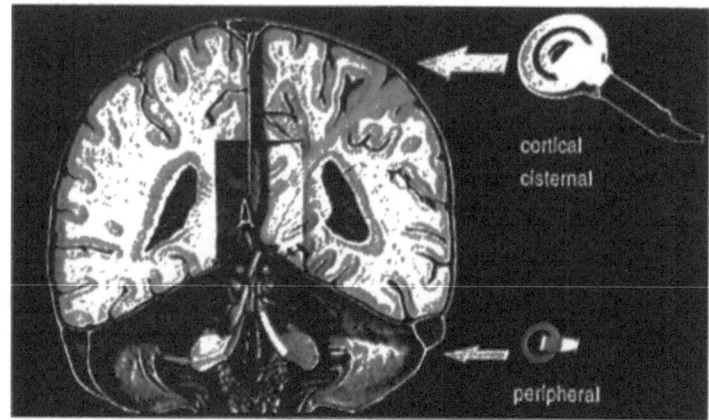

cortical

cisternal

peripheral

Fig. 2 Electrical stimulation at the stylomastoid foramina with surface electrode deduction at the nasolabial fold

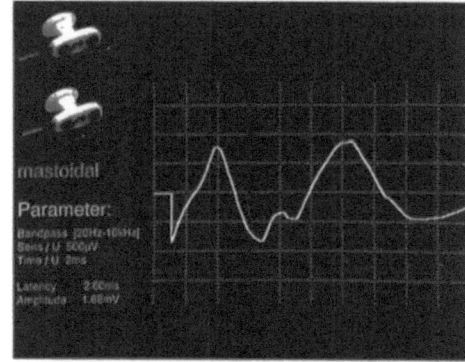

Fig. 3 Magnetic stimulation at the stylomastoid foramina with surface electrode deduction at the nasolabial fold

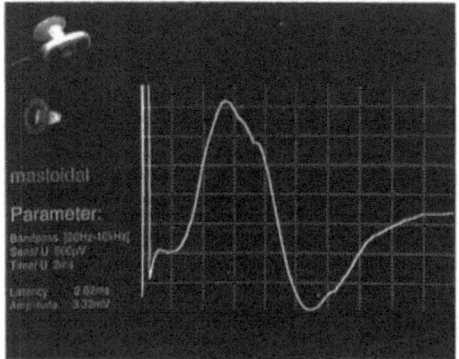

Fig. 4 Electrical stimulation at the stylomastoid foramina with needle electrode deduction at the nasolabial fold

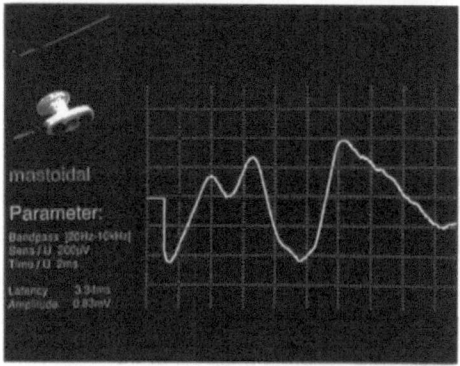

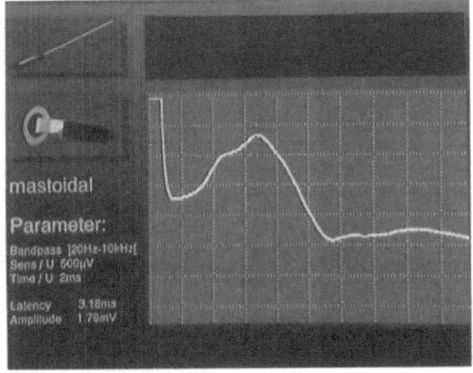

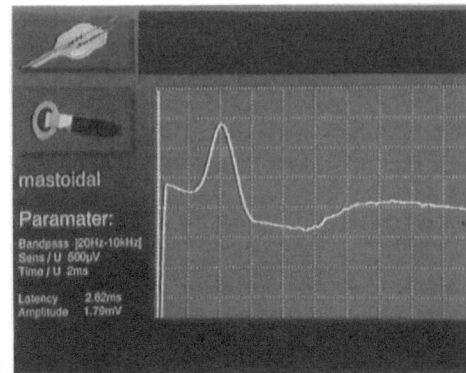

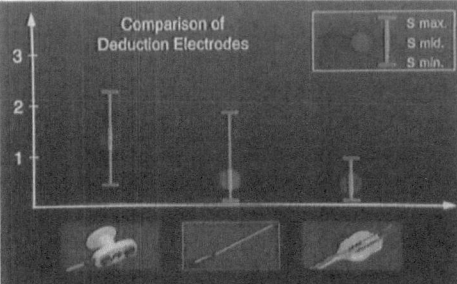

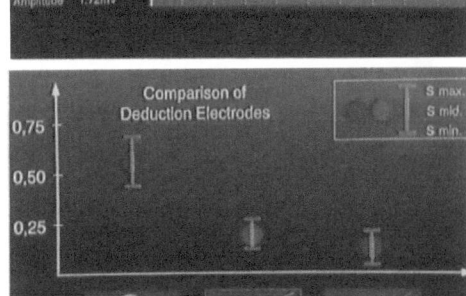

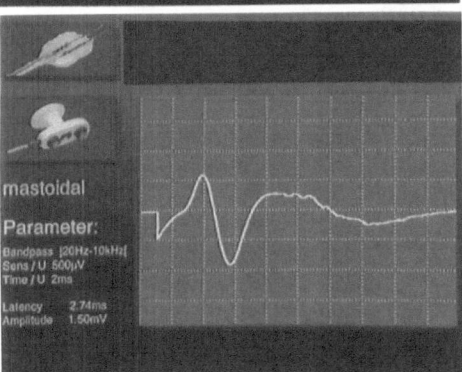

Fig. 5 Magnetic stimulation at the stylomastoid foramina with needle electrode deduction at the nasolabial fold

Fig. 6 Standard deviation of amplitudes using all types of stimulation and stimulation areas

Fig. 7 Double-needle electrodes with electrical stimulus at the stylomastoid foramina

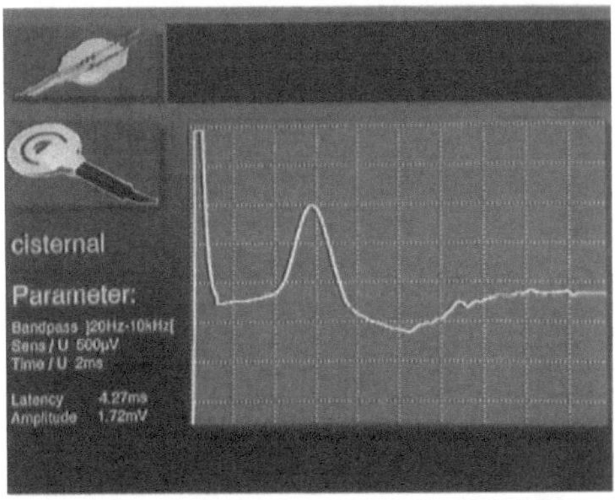

Fig. 8 Double-needle electrodes with magnetic stimulus at the stylomastoid foramina

Fig. 9 Double-needle electrodes with magnetic stimulus in the cerebellopontine area

Fig. 10 Standard deviation of latencies using all types of stimulation and stimulation areas

Using needle electrodes the mean was around 1.7 mV, with limiting values of 0.33 and 3.98 mV; the standard deviation was about 0.5.

Double-needle electrodes showed amplitudes of about 2.2 mV. The limiting values were 1 and 4.3 mV; the standard deviation was about 0.3 (Fig. 6).

No significant differences were seen between double-needle electrodes with electric stimulus at the stylomastoid foramina (Fig. 7), magnetic stimulation at the stylomastid foramina (Fig. 8) and magnetic stimulation in the cerebellopontine area (Fig. 9).

The determination of latencies showed a standard deviaton of about 0.6 using surface electrodes and 0.2 using needle or double-needle electrodes in all types of stimulation (Fig. 10).

Conclusion

Early changes in the muscle answer potentials after onset of palsy, especially after petrous bone traumas, and the possibility of examining the whole nerval course were the main advantages of magnetic stimulation. By allowing precise determination of the potentials, the double-needle electrode turned out to give the most accurate results. Furthermore, they show no susceptibility to other excited cranial nerves, a well-reproducible muscle answer potential, better correlation between muscle function and stimulated response. These electrodes also enable exact positioning. Therefore, they should be used in magnetic stimulation.

References

1. Barker AT, Talinous R, Freeston JL (1985) Non-invasive magnetic stimulation of the human motor cortex. Lancet i (8437): 1106–1107
2. Barker AT, Freeston JL, Jalinous R, Merton PA, Morton HB (1985) Magnetic stimulation of the human brain. J Physiol (Lond) 369: 3 P
3. Barker AT, Jalinous R, Freeston JL, Jarrat A (1987) Magnetic stimulation of the human brain and peripheral nervous system: an introduction and the results of an initial clinical evaluation. Neurosurgery 20: 100–109
4. Benecke R, Meyer B-U, Schönle P, Conrad B (1988) Transcranial magnetic stimulation of the human brain: responses in muscles supplied by cranial nerves. Exp Brain Res 7 1 (3): 623–632
5. Benecke R, Meyer B-U, Schönle P, Conrad B (1988) Beurteilung motorischer Hirnnervenfunktionen mit Hilfe der transkraniellen magnetischen Stimulation. EEG EMG 19 (4): 228–233
6. Kartush JM, Bouchard KR, Graham MD et al. (1990) Magnetic stimulation of the facial nerve. Am J Otol 10 (1): 14–19
7. Mills KR, Murray NMF, Hess CW (1987) Magnetic and electrical transcranial brain stimulation: physiological mechanisms and clinical applications. Neurosurgery 20 (1): 164–168
8. Pototschnig C, Stennert E (1990) Magnetic stimulation: new possibilities in the assessment of facial nerve dysfunction. The facial nerve, international symposium on the facial nerve, 1988, Rio, pp 183–189
9. Pototschnig C, Thumfart WF (1990) Electrodiagnosis of facial nerve palsies. The facial nerve, international symposium on the facial nerve, 1988, Rio, pp 349–350
10. Schriefer TN, Mills KR, Hess CW (1988) Evaluation of proximal facial nerve conduction by transcranial magnetic stimulation. J Neurol Neurosurg Psychiatr 51: 60–66
11. Seki Y, Krain L, Yamada T, Kimura J (1990) Transcranial magnetic stimulation of the facial nerve: recording technique and estimation of the stimulated site. Neurosurgery 26 (2) 286–290
12. Zorowka P, Pototschnig C, Thumfart WF (1989) Magnetic stimulation as a new diagnostic possibility for functional disturbances of the larynx. Annual meeting, European Phoniater, Erlangen

Eur Arch Otorhinolaryngology (1994) [Suppl]: S 253–257

R. Maire and R. Häusler

Evaluation of Peripheral Facial Palsy by Transcranial Magnetic Stimulation

Introduction

An electric impulse in a coil creates an intense transient magnetic field which can pass through organic structures without being modified. This is because different tissues of the body all have the same magnetic permeability and are transparent to the magnetic field. In the body, the magnetic field induces an electric current which causes nerve stimulation. If the coil is placed above the scalp, the intracranial motor pathways are stimulated and the compound action potential of the activated muscles can be recorded.

Many authors [1–6] have recently described transcranial magnetic stimulation of the human brain. This method has opened new investigative perspectives in electrophysiology, allowing a painless and non-invasive examination of the cerebral motor cortex and peripheral nerves. The technique has also been proposed for the evaluation of facial nerve function [7, 8]. For that reason we were interested in studying this new method with a group of patients suffering from peripheral facial palsy and comparing it with classical electroneurography (ENoG). Our goal was to estimate the prognostic value of the magnetic test in acute facial palsy, i. e. the assessment of nerve damage and the usefulness in locating the lesion. Furthermore, we tried to establish whether this technique would replace ENoG. Finally, we compared the results of both methods with the clinical evolution of the patients.

R. Maire
Clinic of Otolaryngology, Head and Neck Surgery,
University Hospital, CHUV, 1011 Lausanne, Switzerland

R. Häusler
Chairmen of the University Clinic of ENT, Head and Neck Surgery,
Inselspital, 3010 Bern, Switzerland

Method

For this study, we used the Magstim 200 (MME, Freiburg, Germany). This apparatus is a high-energy electromagnetic pulse generator with a maximal power of 1500 mT. The duration of the induced electric current in the body is around 200 µs. To stimulate the peripheral facial nerve, the coil is set 5 cm above the ear in the parietal area without touching the scalp. The magnetic energy should be sufficient to cause supramaximal stimulation of the facial nerve with maximal and unvarying muscular compound action potentials. For the Magstim 200, this value corresponds to 750 mT. The data are amplified on a Nicolet CA 2000 equipment usually used for recording auditory evoked potentials. We record the nasolabial muscular response with silver chloride electrodes placed on the alae nasi [7, 9, 10]. This site of recording is also used for ENoG, where the facial nerve is electrically stimulated through the skin at the stylomastoid foramen. The technique and results of ENoG are well described [11–15]: a lack of muscular response indicates full Wallerian degeneration (more than 95% of degenerated nervous fibres), which indicates a serious lesion with reserved prognosis. The persistence of a muscular compound action potential shows neuropraxia (reversible block of nervous conduction) with good prognosis.

The latencies and amplitudes of waves were measured for both electrical and magnetic stimulations. In cases of facial palsy, the healthy side was always tested first to obtain a reference response.

Some precautions must be taken with magnetic stimulation [1, 2, 4, 5, 8]: this method should be avoided in epileptic patients, because it may induce a seizure. It should also be avoided in patients with pacemakers, arterial cerebral clips or metallic implants in the ear (cochlear implants, stapedectomy protheses), which could be displaced.

Patients

We performed transcranial magnetic stimulation of the facial nerve on ten healthy control subjects (five men, five women) with a mean age of 32 years (range, 25–39 years) and 21 patients with peripheral facial palsy (ten men, 11 women) with a mean age of 49 years (range 18–84 years). All these patients were examined between November 1989 and June 1990 at the Clinic of Otolaryngology and Head and Neck Surgery of the University Hospital of Geneva, Switzerland.

In addition to magnetic stimulation, the 31 patients underwent classical transcutaneous ENoG at the stylomastoid foramen. None of the 31 patients had a contraindication to testing. All tests were performed between the fifth day and the tenth month after the onset of facial palsy.

The aetiology of the facial palsy was idiopathic (Bell's palsy) in 13 cases, transverse temporal bone fracture in four cases, herpes zoster oticus in three cases and malignant external otitis in one case.

Results

Healthy Subjects (Control Group)

The latencies and amplitudes of muscular compound action potentials recorded in the ten normal subjects (20 sides) after electrical and magnetic stimulations are given in Table 1. In both tests, the waves are biphasic with similar shapes and amplitudes, as shown in Fig. 1. However, the latency of the response to magnetic stimulation appears with a mean delay of 1 ms when compared with electrical stimulation.

Patients with Peripheral Facial Palsy

Paralysis with Full Axonal Degeneration

After electrical stimulation, a lack of response was observed on the paralysed side of ten patients, indicating full

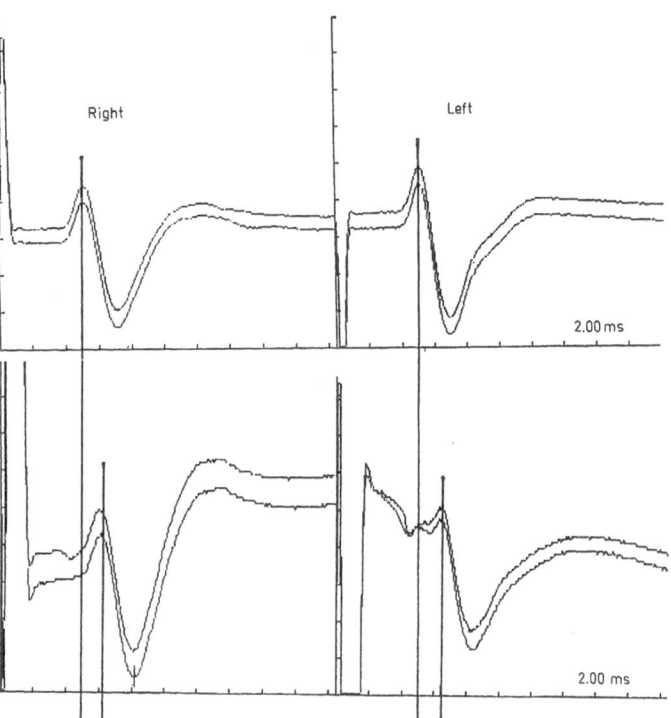

Fig. 1 Example of facial muscular responses recorded in a healthy male subject. *Top*, Waves obtained with electroneurography (ENoG). *Bottom*, Waves obtained with magnetic stimulation. For both methods, the muscular compound action potentials are similar in morphology. Note the latency difference of 1 ms between the onset of responses to electrical and magnetic stimulations

Table 1 Facial muscular responses of 20 healthy sides in ten normal subjects

	± mse Mean latency (ms)	± mse Mean amplitude (mV)
Electrical stimulation (stylomastoid foramen)	5.3 ± 0.1	2.38 ± 0.2
Magnetic stimulation	6.35 ± 0.08	2.54 ± 0.2

Latency difference, 1.05 ms ± 0.13
Amplitude difference, 0.16 mV ± 0.28.

mse, mean standard error.

Wallerian degeneration (Fig. 2a). In all these cases we also noted a flat line after magnetic stimulation. For the healthy side, the muscular compound action potentials obtained with both methods of stimulation were normal in latency and morphology.

In these ten cases of full Wallerian degeneration, the aetiology of the paralysis was Bell's palsy in four cases, temporal bone fracture in three cases, herpes zoster oticus in two cases and malignant external otitis in one case.

The four patients with Bell's palsy and one with herpes zoster oticus began recovering after only a few months. The patient with malignant external otitis and the second patient with herpes zoster oticus were still paralysed after 6 and 12 months, respectively. The two patients with acute facial palsy caused by temporal bone fracture were surgically treated for facial nerve decompression with good postoperative evolution. Unfortunately, we have no follow-up for the last case of temporal bone fracture.

Paralysis with Neuropraxia

In 11 patients, the ENoG displayed an obvious response revealing neuropraxia on the paralysed side (Fig. 2b). In contrast, no response was obtained with magnetic stimulation, as in complete axonal degeneration. Both methods induced normal waveforms on the healthy side.

Among these 11 cases, there were nine Bell's palsies, one herpes zoster oticus and one neglected temporal bone fracture with residual facial paresis.

All the patients recovered rapidly and completely from their palsy in a few weeks, except for the belatedly tested patient with untreated temporal bone fracture, who showed only partial recovery of the paralysis.

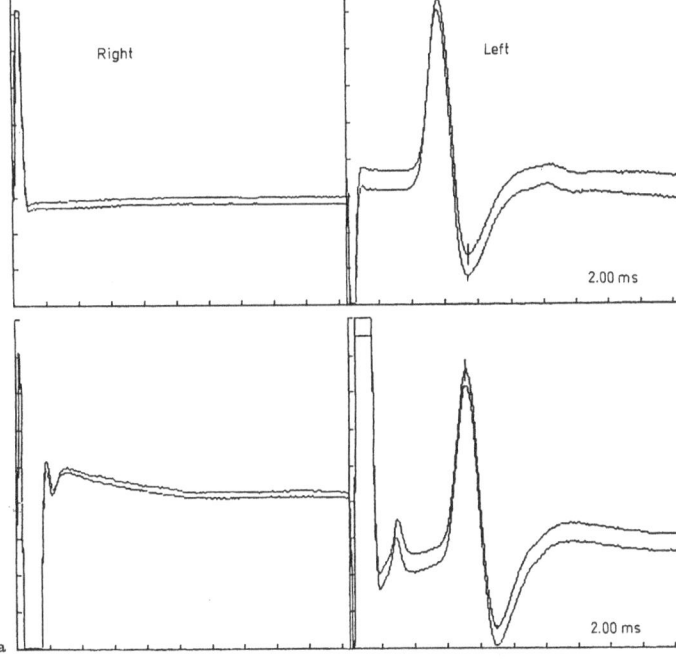

Fig. 2a, b Example of facial muscular responses recorded on patients with peripheral facial palsy in cases of full axonal degeneration (herpes zoster oticus with facial palsy, **a**) and neuropraxia (Bell's palsy, **b**). Right paralysis in both cases. *Top,* Waves obtained with electroneurography (ENoG). *Bottom,* Waves obtained with magnetic stimulation. Normal muscular compound action potentials in response to both electrical and magnetic stimulations are obtained for the healthy left side. In the case of complete degeneration, the two methods induce no response; the little early wave noted on magnetic recording corresponds to the action potential of the upper eyelid levator muscle. In the case of neuropraxia, the electroneurography displays an obvious response where none is induced by magnetic stimulation (in this example, the residual response has an amplitude 80% under the healthy side corresponding to 20% neuropraxia)

For **Fig. 2b** see next page

Fig. 2b. For caption see S. 255

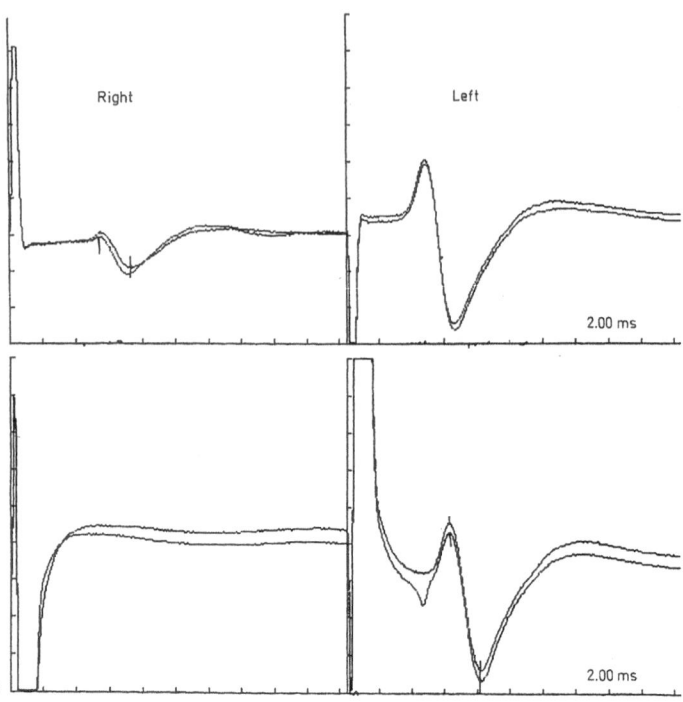

Right   Left

2.00 ms

2.00 ms

b

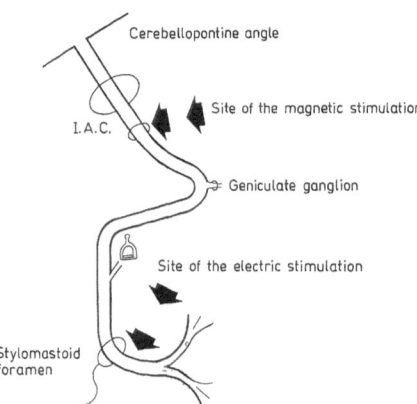

Fig. 3 Magnetic (internal auditory canal, *I.A.C.*) and electrical (stylomastoid foramen) stimulation sites of the facial nerve. The intracranial location of the magnetic stimulation site is estimated from a 1-ms latency difference between the responses to both stimulation methods

Cerebellopontine angle

Site of the magnetic stimulation

I.A.C.

Geniculate ganglion

Site of the electric stimulation

Stylomastoid foramen

In summary, of the 21 patients affected by peripheral facial palsy, no response was obtained on the paralysed side with magnetic stimulation, whereas ENoG induced an obvious response indicating neuropraxia in 11 cases.

Discussion

In normal subjects, both methods of stimulation induce biphasic waves similar in shape and amplitude corresponding to the compound action potential of nasolabial muscles. The major difference is that the latency between the onset of the response to electrical stimulation and the one following magnetic stimulation is 1 ms longer after magnetic stimulation. This value fits with the time required for the action potential of the magnetically excited intracranial facial nerve to reach the transcutaneous electrical stimulation site at the stylomastoid foramen. If we take the facial nerve conduction speed into account, which is around 40 m/s, the latency difference of 1 ms suggests that the magnetic stimulation site of the facial nerve is a few centimeters higher than the stylomastoid foramen at the level of the internal auditory canal (Fig. 3). These findings agree with those of other authors [7, 8]. A magnetic stimulation site on the internal auditory canal is also supported by the observation of normal responses in cases of cerebellopontine angle lesion or central injury of the facial nerve. Furthermore, the cerebrospinal fluid present around the statoacoustic and facial nerves in the internal auditory canal could play a particular role in excitation [7, 8].

In the case of peripheral facial palsy, the results obtained with magnetic stimulation show a lack of response to all conditions of nervous conduction block. This method does not supply information permitting differentiation of neuropraxia from axonal degeneration, since the response is the same in both situations. These findings could be explained by the fact that the magnetic technique stimulates the facial nerve in its internal auditory canal segment above the injury site causing the paralysis. In most cases, as in Bell's palsy, the nervous conduction block is effectively located in the labyrinthine segment of the facial nerve, at the entrance of the Fallopian canal, as proposed by Fisch [16] and recently proved by a histological study of a paralysed facial nerve [17].

In contrast, ENoG displays a persistent muscular compound action potential in the case of neuropraxia, permitting estimation of the seriousness of the nerve damage and establishment of the clinical prognosis of the facial palsy. In our series, the evolution of the paralysis was good in the cases of neuropraxia and in general poor in the cases of full degeneration. These data confirm the prognostic interest in differentiating neuropraxia from axonal degeneration.

Conclusions

Transcranial magnetic stimulation is a new, non-invasive and well-tolerated method for examinatin of the nervous system which will certainly have interesting future developments in neurology. In particular, this technique allows evaluation of the central motor pathways and peripheral nerve conduction.

Regarding peripheral facial palsy, our study did not show any advantage of the magnetic method over classical ENoG. Specifically, transcranial magnetic stimulation does not allow differentiation between neuropraxia and axonal degeneration and therefore cannot be used to establish the clinical prognosis of the paralysis.

With regard to the location of the site of the lesion, our results demonstrate that transcranial magnetic stimulation can provide some precision, indicating that the facial nerve conduction block lies downstream from the internal auditory canal starting at the entrance of the Fallopian canal.

References

1. Barker AT, Freeston IL, Jalinous R, Jarratt JA (1987) Magnetic stimulation of the human brain and peripheral nervous system: an introduction and the results of an initial evaluation. Neurosurgery 20 (1):100–109
2. Bickford RG, Guidi M, Fortesque P, Swenson M (1987) Magnetic stimulation of human peripheral nerve and brain: response enhancement by combined magnetoelectrical technique. Neurosurgery 20 (1):110–116
3. Day BL, Thompson PD, Dick JP, Nakashima K, Marsden CD (1987) Different sites of action of electrical and magnetic stimulation of the human brain. Neurosci Lett 75:101–106
4. Hess CW, Mills KR, Murray NMF (1987) Responses in small hand muscles from magnetic stimulation of the human brain. J Physiol (Lond) 388:397–419
5. Mills KR, Murray NMF, Hess CW (1987) Magnetic and electrical transcranial brain stimulation: physiological mechanisms and clinical applications. Neurosurgery 20 (1):164–168
6. Rothwell JC, Day BL, Thomspon PD, Dick JPR, Marsden CD (1987) Some experiences of techniques for stimulation of the human cerebral motor cortex through the scalp. Neurosurgery 20 (1):156–163
7. Rösler KM, Hess CW, Schmid UD (1989) Investigation of facial motor pathways by electrical and magnetic stimulation: sites and mechanisms of excitation. J Neurol Neurosurg Psychiatry 52:1149–1156
8. Schriefer TN, Mills KR, Murray NMF, Hess CW (1988) Evaluation of proximal facial nerve conduction by transcranial magnetic stimulation. J Neurol Neurosurg Psychiatry 51:60–66
9. Kelleher MJ, Gutnick HN, Prass RL (1990) Waveform morphology and amplitude variability in facial-nerve electroneurography. Laryngoscope 100:570–575
10. Neuwirth-Riedl K, Burian M, Nekahm D, Gstöttner W, Optimizing of electroneuronography of the facial nerve. ENT Clinic, University of Vienna, Austria. ORL (in press)
11. Echapasse P, Dauman R, Cazenave M, Portmann M (1987) Electrophysiological prognosis in facial paralysis. Clin Otolaryngol 12:289–296
12. Esslen E (1977) Electromyography and electroneurography. Facial nerve surgery. Fisch U (ed) Aesculapius, Birmingham, pp 93–100
13. Fisch U (1980) Maximal nerve excitability testing vs electroneuronography. Arch Otolaryngol 106:352–357
14. Fisch U (1984) Prognostic values of electrical tests in acute facial paralysis. Am J Otolaryngol 5:494–498
15. Kartush JM (1989) Electroneurography and intraoperative facial monitoring in contemporary neurotology. Otolaryngol Head Neck Surg 101:496–503
16. Gantz B, Gmür A, Fisch U (1982) Intraoperative evoked electromyography in Bell's palsy. Am J Otolaryngol 3:273–278
17. Jackson CG, Johnson GD, Hyams VJ, Poe DS (1990) Pathologic findings in the labyrinthine segment of the facial nerve in a case of facial paralysis. Ann Otol Rhinol 99:327–329

Eur Arch Otorhinolaryngology (1994) [Suppl]: S258–S260

S. R. Wolf, W. Schneider, M. Berg, and M. E. Wigand

Transcranial Magnetic Stimulation of the Facial Nerve in Small and Medium-sized Acoustic Neurinomas

Introduction

The expanding mass of an acoustic neurinoma in the internal auditory meatus and the cerebellopontine angle induces symptoms dependent on the time period of the tumor growth. Initial signs of acoustic neurinoma are hearing impairment and tinnitus as well as disturbances of equilibrium. The clinician interpretes affections of the facial, trigeminal, or other cranial nerves as indications of a large tumor mass. The size of the tumor and the initial symptoms are not strictly correlated. Patients with small intrameatal tumors can be deaf and vice versa. The subclinical lesions of the facial nerve by tumor growth have been evaluated earlier by stimulation of the extratemporal part of the facial nerve [8, 7]. Transcranial magnetic stimulation (TMS) was first described in 1985 [1] and is now widely used in the diagnosis of neurological disorders [3, 6]. TMS is a noninvasive instrument for stimulation of the facial nerve in its labyrinthine portion, close to the site of the growing tumor [10, 14].

Material and Methods

A total of 60 patients with histologically confirmed acustic neurinomas were examined prior to tumor removal. The tumor size was graded according to Wigand [12]. Class A describes intrameatal tumors, class B tumors with a diameter of up to 15 mm in the cerebellopontine angle, and class C tumors of up to 30 mm. In all patients clinical testing with documentation of the facial function, examination of taste and lacrimation (Schirmer's test), needle electromyography, electroneuronography, and TMS were performed. Magnetic stimulation was carried out with a

S. R. Wolf (✉), W. Schneider, M. Berg, and M. E. Wigand
University Department of Otorhinolaryngology, Waldstr. 1, 91054 Erlangen-Nürnberg, Germany

Magstim 200 (Novametrix) with a 12 cm stimulation coil placed in the occipitoparietal region on the ipsilateral side. The technique has been described by several authors [2, 9, 11, 13]. The site of stimulation is thought to be in the intratemporal course of the facial nerve (own intraoperative measurements, [10, 14]), although discussion regarding the site of stimulation is still going on [4]. The latencies obtained from the orbicularis oris muscle by extracranial electrical stimulation in the area of the stylomastoid foramen in the orbicularis oris muscle (concentric needle electrodes) were subtracted from the latencies after TMS to obtain values independent of the position of the inserted needle electrodes [13].

All patients were operated via the enlarged middle fossa approach [12]. The tumors were removed completely. The intraoperative findings of special vascular abnormalities and the adhesions of the tumor to the facial nerve were documented.

Results

The distribution of tumor sizes is shown in Table 1. Four patients were totally deaf, two in group A and one each in groups B and C (Table 1). Examination of brain stem audiometry (ABR) was normal in five patients. Due to poor hearing, 19 patients had no or inevaluable responses. The comprehensive vestibular examinations [5] revaled just one patient without any pathological signs. In all cases the function of the facial musculature was completely normal.

Single test results such as trigeminofacial reflex, stapedius reflex, needle electromyography with evaluation of fibrillations and further degenerative signs as well as maximal innervation pattern, Schirmer's test, and examination of taste revealed pathological findings only in a few cases, which are not listed separately.

The distribution of the intratemporal conduction time is shown in Fig. 1. We found elongations of more than 0.2 ms

Table 1 Comparison of hearing, brain stem audiometry (ABR), vestibular examination, and function of the face in 60 patients with acoustic neurinomas

Tumor size	Number of patients	Deaf (n)	ABR pathological[a] (n)	Vestibular test pathological (n)	Facial palsy
A	13	2	6/13	13/13	0
B	19	1	11/17	18/19	0
C	28	1	13/24	28/28	0
Total	60	4	30/54	59/60	0

[a] In six patients, no ABR was performed

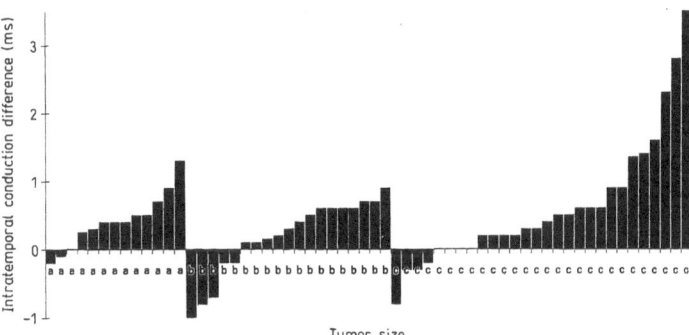

Fig. 1 Intratemporal conduction time in 60 patients with acoustic neurinomas. Difference of the conduction times of the tumor side vs. the unaffected side. Sorted and grouped according to tumor size (see text)

Table 2 Intratemporal conduction time after transcranial magnetic stimulation (median and standard deviations) of the tumor and unaffected sides in 60 patients with acoustic neurinomas

Tumor size	Unaffected side (ms)	Tumor side (ms)	Difference (ms)
A	1.5±0.6	1.9±0.7	0.4±0.4
B	1.5±0.5	1.6±0.7	0.2±0.6
C	1.6±0.5	2.2±1.1	0.6±1.0
Total	1.5±0.5	2.0±0.9	0.4±0.8

in 41 cases. In a further ten cases we observed a shortening of the intratemporal conduction time by more than 0.2 ms (tumor side vs. unaffected side; for details see Table 2). The averaged data are presented in Table 3. There is an obvious difference in the elongation of latencies between the groups with A and B tumors and the group with C tumors.

Discussion

The evaluation of subclinical lesions of the facial nerve due to acoustic neurinomas has been reported earlier [8, 7]. TMS of the facial nerve, with an assumed stimulation site in the labyrinthine segment, was applied preoperatively to

60 patients with acoustic neurinomas. The calculated intratemporal conduction time was generally found to be dependent on the tumor size. The various clinical results in patients with acoustic neurinomas were found with TMS technique, too. Hearing impairment, tinnitus, vestibular disturbances, and subclinical lesions of the facial nerve seem to occur independently of each other.

The observation of decreased intratemporal conduction latencies of the facial nerve after magnetic stimulation in patients with acoustic neurinomas has not yet been reported. Several pathophysiological mechanisms must be considered for these different results. Tumor growth induces direct compression of the nerves in the internal auditory meatus, disturbances in blood supply, and immunological mechanisms, but may cause either changes in the conductivity of the soft tissues by altering the electrochemical constitution, changes in the site of stimulation, or increased irritability of the nerve itself.

Independent of these open questions we found symmetric answers in the facial muscles in this group of 60 patients with acoustic neurinomas in only nine cases (15%).

TMS provides us with an instrument which may help to find subclinical lesions of the facial nerve in patients with acoustic neurinomas. It is independent of hearing, noninvasive (especially if measurements can be successfully made with surface electrodes, which was not performed in this study), and not dangerous. The examination time is short when routinely applied.

Acknowledgement This work was supported by the Wilhelm Sander Foundation, Neustadt Donau (91.021.1).

References

1. Barker AT, Freestone IL, Jalinous R et al. (1985) Magnetic stimulation of the human brain. J Physiol (Lond) 369 :310
2. Benecke R, Meyer BU, Schoenle P, Conrad B (1988) Transcranial magnetic stimulation of the human brain: responses in muscles supplied by cranial nerves. Exp Brain Res 71 : 623–632
3. Claus D (1989) Die transkranielle motorische Stimulation. Fischer, Stuttgart
4. Estrem SA, McCormac T, Haghighi SS, Potter T (1990) A comparison of magnetic and electrical stimulation of facial nerve at the cerebello-pontine angle in the dog. Electroencephalogr Clin Neurophysiol (Ireland) 75 : 558–560
5. Haid CT (1990) Vestibularisprüfung und vestibuläre Erkrankungen. Springer, Berlin Heidelberg New York
6. Hess CW, Mills KR, Murray NM, Schriefer TN (1987) Magnetic brain stimulation: central motor conduction studies in multiple sclerosis. Ann Neurol 22:744–752
7. Kartush JM, Niparko JK, Graham MD, Kemink JL (1987) Electroneurography: preoperative facial nerve assessment for tumors of the temporal bone. Otolaryngol Head Neck Surg 97:257–261
8. Krott HM, Poremba M, Busse M (1969) Latenzmessungen am N. facialis beim Akustikusneurinom. Dtsch Z Nervenheilkd 195:344–355
9. Maccabee PJ, Amassian VE, Cracco RQ, Cracco JB, Anziska BJ (1988) Intracranial stimulation of the facial nerve in humans with the magnetic coil. Electroencephal Clin Neurophysiology 70:350–354
10. Schmid UD, Møller AR, Schmid J (1991) Transcranial magnetic stimulation excites the labyrinthine segment of the facial nerve – an intraoperative electrophysiological study in man. Neurosci Lett 124; 273–276
11. Seki Y, Krain L, Yamada T, Kimura J (1990) Transcranial magnetic stimulation of the facial nerve: recording technique and estimation of the stimulated site. Neurosurgery 26:286–290
12. Wigand ME, Rettinger G, Haid T, Berg M (1985) The removal of VIIIth nerv neurinomas from the cerebello-pontine angle by enlarged middle fossa approach. HNO 33 : 11–16
13. Wolf SR, Goertzen W, Schneider W (1991) Transcranial magnetic stimulation of the facial nerve in patients with acoustic neurinoma. HNO 39 : 482–485
14. Wolf SR, Strauss C, Schneider W (1994) On the site of transcranial magnetic stimulation of the facial nerve: Electrophysiological observations in two cases following transsection of the facial nerve during acoustic neurinoma removal. Neurosurgery (in press)

Eur Arch Otorhinolaryngology (1994) [Suppl]: S261 – S263

FREE PAPERS AND POSTERS

L. Parisi, P. Coiro, G. Valente, M. Terracciano, E. Calandriello, and C. Morocutti

Neurophysiological Evaluation of Bell's Palsy: Electroneurography and Transcranial Magnetic Stimulation

Introduction

Electroneurography (ENOG) is currently the most useful electrophysiological test of facial nerve function [1, 2].

Recently, percutaneous magnetic stimulation has been utilised to stimulate the facial nerve noninvasively, intracranially and to assess conduction in its proximal segment [6].

The purpose of this investigation was to determine the validity of both methods to evaluate the damage and the recovery of facial nerve palsy.

Patients and Methods

Forty-two patients were studied with unilateral Bell's palsy (27 men and 15 women; age range 16 – 66 years, with a mean of 30.1 years). The severity of the facial paralysis was objectively graded (Table 1) [7].

The onset of facial weakness occurred from 2 days to 2 weeks prior to testing. The patients were investigated at various times after onset of idiopathic facial palsy. The surface recording electrodes were taped over the motor region of the superior orbicularis oris muscle and maintained in the same position for electrical stimulation at the stylomastoid foramen and magnetic stimulation transcranially. Responses were amplified with a Medelec MS20 electromyograph machine (bandpass 10Hz to 2 kHz).

For extracranial electrical stimulation, the stimulus was applied through bipolar saline-soaked pad electrodes with an interelectrode distance of 2 cm. The cathode was placed

L. Parisi, P. Coiro, G. Valente, M. Terracciano, E. Calandriello, and C. Morocutti
Istituto II Clinica Neurologica, Universita "La Sapienza", Viale Dell'Universita 30, 00185 Roma, Italy

Table 1 Strength grades of facial muscle

Forehead (voluntary maximal contraction in wrinkling)

- 0: No appreciable movements
- 1: Partial movemets in lateral supraorbital region
- 2: Minimal movements of the whole frontal region
- 3: Appreciable movements, but not equal to the normal side
- 4: Movements equal to the normal side

Eyes (tight and light closure of eyelids)

- 0: 3 mm and more palpebral fissures in tight closure
-    3 mm and more palpebral fissures in light closure
- 1: 3 mm and more palpebral fissures in tight closure
-    Less than 3 mm palpebral fissures in light closure
- 2: Less than 3 mm palpebral fissures in tight closure
-    No palpebral fissures in light closure
- 3: No palpebral fissures in tight closure
-    No palpebral fissures in light closure
- 4: Movements equal to the normal side

Mouth (maximal capacity in showing one's teeth)

- 0: None visible
- 1: First and second superior incissors visible only
- 2: The superior canine visible as well
- 3: Superior and inferior canine visible as well
- 4: Movements equal to the normal side (blown-out cheeks etc.)

The percentage of facial function X (%) was calculated by applying the simple equation $100 : 12 = x : y$ (where y is the sum of the values assigned to the three groups of muscles.

anterior to the mastoid process and the anode positioned so as to minimise stimulus artefact and inadvertent masseter stimulation. Three responses to supramaximal electrical stimuli were recorded. Latency and amplitude of cMAP were measured.

For transcranial peripheral nerve stimulation, a Cadwell MES10 magnetic stimulator was used. The optimal coil position was with the centre 3 cm posterior and 6 cm lateral to Cz, so that the coil lay ipsilateral to the facial nerve being stimulated. This coil position was not rigidly adhered to and it was moved as necessary to produce an optimal response.

The intensity of the magnetic stimulus was gradually increased from subthreshold to supramaximal levels. Five responses to supramaximal stimuli were recorded and averaged. Latency of the responses was analysed. The orbicularis oris muscles were stimulated at rest, and the asymptomatic side was always studied first.

Results

Tables 2–4 summarise latency and amplitude measurement of cMAP recorded from orbicularis oris muscles in 42 Bell's palsy patients following electrical stimulation at the stylomastoid foramen and magnetic stimulation transcranially.

The responses to electrical stimulation were all normal in patients seen within 2 days of the onset of palsy. When the duration of palsy was 8 – 30 days, the responses to electrical stimulation were predominantly abnormal, absent or of prolonged latency. In contrast, responses to magnetic stimulation of the nerve were absent even in those patients examined within the first 2 days, as well as in those examined up to 30 days after onset. Hence, the only direct evidence for the existence of a peripheral nerve lesion within the first few days after onset of palsy was an abnormal response to magnetic stimulation. In patients with facial palsy of longer than 1 month duration, the responses to electrical stimulation were generally obtainable, although with abnormal amplitude. No response to magnetic stimulation could be recorded in any of the patients with Bell's palsy of longer than 2 months duration, in spite of the clinical improvement and of conventional nerve conduction studies.

Table 2 Results from 42 patients with idiopathic facial palsy grouped according to grade of weakness at 2–14 days after onset of palsy

No of patients	Grading (%)	Normal side			Bell's palsy side		
		ENoG		MEP latency	ENoG		MEP latency
		Latency	Amplitude		Latency	Amplitude	
12	20	3.1	1.7	4.4	4.2	0.3	NR
18	35	3.0	2.2	4.3	3.6	0.4	NR
12	45	3.1	1.6	4.4	3.9	0.6	NR

ENoG, electroneurography; MEP, motor evoked potential; NR, not recorded.

Table 3 Results of 30 days after onset of Bell's palsy

No of patients	Grading (%)	Normal side			Bell's palsy side		
		ENoG		MEP latecy	ENoG		MEP latency
		Latency	Amplitude		Latency	Amplitude	
10	35	3.0	1.9	4.3	3.9	0.5	NR
22	45	3.2	2.2	4.5	3.6	0.9	NR
10	60	2.9	1.8	4.2	3.4	1.1	NR

ENoG, electroneurography; MEP, motor evoked potential; NR, not recorded.

Table 4 Results at 60 days after onset of Bell's palsy

No of patients	Grading (%)	Normal side			Bell's palsy side		
		ENoG		MEP latecy	ENoG		MEP latency
		Latency	Amplitude		Latency	Amplitude	
7	50	3.3	1.9	4.6	3.5	0.9	NR
20	60	3.1	2.0	4.4	3.3	1.3	NR
15	75	2.8	2.4	4.1	3.0	1.6	NR

ENoG, electroneurography; MEP, motor evoked potential; NR, not recorded.

Discussion

Electrical stimulation gives a measure of the physiological integrity of the extracranial segment of the facial nerve and an indirect evaluation of its more proximal portion.

The magnetic stimulation can be used to study proximal facial nerve conduction directly and noninvasively. The orbicularic oris cMAP elicited by magnetic stimulation is of similar amplitude and configuration, but shorter latency, to that obtaned by electrical stimulation. If the latency of the magnetic response is subtracted from the latency of the electrical response, a measurament of proximal facial nerve conduction is obtained [4, 5, 10].

We found the mean latency of asymptomatic facial nerve magnetic stimulation to be 4.3 ± 0.7 ms, which was longer than the electrical stimulation, with a mean difference in latency of 1.3 ms.

Our measurements are comparable with results of previous studies [3, 9]. These indicate that the magnetic stimulation of the facial nerve probably occurs between its exit from the brain stem and its entrance in the internal auditory meatus.

The results of this method for Bell's palsy patients are of considerable interest. In fact, 42 patients with recent Bell's palsy had orbicularis oris cMAP elicited by electrical stimulation near the stylomastoid foramen, but none demostrated a response to magnetic stimulation of the facial nerve. This suggests that the site of magnetic stimulation must be proximal to the lesion in facial palsy.

Impossibility to activate facial nerve magnetically in patients persisted 60 days later, even as clinical function returned to near normal.

A demyelinated and still hypoexcitable area would explain the persisting absence of responses to magnetic stimulation, but this does not necessarily portend a worse evolution of palsy [8].

In contrast, magnetic stimulation proves useful for early investigation and for the possibility it offers of studying the proximal portion of facial nerve.

References

1. Esslen E (1977) The acute facial palsies. Springer, Berlin Heidelberg New York
2. Gantz BJ, Gmur A, Fisch U (1984) Electroneurographic evaluation of the facial nerve. Ann Otol Rhinol Laryngol 93
3. Maccabee PJ, Amassian VE, Cracco RQ, Cracco JB, Anzika BJ (1984) Intracranial stimulation of facial nerve in humans with the magnetic coil. Electroencephalogr Clin Neurophysiol 70:350–354
4. Metson R, Rebeiz E, West C, Thornton A (1991) Magnetic stimulation of the facial nerve. Laryngoscope 101:25–30
5. Meyer BU, Britton TC, Benecke R (1989) Investigation of unilateral facial weakness: magnetic stimulation of the proximal facial nerve and of the face-associated motor cortex. J Neurol 236:102–107
6. Murray NMF, Hess CW, Mills KR, Schriefer TN, Smith SFM (1987) Proximal facial nerve conduction using magnetic stimulation. Electroencephalogr Clin Neurophysiol 66:S71
7. Parisi L, Valente G, Mariorenzi R, Dell'Anna C, Amabile G (1986) Paralisi di Bell: studio longitudinale su 120 casi. Riv Neurol 56 (4): 225–235
8. Rosler KM, Hess CW, Schmid UD (1989) Investigation of facial motor pathways by electrical and magnetic stimulation: sites and mechanisms of exitation. J Neurol Neurosurg Psychiatry 52:1149–1156
9. Schriefer TN, Mills KM, Murray NMF, Hess CW (1988) Evaluation of proximal facial nerve conduction by transcranial magnetic stimulation. J Neurol Neurosurg Psychiatry 51:60–66
10. Seki Y, Krain L, Yamada T, Kimura J (1990) Transcranial magnetic stimulation of the facial nerve: recording technique and estimation of the stimulated site. Neurosurgery 26 2:286–290

Conclusion

The results achieved show that magnetic and electrical stimulation are complementary: we consider ENOG to be a useful method for longitudinal electrophysiological evaluation of the recovery of neurotroncular damage and for assessing prognosis in acute facial palsy.

Eur Arch Otorhinolaryngology (1994) [Suppl]: S 264–266

FREE PAPERS AND POSTERS

W. Damenz, R. Laskawi, and P. Roggenkämper

Magnetic Stimulation in Patients with Essential Blepharospasm and Hemifacial Spasm

Introduction

Essential blepharospasm and hemifacial spasm are two different diseases in the group of facial hyperkinesias and are characterized by involuntary spasms of the mimic muscles. The clinical pictures of both diseases show differences in the affected muscles: blepharospasm affects the orbicular oculi muscles bilaterally in most cases, whereas the hemifacial spasm is a spasm of mimic muscles which normally occurs unilaterally.

The origin of both diseases is discussed in the literature differently. In some cases of blepharospasm, the association with organic changes such as tumors and aneurysms is found [2, 4, 11]. In many cases no uniform etiology can be proved [5]. In the discussion about the origin of hemifacial spasm, the most widely accepted theory is that the vessel loop compresses the facial nerve [3].

In order to understand facial hyperkinesias, knowledge about the innervation of facial muscles is important, as it is know that the cortical representation of the frontal muscle has different locations than the other facial muscles. In addition, the trigeminal nerve has afferences to the facial muscles [7–9].

Based on these considerations, we were interested in the examination of facial hyperkinesia patients with magnetic stimulation. With this investigation method we were able to stimulate painlessly both cortical supranuclear structures and the infranuclear cisternal part of the facial nerve.

Material and Methods

As magnetic stimulation appliance the Magstim 200 (Madaus) was used with the large coil. For stimulation 80% of the maximal intensity was used. The latencies of the answer potentials of relaxed muscles were determined in the orbicularis oculi muscle and in the levator labii muscle by repeated stimulation. For registration of answer potentials small surface electrodes were used after establishing standard values of normal individuals (Fig. 1) by repeated investigations of normal persons. In cortical stimulation a normal latency of 12.5 ± 2.9 ms was found; after cisternal stimulation the normal value was determined as 4.6 ± 0.4 ms in the levator labii muscle [1, 6, 10, 12] (Fig. 2). No differences in latencies were found when measuring

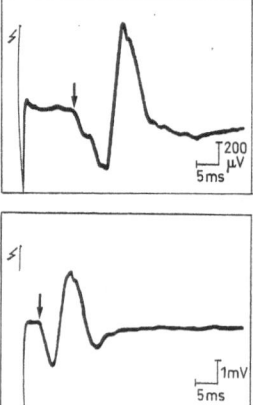

Fig. 1 Answer potentials of a normal individual after transcranial cortical (*top*) and cisternal (*bottom*) magnetic stimulation; registered with surface electrodes

W. Damenz and R. Laskawi
Universitäts-HNO-Klinik Göttingen, Robert-Koch-Str. 40,
37075 Göttingen

P. Roggenkämper
Universitäts-Augenklinik Bonn

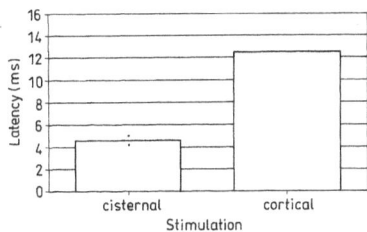

Fig. 2 Mean values and standard deviation of cortical and cisternal stimulation in normal individuals ($n = 13$)

Table 1 Mean latencies after cortical and cisternal stimulation in blepharospasm patients

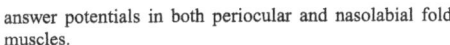

	Mean latencies (ms)	
	Orbicularis oculi	Nasolabial fold
Cortical stimulation	14.4	14.8
Cisternal stimulation	5.2	4.6

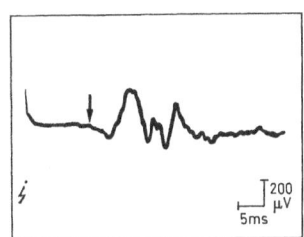

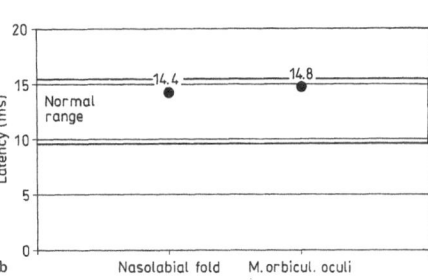

Fig. 3 a Answer potential after cortical stimulation in a blepharospasm patient (*flash symbol* indicates stimulus; *arrow* shows latency). **b** Mean latencies in the nasolabial fold and orbicularis oculi muscle of all blepharospasm patients

answer potentials in both periocular and nasolabial fold muscles.

A total of 59 patients were investigated, 31 patients with a diagnosis of essential blepharospasm and 28 hemifacial spasm patients. Latencies could be measured when an answerpotential could be reached.

Results

Blepharospasm Patients

The results of the magnetic stimulation of 31 blepharospasm patients are shown in Table 1. Both cisternal and cortical stimulation showed values in the normal range with no difference between both muscle groups (Fig. 3).

Hemifacial Spasm Patients

The results of magnetic stimulation of all hemifacial spasm patients are shown in Table 2. In this group a difference between the two investigated muscles was found on the diseased side: whereas in the orbicularis oculi muscle normal latencies (13.1 ms) were found, the latencies in the nasolabial fold were determined as 16.2 ms (Figs. 4, 5). The latencies on the healthy side were found to be normal.

Discussion

In patients with essential blepharospasm, normal latencies were found after cortical and cisternal magnetic stimula-

Table 2 Mean latencies after cisternal and cortical stimulation in hemifacial spasm patients		Mean latencies on healthy side (ms)		Mean latencies on diseased side (ms)	
		Orbicularis oculi	Nasolabial fold	Orbicularis oculi	Nasolabial fold
	Cortical stimulation	12.2	13.2	13.1	16.2
	Cisternal stimulation	–	5.1	–	5.3

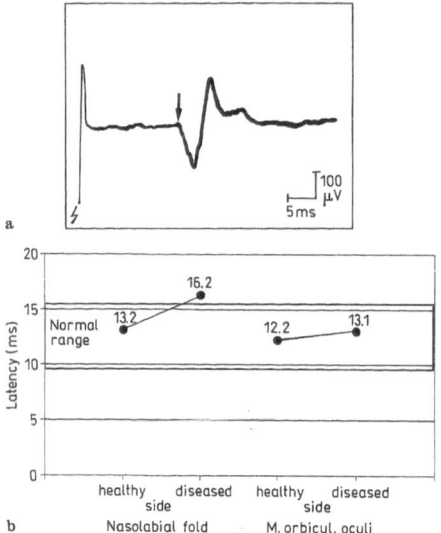

a

b

Healthy diseased · healthy diseased
side   side
Nasolabial fold   M. orbicul. oculi

Fig. 4 a Answer potential determined in the levator labii muscle after cortical stimulation in a hemifacial spasm patient (*flash symbol* indicates stimulus; *arrow* shows latency, here 19.1 ms). **b** Mean latencies in the nasolabial fold and orbicularis oculi muscle of all hemifacial spasm patients

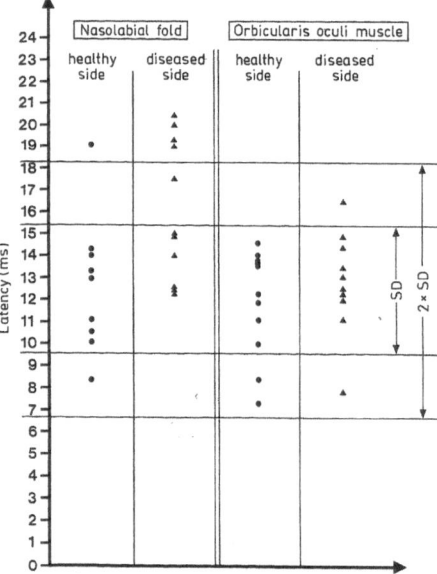

tion with no significant difference between orbicularis oculi muscle and levator labii muscle.

In hemifacial spasm patients, prolonged latencies were found after contralateral cortical stimulation in the nasolabial fold on the diseased side and normal values on the healthy side, whereas in the orbicularis oculi muscle no difference between the two sides was found.

The difference in latencies between two regions of facial muscles may be due to different innervation systems: "eye movement" and "other mimic muscles". Since normal latencies were found in blepharospasm patients, the existence of two different diseases may constitute evidence in this direction.

With the investigative method of magnetic stimulation alone, no statement about the exact location of a lesion is possible; for topodiagnostical investigations additional electrophysiological methods such as neuromyography, blink reflex, and electromyography may help. Further investigatons must be undertaken to establish a complete topodiagnostic tool for the facial nerve by combining all these methods.

References

1. Claus D (1989) Die transkranielle motorische Stimulation. Fischer, Stuttgart
2. Fahn S (1988) Blepharospasm: a form of focal dystonia. Adv Neurol 49 : 125
3. Janetta P (1985) Neurovascular contact in hemifacial spasm. In: Portman M (ed) Facial nerve. Masson, Bordeaux
4. Jankovic J, Havins EW, Wilkins RB (1982) Blinking and blepharospasm. JAMA 23 : 3160–3164
5. Jankovic J, Patel SC (1983) Blepharospasm associated with brainstem lesions. Neurology 33 : 1237–1240
6. Kartush JM, Bouchard KR, Graham MD, Linstrom CL (1989) Magnetic stimulation of the facial nerve . Am J Otol 10 : 14–19
7. Kimura J (1983) Electrodiagnosis in diseases of nerve and muscle: principles and practice. Davis, Philadelphia
8. Kimura J (1988) Blink reflex in facial dyskinesia. Jankovia J, Tolosa E (eds) Facial dyskinesias. Raven, New Yokr (Advances in neurology, vol 49)
9. Laskawi R, Damenz W, Roggenkämper P, Schröder M (1989) Hemispasamus facialis/Blepharospasmus und Botulinus-Toxin – eine elektrophysiologische Untersuchung. Arch. Ohren-Nasen-Kehlkopf-Heilkunde II. 60th annual meeting of the Deutsche Gesellschaft für HNO-Heilkunde, Kopf- und Halschirurgie, Kiel 1989
10. Merton PA, Morton HB (1980) Stimulation of the cerebral cortex in the intact human inject. Nature 285 : 227
11. Walser E, Bebehani AA (1987) Das Krankheitsbild des Blepharospasmus gravis, Ursache und neuratige Behandlungsergebnisse mit Langzeitbeobachtungen. Klin Monatsbl Augenheilkd 190 : 207–212
12. Pototschnig C, Stennert E, Thumfart W (1989) Magnetstimulation. Eine umfassende Methode zur Diagnosik von Schädigungen der kaudalen Hirnnerven. Lecture, 60th annual meeting of the Deutsche Gesellschaft für HNO-Heilkunde, Kopf- und Hals-Chirurgie, Kiel 1989

Fig. 5 Distribution of latencies after magnetic contralateral cortical stimulation in hemifacial spasm patients

Eur Arch Otorhinolaryngology (1994) [Suppl]: S 267–268

FREE PAPERS AND POSTERS

C. Bischoff, B.-U. Meyer, C. Fauth, R. Liscic, J. Machetanz, and B. Conrad

Blink Reflex Investigation Using Magnetic Stimulation

Introduction

The blink reflex (orbicularis oculi reflex) is often used to assess the functional integrity of the facial nerve, the first and second part of the trigeminal nerve, and the brainstem [3, 5, 6]. To evoke a response, an electrical stimulus is usually applied on each supraorbicular nerve. The response of the orbicularis oculi muscle consists of two components, an early R1 on the side of stimulation and a late bilateral R2 component.

Recently, magnetic stimulation has been introduced in clinical neurophysiology and is being used more and more in the investigation of peripheral nerves [1, 2], because magnetic stimuli are less painful and therefore better tolerated by the patients. The aim of the present study was to investigate whether magnetically and electrically evoked blink reflexes show the same characteristics and whether magnetic stimulation can therefore beneficially replace conventional electrical stimulation.

Material and Methods

The blink reflex of 11 healthy persons (six men and five women; mean age, 40.2 ± 6.1 years) was studied. In addition, ten patients (seven men and three women; mean age, 35.2 ± 3.4 years) with (clinically and electromyographically) partial facial nerve palsy in peripheral origin were investigated 2–7 days after the onset of the palsy using both magnetic and electrical stimuli. There were no other motor or sensory abnormalities of cranial nerves or pathological laboratory findings.

C. Bischoff (✉), B.-U. Meyer, C. Fauth, R. Liscic, J. Machetanz, and B. Conrad
Neurologische Klinik und Poliklinik der Technischen
Universität München, Möhlstr. 28, 81675 München

The electrically elicited blink reflex was triggered in a conventional manner using surface electrodes over the supraorbital branch of each side of the trigeminal nerve, and a constant current rectangular pulse of 0.1 ms duration was used. An interstimulus interval of at least 10 s was chosen to avoid habituation of the R2 reflex component.

Magnetic stimulation was performed with the 2.2-T version of the Magstim 200 stimulator (Novametrix), using a small circular coil (outer diameter, 70 mm). The coil windings crossed the supraorbital nerve tangentially, with the center of the coil overlaying the lateral part of the forehead. Stimulation strengths were set at intensities that provided stable responses and were kept constant during the whole investigation. Additionally, the coil was centered in the middle of the forehead with the aim of exciting simultaneously the supraorbital nerves on both sides.

Electromyographic (EMG) recordings were taken of the lower aspects of the orbicularis oculi muscle using surface electrodes; in five of the control subjects, concentric needle electrodes were also used. For each point of stimulation, at least five responses were recorded and the shortest latency was measured.

Results

Reproducible blink reflexes were elicited in all control subjects using electrical and magnetic stimulation (Fig. 1). Stable, magnetically evoked responses were obtained at intensities between 20% and 30% of the maximum output of the stimulation device. The R2 component had lower excitation thresholds than the R1 component. When stimulus intensity was raised, amplitudes of all components increased, but no change of the shortest onset latency occurred. The statistical evaluation using Student's t test did not show any significant difference between the results of the two stimulation techniques concerning onset latencies and interside differences of all components. The direc-

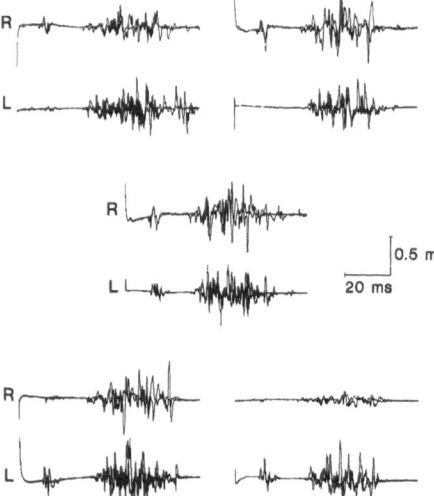

0.5 mV

20 ms

Fig. 1. Blink reflex using unilateral electrical (*left*) and magnetic stimulation (*right*) on the left (*bottom*) and right (*top*) sides and magnetic stimulation in the middle of the forehead (*middle*)

tion of the coil current did not show any influence on the response components.

Applying a magnetic stimulus in the middle of the forehead, a bilateral R1 response was recorded in all healthy subjects. The onset latency of the R1 components did not differ significantly from the response of unilateral electrical and magnetic stimulation (Fig. 1).

In the group of patients with a partial facial nerve palsy, all subjects showed a delayed R1 and R2 on the paretic side, regardless of the side of stimulation. The delayed R1 on the paretic side was also recorded using stimulation in the middle of the forehead, whereas the R2 component was within the normal range.

All subjects investigated with the two methods judged the magnetic stimulation much easier to tolerate than electrical stimulation.

Discussion

The investigation of the blink reflex was possible using both electrical and magnetic stimulation in healthy sub-

jects and patients suffering from peripheral facial palsy. Regarding the shortest latencies of R1, R2, and R2$_c$ and the latency differences in responses following stimulation on the right and left side, no difference between electrical and magnetic stimulation was observed.

Because of the correspondence of onset latencies, it can be assumed that the site of excitation using magnetic stimulation with the coil overlying the supraorbital branch of the trigeminal nerve is approximately the same as using electrical stimulation. The contribution of the excitation of the skin which is covered by the coil to the reflex response cannot be estimated. Such an influence is likely beause R2 components were also elicited with the stimulation coil at positions far away from the supraorbital nerve trunk

The typical response pattern of facial nerve palsy [4] was found using both techniques of stimulation. In lesions involving only the efferent component of the reflex pathway, the delayed R1 can be easily recorded with the magnetic stimulation in the middle of the forehead. This reduces the number of stimuli. Since magnetic stimulation causes less pain, this technique offers a tolerable and reliable method to investigate patients with facial nerve palsies. Especially in follow-up examinations, a stimulation in the middle of the forehead can be used. However, when lesions of the trigeminal nerve or processes within the posterior fossa are suspected, separate examinations of both sides are necessary to delineate the R2 and R2$_c$ components.

Acknowledgement. This work was supported in part by a grant from the Sander Research foundation.

References

1. Bickford RG, Fremming BD (1965) Neuronal stimulation by pulsed magnetic fields in animals and man. Dig of the 6th International Conference on Medical Electronics and Biological Engineering, p 112
2. Britton TC, Meyer B-U, Benecke R (1990) The clinical use of the magnetic stimulator in the investigation of peripheral conduction time. Muscle Nerve 13 : 396–406
3. Kimura J, Lyon LW (1972) Orbicularis oculi reflex in the Wallenberg syndrome: alteration of the late reflex by lesions in the spinal tract and nucleus of the trigeminal nerve. J Neurol Neurosurg Psychiatry 35:228–233
4. Kimura J, Giron LT Jr. Young SM (1976) Electrophysiological study of Bell palsy: electrically elicited blink reflex in assessment of prognosis. Arch Otolaryngol 102 : 140–143
5. Kugelberg E (1952) Facial reflexes. Brain 75 : 385–396
6. Rushworth G (1962) Observations on blink reflex. J Neurol Neurosurg Psychiatry 25 : 93–108

Facial Nerve Lesions: Tumor, Trauma

Eur Arch Otorhinolaryngology (1994) [Suppl]: S271–S273

V. Darrouzet, J. P. Bebear, P. Voyer, S. A. Siddiqui, and M. Papaxanthos

Progressive Facial Palsy and Neurinomas of the VIIth Nerve

Facial nerve neurinomas are rare in comparison to other schwannomas of the base of the skull, notably and especially neurinomas of the VIIIth nerve, but also tumors of mixed nerves expressed in the jugular foramen on in the cervical region. Recent observations have spectacularly illustrated the extremely polymorphous character of the symptomatology encountered and the value of the classification proposed by Sterkers et al. in 1986 [5]. The following is a brief review of that classification.

Classification

Sterkers distinguishes:

- Neurinomas of the cerebellopontine angle (CPA) and the internal auditory canal, which represent 1%–2% of the neurinomas of the CPA and up to 20% of the neurinomas of the internal auditory canal [5]. They appear in the form of a cochleovestibular syndrome and rarely as a facial impairment.
- Neurinomas of the geniculate ganglion, which are characterized by the consistency of progressive, inaugural, facial palsy.
- Tympanomastoidal neurinomas, which are expressed by facial impairment and the existence of a tumoral syndrome of the middle ear and the external auditory canal.

In addition to these three types, there are neurinomas developed on the branches of the facial nerve, often in contact with the nerve itself, from which they sometimes remain cleavable for a long time. These are neurinomas of the intermediate nerve [1], neurinomas of the chorda tympani [3], neurinomas developed on the nerve of the musculus stapedius [3], and, lastly, neurinomas of the greater petrosal nerve [3].

Clinical Cases

Case 1. The first case was that of a 67-year-old woman, consulting for a tumor of the right parotidean region, accompanied by total homolateral deafness. She presented total facial palsy which had appeared progressively 6 years earlier and had been treated palliatively by plastic surgery. MRI made it possible to locate a large tumor occupying the sub- and retrolabyrinthine regions which had caused the explosion of the third portion of the fallopian canal and then continued in the cervical region (Fig. 1).

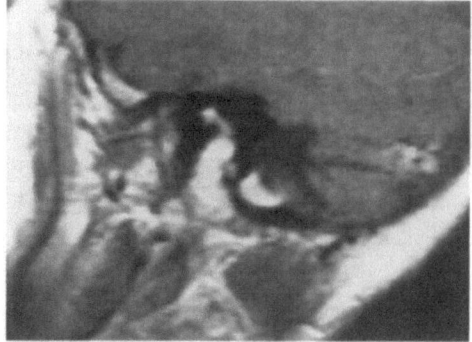

V. Darrouzet, J. P. Bebear, P. Voyer, and M. Papaxanthos
ENT Department, Pellegrin Hospital, Place Amélie-Raba-Léon,
33076 Bordeaux Cedex, France

S. A. Siddiqui
Neurosurgical Department, Pellegrin Hospital,
Place Amélie-Raba-Léon, 33076 Bordeaux Cedex, France

Fig. 1 Neurinoma of the intramastoidal facial nerve. MRI sagittal section with an injection of gadolinium DTPA. Tumor developed in the third portion of the fallopian canal, having caused the osseous structures to explode, and extended into the cervical region

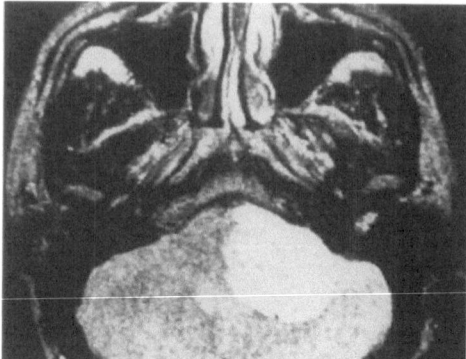

Fig. 2 MRI axial section with an injection of gadolinium DTPA. Substantial neurinoma of the facial nerve, compressive in the CPA. At the center of the petrous part of the temporal bone, a hyperlucency can be seen, corresponding to the extension of the tumor into the middle ear, along the facial nerve in the fallopian canal

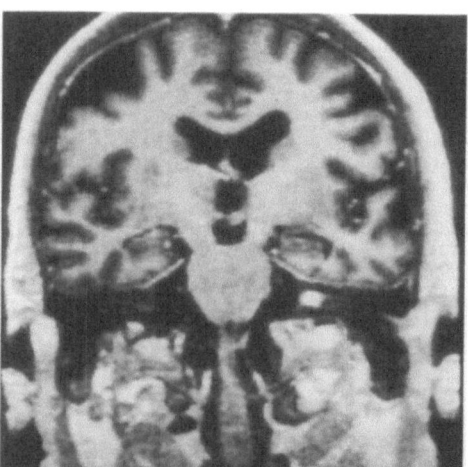

Fig. 3 Three-dimensional MRI frontal section with an injection of gadolinium DTPA. Neurinoma of the intrameatic facial nerve. Small 4-mm tumor occupying the distal portion of the internal auditory canal. The back of the canal appears free

Exeresis was performed through a wide translabyrinthine pathway widened in the cervical region.

Case 2. The second case was that of a 36-year-old man operated on 6 years earlier for a neurinoma of the chorda tympani detected by transmission deafness. No scans were made at the time. The aggravation of his hearing led to MRI, which revealed a very large tumor of the CPA, 4 cm

in diameter (Fig. 2). Exeresis was performed through a wide translabyrinthine pathway. The neurinoma invaded three portions of the fallopian canal and appeared in the middle ear through the ostium of the chorda tympani.

Case 3. The third case was that of a 49-year-old woman who consulted for right-sided cochleovestibular syndrome. She had presented regressive facial palsy 1 year earlier. There was anesthesia of the Ramsay-Hunt zone. MRI detected a stage I tumor which had developed in the internal auditory canal (Fig. 3). Facial electromyography showed few signs of nerve damage and denervation. The auditory evoked potentials were endocochlear, thus eliminating the possibility of auditory pathway compression.

The operation showed a tumor developed in the internal auditory canal at the expense of the intermediate nerve. Hearing was well preserved and the postoperative facial palsy regressed almost completely to HOUSE's grade II.

Discussion

These observations illustrate the extreme symptomatic diversity of neurinomas of the VIIth nerve and of their surgical treatment. They fully support Sterkers' classification.

Since 1970, we have treated ten patients in our department suffering from neurinomas of the VIIth nerve. This group of patients included five men and five women with an average age of 53.3 years. As far as the topography of the lesions was concerned, we encountered four neurinomas of the CPA and the internal auditory canal requiring otoneurosurgical treatment, two isolated neurinomas of the geniculate ganglion, and four tympanomastoidal neurinomas including one expanding into the cervical region.

Clinical Analysis

Evolution of Facial Palsy

Out of the ten patients treated, seven had facial palsy which had a slow onset, either worsening progressively (two cases), worsening by successive stages (three cases), or fluctuating (two cases). Two patients had facial palsy which had a viral or cold appearance. Lastly, one patient only presented a very limited facial deficit. In all the cases, the patients were seen for more than 6 months after the beginning of the facial palsy and up to 5 years afterwards. The average detection was at 18 months. Two of our patients had already undergone palliative plastic surgery. The frequency of the progressive facial impairment was noted and the existence of acute, pseudoviral impairment was striking, notably in the neurinomas developed in the internal auditory canal.

Volume of the Lesion

Surgical exploration made it possible to locate tumors of extremely variable volumes, from 3 mm in the internal auditory canal to 38 mm in the CPA. The tumors which developed in the fallopian canal were very small and therefore more rapidly symptomatic.

Diagnosis

The excellent diagnostic resolution of MRI with an injection of gadolinium currently makes it possible to establish an accurate etiological diagnosis and to eliminate other compressive lesions of the facial nerve, notably and especially intrapetrosal cholesteatomas, but also primary or secondary osseous tumors and tumors developed in the tip of the petrous portion of the temporal bone (chordomas, meningiomas, or chondrosarcomas).

Surgical Treatment

The choice of approach is guided by the location of the tumor on the trajectory of the VIIth nerve, by its size, and, secondarily, by the patient's hearing. The difficulty of these tumors lies entirely in determining the attitude to adopt for a tumor developed in the internal auditory canal at the expense of the intermediate nerve.

In other cases, nerve interruption has been complete and a faciofacial graft performed with the superficial cervical plexus or with a fragment of saphenous nerve (five cases). In one patient, a hypoglossofacial anastomosis proved to be indispensable, as the tumor was developed in the CPA. In two patients, the fact that the facial palsy had existed for a long time and the absence of an underlying muscular bed led to palliative plastic surgery.

Conclusions

In our opinion, all facial palsies with progressive onset justify an "aggressive" surgical attitude based on a very thorough neuroradiological examination, which, if it has negative findings, should not eliminate surgical exploration of the petrous portion of the temporal bone. It may indeed make possible the detection of small schwannomas developed in the fallopian canal, allowing, due to their size, optimal nerve rehabilitation.

References

1. Fuentes JM, Uziel A (1983) Neurinomes intrapétreux du nerf facial et de ses branches. A propos de deux observations. Neurochirurgie 29 : 197–201
2. Portmann M, Bebear JP (1977) A propos des neurinomes du nerf facial intra-pétreux. Rev Laryngol 98 : 21–29
3. Pou J, Chambers C (1974) Neurinoma of the chorda tympani. Laryngoscope 84 : 1170–1174
4. Pulec JL (1972) Facial nerve neuroma. Laryngoscope 82 : 1160–1176
5. Sterkers O, Viala P, Riviere F, Sterkers JM (1986) Neurinomes du nerf facial intra-temporal. Classification anatomo-clinique de 12 cas. Ann Oto Laryngol 103 : 501–508

Eur Arch Otorhinolaryngology (1994) [Suppl]:S274–S276

E. Yamamoto, M. Ohmura, C. Mizukami, H. Oiki, and Y. Muneta

Two Cases of Intratemporal Facial Neurofibroma

Introduction

Intratemporal facial nerve tumors are relatively uncommon, and early diagnosis is difficult because the tumors grow slowly, giving rise to a variety of symptoms, none of which suggest the diagnosis [1]. In this paper, we report two cases of facial neurofibroma developing within the temporal bone, in which a definite diagnosis was made on the basis of CT and MRI findings.

Case Reports

Case 1

A 28-year-old male presented left facial palsy with no improvement following conservative treatment for about 4 years. Examination revealed a moderate degree of facial palsy (palsy score [2], 18/40), and a tumor-like shadow was observed on CT and MRI. On CT, a soft tissue shadow was observed in the horizontal part of the left facial nerve (Fig. 1a, b, arrows). On MRI, there was a slight swelling extending from the horizontal part to the vertical part of the left facial nerve (Fig. 1c, arrow), and the same area was uniformly enhanced after intravenous adminstration of gadolinium (Gd) – diethylene triamine penta-acetate (DTPA) (Fig. 1d, arrow). A left intratemporal facial nerve tumor was suspected and surgery was performed.

Surgery confirmed an intratemporal tumor, which existed between two crura of the stapes in the horizontal portion of the facial nerve. The tumor was totally removed and histologically it was neurofibroma. The nerve was

E. Yamamoto (✉), M. Ohmura, C. Mizukami, H. Oiki, and Y. Muneta
Department of Otolaryngology, Kobe City General Hospital, 4–6, Minatojima-Nakamachi, Chuo-ku, Kobe, 650, Japan

decompressed. During the follow-up period of 12 months, the facial palsy showed remarkable improvement (palsy score, 32/40).

Case 2

A 39-year-old male presented with a 3-year history of right facial palsy. He was treated for Bell's palsy with oral medication by another physician; however, his condition failed to improve.

Examination revealed a moderate degree of facial palsy (palsy score, 20/40). Plain X-rays failed to reveal any abnormalities; however, CT and MRI studies showed a tumor-like shadow. CT revealed a soft tissue shadow from the geniculate ganglion to the horizontal part of the right facial nerve. Figure 2a, b (coronal CT) show the soft tissue shadow in the horizontal area (arrows). MRI images showed mild swelling in the same area (Fig. 2c, arrow), and this was greatly enhanced with Gd-DTPA (Fig. 2d, arrow). A right intratemporal facial nerve tumor was suspected and surgery was performed.

A relatively larger tumor extending from the geniculate ganglion to the horizontal portion of the facial nerve was found during surgery, and was almost completely removed; histologically it was neurofibroma. The palsy improved gradually and the score was 30/40 at 10 months after surgery.

Discussion

Intratemporal facial nerve tumors are rare and can be divided histologically into neurinomas and neurofibromas, with the former comprising the vast majority. Cases of neurofibroma, as reported here, are extremely rare [3]. In case 1, the tumor was small and we were able to resect the tumor alone by separating it from the nerve bundles. In case 2, although the tumor was relatively large and the boundary between the tumor and the nerve bundle was

Fig. 1a–d Case 1. Coronal CT images (**a, b**). Pre- (**c**) and post- (**d**) Gd-DTPA axial T1-weighted MRI

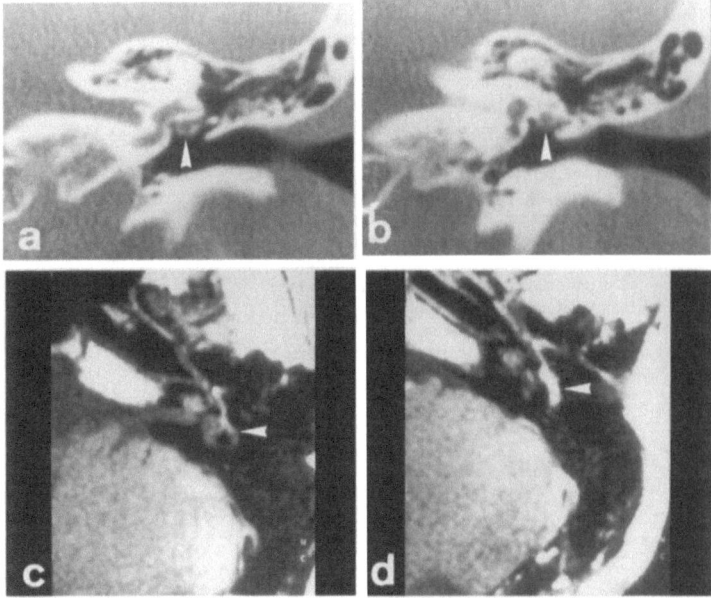

Fig. 2a–d Case 2. Coronal CT images (**a, b**). Pre- (**c**) and post- (**d**) axial Gd-DTPA T1-weighted MRI

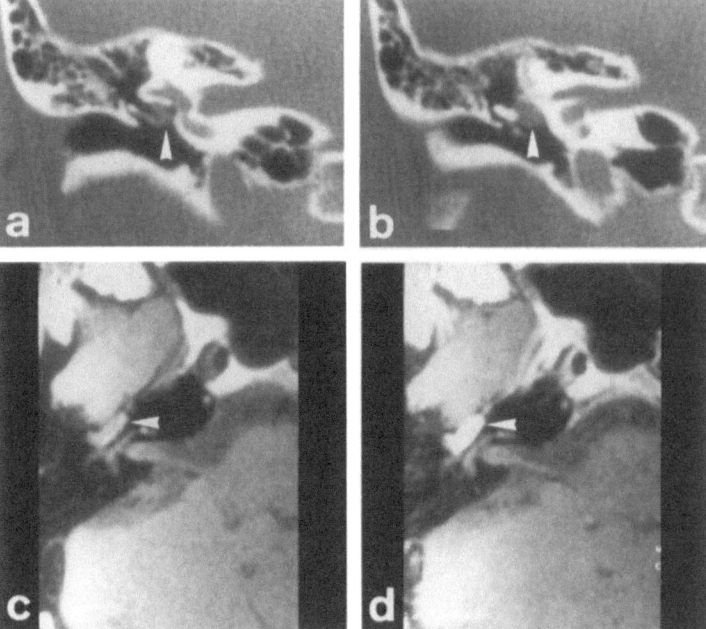

indistinct, in view of the extremely slow tumor growth, and since preoperative palsy was not severe and we did not want to sacrifice the nerve, we removed as much of the tumor as possible. From the standpoint of both ease of resection and the desirability of preserving the nerve, we wish to emphasize the importance of early diagnosis and early surgical treatment.

In both cases of intratemporal facial neurofibroma reported in this paper, the patients received conservative treatment for Bell's palsy when palsy first developed, and when it failed to improve, presented to our clinic 3 or 4 years later. CT and MRI studies were performed, a tumor was suspected, and the diagnosis was confirmed at surgery. When a patient's palsy fails to improve after a considerable period of time, Bell's palsy can be excluded, and other lesions, including tumors, must be considered. When pa-tients fail to show signs of improvement over a period of several months or more and a tumor is suspected, as in the present cases, thorough diagnostic imaging studies, including CT and MRI, should be performed.

References

1. Lipkin AF, Coker NJ, Jenkins HA, Alford BR (1987) Intracranial and intratemporal facial neuroma. Otolaryngol Head Neck Surg 96:71–79
2. Yanagihara N (1985) Grading system for evaluation of facial palsy. In: Portmann M (ed) Facial nerve. Masson, Paris, pp 41–42
3. Wiet RJ, Pyle FGM, Schramm DR (1991) Middle fossa and intra-temporal facial nerve neuromas. Otolaryngol Head Neck Surg 100:141–142

Eur Arch Otorhinolaryngology (1994) [Suppl]: S277–S280

A. J. Gulya

Facial Nerve Neuromas: Diagnosis and Management of the Large Lesion

Introduction

Facial nerve neuromas, or more correctly schwannomas, are unusual lesions. In their review of 600 temporal bone specimens at the Massachusetts Eye and Ear Infirmary, Saito and Baxter [12] found only five such tumors. Symptomatically, facial nerve dysfunction is attributable to a tumor of the facial nerve in only 5% of cases [13] while even less specific symptoms, namely hearing loss and tinnitus, have been cited as the most common presenting complaints [7]. Understandably, historically it has been an infrequent occurrence that the clinician has been able to correctly establish the diagnosis preoperatively, as pointed out by Conley and Janecka [1] in 1974. More recently, however, the evolution of modern imaging modalities has greatly heightened diagnostic accuracy and has also assisted in surgical planning by better delimiting tumor extent.

The patient presented herein exemplifies how diagnostic imaging can facilitate the diagnosis and management of a facial nerve schwannoma, which in this case constituted one of the larger lesions reported in the literature. Additionally, this case presents the challenge of how to optimally reanimate the face when confronted with a facial nerve deficit several centimeters in length.

Case Presentation

A 19-year-old college student complained of left hearing loss, which had progressed over the 3 preceding years, in association with a left lower facial twitch. There was no

A. J. Gulya
Department of Otolaryngology, Head and Neck Surgery, Georgetown University, One Main West, 3800 Reservoir Road, N. W., 2007 Washington, D.C., USA

tinnitus, fluctuation in hearing, otalgia, or history of facial paralysis, although there was some aural fullness. He noted neither xerophthalmia nor dysgeusia. Therapies which had been utilized unsuccessfully included allergy injections and antibiotics; tympanostomy tube insertion had been attempted twice, but on both occasions the tube was "extruded" within 1 week. He was referred to Georgetown University Medical Center after imaging studies revealed a left intracranial and temporal bone mass lesion.

Physical examination documented the Weber to lateralize to the left, while the Rinne was positive on the right and negative on the left. Upon otoscopy a nonpulsatile, slightly erythematous mass lesion appeared to extend through the tympanic membrane to fill the medial portion of the external auditory canal. At rest, the face appeared symmetric, with an intermittent left mental twitch. Upon facial movement, a mild weakness could be appreciated to involve all branches of the facial nerve, approximating a House-Brackmann grade II.

Audiometry showed a 50-dB conductive hearing loss on the left with normal hearing on the right.

The temporal bone computerized tomographic (CT) scan (Figs. 1, 2) showed a soft tissue density filling the tympanic cavity in association with lateral displacement of the malleus and incus. Superiorly, there was tegmental erosion, and laterally the density occupied the medial external auditory canal. The mastoid segment of the fallopian canal was enlarged.

With T_1-weighted magnetic resonance imaging (MRI) (Figs. 3) the lesion displayed a low signal, but brightened both upon gadolinium enhancement and T_2-weighted (Fig. 4) imaging. A 2-cm middle cranial fossa component corresponded to the area of tegmental dehiscence seen on CT. Cerebral arteriography showed the mass to be relatively avascular, with no associated vessel displacement or compression.

The diagnostic imaging findings, in conjunction with the physical findings, supported the diagnosis of a facial nerve neuroma. A combined middle cranial fossa-transmastoid approach, with transection and overclosure of the

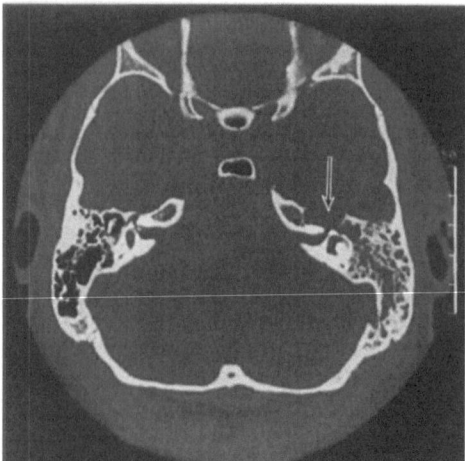

Fig. 1 The axial CT scan shows a lytic lesion at the geniculate ganglion (*arrow*) with dilation of the labyrinthine segment of the facial nerve canal (Reproduced with permission from [14])

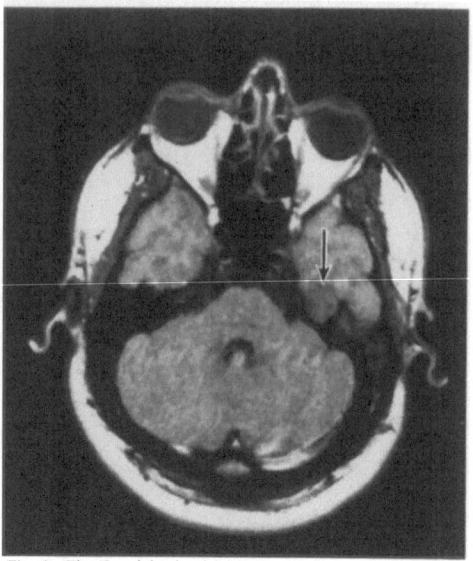

Fig. 3 The T$_1$-weighted axial MR image shows a low-intensity middle cranial fossa mass lesion (*arrow*) with mastoid opacification. (Reproduced with permission from [14])

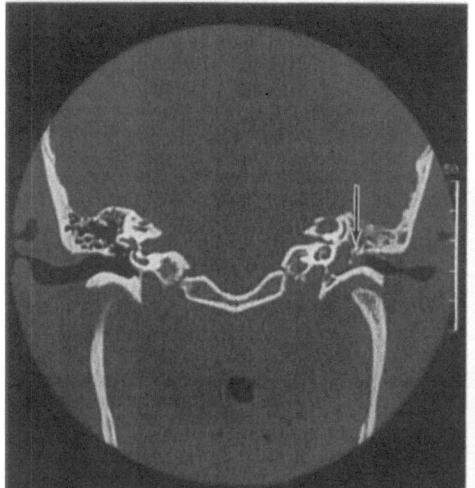

Fig. 2 The coronal CT scan shows the tumor extending into the external auditory canal and displaced the ossicles (*arrow*) laterally. (Reproduced with permission from [14])

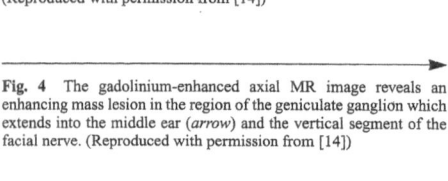

Fig. 4 The gadolinium-enhanced axial MR image reveals an enhancing mass lesion in the region of the geniculate ganglion which extends into the middle ear (*arrow*) and the vertical segment of the facial nerve. (Reproduced with permission from [14])

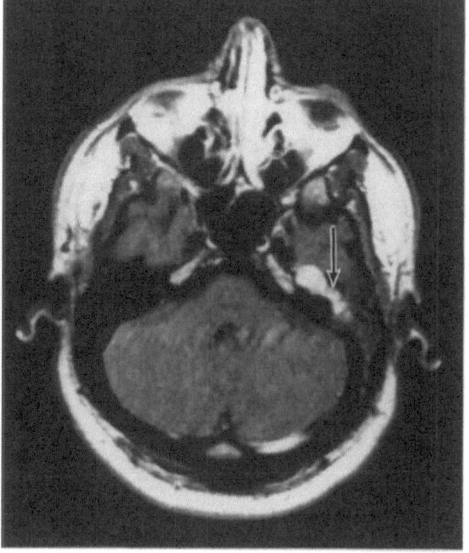

external auditory canal, was selected for tumor extirpation because of the wide-field exposure it afforded. Intratemporally, the tumor was found to engulf the mastoid segment of the facial nerve. The tympanic cavity was filled with tumor which had extended into the external auditory canal, eroded through the stapes crura, and displaced the stapes superstructure, still attached to its tendon, towards the round window. Superiorly, at the anterior aspect of the epitympanum, dehiscent tegmen and tumor were encountered. Through the middle fossa exposure, the intracranial extension was resected, and frozen section margins were clear of tumor only at the most medial aspect of the facial nerve in the internal auditory canal. The tumor did not extend inferiorly beyond the stylomastoid foramen.

A standard VII–XII crossover was carried out, while the tympanomastoid compartment was obliterated.

Postoperatively, facial motion began to appear at $3^1/_2$ months, maximizing at a House-Brackmann grade IV (so categorized because of lack of forehead movement). There was minimal ipsilateral hemitongue atrophy. MRI, approximately 1 year postoperatively, showed no evidence of recurrent tumor.

Discussion

Facial nerve neuromas are unusual lesions, and they most commonly manifest in symptoms – namely, hearing loss and tinnitus [7] – not specific for, or even suggestive of, a facial nerve lesion. Although the anticipated facial paralysis, twitching, or recurrent facial paralysis [4] can occur, they were seen in only 46%, 4.2%, and 19% respectively of 48 patients with facial nerve neuromas reported by the Otologic Medical Group [7].

Clinical findings are misleading in estimating the extent of a facial nerve neuroma. These tumors are notorious for "not following the rules" and both the stapes reflex and tearing may be preserved, even though the vertical segment and the geniculate ganglion are involved with the tumor.

It is understandable then that prior to the advent of modern diagnostic imaging, clinicians had difficulty in correctly establishing the diagnosis prior to surgical intervention [2]. CT findings associated with a facial nerve neuroma vary with its location and extent. The geniculate ganglion in particular seems to have a predilection for tumor involvement [7, 11], and thus bony erosion in the region of the geniculate ganglion is a diagnostic clue. Although ossifying hemangiomas of the facial nerve also occur in the geniculate ganglion region, they more typically manifest "honeycomb" changes in the surrounding bone, in contrast to the sharper bony erosion of the neuroma [5]. The findings of fallopian canal destruction in association with a mass in the tympanomastoid compartment are seen with facial nerve neuromas, as with facial nerve tumors in general. Internal auditory canal widening,

middle fossa extension, contrast enhancement, and cerebellopontine extension are findings of facial nerve neuromas shared with vestibular schwannomas. CT findings specific to facial nerve neuromas are erosion of the anterior-superior face of the internal auditory canal and a middle cranial fossa mass, located at the anterior face of the mid-portion of the petrosa in association with enlargement of the labyrinthine segment of the facial nerve canal [3].

Magnetic resonance imaging has allowed for refinement in determination of tumor extent, the identification of asymptomatic lesions, and differentiation from vestibular schwannomas [8]. Parnes and associates [8] determined gadolinium enhancement of the geniculate ganglion and distal facial nerve to be the most useful MRI features in distinguishing a facial nerve neuroma from a vestibular schwannoma in the patient that presents with an internal auditory canal or cerebellopontine angle mass and retrocochlear findings.

Tumor extirpation comprises definitive management, but the timing of surgical intervention is determined by deterioration of facial nerve function and/or development of an intracranial mass lesion. Even though facial nerve neuromas are thought to arise from the sensory component, in only 23% of cases reported by O'Donoghue and colleagues [7] was it possible to leave at least 50% of the facial nerve in continuity at the time of tumor resection. Thus, surgical planning must also anticipate the need for facial nerve reconstruction, and, since gross nerve distention does not reflect through tumor extent, frozen section margins are advised to assure complete tumor removal [10].

Options available for facial reanimation include end-to-end anastomosis, often after nerve rerouting, interpositional nerve grafting, and crossover procedures – listed in the general order of preference [4]. A VII–XII crossover procedure was selected in this instance. Interpositional graft placement would have required additional posterior fossa exposure, with additional potential for cerebrospinal fluid leakage, and, in view of the length of graft that would have been required, the anticipated time to initial facial movement with the interpositional graft would be anticipated to be several months longer, with little likelihood of substantially better function, than with the VII–XII crossover [9, 13]. The handicap presented by the loss of hypoglossal nerve function is not overwhelming in general, and has been obviated, at least in some series [6], by cable grafting from the partially transected hypoglossal nerve, rather than complete hypoglossal nerve sacrifice.

1. Conley J, Janecka I (1974) Schwann cell tumors of the facial nerve. Laryngoscope 84 : 958–962
2. Conley J, Selfe RW (1981) Occult neoplasms in facial paralysis. Laryngoscope 91 : 205–210
3. Inoue Y, Tabuchi T, Hakuba A, Fukuda T, Nakao T, Nemoto Y, Saiwai S, Miyamoto T, Sato S, Ogata M, Nishimura S, Onoyama

Y (1987) Facial nerve neuromas: CT findings. J Comput Assist Tomogr 11 : 942 – 947

4. Jackson CG, Glasscock ME III, Hughes G, Sismanis A (1980) Facial paralysis of neoplastic origin: diagnosis and management. Laryngoscope 90 : 1581 – 1595

5. Lo WWM, Brackmann DE, Shelton C (1989) Imaging case study of the month: facial nerve hemangioma. Ann Otol Rhinol Laryngol 98 : 160 – 161

6. May M, Sobol SM, Mester SJ (1991) Hypoglossal-facial nerve interpositional-jump graft for facial reanimation without tongue atrophy. Otolaryngol Head Neck Surg 104 : 818 – 825

7. O'Donoghue GM, Brackmann DE, House JW, Jackler RK (1989) Neuromas of the facial nerve. Am J Otol 10 : 49 – 54

8. Parnes LS, Lee DH, Peerless SJ (1991) Magnetic resonance imaging of facial nerve neuromas. Laryngoscope 101 : 31 – 35

9. Pensak ML, Jackson CG, Glasscock ME, III, Gulya AJ (1986) Facial reanimation with the VII – XII anastomosis: analysis of the functional and psychologic results. Otolaryngol Head Neck Surg 94 : 305 – 310

10. Pillsbury HC, III, Jones RO Jr (1986) Surgery of facial nerve neuroma. In: Wiet RJ, Causse J-B (eds) Complications in otolaryngology – head and neck surgery, vol 1, ear and skull base. Decker, Philadelphia, pp 179 – 183

11. Pulec JL (1972) Symposium on ear surgery. II. Facial nerve neuroma. Laryngoscope 82 : 1160 – 1176

12. Saito H, Baxter A (1972) Undiagnosed intratemporal facial nerve neurilemmomas. Arch Otolaryngol 95 : 415 – 419

13. Shambaugh GE Jr, May M (1980) Facical nerve paralysis. In: Paparella MM, Shumrick DA (eds) Otolaryngology, 2nd edn, Saunders, Philadelphia, pp 1680 – 1704

14. Gulya AJ, Stern NM (1993) Imaging case study of the month: facial nerve neuroma. Ann Otol Rhinol Laryngol 102 : 478 – 480

Eur Arch Otorhinolaryngology (1994) [Suppl]: S 281 – S 283

R. Charachon, C. Tixier, J. P. Lavieille, and E. Reyt

End-to-End Anastomosis Versus Nerve Graft in Intratemporal and Intracranial Lesions of the Facial Nerve

There is ongoing debate on the efficacy of end-to-end anastomosis versus nerve graft. The former usually needs at least a partial rerouting of the ends of the nerve with a danger of devascularization and additional traumatism. The latter has the drawback of requiring two sutures instead of one for regeneration of the axons.

Materials and Methods

Thirty patients were operated upon between 1970 and 1990: there were 17 males and 13 females, with a mean age of 43.5 (23 – 71) years. Section of the facial nerve was required for the following lesions: temporal bone fracture (10), middle ear surgery (5), temporal bone cholesteatoma (5), acoustic neurinoma (5), facial nerve neurinoma (4), and tuberculosis (1). The following approaches were used: translabyrinthine (11), middle fossa (7), transmastoidian (5), transmastoidian with exclusion (3), inframtemporal (1), transcochlear (1), and suboccipital (2). Facial nerve reconstruction was performed either with an end-to-end anastomosis (11) or a cable graft (19) with the greater auricular nerve (17) or the sural nerve (2). A partial or total rerouting of the facial nerve was used in 14 cases in addition to these procedures.

The ends of the nerves were approximated either by fibrin glue (13 cases) or by suture (one case). The ends were only fitted together in 16 cases. If fibrin glue was used in the cerebellopontine angle, a piece of lyophylized dura was glued between the internal auditory canal and the brain stem. Then the ends of the rerouted facial nerve or the cable graft were put in position and glued taking care to not place glue between the ends of the nerve.

Results

All the patients but three were followed up for 1 – 10 years. Considering only the cases operated on before the end of the 3rd year of total paralysis and followed up for at least 1 year, we observed a mean grade of 3.3 after end-to-end anastomosis (11 cases) and of 3.7 after a cable (19 cases) graft according to the House-Brackmann grading system. We observed two grade 2 results after a cable graft (one temporal bone fracture and one facial nerve neuroma) (Table 1).

As it may be of interest for a better understanding of the results according to etiology and site of lesion, we have summarized these data in Tables 2, 3, 4, 5, and 6. We notice that one of the best results with grafting was achieved by a surgical procedure performed 18 months after a section of the nerve with a fracture. In contrast, a cable graft performed after 3 years, for a temporal bone cholesteatoma, only achieved a grade IV result. A graft performed after a delay of 7 years was unsuccessful.

Table 1 End-to-end anastomosis versus cable graft with and without rerouting

Grade	EEA	EEA + R	Graft	Graft + R
II			2	
III	1	6	2	2
IV		3	4	3
V			3	
Mean grade		3.3		3.7

EEA, end-to-end anastomosis; R, rerouting.

R. Charachon (✉), C. Tixier, J. P. Lavieille, and E. Reyt
Clinique Universitaire O. R. L. du CHU de Grenoble BP 217x,
38043 Grenoble Cedex 09, France

Table 2 Temporal bone fracture

Type	Site	Approach	Reparation	Grade
Longitudinal: 3 (normal hearing)				
	GG	Middle fossa	EEA + R	Early
	GG	Middle fossa	EEA + R	IV
	GG	Middle fossa	Graft	II
Transversal: 6 (total deafness)				
	T + M	Mastoid	Graft + R	III
	T + M	Translabyrinthine	EEA	III
	L + T	Translabyrinthine	EEA + R	III
	L + T	Translabyrinthine	EEA + R	III
	L + T	Translabyrinthine	EEA + R	III
	IAC + L + T	Translabyrinthine	Graft	V
EAC+mastoid (total deafness)				
	T + M	Mastoid	Graft + R	IV

EEA, end-to-end anastomosis; GG, geniculate ganglion; IAC, internal auditory canal; R, rerouting; L, labyrinthic segment; T, tympanic segment; M, mastoid segment.

Table 3 Middle ear surgery

Site	Approach	Reparation	Delay (years)	Grade
T + M	Mastoid	Graft	0	V
T + M	Rambo	Graft + R	2	IV
T + M	Radical mastoid	Graft	0	III
T + M	Mastoid	Graft + R	0	III
T + M	Mastoid	Graft	1	Early

T, tympanic segment; M, mastoid segment; R, rerouting.

Table 4 Temporal bone cholesteatoma

Site	Approach	Reparation	Delay (years)	Grade
T + M	Translabyrinthine	Graft + R	2	Early
L + T + M	Infratemporal	EEA + R	1	III
IAC + L + T + M	Transcochlear	Graft + R	1/2	IV
IAC + L + T	Middle fossa	Graft + R	3	IV
L + T	Middle fossa	EEA + R	1	IV

L, labyrinthic segment; M, mastoid segment; R, rerouting; T, tympanic segment; IAC, internal auditory canal.

Table 5 Acoustic neuroma

Approach	Reparation	Grade
Suboccipital	Sural	IV
Suboccipital	Sural	III
Translabyrinthine	EEA+R	III
Translabyrinthine	EEA+R	IV
Translabyrinthine	Great auricular	IV

EEA end-to-end anastomosis; R, rerouting.

Table 6 Facial nerve neuroma

Approach	Reparation	Delay (years)	Grade
Translabyrinthine	Great auricular	7	VI
Rambo	Great auricular	2	III
Middle fossa + mastoid	Great auricular	1	V
Middle fossa + mastoid	Great auricular	0	II
No rerouting			

Discussion

End-to-end anastomosis alone is seldom feasible. The actual choice is between end-to-end anastomosis with rerouting and cable graft with or without rerouting. From our short series, it is difficult to draw precise conclusions. We can only observe that there was a better mean grade (3.3) after end-to-end anastomosis than after a cable graft (3.7), but the only grade 2 results were achieved by a graft in two cases.

Spector [5], on a large series of 34 end-to-end anastomosis and 56 cable grafts, observed that voluntary motion and facial reinnervation were decreased and synkinesis increased in the autologous cable graft repairs. Neural cable grafts were associated with more mass movement and less fine precise emotion facial movement. However, cable graft from the internal auditory canal to middle ear or mastoid produced the best results in this group.

Excellent cable graft repair results diminish with time because of continual progressive synkinesis, which may take up to 4 years to develop.

In addition, Spector classified the efficacy of the reparation procedure into four groups:

- Direct facial nerve anastomosis, with the best results.
- End-to-end anastomosis with rerouting, with a delayed recovery period (9–14 months), less total functional recovery, and at least a mild degree of synkinesis.
- Cable graft, with weak voluntary motion and the most severe synkinesis.
- Rerouting and cable graft, with the most synkinesis and the worst results.

The same author observed, in rabbit neural graft repairs, an axonal outgrowth over a wide area at the proximal graft anastomosis site. There were twice as many unmyelinated fibers as in the control. Moreover, there were two distinct myelinated axonal populations: intrafascicular and extrafascicular regenerating axons. The larger population was extrafascicular. The smaller intrafascicular axonal population used the graft as a conduit to innervate the distal transected neural stump. A small population of the extrafascicular axones traversed to enter the distal nerve stump. The others could be eliminated or contribute to abnormal facial movements and synkinesis; however, further studies are needed.

Myelin debris is still present at 5 weeks in the autologous graft conduit. The more myelin debris found in the neural graft, the fewer the intrafascicular axons and the greater the extrafascicular axons. Myelin debris appears to interfere with axonal regrowth through graft endoneural tubes. The mechanism has not been explained: physical blockage or inhibitory substances are possible.

Our series is too small to classify the results according to Spector. Nevertheless, the trend as a whole is the same. We think it is better to perform a graft than an end-to-end anastomosis with extended rerouting. We emphasize that a reconstruction of the facial nerve can achieve a good result if it is performed during the first 2 or even 3 years following the lesion. Nevertheless, results must be studied over the long term because synkinesis may develop at least during the first 3 or 4 years.

Conclusions

- Reconstruction of the facial nerve is possible for at least 3 years following the lesion.
- A cable graft may give as good a result as a suture with rerouting. If a cable graft is performed, rerouting must be minimized.

References

1. Coker NJ, Kendall KA, Jenkins HA, Alford BR (1987) Traumatic intratemporal facial nerve injury: management rationale for preservation of function. Otolaryngol Head Neck Surg 97 (3):262–269
2. Eby TL, Pollak A, Fisch U (1990) Intratemporal facial nerve anastomosis: a temporal bone study. Laryngoscope 100:623–626
3. Janicka IP, Conley J (1987) Primary neoplasms of the facial nerve. Plast Reconstr Surg 79 (2):177–185
4. May M (1983) Trauma of the facial nerve. Otolaryngol Clin North Am 16 (3):661–670
5. Spector JG, Lee P, Peterein J, Roufa D (1991) Facial nerve regeneration through autologous nerve grafts: a clinical and experimental study. Laryngoscope 101:537–554

Eur Arch Otorhinolaryngology (1994) [Suppl]: S284–S286

FREE PAPERS AND POSTERS

A. Sismanis, D. S. Oliver, and G. H. Williams

Primary Facial Nerve Tumors: Diagnostic and Management Dilemmas

Introduction

Primary facial nerve tumors are rare and often present a diagnostic and management dilemma to the otolaryngologist. The vast majority of these lesions are either neurilemmomas (schwannomas) or neurofibromas.

The following three representative cases illustrate these diagnostic and management challenges.

Case 1. A 23-year-old white female presented with a 6-week history of left facial weakness and paresthesias. Otoscopy revealed a mass behind the posterior aspect of the left tympanic membrane and bulging of the posterior external auditory canal wall. Computed tomography (CT) of the temporal bones demonstrated a 1-cm lesion involving the vertical segment of the left facial nerve (Fig..1). Preoperative biopsy of this lesion was compatible with a neurofibroma. A left transcervical, transmastoid resection of facial nerve tumor extending from the distal segment of the horizontal fallopian canal to just proximal to the stylomastoid foramen was accomplished (Fig. 2). A great auricular nerve graft was employed for facial reanimation. Final pathology confirmed the diagnosis of a′ neurofibroma.

Follow-up at 18 months demonstrated satisfactory facial function (House grade, III).

Case 2. A 31-year-old white male was referred to our institution because of a sudden onset of right hearing loss and associated high pitched tinnitus. An erythematous mass of the inferior aspect of the right middle ear protruding into the external auditory canal was identified. A biopsy obtained from this lesion by the referring physician was reported as a glomus tumor. Gadolinium-MRI of the

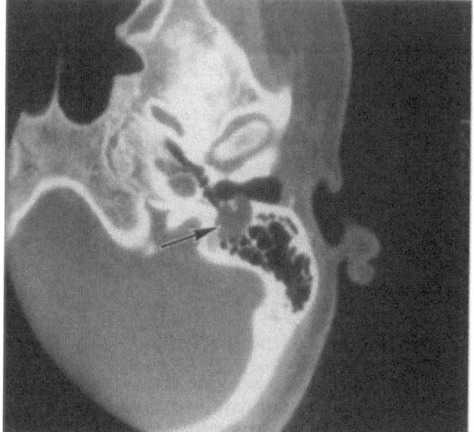

Fig. 1 Case 1. CT scan reveals a 1-cm mass of the vertical portion of the facial nerve. *Arrow* indicates the lesion

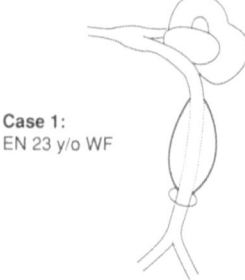

Case 1:
EN 23 y/o WF

Fig. 2 Diagrammatic representation of the extent of the tumor of case 1

A. Sismanis (✉), D. S. Oliver, and G. H. Williams
Department of Otolaryngology, Head and Neck Surgery,
Medical College of Virginia, Richmond, 23298 Virginia, USA

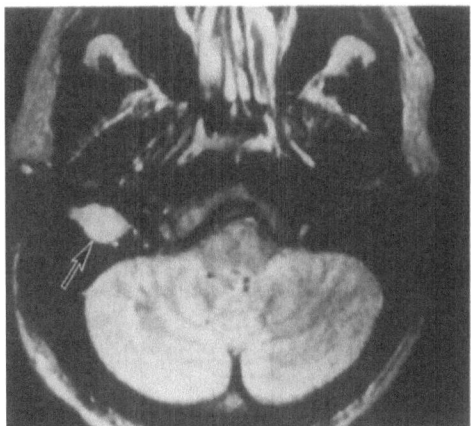

Fig. 3 Case 2. Gad-MRI of the head showing a soft tissue mass protruding from the anterolateral jugular bulb. *Arrow* indicates the lesion

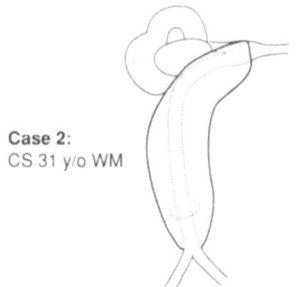

Fig. 4 Diagrammatic representation of the extent of the tumor of case 2

head revealed an enhancing mass protruding from the anterolateral aspect of the jugular bulb (Fig. 3). CT of the skull base revealed erosion of the hypotympanum and floor of the external auditory canal. Carotid angiography showed a poorly vascularized middle ear tumor. With the diagnosis of a glomus tumor, a lateral skull base approach was planned. During mastoidectomy, however, a facial nerve tumor extending from the labyrinthine portion of the nerve to the pes anserinus was identified (Fig. 4). Frozen biopsy was compatible with a neuroma. The lesion was completely excised and a hypoglossal to facial nerve (XII-VII) anastomosis was performed. Final pathology showed a neurilemmoma. At 2 years follow-up there has been satisfactory return of facial nerve function (House grade, III).

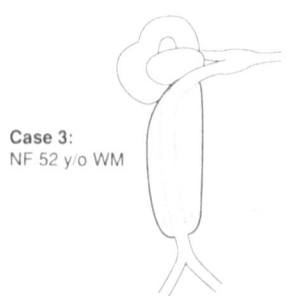

Fig. 5 Diagrammatic representation of the extent of the tumor of case 3

Case 3. A 52-year-old white male was referred to our medical center after two tympanomastoidectomies had been performed to control a right chronic draining ear and facial paralysis. A CT scan of the temporal bones suggested a soft tissue mass involving the middle ear and attic without any bony erosion. Carotid angiography was normal. After appropriate counseling the right ear was reexplored by us. A facial nerve tumor extending from the second genu to just proximal to the pes anserinus was identified (Fig. 5). The tumor was completely resected and a great auricular nerve graft was performed. The final pathology report confirmed the diagnosis of a neurilemmoma.

Discussion

Primary facial nerve tumors are rare, accounting for an estimated 5% of cases of facial paralysis [6]. Asymptomatic facial neuromas have been reported in 0.1%–0.8% of routine autopsy specimens [8].

Facial nerve tumors can arise from any segment of the facial nerve distal to the brain stem [9] several series report the geniculate ganglion as the site of predilection. This is probably related to structural reorganization of this area during embryological development [4]. These tumors are often multicentric involving two to five segments of the nerve [12].

Neurilemmomas arise from the Schwann cell and are commonly solitary, well demarcated, and eccentric in relation to the involved nerve. This eccentricity has led some neurotologists to attempt to salvage the facial nerve by dissecting the tumor from the nerve. Neurofibromas are typically multiple, poorly encapsulated, presenting as concentrically fusiform enlargement of the involved nerve with nerve fibers being entwined within the tumor [12].

Symptoms and signs depend upon the location and size of the tumor along the course of the nerve. Facial palsy is commonly considered the most frequent presentation, yet it can be absent in 25%–50% of cases [13]. In 20% of patients it can be sudden, mimicking Bell's palsy. Hearing loss and tinnitus may be the only manifestations and have been reported as the most common symptoms in other series [13]. Otalgia and aural drainage are rare and are usually due to secondary infection [12].

Evaluation should include a thorough history and complete otoscopic, neurotologic, and head and neck examinations. Audiologic evaluation is essential. Electroneuronography (ENoG) will demonstrate the percentage of facial nerve degeneration. Some investigators have combined ENoG and auditory brain stem responses (ABR) in an attempt to differentiate acustic neuromas from facial neuromas [2].

High-resolution temporal bone CT is a valuable study; however, gadolinium enhanced magnetic resonance imaging (Gad-MRI) is considered by some to be the study of choice [11, 14].

Differential diagnosis should include glomus and acustic tumors, cholesteatomas, primary and metastatic carcinomas to the temporal bone, malignant parotid tumors, meningiomas, hemangiomas, sarcoidosis [1, 5, 7], Lyme disease [10], and idiopathic facial paralysis. Complete excision and immediate facial reanimation by facial nerve grafting or anastomosis to the hypoglossal nerve are the goals of surgery [12]. Hypoglossal to facial (XII-VII) anastomosis should be considered when resection of the facial nerve proximal to the geniculate ganglion is required. Results of this procedure are very gratifying [3].

Conclusions

Primary facial tumors are rare and often present a diagnostic and management dilemma. A high index of suspicion along with detailed neurotologic, head and neck examinations, and audiologic and radiologic testing including Gad-MRI are essential in making a diagnosis.

Complete resection and immediate facial reanimation by grafting or anastomosis to the hypoglossal nerve remain the goals of treatment.

References

1. Brackmann DE (1987) The facial nerve in the infratemporal approach. Otolaryngol Head Neck Surg 97 (1):15–18
2. Brackman DE, House JW, Selters W (1982) Auditory brainstem response in facial nerve neuroma diagnosis. In: Graham MD, House WF (eds) Disorders of the facial nerve. Raven, New York, pp 87–89
3. Clayton MI, Rivron RP, Hanson DR, Fenwick JD (1989) Evaluation of recent experience with cranial nerve XII–VII interpositon. J Laryngol Otol 103 (1): 63–65
4. Fisch U, Ruttner J (1977) Pathology of intratemporal tumors involving the facial nerve. In: Fisch U (ed) Facial nerve surgery. Aesculaptus, Birmingham, pp 448–456
5. Glasscock ME (1990) Facial nerve surgery. In: Glasscock ME, Shambaugh GE (eds) Surgery of the ear, 4th edn. Saunders, Philadelphia, p 445
6. Jackson CG, Glasscock ME, Hughes G, Sismanis A (1980) Facial paralysis of neoplastic origin: diagnosis and management. Laryngoscope 90 : 1581–1595
7. Janecka I, Conley JJ (1984) Facial nerve tumors. In: Portmann M (ed) Proceedings of the 5th international symposium on facial nerve. Masson, New York, pp 423–426
8. Jung TTK, Jun B, Shea D, Paparella MM (1986) Primary and secondary tumors of the facial nerve. A temporal bone study. Arch Otolaryngol Head Neck Surg 112 (12):1269–1273
9. King TT, Morrison AW (1990) Primary facial nerve tumors within the skull. J Neurosurg 72 : 1–8
10. Markby DP (1982) Lyme disease facial palsy: differentiation from Bell's palsy. Br Med J 299 (6699) : 605–606
11. Millen SJ, Daniels DL, Meyer GA (1989) Gadolinium-enhanced magnetic resonance imaging in temporal bone lesions. Laryngoscope 99 : 257–260
12. O'Donoghue GM, Brackmann DE, House JW, Jackler RK (1989) Neuromas of the facial nerve. Am J Otol 10 : 49–54
13. Sharp JF, Kerr AI, Carder P, Sellar RJ (1989) Facial schwannoma without facial paralysis. J Laryngol Otol 103 (1): 973–975
14. Wortham DG, Teresi LM, Lufkin RB, Hanafee WN et al. (1989) Magnetic resonance imaging of the facial nerve. Otolaryngol Head Neck Surg 101:295–301

Eur Arch Otorhinolaryngology (1994) [Suppl]: S287–S289

FREE PAPERS AND POSTERS

D. D. Backous, H. A. Jenkins, and N. J. Coker

Gunshot Injuries to the Intratemporal Facial Nerve

Introduction

The frequency of gunshot injuries is escalating in American urban centers; consequently, the otolaryngologist is confronting increasing numbers of penetrating injuries to the head and neck. The incidence of temporal bone involvement in penetrating head injuries approximates 20% [1], facial nerve paralysis develops in over 50% of these cases [4]. The damage to the intratemporal facial nerve creates major challenges to the restoration of neural continuity and function. The following retrospective study reviews recent experience with this unique form of facial nerve trauma.

Materials and Methods

Between 1986 and 1992 11 subjects sustained gunshot injuries to the intratemporal course of the facial nerve and were treated at the Baylor College of Medicine Affiliated Hospitals (Houston, Texas): Ben Taub General Hospital, The Methodist Hospital, and the Houston Veterans Affairs Medical Center. Only cases of complete facial paralysis with evidence of progressive degeneration by the nerve excitability test (≥ 3.5 mA side-to-side threshold differences) or electroneurography ($\geq 90\%$ amplitude reduction in myogenic compound action potential) were included in the study. The injured segments of the facial nerve were explored via standard otologic approaches – transmastoid, translabyrinthine, middle fossa, and cervicofacial – which were selected on the bases of CT and audiometric findings.

D. D. Backous, H. A. Jenkins, and N. J. Coker (✉)
Department of Otorhinolaryngology and Communicative Sciences, Baylor College of Medicine, One Baylor Plaza, Houston, Texas 77030, USA

The following data were included in the study: patient ages; CT and operative findings; surgical procedures; concomitant cranial nerve, vascular, and intracranial injuries; and, outcome as judged by the House-Brackmann Facial Nerve Grading System [7]. All CT scans were reviewed by the same neuroradiologist to assess the areas of injury to the fallopian canal; radiographic predictions of site of lesion were compared retrospectively to intraoperative findings.

Results

Data are summarized in Table 1. All 11 subjects were males ranging in age from 19 to 46 years (average, 28.9 years). Two subjects had self-inflicted wounds; nine were shot in domestic or criminal assaults. Six bullets entered the temporal bone transversely and five penetrated laterally. Missiles were single projectiles, caliber undetermined. Nine patients presented with immediate facial paralysis, while two presented with pareses and then developed progressive degeneration. Coexisting injuries of the temporal bone included damage to the horizontal semicircular canal (two patients), open fractures into the vestibule (two), ossicular discontinuity (two), and tympanic membrane penetrations (five). Of the five patients with fragments of intracranial bone and shrapnel, only one required craniotomy for removal of the foreign objects and dural repair; this patient (case #1) had a facial nerve interpositional graft repair 5 months postinjury. The remaining ten patients were explored acutely between 6 and 11 days postinjury. One patient (case #2) required a two-stage procedure due to massive contamination of the entry wound.

The primary neural lesions were found at the stylomastoid foramen in seven cases, in the tympanic segment in five, and in the mastoid segment in four. Contiguous segments were often involved. Eight patients had transection or avulsion of the facial nerve and three had severe contu-

Table 1 Data summary of gunshot injuries to the facial nerve

Facial nerve injury			Concomitant injury			Procedure	Outcome
Case	Predicted by CT	Operative findings	Cranial nerve	Vascular	Intracranial		
1	Between GG and SMF	Transection: vertical	IX, X	Cavernous sinus-carotid fistula	FB in posterior fossa; right cerebellar hemisphere injury	TME + TLE + GAIG	Grade V at 18 months
2	Midtympanic to parotid	Avulsion: SMF to pes anserinus Avulsion and severe contusion: GG→SMF	None	None	FB in labyrinth	TME + TLE total parotidectomy; SIG: GG→face	Grade VI at 2 years
3	GG to vertical	Transection: tympanic and vertical	None	None	Midfossa (subdural) bullet tract	TFNE + SIG	Grade V at 13 months
4	Vertical and SMF	Transection: vertical and SMF	None	None	None	TME + GAIG	Grade IV at 1 year
5	Vertical to extracranial	Contusion: tympanic Transection: SMF and vertical	None	None	None	TME + TLE + SIG	LTF
6	Tympanic, vertical, and parotid	Transection: SMF	None	None	None	TME + SIG	Grade IV at 14 months
7	Tympanic and vertical	Transection: SMF	X, XII	Internal jugular vein tear	None	TME + TLE + SIG	LTF
8	CT unavailable	Contusion: SMF	None	None	None	TME + decompression	LTF
9	GG to SMF	Transection: tympanic	None	None	FB in posterior cranial fossa	TME + TLE + RA	Grade V at 4 months
10	No bony defect	Contusion: tympanic and vertical	None	None	None	TME + decompression	Grade III at 11 months
11	Vertical and tympanic	Contusion: SMF	None	None	FB in posterior fossa	TME + decompression	LTF

GG, geniculate ganglion; SMF, stylomastoid foramen; FB, foreign body (metal and/or bone); LTF, lost to follow-up; TME, transmastoid exploration; TLE, translabyrinthine exploration; TFNE, total (middle fossa and transmastoid) exploration; RA, reanastomosis; GAIG, greater auricular interpositional graft; SIG, sural interpositional graft.

sion with bony spicules penetrating the epineurium, a result of fractures through the fallopian canal. Eight patients had anacusis and three had mild-to-moderate mixed (conductive-sensorineural) hearing losses. One patient had deficits of cranial nerves IX and XII; another had a cranial nerve X paralysis. On the basis of bony changes around the facial canal, CT scanning overestimated the extent of damage of the facial nerve in seven patients. Of the eight patients who underwent autograft interpositional repair or rerouting with reanastomosis, six were available for follow-up and facial function ranged from grade IV to VI. The one patient (available for follow-up) with contusion of the nerve in the tympanic and vertical segments had a grade III return of function.

Discussion

Gunshot wounds are epidemic among young, indigent males in urban settings in the United States. Penetrating injuries of the temporal bone by low-velocity projectiles often produce facial paralysis. These penetrating injuries have a predilection for the tympanic and mastoid segments and the stylomastoid foramen area [2, 4]. Lesions of the nerve medial to the geniculate ganglion are rarely encountered, as projectiles passing medial to the otic capsule are most probably lethal [6].

Patients commonly suffer coexisting wounds to the head, neck, thorax, and abdomen. Management of these life-threatening injuries takes precedence over surgery of the ear and facial nerve. Appropriate management of the patient presenting with a gunshot injury to the temporal bone includes a complete head and neck examination with cranial nerve assessment, otologic inspection, CT scanning of the brain and temporal bone, and carotid arteriography; pure-tone and speech audiometry is performed after the patient is stable. Facial nerve testing is reserved for the patient with complete paralysis, and has minimal prognostic value until 3 – 6 days postinjury. In our experience [2, 4] patients with immediate and complete facial paralysis usually have transection of the nerve. Facial nerve exploration and temporal bone debridement of foreign bodies and devitalized tissue are planned, as soon as practical. Preparation for sensory autografts from the greater auricular and sural nerves are a part of preoperative planning.

Recommended CT scanning includes 1.5-mm, thinsection, axial and coronal views using a bone algorithm. Transection of the nerve is suspect if CT demonstrates violation of the fallopian canal. The actual limits of neural damage – contusion, transection, and avulsion – cannot be predicted radiographically. CT can demonstrate associated petrous pyramid fractures which may contribute to the pathogenesis of the facial nerve paralysis.

Those metal fragments easily accessible during facial nerve exploration and repair of the middle ear and mastoid are best removed with devitalized tissue and sequestrated bone. Retention of metal fragments usually do not present foreign body reactions [8], such that those fragments inaccessible or precariously located are best left undisturbed. Because of the highly destructive nature of gunshot injuries to the temporal bone, a radical or modified radical mastoidectomy is frequently performed. For patients with anacusis who require translabyrinthine exploration of the facial nerve, fat or muscle obliteration of the cavity is necessary to seal the communication to the subarachnoid space. A combined middle fossa-transmastoid approach is recommended for total facial nerve exploration of lesions at or proximal to the geniculate ganglion in patients who retain functional hearing thresholds.

Techniques of interpositional grafting are well documented [5]. Sural nerve autografts are most useful in this form of trauma, because of the lengthy and contiguous nature of the injuries. The restoration of facial function is suboptimal compared to grafting for iatrogenic injuries and knife wounds. The kinetic energy dissipated to the temporal bone by the missile is directly related to the mass of the bullet and square of the velocity ($KE = \frac{1}{2} mv^2$). Damage to the facial nerve results from direct impact, fragmentation of bullet or bone, concomitant fractures of the temporal bone, concussion, and ischemia. This extensive injury most likely accounts for the suboptimal outcome of interpositional grafts in these patients, i. e., grades IV – VI.

Acknowledgement The authors greatly appreciate the CT review provided by Michel E. Mawad, M. D.

References

1. Byrnes DP, Crockard HA, Gordon DS, Gleadhill CA (1974) Penetrating craniocerebral missile injuries in the civil disturbances in Northern Ireland. Br J Surg 61 : 169 – 176
2. Coker NJ, Kendall KA, Jenkins HA, Alford BR (1987) Traumatic intratemporal facial nerve injury: management rationale for preservation of function. Otolaryngol Head Neck Surg 97 : 262 – 269
3. Coker NJ, Jenkins HA, Psifidis A (1989) Electrophysiologic prognostication of acute facial nerve trauma. In: Fisch U, Valavanis A, Yasargil MG (eds) Neurologial surgery of the ear and the skull base. Proceedings of the 6th international symposium. Kugler and Ghedini, Amsterdam, pp 355 – 362
4. Duncan NO, Coker NJ, Jenkins HA, Canalis RF (1986) Gunshot injuries of the temporal bone. Otolaryngol Head Neck Surg 94 : 47 – 55
5. Fisch U (1974) Facial nerve grafting. Otolaryngol Clin North Am 7 : 517 – 529
6. Hagan WE, Tabb HG, Cox RH, Travis LW (1979) Gunshot injury to the temporal bone: an analysis of thirty-five cases. Laryngoscope 89 : 1258 – 1272
7. House JW, Brackmann DE (1985) Facial nerve grading system. Bull Am Acad Otolaryngol Head Neck Surg 4 : 4
8. Kerr AG (1967) Gunshot injury of the temporal bone – a histological report. J Irish Med Assoc 60 : 446 – 448

Eur Arch Otorhinolaryngology (1994) [Suppl]: S 290 – S 292

FREE PAPERS AND POSTERS

E. Fernandez, R. Pallini, and L. Lauretti

Microsurgical Selective Removal of Benign Neoplasms of the Parotid Gland

Most of tumors of the parotid gland (about 85%) are benign tumors, especially benign mixed tumors [2]. Surgery of parotid gland tumors is generally performed by otorhinolaryngologists and general surgeons. Conventionally, parotid gland surgery implies the preliminary identification and isolation of the facial nerve and its branches, and then the resection of the parotid gland including the tumor. This procedure is also advocated for the treatment of benign tumors. However, the manipulation of the facial nerve which is performed before decompression of the tumor mass may result in anatomical damage of the neural tissue. Neurosurgeons dealing with peripheral nerve surgery have three aims to pursue, to decompress entrapped nerves, to repair damaged nerves, and to preserve the integrity of undamaged nerves, for example during surgery for removal of intraneural (like schwannomas) or extraneural (e. g., parotid gland tumors) masses. With respect of the latter aim, we treated eight patients with benign mixed tumors of the parotid gland. Selective removal of the tumor was achieved by using microsurgical techniques. In this report we describe the surgical technique of selective microsurgical removal, which has been proved to be effective in the treatment of parotid benign tumors, with functional preservation of the facial nerve in all patients. Compared with the conventional technique, in which lateral and total parotidectomy involve the complete dissection of the facial nerve branches, the selective microsurgical technique requires no manipulation of the facial nerve before tumor decompression, thus greatly minimizing the risk of nerve injury.

E. Fernandez (✉), R. Pallini, and L. Lauretti
Department of Neurosurgery, Catholic University School
of Medicine, Largo A. Gemelli 8, 00168 Rome, Italy

Clinical Material

From 1983 to 1991 eight patients (two males, six females) were treated for benign mixed tumor of the parotid gland. The age of the patients ranged from 15 to 37 years (mean, 24.1 years). Tumor size varied from $2 \times 3 \times 2$ cm to $5 \times 4 \times 3$ cm. In only one case did the tumor involve the deep parotid lobe bulging between the intraparotid facial nerve branches. In this instance, after crossing the thickness of the superfivial lobe, the tumor was approached among the nerve branches and selectively removed. In the remaining cases, the tumor was found in the superficial lobe. In all cases: (a) the great auricular nerve was saved, (b) the tumor was totally and selectively removed, (c) the facial nerve was preserved, (d) the postoperative period was uneventful, and (e) no recurrences were noted during a follow-up ranging from 6 months to 8 years with a mean of 38 months (Fig. 1).

Surgical Technique

The skin incision is centered on the parotid bulging, thus repeating conventional parotid gland skin incision approaches (Fig. 2a). A blunt dissection is used to expose an area of the gland surface over the parotid bulging (Fig. 2b), to recognize and maintain intact the great auricular nerve. Subsequently, with the aid of the operating microscope, the parotid capsule is incised and the parenchyma of the superficial lobe is gradually penetrated until the tumor capsule is reached (Fig. 2c). During these manoeuvers, the parenchyma of the parotid gland is handled extremely carefully during blunt dissection. Sharp dissection with microscissors is used only after having obtained very thin tissue slides, which can be cut with no risk of nerve damage. Then the tumor capsule is incised and the pulp excised piecemeal (Fig. 2d). Hemostasis is obtained with bipolar coagulation. Gradual reduction of the tumor pulp allows dissection and reduction of the tumor capsule from the

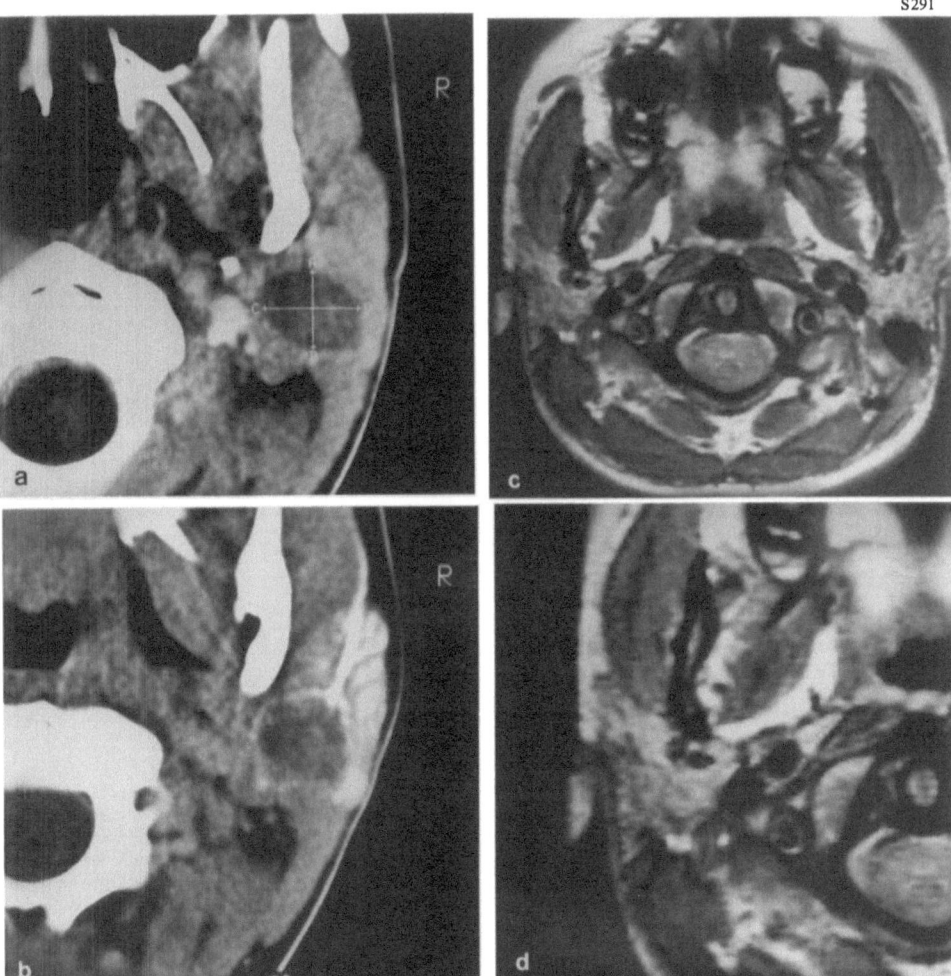

Fig. 1a–d Preoperative CT scan (**a**) and sialo-CT scan (**b**) showing a mixed tumor of the right parotid gland. Postoperative MRI (**c, d**) showing the right parotid gland free of tumor recurrence 6 months after surgery

surroundings and finally complete tumor excision (Fig. 2e).

Discussion

The surgical technique illustrated here is based on the general principles applied in the microneurosurgical removal of benign craniospinal tumors, and these can be summarized as follows: (1) to focus the attention mainly on the tumor mass then on the surrounding neurovascular structures, (2) to incise the tumor capsule and to gradually reduce the mass by piecemeal resection of the tumor pulp, and (3) to dissect free and reduce step by step the tumor capsule from any surrounding neurovascular structures without damaging them. A good combination of the last two principles finally leads to the complete removal of most of the benign tumors along the craniospinal axis with no neurovascular damage. The opposite approach leads to

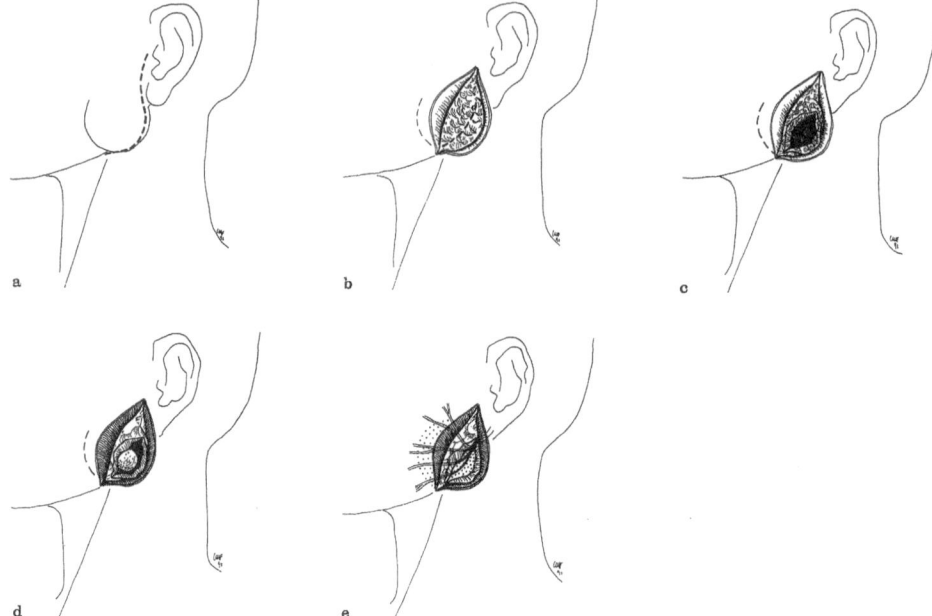

Fig. 2 a Skin incision (*interrupted line*) centered on the parotid tumor bulging. **b** An area of the parotid surface is exposed; the *thick interrupted line* indicates the site of the parotid incision. **c** The *interrupted line* indicates the limits of the tumor; one area of the tumor capsule has been exposed (*in black*) (**d**). A portion of the tumor capsule and pulp have been removed. **e** The tumor has been removed; on the bottom of the tumor bed some facial nerve branches (*in black*) are seen

first isolation of the surrounding neurovascular structures with the aim of protecting them, and subsequently to the approach of the tumor, with the primary aim of resecting it en bloc. Paradoxically, this surgical strategy in neurosurgery would result in marked neurovascular damage especially during removal of large tumors owing to the following two factors: (a) the strong neurovascular retraction manoeuvers used causing neurovascular compression and stretching), and (b) the difficult recognition because of the intact tumor mass of the extremely important cleavage planes between the tumor and surrounding tissues.

Our experience in parotid surgery is limited; nevertheless, we have a consistent experience in peripheral nerve surgery. Using the selective microsurgical technique, we have treated both large parotid tumors more than 4 cm

in diameter and tumors seated in the deep parotid lobe; it is in these conditions that Comoretto and Barzan [1] have recently advocated the use of parotidectomy instead of "enucleation" of the tumor. In our experience neither the size nor the position of the parotid benign tumor pose limits for selective microsurgical tumor excision.

References

1. Comoretto R, Barzan L (1990) Benign parotid tumor enucleation. A reliable operation in selected cases. J Laryngol Otol 104 : 706–708
2. Tucker HM, Olson NR, May M (1986) The facial nerve and extracranial surgery. In: May M (ed) The facial nerve. Thieme, New York, pp 561–577

Eur Arch Otorhinolaryngology (1994) [Suppl]: S293 – S294

W. Schneider, S.R. Wolf, and W.D. Braunwarth

Peripheral Facial Nerve Paresis as the Initial Presenting Manifestation of Tumors of Unknown Origin

Introduction

Leptomeningeal carcinomatosis (LC), which is characterized by the infiltration of the leptomeninges by carcinoma cells and which normally presents with the simultaneous occurrence of neurologial deficits at more than one level of the neuraxis [6], is mostly seen by oncologists taking care of patients terminally ill with cancer. In rare cases the otorhinolaryngologist will be among the first to diagnose a peripheral facial nerve palsy of unknown cause that actually is the initial manifestation of LC. Recently, we have seen two patients in whom the diagnosis of a diffusely metastasizing carcinoma was delayed by the initial symptom of a peripheral facial nerve palsy. The otorhinolaryngologist must be aware of the clinical entity of LC and the modern diagnostic methods of its diagnosis.

Case 1

A 53-year-old male presented to the ORL Department with a 3-week history of right-sided facial palsy. A CT scan of the brain and skull base had been normal, but the patient had noticed a moderate bilateral hearing loss and a mild unsteadiness. He had lost 15 kg of his body weight within 6 months. There was a total paralysis of the right facial nerve with a House index of VI/VI. Electromyography of the facial nerve showed no reaction to electrical or magnetic stimulation and no voluntary motor activity in needle recording from three facial muscles. An audiogram reveal-

ed a profound bilateral sensorineural hearing loss. The caloric responses of the right labyrinth were absent. A cerebrospinal fluid (CSF) sample contained anaplastic malignant cells. Three days later MR examination of the brain showed gadolinium enhancement in the frontal lobe due to a presumed small intracranial metastasis. In a CT scan of the thorax a mass in the upper lobe of the right lung was visible, presumably the malignant primary tumor. Despite repeated palliative intrathecal administration of methotrexate, the patient died 4 months after leptomeningeal carcinomatosis had been diagnosed. An obduction could not be obtained.

Case 2

A 51-year-old male had noted a right-sided facial nerve paresis, which was first diagnosed as idiopathic palsy. No abnormality was found in the cranial CT scan. After complaints of double vision 2 weeks later his general practitioner referred him to the Department of Neurology. Further examination revealed a right oculomotor nerve paresis besides a grade III/VI (House index) dysfunction of the facial nerve. Electromyographically voluntary motor activity was reduced. The compound muscle action potential was increased in latency after electrical mastoidal stimulation and lost after transtemporal magnetic stimulation. A conventional chest X-ray showed bilateral reticulonodular infiltration. Despite several lumbar punctures no raised cell count and no malignant cells in the CSF could be identified. Only once was the glucose concentration lowered and the protein ratio increased. After the sudden occurrence of a profound right sensorineural hearing loss, another cranial CT was taken this time with contrast medium and in high-resolution mode, which showed the posterior ethmoid sinuses and sphenoid sinuses on both sides and the apical parts of the right petrous bone opacified and no contrast enhanced tumor mass. Because of successive pareses of the right cranial nerves I – VIII an emergency

W. Schneider (✉) and S.R. Wolf
Department of Otorhinolaryngology of the University
of Erlangen-Nürnberg, Waldstr. 1, 91054 Erlangen, Germany

W.D. Braunwarth
Department of Neurology of the University of Erlangen-Nürnberg,
Waldstr. 1, 91054 Erlangen, Germany

mastoidectomy and bilateral endoscopic paranasal sinus surgery were performed. In specimens from the ethmoid mucosa, malignant, anaplastic cells were identified in lymph and blood vessels.

A postoperative MR image showed gadolinium enhancement of the meninges at the right skull base, indicating focal leptomeningeal carcinomatosis and a tumorous invasion of the middle cranial fossa, the sella region, and the cavernous sinus. As the primary tumor site an anaplastic gastric carcinoma was detected. The patient died within 3 weeks. Obduction was refused.

Discussion

Leptomeningeal carcinomatosis has rarely been reported by otorhinolaryngologists [4], although they may be faced with its clinical symptoms of isolated cranial nerve palsies. Whereas recently a case of bilateral profound sensorineural hearing loss in LC was published, peripheral facial nerve paresis seems to be a leading symptom of this infrequent disease. Since the results in our two patients showed that there was no characteristic, uniform appearance of the facial nerve paresis itself neither clinically nor electrophysiologically, indicating a metastasizing neoplasm, the occurrence of other cranial base symptoms must make the clinician consider LC. The suspicion of a malignant disease is further aroused by general clinical findings which were obvious in both patients: first a raised erythrocyte sedimentation rate, second a profound weight loss, and third a reticulonodular infiltration on conventional chest X-ray suggesting lymphangiosis carcinomatosa of the lung. In this constellation the next diagnostic step to take is a lumbar puncture, as a neoplasm with metastases to the brain is proven by tumor cells in the cerebrospinal fluid (CSF) [2, 8]. While conventional CT scans with contrast material are efficient in visualizing nodular metastases to the cerebellopontine angle [1] and petrous bone [3], they are of very little benefit in LC [7].

They did not show a contrast-enhanced tumorous mass in our patients with LC. The sheet-like growth pattern of the neoplastic cells along vessels, nerves, and the meninges at the base of the skull [5] produce cranial nerve lesions, which remain undetectable for conventional CT imaging [7]. Only MRI with gadolinium, which has a higher sensitivity in the examination of normal and abnormal meninges, will often show meningeal enhancement [7]. Therefore a contrast-enhanced MRI of the brain and skull base must be performed in all patients with a peripheral facial nerve palsy and additional cranial nerve pareses. This radiological device can be of great help when repeated spinal taps fail to detect tumor cells, which happens in about 10% of autopsy proven LC [2]. Consequently an early lumbar puncture plus MRI with gadolinium must be the golden standard in the further diagnostic workup of a peripheral facial nerve palsy with additional cranial base symptoms to overcome the difficulties in diagnosing LC.

References

1. Brackmann DE, Bartels LJ (1980) Rare tumors of the cerebellopontine angle. Otolaryngol Head Neck Surg 88 : 555–559
2. Boogerd W, Vroom TM, van Heerde P, de la Riviere GB, Peterse JL, van der Sande JJ (1988) CSF cytology versus immunocytochemistry in meningeal carcinomatosis. J Neurol Neurosurg Psychiatry 51 : 142–145
3. Greulich W, Sackmann A, Schlichting P (1992) Garcin-Syndrom: Klinik und Diagnostik eines seltenen Hirnnervensyndroms unter besonderer Berücksichtigung computer- und kernspintomographischer Befunde. Nervenarzt 63 : 228–233
4. Houck JR, Murphy K (1992) Sudden bilateral profound hearing loss resulting from meningeal carcinomatosis. Otolaryngol Head Neck Surg 106 : 92–97
5. Kokkoris CP (1983) Leptomeningeal carcinomatosis – how does cancer reach the pia-arachnoid? Cancer 51 : 154–160
6. Little JR, Dale AJ, Okazaki H (1974) Meningeal carcinomatosis, clinical manifestations. Arch Neurol 30 : 138–143
7. Sze G, Soletsky S, Bronen R, Krol G (1989) MR imaging of the cranial meninges with emphasis on contrast enhancement and meningeal carcinomatosis. AJNR 10 : 965–975
8. Wasserstrom WR, Glass JP, Posner JB (1982) Diagnosis and treatment of leptomeningeal metastases from solid tumors: experience with 90 patients. Cancer 49 : 759–772

Eur Arch Otorhinolaryngology (1994) [Suppl]: S295 – S296

U. Schuss and K. Terrahe

Facial Nerve Neurinoma and Otologic Signs

Introduction

Neurinomas, also called schwannomas according to Batsakis (1979), of the facial nerve are slow-growing, benign tumors [1]. Within the last 60 years abut 200 cases have been reported. Most of the tumors arise from the intratemporal course of the facial nerve, preponderantly at the area of the geniculate ganglion [2, 3] or from the tympanomastoid portion [4, 5].

But the neoplasma can also arise anywhere from the glia-Schwann cell junction through the parotid to the facial muscle [6].

The tumors of the intratemporal portion of the facial nerve cause general but not specific symptoms such as slow progression of paralysis in more than 80% and conductive hearing loss in nearly 50%. These symptoms are more or less independent of the size and the point of origin of the tumor [7]. Even very small-sized tumors can produce unmistakable symptoms [8]; on the other hand, very large tumors may be subtle in their clinical manifestations. Transmission deafness is often associated with an intratympanic tumor visible behind the intact tympanic membrane. The following facultative signs and symptoms, which are according to the literature occasionally present with such tumors, are without diagnostic value: pain, hyperacusis, sensorineural deafness, tinnitus, dizziness, and taste disorders. With the currently available radiodiagnostic techniques, such as high-resolution CT (axial and coronal) and MRI, a detailed visualization of the entire facial nerve would be easy and should be used in all patients with progressive facial weakness and suspected otologic signs [9].

Case Reports

The following two cases are presented because they appeared as showing *pure otologic problems with normal facial nerve function*. It was not at all possible to establish a correct preoperative diagnosis: one was misdiagnosed as otosclerosis the other as tympanic paraganglioma.

Case 1. A 67-year-old man was seen in consultation at our hospital because of progressive hearing loss in his left ear for some years. The pure tone audiogram showed an air-bone gap of 20 – 30 dB. Physical examination revealed an intact tympanic membrane, no mass in the tympanic space was seen, and facial nerve function was normal. With the patient under local anesthesia we performed a tympanotomy and found a tumor that filled the oval niche with contact to the ossicular chain. A biopsy was obtained and the histologic examination showed a facial schwannoma. In a second operaton 1 week later the tumor was totally removed and a graft from the greater auricular nerve was used to repair the defect. The ossicular chain was reconstructed.

Case 2. A 43 year-old woman had developed progressive hearing loss in her left ear for 4 years. But she complained more of a tinnitus that possessed a rhythm corresponding to that of the pulse. Behind the intact ear drum a pulsating reddish mass was seen. Facial nerve function was normal. Postoperatively she told us that she had noticed a rare twitching of the left face for 1 year. High-resolution CT evaluated a tumor extending from the geniculate ganglion to the mastoid segment. Complete tumor removal was obtained via a transmastoidal approach. The nerve was sacrificed and a hypoglossal-facial nerve anastomosis performed. Ten months later facial mobility was very satisfactory. The ossicular chain was reconstructed and hearing was normal.

Comment. In both cases the preoperative diagnosis was wrong. In the first case we clinically expected a fixed

U. Schuss and K. Terrahe
HNO-Klinik, Katharinenhospital, 70174 Stuttgart, Germany

S296

stapes and in the second case we were expecting a vascularized tumor. There was no way possible to establish a correct preoperative diagnosis. These cases are, according to Charachon [10], examples of "unpleasant intraoperative surprises" for which the correct diagnosis of a facial nerve tumor, even when suspected, cannot be made.

Discussion

The purpose of this report was to show how difficult it is to find the right diagnosis of facial neurinomas in view of their extreme rarity and their unspecific symptoms. The two cases of primary facial nerve tumors were both initially misdiagnosed and only after biopsy verified as neurinomas. The main reason for the wrong diagnostic method was *the absence of neurological symptoms* and the exclusive *presence of otologic signs*.

The otologic signs in the above-mentioned cases on the other hand were unspecific and even further tests, for example auditory brainstem response, positional and caloric vestibular tests, topodiagnostic investigations such as Schirmer's test, taste testing, and the stapedius reflex might be helpful in localizing the tumor, but they give no information about the real origin of the disease. Electroneuronography also gives no conclusive evidence.

It was mentioned by many authors that there is also a lower percentage of facial paralysis if the tumor is located extratemporally [7, 9]. Also in these cases it is nearly impossible preoperatively to make the correct diagnosis.

Conclusions

1. Neurinomas may be detected only by radiographic findings or by surgical exploration.

Therefore any case of:

- Progressive facial paralysis
- Unknown intratympanic tumor mass
- Unrecovered Bell's palsy after 1 month

should first be studied radiographically with CT and/or MRI.

2. The surgeon who starts to explore a case with suspicion of facial neurinoma requires experience in transtemporal supralabyrinthine procedures [3]
3. The facial nerve has to be sacrificed and reconstructed in most of cases.

References

1. Batsakis JG (1979) Tumors of the head and neck. Williams and Wilkins, Baltimore
2. Horn KL, Crumley RL, Schindler RA (1981) Facial neurilemmomas. Laryngoscope 91:1326–1331
3. Fisch U, Rüttner J (1977) Pathology of intratemporal tumors involving the facial nerve. In: Fisch U (ed) Proceedings of the 3rd international symposium of facial nerve surgery, Zürich. Aesulapius, Birmingham/USA, pp 448–456
4. Fuentes JM, Uziel A (1983) Neurinomas intra-petreux du nerf facial et de ses branches. A propos de deux observations. Neurochirurgie 29:197–201
5. Pellet W, Cannoni M, Pech A (1990) Otoneurosurgery. Springer, Berling Heidelberg New York
6. Sneige N, Batsakis JG (1991) Primary tumors of the facial (extracranial) nerve. Ann Otol Rhinol Laryngol 100:604–606
7. Balle VH, Greisen O (1984) Neurilemmomas of the facial nerve presenting as parotid tumors. Ann Otol Rhinol Laryngol 93:70–72
8. Iwanaga M, Yamamoto E, Yamaguchi M, Fukumoto M, Uchino R, Sawada S (1984) Facial nerve neurinoma: two cases located in the horizontal portion. Laryngoscope 94:938–941
9. Janecka IP, Conley J (1987) Primary neoplasms of the facial nerve. Plast Reconstr Surg 79 (2):177–183
10. Charachon R, Roux O, Dumas G (1978) Tumeur du nerf facial. A propos de trois observations. Ann Oto Laryngol (Paris) 95:777–784

Eur Arch Otorhinolaryngology (1994) [Suppl]: S 297 – S 298

FREE PAPERS AND POSTERS

J. P. Diard, M. Borsik, M. Wassef, and G. Freyss

Facial Paralysis Induced by Tumors

Introduction

In the case of malignant tumors in the parotid area with facial paralysis, the classical treatment is resection of the facial nerve. The resection around the tumor must be as substantial as justified by the extent of the tumor "in order to obtain a sufficiently wide safety margin around the tumor" (Eneroth 1977 [3]).

Materials and Methods

This study examined 12 cases of facial paralysis caused by tumors involving the parotid area. These cases were observed between 1982 and 1991. Most patients underwent complete examination of the facial nerve, including: (a) cochleovestibular examination, (b) testing according to Pr. Freyss' method, (c) computed electromyography, (d) Esslen's neurography, and Schirmer's test.

The approach was classical parotidectomy with the patient under total anesthesia. The surgical act was sometimes extended as a function of per surgical examination and extratemporaneous frozen sections.

Results

The population consisted of patients aged between 20 and 76 years (mean age, 55 years) including seven men and five women. The pathological condition affected the right

J. P. Diard
Medical Aircrew Examination Center, 00460 Armées, France

M. Borsik and G. Freyss
ENT Department Lariboisiere Hospital

M. Wassef
Pathological Anatomy Department Lariboisiere Hospital

side in five cases and the left side in seven cases. Facial paralysis gradually developed in four cases, was sudden in four cases, and undetermined in another four cases. The time necessary for the disease to fully develop prior to surgery ranged between 15 days and 1 year, with an average of 4 months.

Tumoral paralysis was total in ten cases. It was severe, test results ranging between 0 and 19 out of 30. In two cases it was partial, affecting the lower part of the face in one case, and the upper part in the other. The presurgical topographic diagnosis with Schirmer's test was performed in five cases and was normal in all five. The stapedian reflex was tested for in seven cases. It could not be tested for in one case due to tumor proliferation of the canal, and in another case because of suffusion into the middle ear. It was positive in four cases, negative in three. Correlation with the tumors spread to the nerve in the third portion was: consistent results, 4; reflex present and proliferation, 1; reflex absent, no lesion, 2.

Surgery always included total parotidectomy with total resection of the facial nerve in ten cases and resection of one branch in two cases. The histologic diagnosis was: adenoid cystic carcinoma, 4; adenocarcinoma, 2; actinic cell carcinoma, 2; muco-epidermoid tumor, 1; differentiated keratinizing squamous cell carcinoma, 1; skin squamous cell carcinoma, 2.

The facial nerve was macroscopically invaded in all cases. Resection was extended under eye control to areas apparently healthy under macroscopic observation. An extratemporaneous histological examination was performed in ten cases. It confirmed this diagnosis in six cases, but in four cases the histological result required extension of surgery. Resection had to be extended to the first portion in two cases. In one case the geniculate ganglion was invaded. Invasion of the first portion has never been observed. Nerve invasion affected the perineurium, the endoneurium, or sometimes the epineurium. Lymph node invasion was observed in four cases, with extracapsular spread in three. There was no relationship between the tumor extension into the nerve and the presence

S298

of invaded nodes. We observed one case of local recurrence in a patient treated for a muco-epidermoid tumor with mastoid bone invasion. Supraclavicular metastases, followed by lung metastases 1 year after surgery, were observed in the case of an actinic cell carcinoma.

Discussion

We observed 12 cases of tumoral spread into the facial nerve. The prevalence of malignant tumors in parotid tumors varies from 29% (5), to 25% (7), to 2.5% (6), depending on the author. The frequency of facial paralysis is estimated to be 34.7% by Katoh et al. [5]. From a clinical standpoint, the concept of gradual tumoral paralysis must be reviewed. In four of our cases paralysis developed very suddenly. Some authors [6, 9] underline the possibility that facial paralysis may be recurrent in 23%–33% of cases of neoplasic facial paralysis. It is striking to observe the histological diversity of the various types of tumors. The adenoid cystic carcinoma is not the only tumor with nerve tropism. This has already been observed by May [8]. In our group of patients we have not observed any carcinoma developing on a recurrent pleomorphous adenoma. The histological examination showed that tumoral cell groups could progress within nerve tissue. This explains that the nerve has a normal aspect or that its function is preserved although it is already invaded by tumoral cell groups. Some authors [2] report that facial paralysis can be caused by compression or by perineural infiltration. Perineural infiltration makes the prognosis more severe as it is the manifestation of a very aggressive tumor.

Regarding the surgical technique in the case of adenoid cystic carcinoma, Tran Ba Huy recommended in 1987 posterior exploration of the facial nerve if it was affected by the tumor. It seems that his approach should be suggested in the case of other malignant tumors which have reached the nerve. This should call for the greatest circumspection before grafting or attempting facial rehabilitation in cases of invasive cancers [8, 9].

Five-year survival in the case of parotid tumor with facial paralysis seems to diminish by half for Katoh et al. [5]. For Haruto et al. [6], 24% of patients developed petrous metastases, i.e., 37% of patients died from their tumors. This again should attract our attention to the risk of dissemination along a preformed pathway [11]. It would be interesting to perform patient exploration using MRI with injection of gadolinium to show the tumoral extension in the facial nerve.

Conclusion

These results provide more accurate information on the frequency of tumoral facial paralysis, on the nature of tumors, on presurgical evaluation, and on the strategy during surgery, fitting treatment into a coherent carcinological approach. It sometimes requires resection of the first, second, and third portions of the facial nerve in the petrous bone. An extemporaneous histologic examination has to be performed in all cases when exeresis of a parotid tumor is under consideration in the case of facial paralysis.

References

1. Conley J (1981) Occult neoplasm in facial paralysis. Laryngoscope 91:205–210
2. Dean A, Naval L (1990) Tumeur occulte de la parotide et paralysie faciale, un problème diagnostique. Rev Stomatol Chir Maxillofac 91 (5):390–394
3. Enroth CM (1977) Classification and management of parotid gland tumours. In: Fish U (ed) Facial Nerve Surgery. Aesulapius, Birminham/ZSA, pp 186–192
4. Hickman RE, Cawson RA (1984) The prognosis of specific types of salivary gland tumors. Cancer 54:1620–1624
5. Katoh T, Ishige T (1984) Malignant parotid gland tumors and facial nerve paralysis. Arch Otolaryngol 240:139–144
6. Haruto S (1988) Facial paralysis of neoplastic origin. In: Castro D (ed) The facial nerve. Kugler and Ghedini, Amsterdam
7. Harvey M, Tucker A (1977) Indications for irradiation in malignancy of parotid gland. In: Fish U (ed) Facial nerve surgery. Aesulapius, Birmingham/USA
8. May M (1986) Tumors involving the facial nerve. Thieme, Stuttgart, pp 455–467
9. Miehlke A (1977) General management of extra temporal lesions. In: Fisch U (ed) Facial nerve surgery, Aesulapius, Birmingham/USA, pp 198–203
10. Naval L et al. (1989) La dissémination perineurale dans le carcinome labial. Rev Stomatol Chir Maxillofac 90:5–9
11. Romain P, Desphieux JL (1989) Adénocarcinomes occultes de la parotide. A propose de deux cas. Rev Stomatol Chir Maxillofac 90:123–130
12. Tran Ba Huy P, Brette M-D (1987) Les parotidectomies. Encycl Med Chir Techniques chirurgicales thorax, pp 42030

Eur Arch Otorhinolaryngology (1994) [Suppl]: S299–S301

R. A. Jahrsdoerfer and A. M. Gillenwater

The Facial Nerve in Congenital Ear Malformations

Introduction

The facial nerve is the nerve of the second branchial arch and is intimately related to the temporal bone. Knowledge of facial nerve anatomy is critical to the success of any otologic or neurotologic surgical procedure. While this is true of normal temporal bone anatomy, it is of even greater significance for congenital ear malformations.

It is convenient to classify congenital ear malformations into major and minor categories. Minor malformations are those in which there is a patent external ear canal and the presence of an eardrum. In minor malformations, the abnormality is largely limited to the middle ear. Major malformations have as their hallmark congenital atresia or stenosis of the external ear canal. There is usually microtia of the external ear, although on occasion it may be well formed. Although the facial nerve may be abnormal in either category, it is our contention that in minor malformations the course of the facial nerve is less predictable and therefore surgery is more dangerous.

The Facial Nerve in Minor Malformations of the Ear

The most compelling reason why the facial nerve is at greater risk of injury in minor malformations is because the surgeon may be unaware that he or she is dealing with a congenital ear problem. An adult patient with a well-formed auricle and a flat conductive hearing loss will very likely be diagnosed as having otosclerosis or an ossicular discontinuity. Only after raising a tympanomeatal flap and

R. A. Jahrsdoerfer (✉) and A. M. Gillenwater
Department of Otolaryngology, Head and Neck Surgery,
University of Texas Medical School, 6431 Fannin Suite 6.132,
Houston, Texas 77030, USA

entering the middle ear will the astute surgeon realize that a congenital anomaly exists. Failing to recognize this invites a surgical disaster.

How is one forewarned of this potential catastrophe? There are subtle clues which may be apparent preoperatively that will alert the surgeon to the fact that he or she is dealing with a congenital ear malformation. Is the external ear oddly shaped? Are there preauricular skin tags? A preauricular pit? Does the ear canal slant superiorly? Is the eardrum smaller than normal? What is the status of the malleus handle? Short and blunt? Curved like a boomerang? Does it encroach on the anterior bony annulus? Any of these may be faint warning signals that the patient has a congenital ear malformation.

Even if none of the above clues are noted preoperatively, other signs noted intraoperatively may warn of a middle ear malformation. On occasion the chorda tympani nerve may be found exiting the bony posterior canal wall *lateral* to the annulus, but still covered by skin. Also, attention should be paid to the large chorda tympani nerve. It may not be the chorda tympani at all, but a bare facial nerve suspended across the middle ear. The presence of fat or salivary gland tissue (choristoma) in the middle ear should give one pause. Soft tissue of this sort in the middle ear indicates faulty embryogenesis. The real significance, however, is that his tissue, or other primitive tissue, may envelope a bare facial nerve which may then be irreparably harmed by careless dissection.

If the otologic surgeon suspects that the conductive hearing loss may be congenital in nature, it is wise to obtain an imaging study of the temporal bone. The preferred study is high-resolution computed tomography of the temporal bone in the 30° axial and 105° coronal views. These views will best show the course of the facial nerve in relation to the ossicles, labyrinthine windows, and inner ear. More recently, three-dimensional computed tomographic reconstructions of the temporal bone in congenital ear malformations have successfully plotted the course of the facial nerve [1]. Magnetic resonance imaging also has promise for facial nerve mapping, although this is more difficult in malformed ears than in normal temporal bones because of the failure to image bony structures. A second reason why suspected congenital ear malformations should be imaged is to identify, if present, any widening of temporal bone structures – internal auditory canal, cochlear aqueduct, semicircular canals, vestibule – which may indicate an abnormal communication between the labyrinth and the subarachnoid space. These findings may warn of a perilymphatic gusher.

Surgery of Minor Malformations

It is our contention that surgery of minor malformations is more dangerous to the patient than is surgery of major malformations. The middle ear problem in minor malformations often involves the stapes/facial nerve axis. The bony facial canal is derived from both the second branchial arch and the otic capsule. Any failure in development may prevent the facial nerve from being "locked in" against the otic capsule. In the absence of a bony canal the bare facial nerve is free to migrate anteriorly and inferiorly and will do so independent of the stapes. The analage of the stapes does not act as a barrier. It is sufficient only that the developing facial nerve pass through the blastema of the stapes to cause this ossicle to be malformed or absent. The development of the oval window is likewise affected and may be hypoplastic or absent.

The reported positions of the facial nerve relative to the oval window area are: (a) crossing at the level of the oval window, (b) crossing inferior to the oval window, (c) pressing against the stapes superstructure, (d) bifurcating to branch around the facial nerve (may or may not rejoin), (e) crossing the promontory vertically, and (f) suspended in midair.

By far the most dangerous situation in which to find the facial nerve is bare and running in a bony trough across the promontory. In this situation the nerve is often covered with respiratory mucosa and is disguised or effectively hidden. A small or hypoplastic stapes remnant may end blindly in the substance of the nerve. If this goes unrecognized, the nerve is vulnerable and subject to permanent injury. We have noted this in two of our patients operated elsewhere. This mode of injury has been recently reported in three patients, all of whom had a "soft tissue band" dissected to improve exposure of the oval window [3].

The Facial Nerve in Major Malformations

In major malformations of the ear there is always atresia/stenosis of the external ear canal. There is usually some degree of microtia. In our opinion, the course of the facial nerve is more predictable in this category than in minor malformations. This statement implies *operated*

cases in which the course of the facial nerve preoperatively was tracked by imaging and the pathway confirmed intraoperatively. We recognize that there are patients with severe temporal bone malformations in whom the course of the facial is markedly altered. However, these patients infrequently come to surgery because they are poor candidates. Their middle ear anatomy is so distorted that the chance of achieving a satisfactory hearing result does not warrant the risk of injuring the facial nerve. We have developed a preoperative rating scale to better select those patients who have the greatest chance of success through surgery [2]. While the facial nerve factors into the final grade assigned to the patient, by itself it does not disqualify the patient for surgery.

In ear malformations, the most common anomalies of the facial nerve are displacement and lack of a bony cover. In congenital atresia, the most common nerve problem is displacement. In approximately 25% of patients, the facial nerve makes a sharp bend (60°) at the second genu to cross the middle ear at the level of the promontory and exit into the temporomandibular joint. While the nerve in this situation may be bare in its horizontal portion, it is encased in bone thereafter as it curves its way to the glenoid fossa. Herein lies the risk of injury, because the nerve does not run in the same plane through the atretic bone. From the horizontal segment above the oval window to the temporomandibular joint, the course of the nerve is progressively more lateral. The significance of this is that at the level of the round window the nerve may be 2–3 mm lateral to where one would find a hypothetical bony annulus. If the surgical approach is low and does not hug the tegmen, the nerve may be severely traumatized by the cutting burr even before the middle ear is reached.

There are subtle signs to forewarn of this potential disaster. As one is drilling through atretic bone, the proximity of the facial nerve can be appreciated as a whitish linear structure highlighted against the pale yellow hue of the atretic bone. Moreover, the facial nerve often has small parallel blood vessels running on its surface which may become apparent as the bone overlying the nerve is thinned by drilling. The surgeon should never be comfortable with the progress of the operation until he has positively identified the facial nerve. Only then can it be protected with confidence.

A second location in which the nerve is vulnerable to injury is the glenoid fossa. We advocate that a tympanic bone remnant be searched for as this will point the way to the middle ear. On rare occasions, the tympanic bone remnant will be found deep in the glenoid fossa on the anterior surface of the mastoid bone. As the facial nerve exits the temporal bone into the temporomandibular joint in 25% of cases, soft tissue dissection in this area should be performed with great care. We now have tempered our recommendation and do not routinely dissect deep into the glenoid fossa.

Since we began using preoperative high-resolution CT scanning in 1982, we have been surprised only once by a postoperative facial paralysis. This occurred in an adult male in whom the facial nerve pursued a vertical course through the middle ear, without bending, and was bruised by the drill. The paralysis was temporary and there was full recovery of facial function in 1 month.

Facial Nerve Monitoring

The advent of reliable methods to monitor the function of the facial nerve intraoperatively has greatly aided the ear surgeon. Most neurotologic, and many otologic procedures, are now performed with facial nerve monitoring. Although we do not routinely monitor the facial nerve in atresia operations, we nonetheless have the Nerve Integrity Monitor II (NIMS, Xomed) available in the operating room at all times. When we know beforehand that the nerve is displaced and the middle ear structures are poorly developed, we routinely monitor. We monitor patients with Treacher Collins syndrome and hemifacial microsomia. In Treacher Collins syndrome, the nerve often exits the temporal bone through a bony cleft on its lateral surface. In this location the nerve may be injured by indiscreet soft tissue dissection before drilling has even begun. We believe the monitor is an important adjunct to ear surgery and we have no objection to its routine use in congenital ear malformations.

Facial Nerve Rerouting

One of the major advantages of a preoperative rating system for patients with congenital atresia is that it allows a reasonable prediction of hearing outcome [2]. However, in those patients who are "poor" or "marginal" candidates for surgery, the facial nerve is often displaced over the oval window area. In this location, it may be impossible to determine whether a stapes is present or whether the oval window is patent.

In select circumstances we carefully decompress the nerve and displace it inferiorly. This allows exposure of the stapes/oval window area. Careful assessment will determine whether ossiculoplasty is feasible. The method of choice is usually a total ossicular replacement prosthesis (TORP) from a mobile footplate to the new fascia graft tympanic membrane. Occasionally a stapedectomy is done.

Decompression and rerouting of the facial nerve is a delicate task. We limit the length of the facial nerve decompression to 5–6 mm. The decision to reroute often depends on the size of blood vessels feeding the nerve at that level. If the blood vessel is small and amenable to bipolar cautery, it is sacrificed. If the blood vessel is large (>0.5 mm in diameter), we usually elect to leave the nerve in place. To date, there have been no instances of facial nerve paresis or paralysis following rerouting of the nerve in the middle ear.

References

1. Andrews J, Anzai Y, Mankovich N, Favilli M, Lufkin R, Jabour B (1992) Three-dimensional CT scan reconstruction for the assessment of congenital aural atressia. Am J Otol 13 : 236–240
2. Jahrsdoerfer R, Yeakley J, Aguilar E, Cole R, Gray L (1992) A grading system for the selection of patients with congenital aural atresia. Am J Otol 13 : 6–12
3. Welling D, Glasscock M, Gantz B (1992) Avulsion of the anomalous facial nerve at stapedectomy. Laryngoscope 102 : 729–733

Eur Arch Otorhinolaryngology (1994) [Suppl]: S 302

POSTERS

J. T. Roland, P. E. Hammerschlag, W. Lewis, and A. Berenstein

Management of Traumatic Facial Nerve Paralysis with Carotid Artery Cavernous Sinus Fistula

Massive skull base injuries require detailed preoperative neurologial and neurovascular assessment prior to undertaking surgical repair of isolated cranial nerve deficits. We present the management of a traumatic facial paralysis, cerebrospinal fluid leak, and carotid artery cavernous sinus fistula from a gunshot wound to the skull base. The carotid artery cavenous fistula was ultimately controlled with a superselective embolization via the vertebral artery. The facial nerve injury was then safely treated with mobilization of the labyrinthine and vertical segments to allow a primary anastomosis. This illustrative case with pertinent radiological studies is presented and discussed.

J. T. Roland, P. Hammerschlag (✉), W. Lewis, and A. Berenstein
Department of Otolaryngology, NYU School of Medicine New York,
New York, USA

Eur Arch Otorhinolaryngology (1994) [Suppl]: S 303 – S 304

POSTERS

R. Ferreira Bento, P. Bogar, and A. Miniti

Facial Nerve Neuroma

Introduction

The tumors that affect the facial nerve account for 5 % of all cases of facial palsy; they can be intrinsic or extrinsic. Neuroma of the facial nerve extremely rare and plays only a small part among all the tumors that affect the nerve, although it accounts for 90 % of primary tumors of the facial nerve. In the literature, about 240 cases have been described, the majority in the last 14 years because of the development of radiological examinations. We present three cases of intratemporal neuroma of the facial nerve diagnosed only by surgical procedure. We review the histology, diagnosis, and treatment of this tumor. The aim of the paper is to alert otolaryngologists to the importance of early diagnosis and surgical treatment, which is directly proportional to a good functional result.

Case 1

A 38-year-old man suffered a sudden right facial palsy after otologic surgery (stapedectomy) in an other hospital. According to the surgeon, in the tympanotomy he found a white mass occupying the middle ear, so he opened the mastoid and found the mass in the antrum too; he then made a biopsy. The patient developed facial palsy and neurosensorial hearing loss, with vertigo and tinitus. Postoperative tomography showed a lesion in the second portion of the facial nerve. Histopathological examination revealed a neurinoma. In the transmastoid approach a large exposition of the dura of the middle fossa was found with herniation to the antrum and a mass coming from the second portion of the facial nerve occupying the middle ear. It was necessary to perform a labyrintectomy to remove the mass, and during this procedure it was noted that the tumor affected the geniculate ganglion; this was also removed. With no possibility of rerouting, a hypoglossal-facial anastomosis was made. Histopathological examination confirmed the facial neuroma diagnosis.

Case 2

A 22-year-old woman presented with right progressive facial palsy and underwent to neurologic treatment with cortisone for Bell's palsy. After 3 months the patients began to go deaf and was sent to an otolaryngologist. A white – yeollow mass was found occupying the external auditory canal and a transmission hearing loss of 30 dB. Conventional tomography demonstrated a mass in the mastoid, erosion of the posterior portion of the auditory external canal, and enlargement of the stylomastoid foramen. CT scan showed the same, as well as a prolongation of the mass to soft tissues of the neck. In a transmastoid approach a mass was found in the site of the third segment of the facial nerve, eroding the external auditory canal, coming out of the neck through the stylomastid foramen, and invading the parotid gland as far as the mandibular branch. After removing the tumor, which involved the second and third portions, the facial nerve was reconstructed with sural nerve. The external auditory canal was reconstructed with bone and fibrin glue. The ossicular chain and the tympanum were intact. Histopathological examination revealed a neurinoma without signs of malignancy. The patient woke up with total facial palsy that recovered partially in 18 months.

R. Ferreira Bento, P. Bogar, and A. Minit
ENT Department Faculdade de Medicina da USP, LIM 32, Brazil, AV Eneas de Carvalho Aguiar, 255, 6²andar, sala 602, CEP 05403, Saõ Paulo, SP, Brazil

Case 3

A 37-year-old woman presenting with a 3-cm mass below the right mastoid, underwent excision of the mass for diagnosis. The patient developed total facial palsy, and histopathological examination revealed neurinoma. The surgeon treated the patient with cortisone, affirming that the neurinoma was due to manipulation of the nerve. Eight months later, the patient underwent exploration of the facial nerve in order for a nerve graft to be made. The surgeon found a mass in the stylomastoid foramen, originating in the mastoid. Surgery was interrupted for investigations. CT scan showed a mass originating in the third portion of the fallopian Canal, with bone erosion of the external auditory canal. The audiogram was normal. In a transmastoid approach a mass was found occupying the mastoid and eroding the posterior portion of the external auditory canal, probably originating in the third portion of the facial nerve. The tumor was completed removed and the facial nerve was reconstructed with sural nerve; the external auditory canal was reconstructed with bone powder and fibrin glue. The ossicular chain and the tympanum were intact. Histopathological examination confirmed the diagnosis of neurinoma.

Discussion

The term neurinoma is used for benign tumors originating from Schwann's cells [10]. They can occur at any age, though mainly in the third and fourth decades [3] and in females [7, 10]. These tumors can be intratemporal, intracranial, or extratemporal. The locations most frequently found are the second and third portions or the extratemporal portion. Symptoms depend on the site of the tumor. The majority of patients develop sudden or progressive facial palsy. Deafness can be the first manifestation, neurosensorial hearing loss can be due to a tumor originating in the internal auditory canal, and a transmission hearing loss is found in tumors in the middle ear. Mixed types are also sometimes observed. Tumors in the parotid region are only expressed as a mass in the neck or face. Some patients develop hemifacial spasm, and others may have a yellow mass visible in the middle ear by otoscopy. At microscopy, the tumor consists of small and elongated cells, with nuclei with little chromatin. Positional changes in the palisade of the nucleus or files of cells separated by fibers or hyaline substance are well known,

but infrequent. Conjunctive tissue is found among this organization. The definitive diagnosis is histopathological, and the tumor can be classified as a glioma, schwannoma, ganglioneurofibroma, neurinoma, or schwannoglioma. The differential diagnosis includes the other intrinsic facial tumors, as well as tumors that occur sideways in the nerve such as acoustic neurinomas, meningiomas, and parotidean tumors. Bell's palsy, chronic otitis media, and cholesteatoma should be included in the differential diagnosis.

Conclusions

The possibility of facial nerve neurinoma, as was shown in the case reports, always has to be considered and investigated by specialist, in spite of it being a rare disease. The treatment and prognosis depend directly on early diagnosis and adequate surgical procedure. Analyzing cases 1 and 3 we can verify that the final result would have been much better if the surgical intervention had been made after a well-established diagnosis. Concentional tomography of the temporal bone was more useful than CT scan in establishing the limits of the tumor and planning the surgical approach. Based on these observations we concluded that conventional tomography is an examination that should be considered in ear pathologies.

References

1. Neely JG (1974) Neoplastic involvement of the facial nerve. Otolaryngology Clin North Am 7/2 : 385–396
2. Yamamoto E et al. (1984) Facial nerve neurinoma: two cases located in the horizontal portion. Laryngoscope 94 : 938–941
3. Bento RF et al. (1985) Traumatic peripheral facial palsy diagnosis. In: Portmann M (ed) The facial nerve. Masson, Paris, p 299
4. Ferrara O (1985) Neurinoma of the facial nerve. In: Portmann M (ed) The facial nerve, masson, Paris, p 432
5. Formigoni LG et al. (1980) Neurilenome du nerf facial en trajet intraparotidien: presentation d'un cas. Rev Laryngol Otol Rhinol 101 : 23–26
6. Contravreux C et al. (1986) Isolated facial palasilis caused by intrapetrous facial neurinoma. Presse Med 15 : 888–889
7. Schneck SA et al. (1960) Facial nerve tumors and progressive facial palsy. Arch Neurol 2 : 452
8. Pulec JL (1972) Facial nerve neurinoma. Laryngoscope 82 : 1160–1172
9. Conley J, Janecka I (1974) Schwann cell tumors of the facial nerve. Laryngoscope 84 : 958–962
10. Citobaut JC (1985) Intratemporal facial nerve tumors. In: Portmann M (ed) The facial nerve. Masson, Paris, p 417

Eur Arch Otorhinolaryngology (1994) [Suppl]: S305 – S306

POSTERS

P. Quesada, M. L. Navarrete, J. L. Quesada, F. Galletti, and M. Garcia

The Acoustic Trauma in Decompression Surgery of Facial Nerve

Introduction

The cochlear damage produced by facial nerve decompression surgery, which results in a neurosensorial hearing loss, is not well understood. There are few bibliographic references on this subject and the studies which have been written on facial nerve pathology report a possible etiopathogenic relation with the acoustic trauma brought about by drilling near to the labyrinthine area.

Material and Methods

We studied two groups of patients treated by transattical decompression of the facial nerve.

Group 1 was composed of seven patients (five Bell's palsies, one cholesteatoma, and one temporal bone fracture) who had been operated using a cleansing serum irrigation at room temperature (20 °C). They were studied before and after surgery by means of audiometry and vestibular caloric test.

Group 2 consisted of 24 patients (15 Bell's palsies, five otic zones, two temporal bone fractures, one Melkersson Rosenthal syndrome, and one facial nerve angioma) operated with a cleansing irrigation during drilling at body temperature (37 °C). They were studied before and after surgery by means of audiometry, caloric test, and evoked auditory potentials.

Results

The audiometric results in comparison to the study before operation were as follows: group 1 showed an average

P. Quesada, M. L. Navarrete, J. L. Quesada, F. Galletti, and M. Garcia
Department of Otorhinolaryngology and Neuroradiology,
Autonomous University of Barcelona, Spain

hearing loss of 30 db at 2000 Hz, 45 db at 4000 Hz, and 55 db at 8000 Hz. In group 2, the hearing loss average was 5 db at 2000 Hz, 25 db at 4000 Hz, and 10 db at 8000 Hz.

The results for the caloric test in group 1 showed one case of ipsilateral vestibular irritability which disappeared at the time of a new control test after 3 months of evolution. In group 2, we did not notice any type of secondary vestibular failure.

In group 1, evoked auditory potentials were not used before operation, but after 3 months of evolution. They allowed us to see an endocochlear pattern. In group 2, the altered evoked auditory potentials were slightly so and had disappeared at the time of the control test performed after 3 months of evolution.

Discussion

There are few bibliographic references on secondary cochlear lesions in facial nerve decompression. There are only the comments of Olson [1], who notices, among 21 decompressions, seven cases of cochleovestibular lesions. Salaverry reported four cases of conduction hearing loss by lesion of the ossicular chain out of 22 transattical decompressions [2]. Charachon [3] observed two neurosensorial hearing losses out of 38 transmastoid decompressions.

On the other hand, there are numerous references on secondary neurosensorial hearing loss after surgery of the cholesteatoma [4, 5]. These authors give percentages between 1.7% and 4.5%. They explain that its etiopathogenesis could be caused by the acoustic trauma of drilling associated with movements of the ossicular chain. They also notices that the noise produced by drilling caused a neurosensorial hearing loss for high frequencies, particularly at 4000 Hz.

Experimentally, Helms [6] has demonstrated that drilling produces a damage of 130 db ipsilaterally.

Palva's studies refer to the presence of a contralateral neurosensorial hearing loss, but this is not corroborated by others [7].

Parkin [8] adds the noise effect produced by the suction-irrigation system to the etiopathogenesis of the acoustic trauma.

In fact, it seems obvious that the acoustic trauma brings about an ipsilateral neurosensorial hearing loss and a less important contralateral one. However, there are some authors who do not report similar results. We infer that the drilling acoustic trauma might not be the only cause of this sequela. This idea is founded on our previous studies [9], through which we established the nonalteration of the ciliated cells of guinea pigs subjected to mastoid drilling with irrigation at 37 °C. However, there were frequent alterations of the ciliated cells, particularly when irrigation was done at 20 °C. These experimental data are confirmed clinically by our present study.

Though we agree our cases of neurosensorial hearing loss might be due to the acoustic trauma, we think the appearance of the vestibular alteration is not caused by it. This is the reason why we watched the irrigation temperature systematically. We observed that using irrigation at body temperature (37 °C), there was no vestibular failure. Moreover, hearing losses were always less severe than those which appeared previously. We explain this phenomenon by the hypoxia following a secondary vasoconstriction using an irrigation at a temperature lower than body temperature.

In fact, clinical and experimental studies report the preventive effect of oxygen therapy using an mixture of 95% oxygen and 5% CO_2 because of the vasodilatation effect of the latter [10].

Conclusions

Though the Corti organ does not receive blood nutriment directly, its nutrition is supplied through endolymph, the metabolism of which is regulated by the vascular stria. We think that the acoustic trauma produced by drilling in addition to the vasoconstriction which can be caused by an irrigation at a temperature lower than body temperature results in poor local microcirculation. This may create difficulties in relation to the oxygen supplied to the ciliated cells by causing a state of hypoxia.

In support of this hypothesis, we noticed that the area of the cochlea where the 4000-Hz receptors are located is injured more easily. This zone is known for its poor irrigation.

In addition, there is no contralateral neurosensorial hearing loss, because there is no hypoxia to foster a cochlear lesion due to the acoustic trauma.

References

1. Olson N, Goin D, Nichols R (1973) Adverses effects of facial nerve decompression for Bell's palsy. Trans Am Acad Ophtalmol Otolaryngol 77 : 67–71
2. Salaverry MA (1982) Transattical approach to the labyrinthine segment of the facial nerve. In: Graham M, House WF (eds) Disorders of the facial nerve. Raven, New York, pp 423–430
3. Charachon R, Roux C, Gratacap B (1985) Comparative analysis of medical and surgical treatment of Bell's palsy in a series of severes palsies. In: Portmann (ed) Facial nerve. Masson, pp 264–268
4. Schuknecht HF, Tondorf J (1960) Acoustic trauma of the cochlea from ear surgery. Laryngoscope 70:4479–4505
5. Tos ML, Plate S (1984) Sensorineural hearing loss following chronic ear surgery. Ann Otol Rhinol Laryngol 93 : 403–409
6. Helms J (1976) Acoustic trauma from the bone cutting burr. J Laryngol 90 : 1143–1149
7. Palva A, Sorri M (1979) Can an operation on a deaf ear be dangerous for hearing? Acta Otolaryngologica Suppl 360: 155–157
8. Parkin J, Wood R, McCandless G (1980) Drill and suction-generated noise in mastoid surgery. Arch Otolaryngol 106 : 92–96
9. Ciges M, Quesada P (1970) Estudio vital de la cóclea del cobaya. Acta ORL Iber Am 21 5 : 504–521
10. Joglekar SS, Lipdscomb B, Shambaugh GE (1977) Effects of oxygen inhalation on noise-induced threshold shifts in humans and chinchillas. Arch Otolaryngol 103 : 574–581

Eur Arch Otorhinolaryngology (1994) [Suppl]: S307

ABSTRACTS

S. Harris and L. Salemark

Recovery of Total Facial Palsy after Neuroma Surgery

Facial palsy after neuroma surgery with an anatomically intact VIIth nerve can be expected in about 10%–20% of the cases operated on. In most instances the palsy is partial and temporary. In total palsy function often does not return. However, in several cases with neurophysiologically documented total palsy with denervation signs facial function has returned after 6–18 months. Immediate anastomoses with hypoglossus or accessorius nerves in these cases therefore can be questioned. A strategy including gold weights in the eyelid, suspension of the chin, and a partial crossover grafting gives the patient an immediate improvement and a chance of natural recovery.

S. Harris and L. Salemark
ENT Clinic, University of Lund, 22185 Lund, Sweden

Facial Nerve Monitoring

Eur Arch Otorhinolaryngology (1994) [Suppl]:S311–S313

F. Soldner, L. Papavero, T. Wallenfang, and F. Schnorpfeil

Intraoperative NIM-2™ Monitoring for Facial Nerve Preservation in Acoustic Neurinoma Surgery

Introduction

Since the early 1980s intraoperative monitoring of the facial nerve during CPA (cerebellopontine angle) tumor operations has been routinely used in the United States. In several European countries the value of this tool is still questioned. The intraoperative stimulation of the facial nerve was described as early as 1898 [1]. A highly sophisticated and clinically reliable technology has since then developed [2–4]. Today it is possible to identify the facial nerve and obtain data about its neural integrity during and at the end of the surgical procedure. An EMG-based system with quantitative measuring of compound muscle action potentials has been used in our department since 1991.

Patients and Methods

This study was performed in 14 patients with acoustic neurinoma. There were 6 men and 8 women, aged from 16 to 76 years. The tumors were removed via the retromastoidal approach with the patient in the sitting position. Eight patients were given intraoperative monitoring of the facial nerve using the Nerve Integrity Monitor "NIM-2™". They underwent brainstem auditory evoked potential (BAEP) monitoring during resection of the tumor. In the monitored group preoperative electrodiagnostic testing of the facial nerve (facial nerve conduction, blink reflex, needle EMG) and an otoneurological evaluation was performed. The facial nerve function was assessed in all cases according to the House 6-point scale [5]. The tumor size was assessed according to the Koos classification. In four

F. Soldner, L. Papavero, T. Wallenfang, and F. Schnorpfeil
Department of Neurosurgery, City Hospital Fulda,
36043 Fulda, Germany

cases a CT-guided volumetric estimation was added. The stimulus parameters of the NIM-2™ included a constant current electrical source set between 0.05 and 1.00 mA with a frequency of 4 cycles/s and a 100-µs pulse duration. We used several monopolar insulated stimulus dissectors.

A pair of subdermal needle electrodes were inserted in the nasolabial groove and in the lateral m. orbicularis oculi. A separated needle electrode was inserted in the top of the forehead (Fpz) to act as the ground for the two recording channels. An additional electrode was placed near to Fpz as an anode for the monopolar stimulator. The system provided a visual (oscilloscope) and acustic (loudspeaker) representation of the facial response. An effective muting system that automatically attenuated the output of the loudspeaker during electrocautery was included.

Difficulties

Muscle relaxants obviously influence the responses to electrical stimulation. Therefore these agents were given only during induction of anesthesia. In only one patient were several doses of pancuronium necessary during the operation. A technical problem relating to the use of NIM-2™ occurred during the intraoperative monitoring of BAEPs. Two types of artifacts, disturbing considerably the brainstem evoked responses, could be identified. To eliminate the artifacts we found it was necessary (1) to reset the stimulus intensity to 0.00 mA and (2) not to use the status check during the averaging of the brainstem evoked potentials.

Results

Using the system of Prass and Luders [3], we classified the responses into trains and bursts. "Bursts" are single synchronized potentials and can be caused by an electrical or mechanical stimulus. The "trains" are multiple asyn-

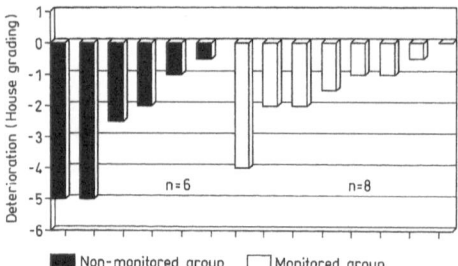

Fig. 1   Facial nerve function pre- and postoperatively

Values higher than 2000 µV indicate no deterioration and we expect good facial nerve function postoperatively. Nevertheless low amplitudes are not necessarily the expression of functional damage because after prolonged dissection and stimulation the facial nerve can be exhausted.

Comparing the facial nerve function pre- and postoperatively (Fig. 1), the early postoperative examination showed in 50% of the monitored patients none or only a slight deterioration (a maximum of one point on the House 6-point scale). Complete facial nerve palsy did not occur, whereas this deficit was observed in two cases of the non-monitored group.

Case Report.   A 15-year-old girl presented cranial nerve deficits: VII (House grade, I–II), VIII, IX, X, and cerebellar symptoms. The MRI and CT scan showed a right-sighted CPA tumor (4 cm in diameter, 31 ml in volume) compressing the brainstem. The operation was monitored by the NIM-2™ (Fig. 2). In the beginning train potentials occurred, being generated by traction of a retractor. The stimulation of the tumor mass even with an intensity of 0.40 mA did not evoke electrical responses. After a prolonged dissection the facial nerve could finally be identified by stimulation. Burst potentials of more than 1000 µV were recorded after stimulation with 0.20 mA. The tumor was extremely adherent to the facial nerve, so that only a subtotal removal could be performed. At the end of the operation we stimulated the facial nerve at the brainstem to assess the integrity of the nerve. Postoperatively we found a facial nerve palsy II–III according to the House scale, which improved in the following 4 months to nearly I.

chronous potentials resulting from mechanical stimulus like traction or pressure during tumor removal or after retractor manipulation. We often recorded train potentials following irrigation with cold saline. The values of these potentials never exceeded 500 µV. In patients with a preoperative facial nerve palsy they could not be observed.

An effective facial nerve stimulation results in a single compound muscle action potential. We compared the maximum values of these potentials with the preoperative facial nerve function. Four patients had no facial nerve palsy preoperatively and showed responses between 2500 and 3600 µV. In patients with a preoperative deficit of the facial nerve function we found reduced amplitudes of less than 1500 µV.

At the end of the operation we stimulated the facial nerve at the brainstem in order to assess its integrity.

Fig. 2   Case report: acoustic neurinoma, 15-year-old girl, 31 ml, Koos grade IV

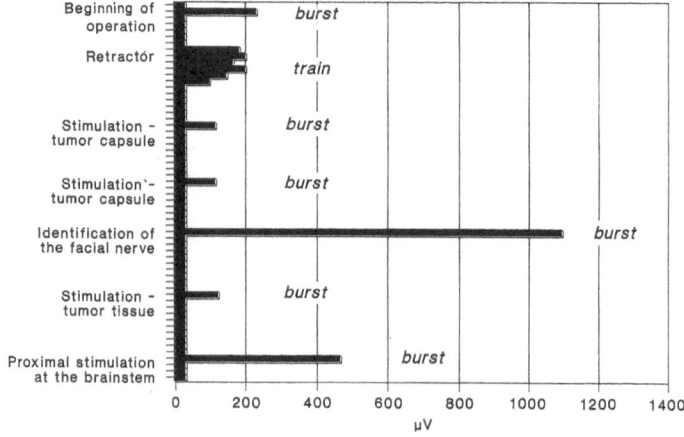

Discussion

The main advantages of the NIM-2™ monitoring are: (1) early identification of the facial nerve, (2) differentiation from other cranial nerves (3), differentiation from tumor tissue, and (4) the data at the end of the surgical procedure about neural integrity for prognosis of facial nerve function. The different artifacts produced by NIM-2™ which influence other monitoring systems like brainstem auditory evoked potentials (BAEP) should be kept in mind. The nerve-integrity monitoring represents a dependable and easy method for monitoring the facial nerve function during CPA-tumor operation. It is still necessary to obtain more experience in the field of neurophysiology of the facial nerve. Monitoring is a very important tool in the procurement of better postoperative results, but it does not replace surgical experience. NIM-2™ monitoring enables us to shorten the operating time when dealing with small tumors and to preserve facial nerve function when resecting huge tumors.

References

1. Krauze F (1912) Surgery of brain and spinal cord, 1st Englisch edn. Rebman, pp 738–743
2. Jako G (1965) Facial nerve monitor. Trans Am Acad Opthalm Otolaryngol 69:340–342
3. Prass R, Luders H (1986) Acoustic (loudspeaker) facial electromyographic monitoring: part I. Evoked electromyographic activity during acoustic neuroma resection. Neurosurgery 19:392–400
4. Kartush JM (1989) Electroneurography and intraoperative facial monitoring in contemporary neurotology. Otolaryngol Head Neck Surg 101:496–503
5. House JW, Brackmann DE (1985) Facial nerve grading systems. Otolaryngol Head Neck Surg 93:146–147

Eur Arch Otorhinolaryngology (1994) [Suppl]:S314–S315

G. Magliulo, R. Petti, G. M. Vingolo, R. Ronzoni, and P. Cristofari

Facial Nerve Monitoring of Skull Base and Cerebellopontine Angle Lesions

Introduction

The object of the present paper is to compare pre- and postoperative facial nerve function results between unmonitored and monitored surgical cases of cerebellopontine angle and skull base lesions.

Material and Method

The cases of 45 patients undergoing surgery for tumors in the cerebellopontine angle and lateral skull base were analyzed retrospectively. There were 27 women and 18 men, ranging in age from 25 to 71 years (mean, 42.7 years). Twenty patients underwent infratemporal approaches (type A and type B) by the same surgeon (G.M.) [2]. The other 25 patients suffering from acoustic neuroma were operated on using different surgical approaches dictated by the clinical and radiologic criteria (translabyrinthine or retrosigmoid approach). In all cases facial nerve function was assessed according to the House 6 point scale [4]. Twenty patients had intraoperative monitoring using evoked electromyography (EMG, nerve integrity monitor, Xomed-Treace, Jacksonville, FL) [5–7]. The patients were recalled and assessed at various times after surgery, which ranged from 6 to 47 (mean, 15.8) months.

Results

The data from the monitored and unmonitored cases of cerebellopontine angle and lateral skull base tumors

G. Magliulo (✉), R. Petti, G.M. Vingolo, R. Ronzoni,
and P. Cristofari
IV ENT Clinic-University "La Sapienza", Piazza Pio XI, 13,
Roma 00165, Italy

regarding tumor pathology and tumor size are listed in Table 1 and Table 2. Preoperative facial function of the skull base lesions is summarized in Table 3. Three patients (two unmonitored; one monitored group) and a grade VI function preoperatively. One of these patients had undergone previous surgery, while in the others the facial nerve was invaded by the tumor in its mastoid portion. Table 4 shows the preoperative facial function in the acoustic neu-

Table 1 Tumor type

Histology	Unmonitored	Monitored
Skull base		
Glomus	6	5
Cholesteatoma	2	2
Basal cell		
Carcinoma	1	–
Cranial nerve		
Neuroma	–	1
Adenoid cystic	–	1
Carcinoma		
Meningioma	1	–
Epidermal carcinoma	–	1
Cerebellopontine angle		
Acoustic neuroma	15	10

Table 2 Tumor size

	Unmonitored	Monitored
Skull Base Tumors		
<2 cm	2	1
3–5 cm	6	7
>5 cm	2	2
Cerebellopontine angle tumors		
<1.5 cm	7	5
1.5–3 cm	4	1
>3 cm	4	4

Table 3 Skull base tumors: preoperative facial function

House grades	Unmonitored	Monitored
I	7	8
II	1	–
III	–	1
IV	–	–
V	–	–
VI	2	1

Table 4 Cerebellopontine angle: preoperative facial function

House grades	Unmonitored	Monitored
I	14	9
II	1	–
III	–	1
IV	–	–
V	–	–
VI	–	–

Table 5 Skull base tumors. Postoperative facial function

House grades	Unmonitored	Monitored
I	2[a]	5[a]
II	2[a]	2[a]
III	2	1
IV	–	1[a]
V	1[a]	–
VI	3[a](1)	1

[a] Normal preoperative function with nerve rerouted.

Table 6 Cerebellopontine angle tumors. Postoperative facial function

House grades	Unmonitored	Monitored
I	5[a]	4[a]
II	1[a]	2[a]
III	4[a]	3[a](1)
IV	1	–
V	2[a]	–
VI	2[a]	1[a]

[a] Normal preoperative facial function.

roma group. Postoperative facial function for skull base and cerebellopontine angle lesions are presented respectively in Table 5 and in Table 6. In the unmonitored group of skull base tumors a grade I or II function was noted in four patients (40%). Four patients (40%) complained of poor or no function (grade V or VI). In contrast the findings of the monitored group revealed a greater incidence of

grade I and II function which was achieved by seven patients (70%). This favorable outcome was substantiated by no development of grade V or VI facial nerve dysfunction. Similar results were observed in the cerebellopontine angle lesions.

Discussion

Data from this study, which compares monitored cases with unmonitored cases, support the use of continuous evoked EMG monitoring for any procedure involving the facial nerve. The advent of acoustic EMG facial monitoring enhanced our preservation rate of the seventh nerve and maximized postoperative function both in cerebellopontine angle and skull base lesions. In the latter, favorable facial nerve function (grade I or II) was noted in 87% of the patients with normal preoperative function, who were monitored intraoperatively. This is compared to only 50% of the unmonitored group. In addition, none of the monitored patients developed grade V or VI function, while 25% of the unmonitored patients showed these unfavorable sequelae. Analogous findings were observed in acoustic neuromas. Facial nerve preservation was achieved in 66% of the EMG patients with normal preoperative facial function. In contrast a grade I or II result was obtained in only 40% of the cases with no facial nerve monitoring. Furthermore, 26.6% of the unmonitored group progressed to a dramatic result (grade V or VI) compare with 11% sustained by the EMG monitored group.

These observations parallel the experiences from other studies [1, 3, 6].

References

1. Benecke JE, Calder HB, Chadwick G (1987) Facial nerve monitoring during acoustic tumor removal. Laryngoscope 97 : 697–700
2. Fisch U (1982) Infratemporal fossa approach for glomus tumors of the temporal bone. Ann Otol Rhinol Laryngol 91 : 474–481
3. Harner SG, Daube JR, Beatty CW (1988) Intraoperative monitoring of facial nerve. Laryngoscope 98:209–212
4. House JW, Brackmann DE (1985) Facial nerve grading system. Otolaryngol Head Neck Surg 93 : 146–147
5. Kartush JM (1989) Electroneurography and intraoperative facial monitoring in contemporary neurology. Otolaryngol Head Neck Surg 101 : 496–503
6. Leonetti JP, Brackmann DE, Prass RL (1989) Improved preservation of facial nerve function in the infratemporal approach of the skull base. Otolaryngology – Head and Neck Surgery 101 : 74–78
7. Prass RL, Luders H (1986) Acoustic (loudspeaker) facial electromyographic monitoring: evoked electromyographic activity during acoustic neuroma resection. Neurosurgery 19 : 392–400
8. Silverstein H, Smouha E, Jones R, Sarasota FL (1989) Routine identification of the facial nerve using electrical stimulation during otological and neurotological surgery. Laryngoscope 98 : 726–730

Eur Arch Otorhinolaryngology (1994) [Suppl]: S316–318

T. Yokoyama, K. Uemura, H. Ryu, K. Sugiyama, S. Nishizawa, I. Shimoyama, and M. Nozue

Intraoperative Facial Nerve Monitoring
by Monopolar Low Constant Current Stimulation
and Postoperative Facial Function in Acoustic Tumor Surgery

Introduction

Among the several methods of intraoperative facial nerve monitoring in acoustic neurinoma surgery, the evoked facial muscle responses (EFMR) by electrical stimulation of the nerve have been most commonly and effectively used [2, 4]. However, the most effective stimulus parameters during surgery have not yet been defined. In the past 9 years, monopolar low constant current stimulation (0.5–0.6 nA) was applied in 52 cases. We report intraoperative findings of the EFMR and their relations to postoperative facial functions.

Materials and Method

In the past 9 years (1984–1992) 64 patients were operated upon and the facial nerve was identified and monitored by the EFMR in 52 cases (male 21 and female 31 cases). The tumor size was small (≤ 1 cm) in 13, medium (1–3 cm) in 15, and large (> 3 cm) in 24 cases.

The tumor was approached through the suboccipital route and the stimulation was applied periodically to identify the nerve and to monitor its function. The stimulation was delivered through a handmade bayonet-shaped electrode consisting of a stainless pipe (2 mm in diameter) and of a tungsten rod (0.6 mm in diameter). It was insulated by Epoxylite except for 0.5 mm from the tip (resistance less

T. Yokoyama (✉), K. Uemura, H. Ryu, K. Sugiyama, S. Nishizawa, and I. Shimoyama
Department of Neurosurgery, Hamamatsu University School of Medicine, 3600 Handa, Hamamatsu, 431-31 Japan

M. Nozue
Department of Otorhinolaryngology, Hamamatsu University School of Medicine, 3600 Handa, Hamamatsu, 431-31 Japan

than 1 K ohms). The stimulating condition was adjusted to deliver a 0.1-ms duration square wave with the intensity of 0.5–0.6 mA at 3 Hz [8, 9]. The EFMR obtained by stimulation of the nerve in the internal auditory meatus (IAM), at the porus, and over the pons were compared each other.

The amplitudes of the EFMR recorded immediately after the tumor removal were compared to postoperative facial functions (followed up for 6–24 months). Facial functions were evaluated with the facial score, proposed by the Japan Soiety of Facial Nerve Research [7], and total scores of 0–10 (House-Brackman grade V–VI), 12–20 (grade IV), 22–32 (grade II–III), 34–40 (grade I) were classified as poor, fair, good, and excellent recovery of function, respectively.

Results

Case Presentation

Figure 1 shows the facial nerve after total tumor removal in a 41-year-old female who had a large tumor 4.2 cm in diameter on the left side. The facial nerve was not severely damaged by tumor compression over the pons and in the IAM, and it was preserved well in these areas. However, at the porus the nerve was elongated by tumor compression and was hardly identified under microscope. Figure 2 shows the intraoperative EFMR obtained by stimulation in the respective areas. Those obtained by stimulation in the IAM were fairly constant throughout the operation. At the porus, the wave forms were quite small compared to those in the IAM. Among the EFMR obtained by stimulation over the pons, the bottom one was recorded immediately after the tumor removal. Although the nerve at the porus was not recognized as a strand, the EFMR clearly showed the anatomical continuity of the nerve. However, the amplitudes reduced to 53 μV. Her facial functions were excellent, with a facial score of 36 at 18 months after the operation.

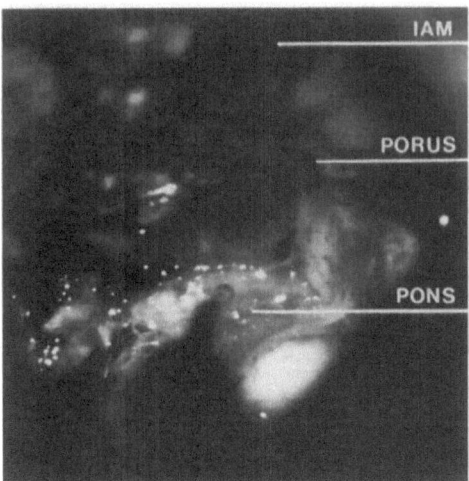

Fig. 1 Photograph shows the facial nerve in the internal auditory meatus, at the porus, and over the pons. The nerve at the porus was elongated by the tumor compression and was not recognized as a strand under the microscope

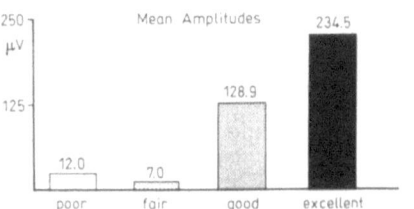

Fig. 3 Mean amplitudes of EFMR to stimulation of the nerve over the pons after removal of the tumor in patients who showed poor, fair, good, and excellent facial recovery

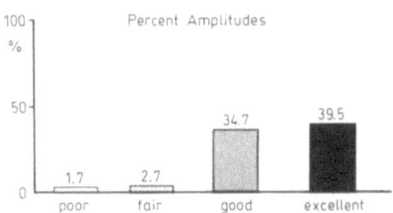

Fig. 4 Mean percentage of amplitudes (the amplitude of responses over the pons was divided by that in the internal auditory meatus) in patients who showed poor, fair, good, and excellent facial recovery

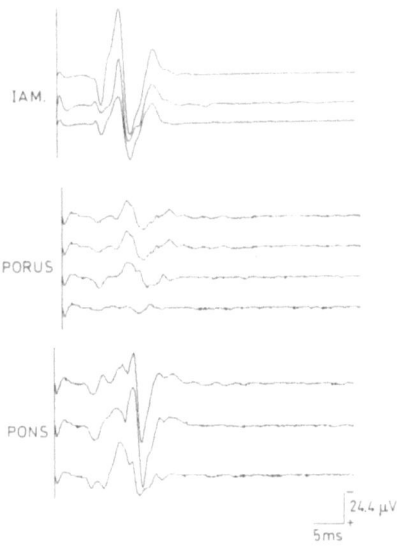

Fig. 2 Intraoperative EFMR obtained by stimulation of the nerve in the IAM, the porus, and over the pons

The facial nerve was preserved in 13 small tumors (100%), in 14 medium-sized tumors (93%), and in 18 large tumors (75%). Of the small tumors, all cases showed good (8%) or excellent (92%) facial functions. Of the medium-sized tumors, only one (6%) showed poor and the others showed good (20%) or excellent (74%) facial recoveries. Of the large tumors, ten were poor (42%), one was fair (4%), eight were good (33%), and five were excellent (21%). In total, 11 were poor (23%), 1 was fair (2%), 12 were good (24%), and 28 were excellent (54%).

The EFMR in the IAM were fairly constant throughout the operation but those over the pons usually decreased in amplitude as the operation proceeded. The mean amplitudes of EFMR to stimulation of the nerve over the pons after total tumor removal were 12.0 ± 26.1 in poor, 7.0 in fair, 128.9 ± 122.1 in good, and 234.5 ± 188.7 µV in excellent cases (Fig. 3). The percentage of amplitudes (the amplitude of responses to stimulation over the pons was divided by that to stimulation in the IAM) was $1.7\% \pm 3.4\%$ in the poor, 7.0% in the fair, $34.7\% \pm 26.7\%$ in the good, and $39.5\% \pm 23.1\%$ in the excellent group (Fig. 4). It was noted that the amplitudes were statistically significantly lower in poor and fair cases compared to good and excellent cases (t test, $p < 0.01$). However, there was no significant difference between good and excellent cases.

Discussion

In facial nerve monitoring, it is essential to refine stimulus parameters for accurate anatomical orientation of the nerve. For this, spreading current form the electrode should be as low as possible. Otherwise, the nerve will be excited even if the electrode is not in contact with the nerve. This will confuse the orientation of the nerve and make it difficult to preserve the nerve, especially at the porus. The extent of spreading current is strongly related to the given current intensity. In our previous studies, the current spread for about 1 mm from the electrode with an intensity of 0.6 mA, and 5 mm with an intensity of 1.8 mA. Therefore, the intensity should be 0.5–0.6 mA or less if a stimulator can provide a reliable intensity below 0.5 mA [5, 8, 9]. Another important thing is that the electrode should be insulated to prevent the changes of electrode impedance in CSF. This also contributes to minimizing the current spread from the electrode. Our stimulating electrode is 0.6 mm in diameter and is insulated with Epoxylite, except for 0.5 mm from the tip. These stimulation parameters provided us reliable data to precisely identify the nerve and to achieve better preservation rates. The facial nerve preservation rates had been reported to be 80%–100% in small or medium-sized tumors, and 20%–57% in large tumors [1, 3, 6]. Our results were 100% in small tumors, 90% in medium-sized tumors, and 75% in large tumors.

The amplitudes of EFMR in this area are sometimes small compared to those in the IAM. This may be due to the difference in the stimulated nerve fibers. Many fibers are stimulated in the IAM but only a few at the porus, because the amplitudes of EFMR are assumed to reflect the number of intact fibers. Over the pons, EFMR decreased in amplitude as the operation proceeded. This attenuation in amplitude indicated that the facial nerve fibers were being damaged as the dissection of the tumor from the nerve pro-

ceeded. This means that stimulation of the nerve over the pons was quite useful to check the extent of damage to the nerve during operation. The EFMR obtained immediately after the tumor removal predicted some functional prognosis of the nerve after operation. The mean amplitudes of these were 128.9 ± 122.1 with good and 234.5 ± 188.7 μV with excellent recovery of facial functions. We think that if the amplitudes were more than 100 μV of the precentage amplitudes were more than 30%, good or excellent facial functions would be excepted after surgery.

References

1. Bentivoglio P, Cheeseman AD, Symon L (1988) Surgical management of acoustic neurinomas during the last five years, part II: results for facial and cochlear nerve function. Surg Neurol 29 : 205 – 209
2. Delgado TE, Buchheit WA, Rosenholtz HR, Chrissian S (1980) Intraoperative monitoring of facial muscle evoked responses obtained by intracranial stimulation of the facial nerve: a more accurate technique for facial nerve dissection. Neurosurgery 4 : 418 – 421
3. Olivercrona H (1967) Acoustic tumor. J Neurosurg 26 : 6 – 13
4. Redhead J, Mugliston T (1985) Facial electroneuronography: action potential amplitude and latency studies in 50 normal subjects. J Laryngol Otol 99 : 369 – 372
5. Silverstein H, Smouha EE, Jones R (1988) Routine intraoperative facial nerve monitoring during otologic surgery. J Otol 9 : 269 – 275
6. Smith DL Gordon DS, Campbell R, Kerr AG (1982) The facial nerve in acoustic neuroma surgery. J Laryngol Otol 96 : 335 – 346
7. Yanagihara N, Kishomoto M (1972) Electrodiagnosis in facial palsy. Arch Otolaryngol 95 : 376 – 382
8. Yokoyama T, Ryu H, Uemura K, Miyamoto T, Sugiyama K, Ninchoji T, Nakajima S, Yamamoto T, Yamamoto S (1987) Monitoring of facial nerve with electroneuronography in surgery of acoustic tumor. Facial N Res Jpn 7 : 23 – 26
9. Yokoyama T, Uemura K, Ryu H (1991) Facial nerve monitoring by monopolar low constant current stimulation during acoustic neurinoma surgery. Surg Neurol 36 : 12 – 18

Eur Arch Otorhinolaryngology (1994) [Suppl]: S319–S320

FREE PAPERS AND POSTERS

T. Lenarz, A. Ernst, and P. Plinkert

Intraoperative Facial Nerve Monitoring in the Infratemporal Fossa Approach: Improved Preservation of Nerve Function

Introduction

The infratemporal fossa approach [1] provides an excellent exposure of the lateral skull base with safe handling of crucial anatomical structures. However, the necessary transposition of the facial nerve (anterior rerouting) caused a transient or permanent paresis in most cases due to surgical trauma and disrupted blood supply. Intraoperative monitoring (IOM) is one tool to assess the nerve function intraoperatively by recording the spontaneous as well as evoked electric activity of the facial muscles. The aim of this study was to evaluate the possible benefit of IOM for the postoperative functional outcome in the infratemporal fossa approach.

Methods

The infratemporal fossa appraoch type A was performed in 41 patients (34 glomus jugulare tumors type C and D, 7 neurinomas of the jugular foramen) between 1986 and 1991 by the same surgeon (T.L.). The patients were divided into two groups with comparable tumor locations and sizes: the monitored group (19 cases) and the unmonitored group (22 cases). Postoperative facial nerve function was evaluated according to the criteria of House and Brackmann [2]. Monitoring was performed with Nicolet Viking II equipment. The electromyograhic activity was recorded in two channels bipolarly with monopolar needle electrodes into the orbicularis oris and oculi muscles. The spontaneous activity and the mechanically or thermically elicited

activity were both evaluated for the occurrence of burst and train activity as signs of nerve irritation (burst) and nerve impairment (train). For electrical stimulation of the exposed nerve either a monopolar bendable electrode with a ball-shaped tip or a bipolar forceps electrode was used. Constant current rectangular biphasic pulses of 100 µs duration were delivered, with a current strength between 0.05 and 0.8 mA. The threshold current was estimated and followed during the operation.

Results

The mechanically or thermically elicited muscle activity obtained by drilling, direct surgical manipulation, or coagulation consisted of bursts and trains. The number of train events was correlated to the degree of the postoperative nerve paresis. When the intensity of train activity diminished and/or no bursts could be elicited, a postoperative total paresis (House and Brackmann grade V or VI) could be predicted. Due to these experiences the surgical technique was changed so as to avoid train activity. The main manipulations were traction and squeezing of the nerve or coagulation without sufficient irrigation and cooling. The threshold current increased in all patients, but significantly more in patients with a postoperative paresis (0.73 vs. 0.25 mA). The electrically evoked activity was especially useful for the identification of the nerve at the cerebellopontine angle and in large cases with erosion of the fallopian canal. Short- and long-term results showed an improved outcome for monitored patients versus unmonitored patients (Table 1). This held true for all grades of paresis.

Discussion

Transient or permanent facial nerve paresis is a common finding in patients who undergo an infratemporal fossa

T. Lenarz (✉)
Medizinische Hochschule Hannover, Department of Otolaryngology, Konstanty-Gutschow-Str. 8, 30625 Hannover, Germany

A. Ernst and P. Plinkert
Department of Otolaryngology, University of Tübingen

Table 1 Postoperative outcome/long-term results (1 year)

Facial nerve function (House and Brackmann)	Unmonitored	Monitored
I, II	49%	63%
III, IV	31%	22%
V, VI	26%	15%
Total	100%	100%

approach due to the required anterior rerouting procedure [4]. The loss of nerve function can be attributed to two factors, the surgical manipulation and the loss of blood supply. Whereas the impaired vascularization can hardly be avoided the surgical procedure might be a matter of modification. Intraoperative monitoring (IOM) may help to identify harmful surgical manipulations which lead to nerve impairment and identify the nerve in its course along the cerebellopontine angle and across or within the tumor.

The results of this comparative study show a benefit from IOM. A high number of train events and their decline during operation as well as a major increase of threshold current are signs of intraoperative nerve impairment. The increase in threshold is due to the impaired nerve sheaths. It can be related to a functional conduction block because the threshold peripheral to the site of manipulation stays in a normal range. The surgical procedure was modified to avoid train activity which occurred with traction or squeezing of the nerve or improper coagulation.

Short- as well as long-term results of facial nerve function exhibited a better functional outcome for monitored patients. Especially the rate of severe paresis could be reduced. Therefore, IOM should be used as an essential tool in the infratemporal fossa approach to improve facial nerve function. The same has been established also for other surgical procedures of the lateral skull base [3].

References

1. Fisch U (1977) Infratemporal fossa aproach for extensive tumors of the temporal bone and base of the skull. In: Silverstein H, Norell H (eds) Neurological surgery of the ear. Aesculapius, Birmingham/USA, p 34
2. House JW, Brackmann DE (1985) Facial nerve grading system. Otolaryngol Head Neck Surg 93 : 146–147
3. Lenarz T, Ernst A (1993) Intraoperative facial nerve monitoring in cerebello-pontine angle tumors. ORL (in press)
4. Lenarz T, Plinkert PK (1992) Glomustumoren des Felsenbeines – Operatives Konzept und Ergebnisse. Laryngol Rhinol Otol 71 : 149–157
5. Oldring D, Fisch U (1979) Glomus tumors of the temporal region: surgical therapy. Am J Otol 1 : 7–18

Eur Arch Otorhinolaryngology (1994) [Suppl]: S 321

ABSTRACTS

F.X. Glocker, M.R. Magistris, K.M. Rösler, and Ch.W. Hess

Electrical Stylomastoidal and Magnetic Transcranial Stimulation of the Facial Nerve in Bell's Palsy: Time Course of Electrophysiological Parameters

Facial nerve motor neurographies were performed at various time intervals after onset of Bell's palsy in 75 patients. Amplitudes and onset latencies of the compound muscle action potential (CMAP) of m. nasalis and/or mentalis were measured after electrical extracranial (fossa stylomastoidea; ElStim) and magnetic transcranial (intracranial; MagStim) stimulation of the facial nerve, and in some patients also after magnetic cortex stimulation. Onset latencies were on average slightly increased on the side of the palsy: MagStim 109.8% (SD 19.8), ElStim 107.2% (SD 15.2). The time course of CMAP amplitudes was characterized by an early and marked reduction after MagStim as compared to ElStim (in 68% of patients MagStim evoked no response). Mean amplitudes (as percentages of the healthy side) versus days of palsy were:

The reduction of amplitude after ElStim in Bell's palsy is generally believed to be due to axonal loss. The marked additional decrease of amplitude, or lack of response, after MagStim is a highly sensitive parameter in Bell's palsy: it is observed very early, does not parallel the severity of the weakness (often MagStim evokes no response while paresis is incomplete), and tends to persist, sometimes long after clinical recovery is achieved. This discrepancy between the clinical and electrophysiological time course was corroborated by the observation in some cases that cortex stimulation could evoke CMAPs, whereas MagStim could not. This suggests that, in Bell's palsy, the additional decrease of amplitude after MagStim is mostly related to a localized increased threshold of the facial nerve to MagStim, rather than to conduction block within the facial canal.

Days	0-4	5-14	15-42	43-182	183-730	>730
MagStim	28.1%	7.7%	14.3%	10.9%	48.9%	84.3%
(SD)	(42.0)	(17.0)	(27.4)	(17.9)	(36.0)	(27.5)
ElStim	84.6%	56.6%	51.8%	38.0%	67.9%	91.1%
(SD)	(30.0)	(27.5)	(32.3)	(34.9)	(31.6)	(29.8)

F.X. Glocker, M.R. Magistris, K.M. Rösler (✉), and Ch.W. Hess
Department of Neurology and Division of Clinical Neurophysiology,
Universities of Berne and Geneva, Switzerland

Facial Nerve Imaging

Eur Arch Otorhinolaryngology (1994) [Suppl]: S 325 – S 326

FREE PAPERS AND POSTERS

H. Tanaka, K. Murata, M. Ishikawa, and K. Tanaka

Gadolinium-DTPA-Enhanced MRI of the Facial Nerve

Introduction

Gadolinium(Gd)-DTPA-enhanced magnetic resonance images (MRI) of facial nerves in the temporal bone were evaluated to ascertain the relation between the duration of the disease and the sites of enhancement.

Subjects and Methods

The sujects consisted of 26 patients with peripheral facial nerve paralysis (11 with Bell's palsy, 8 with Hunt's syndrome, and 7 with traumatic paralysis) on whom MR imaging diagnoses were performed from March 1990 to March 1991. The MR imaging instrument used was a 0.5-Tesla Shimazu SMT-50. T1-weighted images were obtained by the spinecho method. Axial images and sagittal oblique images were obtained by the 3D-gradient echo method. MR imaging was performed before and after enhancement with Gd-DTPA, 0.1 mmol/kg. For each disease, the images were evaluated in relation to the duration of paralysis after the onset. The effect of facial nerve enhancement was judged as positive when a higher signal intensity was transmitted from the facial nerves in the axial images than from the cerebral parenchyma.

H. Tanaka (✉), K. Murata, M. Ishikawa, and K. Tanaka
Department of Otolaryngology, Kinki University School
of Medicine, 377-2 Ohnohigashi Osakasayama-shi, 589 Osaka,
Japan

Results

Relationship Between Duration of Disease and Sites of Facial Nerve Enhancement

The relationship between the duration of the disease and the sites of enhancement was investigated by dividing the times of MR imaging into three periodes: within 10 days after the onset, 11 – 30 days after the onset, and more than 31 days after the onset (Table 1). In MR imaging within 10 days after the onset, the geniculate ganglion and horizontal segment were enhanced very frequently. In MR imaging at 11 – 30 days after the onset, the horizontal and vertical segments were enhanced very frequently. In MR imaging at more than 31 days after the onset, the vertical segment was enhanced very frequently.

Presentation of MR Images

Magnetic resonance images in a 59-year-old woman with right Bell's palsy at 33 days after the onset are seen in Fig. 1. Routine topographic diagnosis by neurological method suggested local lesion above the stapedial muscle. Figure 1, upper left shows an image before enhancement and Fig. 1, lower left after enhancement. The facial nerves which had not been clearly visualized before enhancement were uniformly and distinctly visualized from the internal acoustic meatus to the horizontal segment after enhancement with Gd-DTPA. Figure 1, right shows MR images rephotographed in the same patient at 1 year after the onset when the paralysis was improved. Figure 1, upper right shows an image before enhancement and Fig. 1, lower right after enhancement. The enhancement effect which had been manifested previously could no longer be recognized in these images.

Table 1 Relationship between duration of disease and sites of facial nerve enhancement

Days from onset to MR scan	No. of cases	IAC segment	Labyrinthine segment	Geniculate ganglion	Horizontal segment	Vertical segment	Enhancement	
							+	-
~ 10 days	10	1	2	4	5	2	7	3
11 ~ 30 days	9	0	2	3	4	5	7	2
31 ~ days	7	1	2	2	2	5	6	1

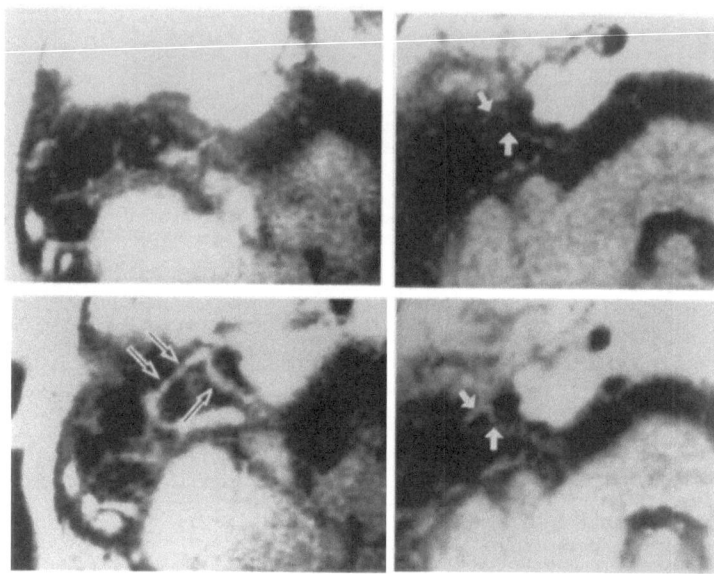

Fig. 1 Magnetic resonance imaging in a 59-year-old man with right Bell's palsy

Discussion

Yanagida et al. [1] performed enhancement MR imaging on 41 patients with facial nerve paralysis and discussed the relationship between the sites of enhancement an the time when MR imaging was performed. They obtained an enhancement effect at the segment of the internal acoustic meatus in many of their patients on whom MR imaging was performed very early after the onset and mainly at the vertical segment in patients on whom MR imaging was performed after a considerable lapse of time after the onset. In the MR imaging of our patients on whom MR imaging was performed within 10 days after the onset, the horizontal segment and the segment of the geniculate ganglion were clear very frequently, while the internal acoustic meatus was enhanced in ony one patient. Both reports suggest that sites of enhancement are proximal in the early days after onset and distal in the late days after onset. In a review of earlier reported histopathological characteristics of the temporal bones of patients with Bell's palsy Yanagihara [2] described that the facial nerves were more strongly degenerated at the distal segment than at the segment of the geniculate ganglion in all cases examined. Further investigation is necessary to learn the time course of the appearance and site of enhancement effect and to thereby determine whether the change in the site of appearance of the enhancement effect may reflect, in some form or other, the histological change of the facial nerves.

References

1. Yanagida M et al. (1990) Depicting of affeced facial nerve with Gd-DTPA (Jpn). Facial N Res 10:123–128
2. Yanagihara N (1986) Intratemporal facial nerve paralysis: pathophysiology and treatment (Jpn). Department of Otolaryngology, Ehime University School of Medicine, Ehime, Japan

Eur Arch Otorhinolaryngology (1994) [Suppl]: S327 – S329

M. Engström, L. Jonsson, K.-Å. Thuomas, A. Lilja, and M. Bergström

Gadolinium-Enhanced MRI and Positron Emission Tomography in Bell's palsy: A Preliminary Report

Introduction

An inflammatory edema with secondary ischemia of the facial nerve may be the cause of Bell's palsy [1, 5]. This may accord with the transient facial nerve enhancement on gadolinium-enhanced magnetic resonance imaging (GadMRI) that we recently have reported [4]. In this previous study [4] we used carbohydrate and gadolinium in an attempt to improve the GadMRI technique. The aim of the present preliminary study was to see if readministration of gadolinium may give additional information when examining patients with Bell's palsy on high-Tesla MR equipment. Furthermore, we report our limited experience from three investigations using positron emission tomography (PET), a unique imaging technique which allows in vivo measurements of the anatomical distribution and rates of specific biochemical reactions [9].

Patients and Methods

Ten patients with Bell's palsy, aged 21 – 60 years, have been examined so far (February 1991 to April 1992). The MRI and PET examinations were performed within 10 days after the onset of the palsy. Follow-up MRI has so far been performed in five patients (2 – 5 months after the onset). MRI (nine patients) was performed on a 1.5-T unit (Signa, General Electric) using spin echo (SE) and gradient echo (GRE) sequences. T1-weighted images were

M. Engström (✉), L. Jonsson
Departments of Oto-Rhino-Laryngology and Head & Neck Surgery
Uppsala University, 75185 Uppsala, Sweden

K.-Å. Thuomas
Diagnostic Radiology

A. Lilja and M. Bergström
PET-Centre, Uppsala University, Sweden

obtained with fat suppression, 500/12/4 (TR/TE/excitations), contiguous 2-mm slice thickness 20-cm field of view, and 256×192 acquisition matrix as previously described [4]. After pre-contrast MRI, gadolinium (0.2 ml GdDTPA/kg body weight) was administered intravenously and images were immediately obtained in the axial and coronal planes. A second dose of gadolinium was given after 30 min (four patients) or 2 h (five patients) and new images were obtained.

Positron emission tomography (three investigations) was performed on an 8-ring camera (2048B, GEMS, Uppsala, Sweden) producing 15 slices simultaneously of approximately 6 mm thickness with an in-plane resolution of about 5 mm. For estimation of the glucose metabolism, approximately 200 MBq ^{18}F-fluoro-2-deoxy-D-gluose (FDG) was administered intravenously in two patients at the start of continuous scanning during a period of 50 min. Images obtained 30 – 50 min postinjection were used for visual estimation of FDG uptake. For further evaluation of inflammatory activity, ^{11}C-D-Deprenyl was used in one patient as a lysosomotrophic marker. Basically, a similar scanning and sampling technique was used as for FDG.

Results

Pre-contrast T1-weighted images of the facial nerve were considered to be normal in the nine patients (both for the "acute" and the follow-up MRIs). After the first administration of gadolinium, seven of the nine patients demonstrated ipsilateral facial nerve enhancement: five in the meatal (Fig. 1), one in the labyrinthine, and one in both the labyrinthine and the meatal segments. A significant change of the signal pattern after the readministration of gadolinium (after 30 min or 2h) was not demonstrated. In the five patients who had follow-up scan, enhancement was no longer present 2 – 5 months after the onset of the palsy. Contralateral facial nerve enhancement was not demon-

S328

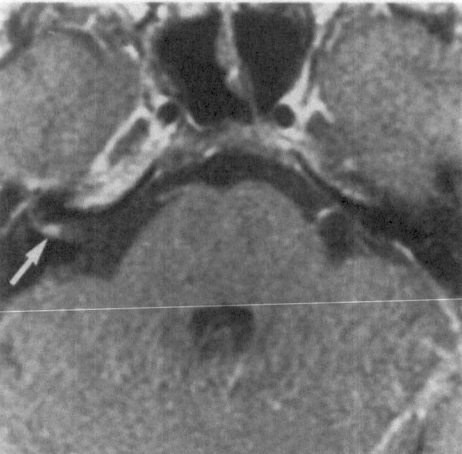

Fig. 1 A woman aged 34 years with right-sided Bell's palsy. T1-weighted axial magnetic resonance imaging with gadolinium on day 13 shows ipsilateral facial nerve enhancement in the meatal portion (*arrow*)

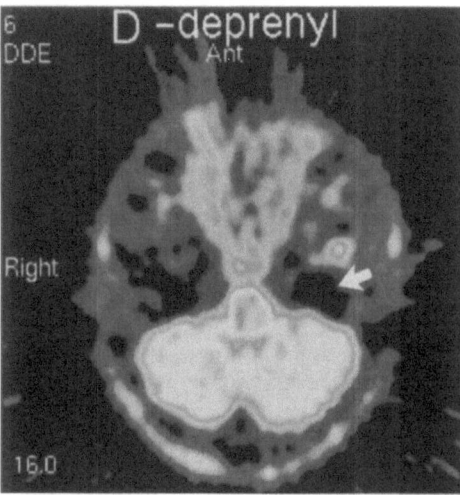

Fig. 2 Positron emission tomography of the brain stem and the temporal bone (*arrowed*) using ^{11}C-D-Deprenyl in a 25-year-old male 9 days after the onset of complete left-sided Bell's palsy. A difference in radioactivity between the affected and nonaffected side was not demonstrated

strated. The brain stem was visualized on PET but a side difference was not present. A difference in glucose utilization (FDG) of the temporal bones, in the region of the facial nerve, between the paretic and nonparetic side was not demonstrated (Fig. 2). Similar to this finding, we were unable to demonstrate a difference between the two sides when ^{11}C-D-Deprenyl was used.

Discussion

In the present preliminary report, ipsilateral facial nerve enhancement was demonstrated on GadMRI in the early stage of Bell's palsy in seven of nine patients. This accords with the results of previous workers [3, 4, 7, 8, 10, 12]. Accumulation of gadolinium indicates an inflammatory process [3] and the present findings in addition to our previous MRI results [4, 11] support the view that a transient viral inflammatory process [2, 6] may be the cause of the nerve injury in Bell's palsy. High-Tesla (1.5 T) equipment with readministration of gadolinium was used in the present study. Our preliminary results indicate that, when examining patients with Bell's palsy on this type of MR unit, it is sufficient to use a single dose of the contrast agent. FDG is a marker of tissue glucose metabolism and ^{11}C-Deprenyl is an indicator of an inflammatory reaction (Bergström and coworkers, personal communication). The brain stem was equally visualized on both sides and a difference in the radioactivity between the affected and nonaffected temporal bone was not demonstrated. Hence, we were unable to demonstrate a specific biochemical reaction on PET. The in-plane resolution of the PET method used was about 5 mm. Further improvements of the technique and earlier investigation during the course of the disease (when an inflammatory response might be more predominant) will hopefully help to find evidence of specific metabolic changes of the facial nerve in Bell's palsy.

Acknowledgements This study was supported by grant 7503 (L.J.) from the Swedish Medical Research Council, Stockholm.

References

1. Adour KK, Byl FM, Hilsinger RL Jr, Kahn ZM, Sheldon MI (1978) The true nature of Bell's palsy: analysis of 1,000 consecutive patients. Laryngoscope 88 : 787–801
2. Aviel A, Ostfeld E, Burstein R, Marshak G, Bentwich Z (1983) Peripheral blood T and B lymphocyte subpopulations in Bell's palsy. Ann Otol Rhinol Laryngol 92 : 187–191
3. Daniels DL, Czervionke LF, Millen SJ, Haberkamp TJ, Meyer GA, Hendrix LE, Leighton PM, Williams AL, Haughton VM (1989) MR imaging of facial nerve enhancement in Bell's palsy or after temporal bone surgery. Radiology 171 : 807–809
4. Engström M, Thuomas K-Å, Naeser P, Stålberg E, Jonsson L (1993) Facial nerve enhancement in Bell's palsy demonstrated by different gadolinium-enhanced MRI techniques. Arch Otolaryngol Head Neck Surg 119 : 221–225

5. Fisch U, Esslen E (1972) Total intratemporal exposure of the facial nerve. Arch Otolaryngol 95 : 335 – 341
6. Jonsson L, Sjöberg O, Thomander L (1988) Depression of T cells in Bell's palsy. Ann Otol Rhinol Laryngol 97 : 138 – 141
7. Korzec K, Sobol SM, Kubal W, Mester SJ, Winzelberg G, May M (1991) Gadolinium-enhaned magnetic resonance imaging of the facial nerve in herpes zoster oticus and Bell's palsy: clinical implications. Am J Otol 12 : 163 – 168
8. Murphy TP, Teller DC (1991) Magnetic resonance imaging of the facial nerve during Bell's palsy. Otolaryngol Head Neck Surg 105 : 667 – 674
9. Phelps ME, Mazziotta JC (1985) Positron emission tomography: human brain function and biohemistry. Science 228 : 799 – 809
10. Schwaber MK, Larson TC, Zealer DL, Creasy J (1990) Gadolinium-enhanced MRI in Bell's palsy. Laryngoscope 100 : 1264 – 1269
11. Stenquist M, Engström M, Thuomas K-Å, Jonsson L (1993) Inflammatory paranasal sinus disease in Bell's palsy demonstrated by MRI. Am J Otol 14 : 295 – 300
12. Tien R, Dillon WP, Jackler RK (1990) Contrast-enhanced MR imaging of the facial nerve in 11 patients with Bell's palsy. AJNR 11 :(AJR 155) : 735 – 741

Eur Arch Otorhinolaryngology (1994) [Suppl]: S 330 – S 331

L. Jonsson, M. Engström, K.-Å. Thuomas, and E. Stålberg

Correlation Between Gadolinium-Enhanced MRI and Neurophysiology in Bell's Palsy: A Preliminary Study

Introduction

Fifty percent of patients with clinically complete Bell's palsy run the risk of suffering from sequelae, including persisting muscle weakness and dyskinesia (abnormal facial muscle movements). The pathophysiological event that causes facial dyskinesia and the location of the primary nerve injury in Bell's palsy is unknown. It has been speculated that central (facial nucleus) hyperexcitability, ephaptic transmission along the facial nerve, or defect reinnervation (to false muscle) of the nerve fibers may be responsible for facial dyskinesias [2]. In the present study, gadolinium-enhanced MRI (GadMRI) and refined neurophysiological methods were used in an attempt to locate the primary nerve injury and get more information on the pathogenesis of facial dyskinesias in Bell's palsy.

Patients and Methods

GadMRI was performed in 28 patients with complete Bell's palsy (median, 42 years) using a 0.5-T (Siemens Magnetom) or 1.5-T (Signa, GE) MRI unit (13 patients) as previously described [1]. After pre-contrast MRI, gadolinium (0.2 ml GadDTPA/kg body weight) was administered intravenously and T1-weighted images were immediately obtained in the axial and/or coronal planes. GadMRI was performed within 3 weeks after the onset of palsy and so far 22 patients have had a follow-up MRI after 2 – 6 months.

L. Jonsson (✉) and M. Engström
Departments of Oto-Rhino-Laryngology and Head & Neck Surgery
Uppsala University, 75185 Uppsala, Sweden

K.-Å. Thuomas
Diagnostic Radiology

E. Stålberg
Clinical Neurophysiology, Uppsala University, Sweden

Fifteen patients (median, 43 years) who were randomly chosen from a group of 63 patients, were in addition to electroneurography and blink reflex studies examined for the presence of facial synkinesias usually at 1, 2–3, and 10–12 weeks after the onset of the palsy. The presence of synkinetic facial movements was recorded clinically and electrophysiologically. Synkinesia was considered present if there were contractions in other facial muscles than the orbicularis oris muscle when blinking, if the R1 of the blink reflex could be recorded outside the orbicularis oculi muscle (extended blink reflex) or if electrical stimulation of zygomatic or mental nerves evoked muscle responses in the orbicularis oris or orbicularis oculi muscle, respectively. In order to find signs of abnormal excitablity along the facial nerve or in the facial nucleus, peripheral branches of the facial nerve were stimulated by means of monopolar electrodes, either the upper and lower zygomatic nerve or the upper zygomatic and mental nerve branches. Needle EMG recordings were performed from the orbicularis oculi and orbicularis oris muscles. Latencies to the responses were measured.

Results

T1-weighted GadMRI within 3 weeks after the onset of palsy demonstrated ipsilateral facial nerve enhancement, most consistently in the meatal and labyrinthine portions, in 17 of the 28 patients (cf. Fig. 1 in the paper by Engström et al. in the present supplement). At follow-up examination after 2–6 months, the enhancement had disappeared in 14 of the 17 positive patients and persisted in 2 of the patients (1 positive patient has not been followed-up). Contralateral enhancement was found in one patient. The GadMRI findings were not significantly correlated to the severity and outcome of the palsy.

Neurophysiologically, the vast majority of the 15 selected patients suffered from a moderate to severe axonal degeneration (as judged from electroneurography). After more than 30 days, all except for 2 patients showed electrophysiological signs of synkinesia. In one examination performed at day 57, we were unable to find abnormalties although such abnormalities were present both before (day 36) and after (day 115) this examination. In the other case with complete palsy, but only neurophysiological signs of neurapraxia, abnormalities were seen at day 10 (complete palsy) but not at day 120 (no palsy). On the other hand, none of the patients who were examined before day 13 showed signs of hyperexcitability, except for the one mentioned above. In some cases, where the extended blink reflex was obtained, the nerve branch stimulation demonstrated normal findings. The reverse was not demonstrated. In those patients in whom the neurophysiological recordings were positive, the latency time from stimulus to response in a remote muscle was 4 – 8 ms. Only in one case did we obtain a latency of 38 ms, but it cannot be excluded that this was a recorded blink reflex.

Discussion

The transient facial nerve enhancement on T1-weighted GadMRI on the affected side may indicate that an inflammatory reaction with edema is part of the nerve injury in Bell's palsy. Our GadMRI findings accord with those recently reported [4].

The results of the present preliminary study suggest that ephaptic transmission between abnormal axons, a possible cause of hemifacial spasm [3], may be responsible for dyskinesias in Bell's palsy. It is abnormal to obtain responses in muscles others than those innervated by the stimulated nerve branch. The latency to the response carries information about the site where the traveling volley turns from an antidromic to an orthodromic direction. Our results with latencies of 4 – 8 ms should be compared with a latency of 2 – 3 ms from the stylomastoid foramen to the nasalis muscle and studies of so-called F-responses (recurrent responses from the facial nucleus) and cortical stimulation, which show a conduction time of about 11 ms from the stylomastoid foramen to the facial nucleus. Hence, in most cases, the hyperexcitable site seems to be located along the facial nerve proximal to the foramen.

Our findings may be of importance in the discussion regarding the site for the lesion in Bell's palsy. It seems reasonable to assume that the primary site for the lesion and the subsequent hyperexcitable region which gives ephaptic cross talk, should be the same or at least closely related. The results of the GadMRI indicate that the lesion in Bell's palsy is located in the meatal/labyrinthine portions of the facial nerve, a finding which may be compatible with the neurophysiological results.

Acknowledgements This study was supported by grants 135 (E. S.) and 7503 (L. J.) from the Swedish Medical Research Council, Stockholm, and from the Swedish Society of Medicine, Stockholm.

References

1. Engström M, Thuomas K-Å, Naeser P, Stålberg E, Jonsson L (1993) Facial nerve enhancement in Bell's palsy demonstrated by different gadolinium-enhanced MRI techniques Arch Otolaryngol Head Neck Surg 119:221–225
2. Jankovic J (1988) Cranial-cervical dyskinesias. An overview. In: Jankovic J, Tolosa E (eds) Facial dyskinesias. Raven, New York, pp 1–13 (Advances in neurology, vol 49)
3. Kamp Nielsen V (1985) Electrophysiology of the facial nerve in hemifacial spasm: ectopic/ephaptic excitation. Muscle Nerve 8:545–555
4. Schwaber MK, Larson TC, Zealar DL, Creasy J (1990) Gadolinium-enhanced MRI in Bell's palsy. Laryngoscope 100: 1264–1269

Eur Arch Otorhinolaryngology (1994) [Suppl]: S 332 – S 335

Y. Matsumoto, N. Yanagihara, M. Sadamoto, and K. Sadamoto

Gadolinium-DTPA-Enhanced MRI in Facial Palsy

Introduction

We evaluated the specificity of facial nerve enhancement on magnetic resonance imaging (MRI) using contrast agent gadolinium-DTPA (Gd-DTPA) for the diagnosis of facial nerve lesions.

Materials and Methods

Magnetic resonance imaging was performed 124 times in 116 cases with facial palsy from February 1990 (Table 1). Ninety-seven cases were Bell's palsy. 14 were Hunt's syndrome, 4 were traumatic, and 1 was a central nervous system lesion. Three cases of recurrent palsy and two of alternative palsy were involved in Bell's palsy. MRI was performed with a 0.5-T superconductive system (Hitachi G-50) and a head coil. Axial (oblique), coronal, and (oblique) sagittal T1-weighted spin echo images were obtained before and after Gd-DTPA administration. Technical details were repetition times of 500 ms, echo times of 25 – 33 ms, 2 (or 4) excitations, 256×256 matrix, 22 – 24 cm field of view, and 5-mm-thick gapless sections. Gd-DTPA was administered by intravenous injection at a dose of 0.1 mmol/kg. If there was a clear difference in the affected facial nerve between before and after Gd-DTPA administration or between the affected facial nerve and the contralateral facial nerve after Gd-DTPA aministration in more than two images in different directions, it was judged as positive enhancement.

Y. Matsumoto (✉) and N. Yanagihara
Department of Otolaryngology, Ehime University School of Medicine, Shigenobu-cho, Onsen-gun, Ehime, 791-02 Japan

M. Sadamoto
Department of Otolaryngology, Sadamoto Hospital

K. Sadamoto
Department of Neurosurgery, Sadamoto Hospital

Table 1 Cause of facial paralysis (February 1990 – March 1992)

	Patients	Times MRI performed
Bell's palsy	97	103
Hunt's syndrome	14	16
Traumatic	4	4
CNS	1	1
	116 cases	124 ex.

CNS, central nervous system.

Four items were evaluated: (1) MRI specificity in different types of facial palsy; (2) correlation between the enhancement pattern and the timing of MRI study; (3) the interval change of repetitive MRI in the same case; and (4) correlation between the enhanced pattern and the presence of acoustically evoked stapedius reflex.

Results

1. An enhancement was seen in various segments of the affected-side intratemporal facial nerve in Bell's palsy and Hunt's syndrome (Table 2). An enhancement was most frequently observed at the geniculate ganglion (Figs. 1, 2). The total enhancement incidence at the geniculate ganglion was 82% in Bell's palsy and 94% in Hunt's syndrome. In Hunt's syndrome, the incidence

Table 2 Gadolinium-enhanced segment of facial nerve in 124 MRI studies of 116 cases

	IAC	Labyrin-thine	Geni-culate	Tym-panic	Mastoid
Bell's palsy	47%	34%	82%	68%	61%
Hunt's syndrome	56%	63%	94%	87%	75%
Traumatic	0%	0%	0%	0%	25%
CNS	0%	0%	0%	0%	0%

IAC, internal auditory canal.

Table 3 Time-related Gd-enhanced MRI characteristics in Bell's palsy and Hunt's syndrome. Intervals from onset of palsy are shown in the first column

		IAC	Labyrinthine	Geniculate	Tympanic	Mastoid
Bell's palsy						
< 10 days	(n = 36)	50%	10%	81%	61%	53%
< 1 mos.	(n = 51)	57%	45%	88%	76%	69%
< 3 mos.	(n = 9)	22%	22%	89%	78%	78%
> 3 mos.	(n = 7)	0%	0%	43%	29%	29%
Hunt's syndrome						
< 10 days	(n = 6)	83%	67%	100%	83%	67%
< 1 mos.	(n = 2)	50%	50%	100%	100%	100%
< 3 mos.	(n = 7)	43%	71%	100%	100%	100%
> 3 mos.	(n = 1)	0%	0%	0%	0%	0%

IAC, internal auditory canal.

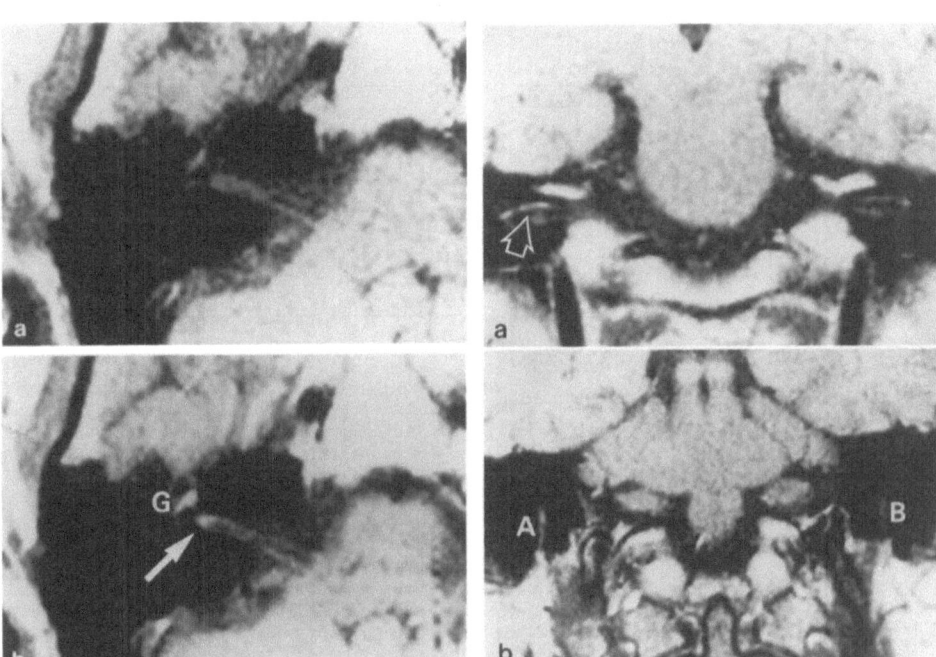

Fig. 1a, b Right-sided Bell's palsy. Case #73, 39-year-old female. MRI was performed 16 days after onset. **a** Axial plain T1-weighted (TR500/TE26) MRI of the right facial nerve. **b** Axial Gd-enhanced T1-weighted MRI. Enhancement of the nerve was demonstrated at the meatal foramen (*arrow*), labyrinthine, geniculate ganglion (*G*), and proximal horizontal segment

Fig. 2a, b Right-sided Bell's palsy. Case #74. 31-year-old male. MR was performed 20 days after onset. **a** Coronal Gd-enhanced T1-weighted (TR500/TE32) MRI. Enhancement of affected internal auditory canal segment (*large arrow*) and geniculate ganglion of right facial nerve was demonstrated. No enhancement of unaffected nerve (*small arrow*) was visualized. **b** Enhancement of affected mastoid portion of the nerve (*A*) was demonstrated as well. No enhancement of unaffected nerve (*B*) was visualized

Table 4 Intervals of repetitive Gd-enhanced MRI in eight patients. Intervals from onset of palsy are given in the first column

		IAC	Labyrinthine	Geniculate	Tympanic	Mastoid
Bell's palsy						
Case #23	21 days	−	−	+	+	+
	45 days	−	−	+	+	+
#60	5 days	+	+	+	+	−
	73 days	−	−	+	+	+
#72	20 days	+	−	+	+	+
	57 days	−	−	+	−	−
#80	12 days	+	−	+	+	+
	33 days	+	−	+	+	+
#82	21 days	+	+	+	−	−
	39 days	+	+	+	+	+
#96	13 days	+	+	+	+	+
	27 days	−	−	+	+	+
Hunt's syndrome						
Case #5	5 days	−	−	+	−	−
	56 days	−	−	+	+	−
#12	9 days	+	+	+	+	+
	70 days	+	+	+	+	+

IAC, internal auditory canal.

Tab. 5 Gadolinium enhancement at the geniculate ganglion and stapedius reflex

	Geniculate ganglion
Bell's palsy	
Rx. (−) = 38 cases	Gd-enhancement (+) = 87%
Rx. (+) = 22	Gd-enhancement (+)= 77%
Hunt's syndrome	
Rx. (−) = 8	Gd-enhancement (+) = 100%
Rx. (+) = 0	

of enhancement in every segment was always more than in Bell's palsy. An enhancement was only seen at the mastoid segment in one of four cases of traumatic facial palsy. There was no enhancement in a case with palsy of a central nervous system lesion. A clear enhancement of the contralateral facial nerve was not observed in the cases evaluated in this paper.

2. The timings of the MRI studies are shown in Table 3. The main enhancement was always seen at the geniculate ganglion in both Bell's palsy and Hunt's syndrome. There was no clear correlation between the enhanced area and timing of the MRI within 3 months of the onset.

3. Repetitive MRI study was carried out in eight cases (Bell's palsy, six, Hunt's syndrome, two) at various intervals. The result was that the main enhancement was seen at the geniculate ganglion all the time in these cases. A minimal interval change was seen in the other segments (Table 4).

4. The stapedius reflex was measured in 60 cases of Bell's palsy and 8 cases of Hunt's syndrome (Table 5). And it was preserved in 22 cases (36.7%) of Bell's palsy.

Among them, 77% had an enhancement at the geniculate ganglion. There was no correlation between the enhancement pattern and the presence of stapedius reflex.

Discussion

The etiology of Bell's palsy is still unknown. Some investigators suggest that Bell's palsy is a self-limited geniculate ganglionitis caused by herpes simplex virus [6]. On the other hand, some investigators suggest that the cause of Bell's palsy is multiple and may be vascular or degenerative [1, 3]. Gd-DTPA is distributed in the extracellular spaces. The influence of T1 relaxation time is most pronounced in regions with increased extracellular fluid, including areas of inflammation, edema, or tumors [4]. The mechanism of enhancement of the facial nerve in Bell's palsy after Gd-DTPA administration is uncertain but may relate to either hypervascularity of the perineural structures of the nerve or actual disruption of the blood-nerve barrier [5].

The site of the main lesion in Bell's palsy is also controversial. Our results using Gd-DTPA-enhanced MRI showed that the most frequent enhanced area was at the geniculate ganglion despite preservation of the stapedius reflex, which was used for topodiagnosis of infrastapedial lesions. Hunt's syndrome is a geniculate ganglionitis caused by reactivated varicella-zoster virus. Surgical observations of Fisch et al. [2] suggest that the greatest amount of inflammation in Bell's palsy and Hunt's syndrome is at the "physiologic bottleneck" created by the constricting meatus of the fallopian canal. A similar enhancement pattern was obtained in both Bell's palsy and Hunt's syndrome in this study. Our results are compatible with the bottleneck entrapment theory.

It is controversial whether there is an enhancement in the contralateral facial nerve or not. Tien et al. [6] reported that there was moderate enhancement in some cases. Millen et al. [4] reported that no enhancement was noted in normal temporal bone strutures such as the seventh and eighth cranial nerves. In our cases, a clear enhancement was not obtained in the clinically normal contralateral facial nerve. The image in every direction should be evaluated very carefully if there is a case which is difficult to judge. Further study is needed in this regard.

References

1. Daniels DL, Czervionke LF, Millen SJ, Haberkamp TJ, Meyer GA, Hendrix LE, Mark LP, Williams AL, Haughton VM (1989) MR imaging of facial nerve enhancement in Bell's palsy or after temporal bone surgery. Radiology 171 : 807 – 809
2. Fisch U, Felix H (1983) On the pathogenesis of Bell's palsy. Acta Otolaryngol 95 : 532 – 538
3. May M (1986) The facial nerve. Thieme, New York, p 370
4. Millen SJ, Daniels DL, Meyer GA (1989) Gadolinium-enhanced magnetic resonance imaging in temporal bone lesions. Laryngoscope 99 : 257 – 260
5. Osumi A, Tien RD (1990) MR findings in a patient with Ramsay-Hunt syndrome. J Comput Assist Tomogr 14 : 991 – 993
6. Tien R, Dillon WP, Jackler RK (1990) Contrast-enhanced MR imaging of the facial nerve in 11 patients with Bell's palsy. AJR 155 : 573 – 579

Eur Arch Otorhinolaryngology (1994) [Suppl] : S 336

FREE PAPERS AND POSTERS

P. Brändle, S. Schefer, W. Wichmann, V. Gallati, D. Huber-Gut, and U. Fisch

Correlation of MRI, Clinical, and Electroneuronographic Findings in the Natural Course of Acute Facial Nerve Palsies

Seven patients (six with Bell's palsy, one with herpes zoster oticus) were examined over a period of 3 months by repeated MRI (surface coil, interleaved overlapping technique), electroneurography (ENoG), and clinical observation. Ten reference MRIs of normal persons showed mild enhancement of gadolinium-DTPA from the distal labyrinthine segment of the facial nerve to the stylomastoid foramen. The proximal labyrinthine and meatal segments showed no enhancement. In patients with facial palsy the distal segments of the facial nerve showed a nonquantifiable enhancement with no correlation to the etiology or degree of the palsy. In the proximal segments of all patients with facial palsy, there was a marked enhancement of the facial nerve in the meatal fundus. The meatal enhancement was limited to the superior compartment in Bell's palsy and extended also to the inferior compartment in the herpetic involvement. There was no correlation between intensity and extent of enhancement and the electrical and clinical degree of facial palsy over the whole observation time of 3 months, during which a decrease of enhancement could be seen only in one case. The observed localization of facial nerve enhancement in acute facial palsy is in good agreement with the previous surgical findings of Fisch and Esslen [1].

Reference

1. Fisch U, Esslen E (1972) Total intratemporal exposure of the facial nerve. Arch Otolaryngol 95 : 335–341

P. Brändle (✉), V. Galleti, D. Huber-Gut and U. Fischer
Department of Otorhinolaryngology, Head- and Neck Surgery,
University Hospital, Rämistr. 100, 8091 Zürich, Switzerland

S. Schefer and W. Wichmann
Department of Neuroradiology, Head- and Neck Surgery,
University Hospital, Zürich, Switzerland

Eur Arch Otorhinolaryngology (1994) [Suppl]: S 337 – S 342

R. J. Wiet, S. A Harvey, C. Z. Jin, and G. Dobben

Hemifacial Spasm: Evaluation and Management Options

Vascular loop compression syndrome of the facial nerve is well documented as a cause of hemifacial spasm (HFS). These unilateral synchronous contractions of facial musculature are a cause of cosmetic defomity, social embarrassment and often mild facial weakness in longstanding cases. However, other documented causes of HFS include tumor infiltration, aneurysms, primary congenital cholesteatoma, herpes zoster oticus and primary facial nerve neuromas. Therefore, a knowledgeable diagnostic evaluation is necessary to avoid pitfalls of improper management. Advances in imaging techniques that aid in uncovering the etiology of HFS are reviewed. We now combine three modalities – computed tomography (CT), magnetic resonance imaging (MRI) and magnetic resonance angiography (MRA) – to avoid pitfalls in the management of this uncommon disabling condition. We also present 11 cases of hemifacial spasm; five patients did not have vascular loop compression as the underlying cause for their spasm.

Introduction

Vascular loop compression of the facial nerve at the cerebellopontine angle (CPA) causing HFS has been well documented [1 – 3]. However, misdiagnosis of the precise etiology of HFS has caused the authors to rephrase Cawthorne's words, "All that spasms is not vascular loop." Therefore, careful workup of the cause of the spasm and effective screening techniques are required. Surgical management is considered the mainstay of treatment as medical therapy in general is often ineffective. Muscle relaxants, sedatives, and anticonvulsants are only occasinally beneficial. Phenol injection into peripheral branches may be temporarily beneficial, but recurrence of spasm is common within several months [4]. Botulinum toxin injections have also been used, but this is most effective for the tonic contractions and has less effect on the clonic spasms [5].

R. Wiet
Professor of Clinical Otolaryngolog, Director of Otology and Neuro-
tologic-Skull Base Surgery Fellowship, Northwestern University
Medical School, Chicago, Illinois, USA

S. A. Harvey
Fellow in Otology and Neurotologic-Skull Base Surgery, Northwestern University Medical School, Chicago, Illinois, USA

C. Z. Jin
Associate Profeesor of Otolaryngology, Tianjin Medical School,
Tianjin, China

G. Dobben
Professor of Radiology, University of Illinois, Chicago, Illinois, USA

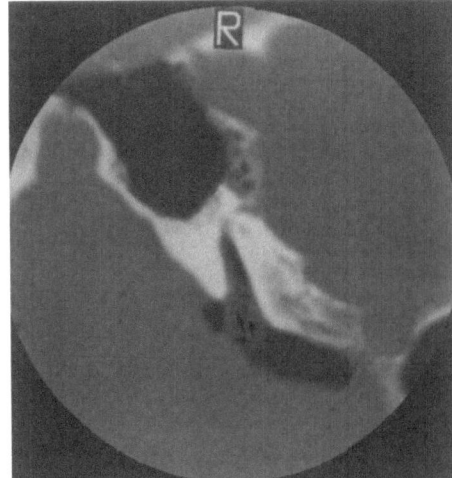

Fig. 1 Air-contrast CT scan of right temporal bone demonstrating the relationship of the VII – VIII nerve complex to surrounding vasculature (*arrows*)

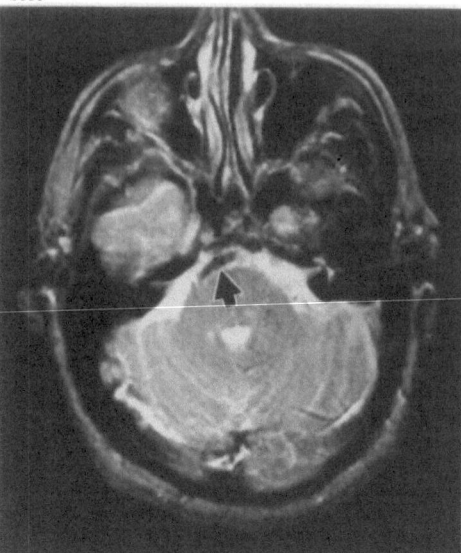

Fig. 2 Axial MRI of 80-year-old male who underwent selective peripheral facial neurolysis. Tortuosity of basilar artery can be seen (*arrow*)

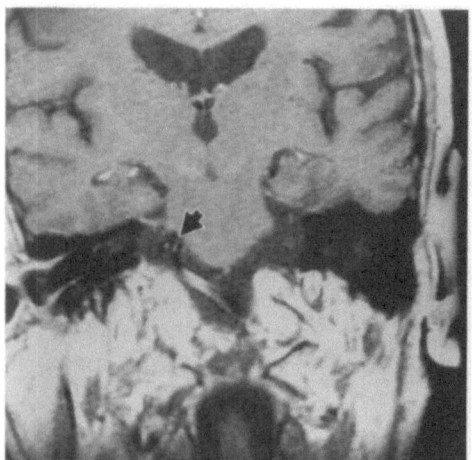

Fig. 3 Coronal MRI of same patient as in Fig. 2. Tortuosity of basilar artery seen near exit of facial nerve from brainstem (*arrow*)

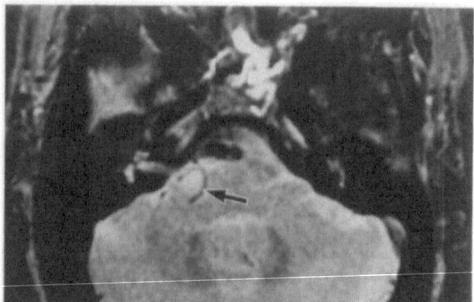

Fig. 4 Axial MRI demonstrating vascular loop near right CPA (*arrow*)

In general, when a patient presents with HFS the imaging modality of choice is MRI of the CPA, temporal bone, and parotid gland to search for the underlying cause. If the study is completely negative and suspicion for vascular compression is high, thin-section CT of the temporal bones is ordered with air contrast (CT pneumoencephalography). The CT will rule out intratemporal pathology such as cholestatoma, osteopetrsis, etc., that may lead to HFS. Air contrast allows for delineation of nerve/vessel relationships within the CPA (Fig. 1). Our experience, and confirmed by others, shows that vascular loop compression leading to HFS occurs in the root entry zone (REZ) of the nerve located just distal to its exit from the brainstem. Only recently, has MRI been employed to demonstrate cerebrovascular ectasia (Figs. 2–4).

Materials and Methods

Data from 11 patients seen over the past 7 years (1985–1991) were retrospetively reviewed. Each patient presented with a chief complaint of HFS; extensive workup included medical history, physical examination, and neurootological evaluation. A CT scan with or without pneumocisternography, MRI, and/or MRA is routine. Conventional MR parameters such as TR, FOV, NEX, and flip angle play important roles. In addition, time of flight (TOF) and phase contrast (PC) may be manipulated to formulate appropriate images. Three-dimensinal (3) TOF has the advantage of improved resolution and detail. One disadvantage of MRI or MRA is that neither study will demonstrate in detail both nervous and vascular structures (MRI delineates nervous tissue best; MRA demonstrates only vascular structures), and thus the relationship between these two can be difficult to assess. Air-contrast CT will better define this relationship. All of the patients underwent surgical treatment. General characteristics of the 11

Table 1 General characteristics of HFS due to vascular loop compression in six patients

No.	Age/sex	Presentation	Symptom Duration	Surgery	Surgical findings
1	34/M	R HFS	< 1 yr	Retrolabyrinthine microvascular decompression	Vertebral artery compression at REZ
2	62/M	R HFS	3½ yrs	Retrolabyrinthine microvascular decompression	AICA loop compression at REZ
3	51/M	L HFS	12 yrs	Retrolabyrinthine microvascular decompression	AICA loop compression at REZ
4	80/M	R HFS	4 yrs	Facial nerve neurolysis (extratemporal)	MRA demonstrated basilar artery ectatic vessels at brainstem
5	46/F	L HFS	5 yrs	Retrolabyrinthine microvascular decompression	AICA loop compression at REZ
6	52/F	L HFS	9 yrs	Retrolabyrinthine microvascular decompression	AICA loop compression at REZ

Table 2 General characteristics of HFS without vascular loop compression in five patients

No.	Age/sex	Presentation	Symptom Duration	Surgery	Surgical findings
1	34/F	R HFS	1 yr	Middle cranial fossa approach	5×3-mm facial nerve neuroma in IAC
2	24/M	L HFS and progressive paresis	4 yrs	Transmastoid and middle cranial fossa approach	1×1.5-cm cholesteatoma at geniculate ganglion
3	78/F	L HFS	2 yrs	Translabyrinthine approach	2.5×3.0-cm acoustic neuroma in IAC and CPA
4	54/M	R HFS	8 yrs	Total parotidectomy facial nerve resection, neck dissection	3-mm lesion at stylomastoid foramen involving facial nerve
5	72/F	R HFS then slow, progressive paresis	2 yrs	Total parotidectomy, facial nerve resection with interposition graft, neck dissection. Postoperative radiation	1.0-cm lesion at stylomastoid foramen involving facial nerve

Cases 2 and 3 submitted by Dr. Zhao, China.

Fig. 5 Axial CT scan of
patient with large acoustic
neuroma who presented
with HFS

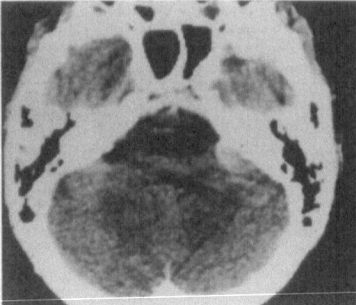 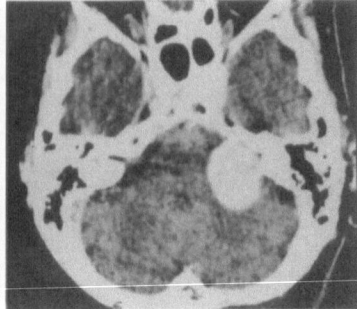

patients are listed in Tables 1 and 2; ages ranged from 24 to 80 years, with a male/female ratio of 6/5.

Results

In patients with underlying vascular loop compression, the spasm initially began in the inferior orbicularis oculi region and gradually spread to involve the lower face. Duration of spasm ranged from 2 months to 12 years prior to evaluation. The six patients with vascular loop compression underwent diagnostic air-contrast CT or MRI with MRA. Five patients underwent microvascular decompression for demonstrated vascular loop indentation of the facial nerve at the REZ. In four patients the anomalous vessel was the anterior-iinferior cerebellar artery (AICA), while in one patient the vertebral artery was causing compression. One patient was advised against posterior fossa surgery but underwent peripheral facial nerve neurolysis.

The spasm in the patient with acoustic neuroma did not originate in an isolated area then subsequently spread, but rather presented as generalized contractions on the side of involement Voluntary muscle contractions led to exacerbation of the spasm, with sustained activity lasting up to 5 min in duration. This patient, along with those suffering vascular compression, demonstrated spasms while sleeping. Spasm in the patients with facial neuroma and primary cholesteatoma was similar in character to that caused by vascular loop. CT revealed an acoustic neuroma in the internal auditory canal (IAC) extending into the CPA (Fig. 5) that resulted in HFS. This patient underwent a translabyrinthine approach for excision of the lesion. The facial nerve was adherent to the tumr and compressed paper-thin. Comlete removal of the tumor was achieved, and the facial nerve was anatomically preserved. Two patients had undetectable (on palpation) adenoid cystic carcinoma of the deep lobe of the parotid gland involving the facial nerve near the stylomastoid foramen.

In one patient a primary cholesteatoma was located medial to the malleus and incus, occupying the region in-

ferior to the geniculate ganglion. This forced the labyrinthine segment of the nerve, which was attenuated superiorly just beneath the dura of the middle cranial fossa. The tympanic segment was displaced inferiorly and laterally. Intraoperatively it was revealed that one patient had a 5×3-mm facial neuroma at the anterior genu of the nerve.

The patients with vascular loop compression have had careful follow-up postoperatively. HFS has not recurred in any of the five patients who underwent posterior fossa decompression and insertion on Teflon sponge between the nerve and offending vessel. After 6 months, the patient with HFS due to an acoustic tumor required facial reanimation with a VII–XII anastomosis. The patient with a facial neuroma underwent interposition cable grafting after tumor removal. A significant return of function (House grade III) was noted. One patient with adenoid cystic carcinoma has survived surgery and radiation; another died from metastatic disease.

Discussion

Schultze, in 1875, was the first to report autopsy findings in a patient with HFS. He found a vertebral artery aneurysm compressing the facial nerve [6]. Gardner described facial neurolysis (along with vessel mobilization in selected cases) for the treatment of HFS in 19 patients. He suggest that this disorder is a reversible pathophysiologic state due to transaxonal short-circuiting or "cross talk'" [7]. Jannetta found the etiologic factor for HFS to be vascular compression at a right angle to the REZ of the facial nerve and developed the technique of microvascular decompression through a retrosigmoid craniectomy [1]. Since then, microvascular decompression has become the standard surgical treatment for HFS. Nagahiro et al. reported on 32 patients with HFS who underwent microvascular decompression; 36 months postoperatively 76% had excellent relief of spasm [8]. Auger reported on 54 patients with 10-year follow-up; total resolution of HFS occurred in 70% [9]. Loeser and Chen reviewed the literature through 1982 and reported a mean cure rate of 84% in surgery for HFS [10]. At the present time, microvascular decompression has been widely accepted as the most effective management for this disorder.

To date the diagnosis of vascular loop compression of the facial nerve is based primarily on medical history and physical examination. Air-contrast CT and digital subtraction angiograaphy (DSA) occasionally are sufficient to diagnose CPA the IAC lesions that can be ascribed as the cause of hemifacial spasm [11]. However, the invasive nature of air-contrast CT and DSA limit their usefulness for screening purposes. Evidence from surgical and experimental studies using imaging and anatomical techniques have demonstrated the most frequently responsible vessels compressing the facial nerve and causing HFS are AICA, the posterior-inferior cerebellar artery (PICA), the vertebral artery, and the internal auditory artery [9, 12], which, except for the vertebral artery, are beyond the resolution capabilities of MRI. In patients with HFS, an accurate and detailed delineation of the neurovascular structures in the CPA is always necessary before proper treatment can be prescribed. Magnetic resonance gradient echo imaging techniques (MRA) have rendered clear delineation of the vascular structures in the CPA. Their disadvantage is the elimination of signals from surrounding tissues, specifically the brainstem and exiting cranial nerves. Thus, the neural strutures and their relationship to surrounding vessels cannot be assessed. Also, artifact from turbulent flow, patient motion, or technical problems may exist [13]. We use MRA in conjunction with conventional MRI for preoperative assessment of larger ectatic vessels.

Further information regarding the underlying etiology of HFS may be provided by electrmyography (EMG). It is well known that a characteristic EMG pattern is seen in patients with HFS due to vascular compression at the REZ which consists of synchronized firing of the involved motor units at high rates (up to 350/s) in contrast to firing rates of 50–70/s in normal motor units [14]. Dobie and Fisch have noted, however, that HFS due to other causes such as tumor, cholesteatoma, etc., Jacks this high-frequency, synchronous firing pattern n EMG and may be used to differentiate vascular loop compression from other various underlying etiologies [4]. They feel that the discharge rate of motor units in HFS due to causes other than vascular compression at the REZ is within the normal range.

Hemifacial spasm due to tumor is rare. One series reported a single tumor (CPA) epidermoid in 425 cases of HFS (0.24%), and a literature review indicates HFS caused by tumrs to be 1.2%. CPA epidermoids may cause HFS in about 10% of cases [15] and 7.8% of cholesteatomas or meningiomas [16]. Even more uncommon is HFS due to acoustic neuroma, having been noted in 2.5% of cases [17]. We encountered 1 case out of 300 referred patients with acoustic neuroma; Sugiura et al. reported 2 cases [18], and Morita reported 1 case [19]. The most interesting case was reported by Nishi [20], a patient with a large acoustic

neuroma who exhibited contralateral HFS. A CT scan indicated the brainstem was markedly displaced and distorted by the tumor. After total removal of the tumor, the spasm completely disappeared.

Two theories regarding the cause of HFS have been advocated – the central nucleus and the peripheral nerve hypothesis. The central nucleus hypothesis states that reorganization of functional connections takes place in the facial motor nucleus secondary to regressive medullary changes [21, 22]. The peripheral nerve hypothesis states that the impulses are due to ectopic excitation and ephaptic transmission. Ectopic excitation of nerves can be triggered by (1) mechanical irritation or compression [23], (2) biochemical changes in the environment that lower the threshold of firing (i.e., reduction of calcium concentration in the paranodal area [24] or (3) extra-axonal current flow to adjacent fibers [25]. This extra-axonal current can lower the threshold of normal surrounding fibers, but not usually to the point of excitation. However, in fibers with a pre-existing low threshold for firing (such as a partially demyelinated nerve fiber), this polarity change may be sufficient for activation – leading to ephaptic transmission [26]. This transmission occurs from a severely demyelinated, slowly conducting fiber to a less demyelinated, faster conducting fiber. Considerable research in the last 2 decades has lent support to the peripheral nerve hypothesis.

References

1. Jannetta PJ (1975) The cause of hemifacial spasm: definitive microsurgical treatment at the brainstem in 31 patients. Trans Am Acad Ophthalmol Otolaryngol 80 (3/1): 319–322
2. Ruby JR, Janetta PJ (1975) Hemifacial spasm: ultrastructural change in the facial nerve induced by neurovascular compression: Surg Neurol 4: 369–370
3. Maroon JC (1978) Hemifacial spasm: a vascular cause. Arch Neurol 35: 481–483
4. Dobie RA, Fisch U (1986) Primary and revision surgery (selective neurectomy) for facial hyperkinesia. Arch Otolaryngol Head Neck Surg 112: 154–163
5. Biglau AW, May M, Bowers RA (1988) Managemen of facial spasm with clostridiom botulinum toxin, type A (oculinum). Arch Otolaryngol Head Neck Surg 144: 1407–1412
6. Schultze F (1875) Linksseitieer fatialiskrampf in folge cines aneurysma der arterid verteralis sinistra. Virchows Arch 65: 385–391
7. Gardner WJ, Sara GA (1962) Hemifacial spasm – a reversible pathophysiologic state. J Neurosurg 19: 240–247
8. Nagahiro P, Takada A et al. (1991) Microvascular decompression for hemifacial spasm: patterns of vascular compression in unsuccessfully operated patients. J Neurosurg 75: 388–392
9. Auger RG, Piepgras DG, Laws ER (1986) Hemifacial spasm: results of microvascular decompression of the facial nerve in 54 patients. Mayo Clin Proc 61: 640–644
10. Loeser JD, Chen J (1983) Hemifacial spasm: treatment by microsurgical facial nerve decompression. Neurosurgery 13: 141–146
11. Applebaum EL, Valvassori GE (1984) Auditory and vestibular system findings in patients with vascular loop in the internal auditory canal. Ann Otol Rhinol Laryngol 92 [Suppl 112]: 63–69

12. Nagahiro S, Takada A et al. (1991) Microvascular decompression for hemifacial spasm – patterns of vascular compression in unsuccessfully operated patients. J Neurosurg 75 : 388 – 392
13. Edelmen RR, Mattle HP et al. (1990) MR angiography. A J R 154 : 937 – 946
14. Esslen E (1977) Facial hyperkinesia. In: Fisch U (ed) Facial nerve surgery. Aesculapius, Birmingham/USA, pp 477 – 484
15. Miyazaki S, Fukushima T (1983) Cerebellopontine angle epidermoid presenting as hemifacial spasm. No To Shinkei 35 : 951 – 955
16. Revilla AG (1948) Differential diagnosis of tumors at the cerebellopontine recess. Bull John Hopkins Hosp 83 : 187 – 212
17. Revilla AG (1942) Neurinomas of the cerebellopontine recess. Bull John Hopkins Hosp 80 : 254 – 296
18. Sugiura Y, Yokyama T et al. (1988) Clinical and electromyographic features of "intermittent tonic facial spasm" due to acoustic neuroma. Report of two cases. Neurol Med Chir 28(12) : 1198 – 1202 (Japanese-English abstract)
19. Morita, Fukushima T et al. (1987) Management of acoustic neuroma with preserved hearing. No Shinken Geka Neurol Surg 15(8) : 821 – 829 (Japanese-English abstract)
20. Nashi T, Matsukado Y et al. (1987) Hemifacial spasm due to contralateral acoustic neuroma: case report. Neurology 37(2): 339 – 342
21. Wartenberg R (1952) Hemifacial spasm: a clinical and pathophysiological study. Oxford University Press, New York
22. Ferguson JN (1978) Hemifacial spasm and the facial nucleus. Ann Neurol 4 : 97 – 103
23. Smith KJ, McDonald WI (1980) Spontaneous and mechanically evoked activity due to central demyelinating lesion. Nature 286 : 154 – 155
24. Katz B, Schmitt DH (1940) Electrica interaction between two adjacent nerve fibers. J Physiol 97 : 471 – 488
25. Arvomitaki A (1942) Effects evoked in an axon by the activity of a contiguous one. J Neurophysiol 5 : 89 – 108
26. Nielsen VK (1985) Electrophysiology of the facial nerve in hemifacial spasm: ectopic/ephaptic excitation. Muscle Nerve 8 : 545 – 555

Eur Arch Otorhinolaryngology (1994) [Suppl]:S343–S345

C. Wagner-Manslau and V. Bonkowski

Idiopathic Facial Nerve Palsy (Bell's Palsy): Morphological Changes in MRI

Purpose

Magnetic resonance imaging (MRI) has already proved to be superior to CT for visualization of cranial nerves. MRI becomes the diagnostic procedure of choice for evaluation of nerve pathology. We developed a morphological MRI protocol to evaluate idiopathic facial nerve palsy, so-called Bell's palsy. Focal nerve enhancement in facial paralysis has been reported from LaBagnara, Doringer, Haberkamp, Millen, Schwaber, Tersi, Traxler, and Wortham [2, 4, 5, 7, 8, 10–13]. MRI is proposed to add to our knowledge about Bell's palsy. The facial nerve is thought to have a reactive edema, for example, reactivation of herpes simplex virus located in the Ganglion geniculi or in peripheral facial nerve. Does MRI show pathomorphological changes in virological and immunological positive cases? Is there prognostic significance to facial nerve enhancement?

Material and Method

A control group of 50 patients was studied who underwent MRI investigations for other reasons such as tumor diagnosis in the pontocerebellar region. We investigated 25 patients, 7 females and 18 males in the age range 22–71 years, median age 34 years, within 24 h of the onset of Bell's palsy and before corticosteroid therapy. Two patients were examined after restitutio ad integrum of Bell's palsy and three patients with residual and chronic facial nerve palsy. MRI was performed on a 1.5-Tesla system (Philips Gyroscan S15) with a head coil. A transversal and sagittal T1-weighted SE image was used for localization; subsequently sagittal T1-weighted SE images were obtained on the pathological side. The mastoideal part of the facial

C. Wagner-Manslau and V. Bonkowski
Nuklearmedizinische Klinik, TU München, Ismaninger Str. 22, 81675 München, Germany

nerve is best seen on these sagittal views. Coronal images are then planned over the mastoidal course of the facial nerve. The following modes were used: SE-T2 (TR 2000/TE3 0, 100), SE-T1 (TR 500/TE 20). Gd-DTPA was administered by means of slow intravenous injection in a dose of 0.1 mmol/kg. The following scans were obtained within 12 min of the Gd-DTPA injection. Technical details: two excitations, 256×256 matrix, 250-mm field of view 3-mm-thick contiguous sections. Special attenuation was given to enhancement patterns of facial nerve. The sagittal orientation was suitable for planning coronal slices on the facial nerve course. The angulation of nerve transit through the temporal bone was not always perpendicular to the ac-pc-line (commissura anterior/commissura posterior). Facial nerve was completely visualized mostly by planning in this way.

Results

Anatomy

The nerve through the anterosuperior part of the internal auditory meatus, swings anteriorly above the cochlea, and pit the ganglion geniculi. In comparison to transversel slices this labyrinthine part is best seen in coronal slices due to the superior localization. Passing the ganglion geniculi the nerve turns sharply backwards and downwards into the second and third part of the facial canal. The tympanic part has an oblique course below the canalis semicircularis lateralis and is in this short section best seen in axial projections. The third part of the nerve, the mastoidal or descending part, runs downwards to the foramen stylomastoideus, lateral to the fossa jugularis. Sagittal orientation provides good discrimination of the mastoidal section of the facial nerve in its entire course as well as the ganglion geniculi. Coronal slices show the passage of the facial nerve along the fossa jugularis. None of the 50 patients of the control group and none of the facial

Table 1 Results of physiological and pathological enhancement in the facial nerve	n	Meatal section	Labyrinthal section	Ganglion geniculi	Mastoidal section
Anatomy	50	No E	No E	No E 8 T2+	No E 2 T2+
Bell's palsy	25	1 Gd+ 3 Gd (+)	8 Gd+ 3 Gd (+)	19 Gd+ 1 Gd (+)	14 Gd+ 3 Gd (+)
Restitution ad integrum of Bell's palsy	2	No E	No E	No E	No E
Residual or chronic palsy	3	No E	No E	No E	2 Gd (+)

No E, no enhancement; +, high enhancement after i.v. Gd-DTPA; (+), slight enhancement; T2+, hyperintense in T2.

nerves of the nonpathological sites showed an enhancement after intravenous Gd-DTPA in a dose of 0.1 mmol/kg (see Table 1).

Pathology

T2-weighted images do not show demarcation of edema in facial nerve as exact as T1-weighted SE sequences. In 8

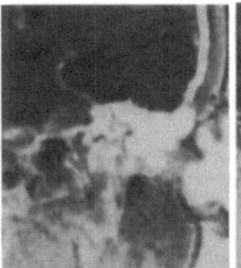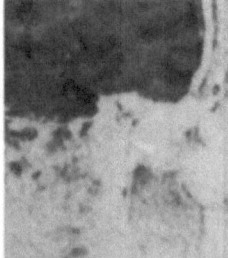
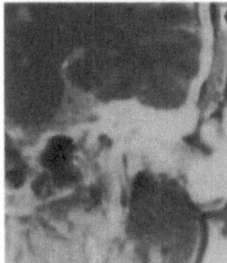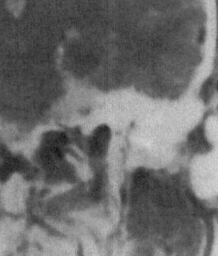

Fig. 1a–d Coronal slice through the temporal bone showing the peripheral facial nerve. Gd-DTPA enhancement and hyperintense signal in the ganglion geniculi (➤) and mastoidal part of the facial nerve are seen. **a** SE-T2 (TR2000/TE30); **b** SE-T2 (TR2000/TE100); **c** SE-T1 (TR600/TE30); **d** SE-T1 (TR600/TE30) with Gd-DTPA (0.1 mmol/kg)

cases out of 20 (40%) a pronounced signal intensity was seen (Fig. 1). In all patients after acute onset of Bell's palsy the facial nerve showed unilateral enhancement on the side of paralysis. The enhancement was globaly seen over the facial nerve only in 16% of cases, always pronounced in one to two sections, the ganglion geniculi and/or mastoidal section. Mostly only sectional involvement was seen: the ganglion geniculi was affected in 80% of cases, less often the mastoidal section in 68% of cases the labyrinthal section in 44% of cases and the meatal section in 16% of cases (see Table 1). Enhancement patterns of the facial nerve on both sides were compared. They were subdivided into two groups, the first one with high, the second with slight and measurable enhancement (see Table 1).

Discussion

Magnetic resonance imaging has significantly contributed to improving imaging of the facial nerve. In MRI the facial nerve is visualized as bone is washed out and soft tissues become the imaged structure. Bell's palsy, in acute idiopathic peripheral facial palsy, involves distal branches of the facial nerve. The diagnosis is based on clinical findings with a rapid onset and subsequent spontaneous recovery. In our study group, with the exception of two patients all recovered within 6 months.

Possible causes include viral inflammation, polyneuropathy, and immunologic or ischemic factors [3, 6]. In all our cases appropiate laboratory parameters with a positive herpes titer was determined. The theory of herpes reactivation in the ganglion geniculi is supported by the MRI data showing accentuated enhancement in the ganglion geniculi in 80% of all cases. The presence of enhancement in the ganglion geniculi is consistent with the works of Fisch [3] and Murphy [9]. Fisch found the meatal foramen to be the narrowest bony constriction of the nerve. Another important factor seems to be the capillary density [1]. The labyrinthal segment of the human facial nerve contains fewer and smaller intrinsic blood vessels than do the mastoid and tympanic segments.

An edematous nerve as a result of inflammation and pronounced perfusion should demonstrate enhancement; in all studied cases having an examination within 24 h of acute onset of Bell's palsy enhancement was proved, the gadolinium scan confirming the clinical diagnosis. Recovery of paralysis in our 25 cases was not dependent on Gd-DTPA enhancement patterns, like expansion and intensity, but 2 of 3 patients with residual and chronic palsy did show further enhancement. Gd-DTPA seems to be a parameter of floride inflammation.

Many questions remain unanswered, but the information provided through MRI gives additional information in facial nerve disorders that may prove clinically useful. MRI has been proved as a new topographic method but not yet as a prognostic test. Further investigations are necessary.

References

1. Balkany T, Fradis M, Jafek B, Rucker N (1991) Intrinsic vasculature of the labyrinthine segment of the facial nerve – Implications for the site of lesion in Bell's palsy. Otolaryngol Head Neck Surg 104 (1): 20 – 23

2. Doringer E, Albegger K, Sinzinger G, Schmoller H (1991) Ideopathische Facialisparese and MRT. HNO 39 : 362 – 366
3. Fisch U (1981) Surgery of Bell's palsy. Arch Otolaryngol 107 : 1 – 11
4. Haberkamp T, Harvey S, Daniels D (1990) The use of Gd-enhanced MRI to determine lesion site in traumatic facial paralysis. Laryngoskope 100 : 1294 – 1300
5. LaBagnara J, Jahn A, Habif D, Solomon E (1989) MRI findings in two cases of acute facial paralysis. Otolaryngol Head Neck Surg 101 (5): 562 – 565
6. May M, Hughes G (1987). Facial nerve disorders: update 1987. Am J Otol 8 : 167 – 180
7. Millen S, Daniels D, Meyer G (1989) Gadolinium enhanced MRI in temporal bone lesions. Laryngoskope 99 : 257 – 260
8. Millen S, Daniels D, Meyer G (1990) Gadolinium enhanced MRI in facial nerve lesions. Otolaryngol Head Neck Surg 102 : 26 – 33
9. Murphy T (1991) MRI of the facial nerve during paralysis. Otolaryngol Head Neck Surg 104 (1): 47 – 49
10. Schwaber M, Zealear D, Netterville J, Seshul M, Ossoff R (1989) The use of MRI and HRCT in the evaluation of facial paralysis. Otolaryngol Head Neck Surg 101 (4): 449 – 458
11. Tersi L, Lufkin R, Wortham D, Flannan B, Reicher M, Halbach V, Bentson J, Wilson G, Ward P, Hanafee W (1987) MRI of the intratemporal facial nerve using surface coils. AJR 148 : 589 – 594
12. Traxler M, Gritzmann N, Kramer J, Grasl M, Hajek P (1989) Der intratemporale Verlauf des N. facialis im MR. HNO 37 : 19 – 22
13. Wortham D, Teresi L, Lufkin R, Hanafee W (1989) MRI of the facial nerve. Otolaryngol Head Neck Surg 101 : 295 – 301

Eur Arch Otorhinolaryngology (1994) [Suppl]: S 346 – S 348

FREE PAPERS AND POSTERS

Y. Koike, H. Tojima, H. Maeyama, and M. Aoyagi

Contrast-Enhanced MRI of the Facial Nerve in Patients with Bell's Palsy

Magnetic resonance imaging (MRI) enhanced by Gd-DTPA has been one of the recent topics under discussion for imaging diagnosis. However, the clinical evaluation of MRI in facial palsy has not yet been established. In this report, the diagnostic value of enhanced MRI in patients with Bell's palsy was investigated.

Subjects and Methods

Twenty-two affected sides and 19 normal sides of 22 patients with early stage Bell's palsy and 14 sides of 7 normal volunteers were involved in this study. In all subjects, an MRI scan was taken within 6 – 43 days after onset of palsy, with a 1.5-T superconducting maget (Siemens, MAGNE-TOM H15), under the following conditions: 600/20 (TR/TE), 2 mm slice thickness, absence of an interslice gap, a 256×512 matrix, a 190 – 210 mm field of view, five excitations, and an imaging time of about 13 min. For all the subjects, the T1-weighted MRI scans were taken before and after intravenous injection of Gd-DTPA (0.1 mmol/kg). The contrast enhancement was objectively determined, based on the value of the signal intensity ratio, which was calculated according to the following equation: signal intensity ratio = (signal intensity in the facial nerve – the background noise)/(signal intensity in the brainstem – the background noise). If the signal intensity ratio was above the value of 1.0, the contrast enhancement of the MRI scan was evaluated as positive.

Results

Figures 1 and 2 show axial and coronal images of T1-weighted Gd-enhanced MRI on one patient with Bell's palsy. The enhanced MRI scan showed intense enhancement of the internal acoustic meatal segment, the labyrinthine segment, the geniculate ganglion, the tympanic segment, and the mastoid segment.

Table 1 shows the number and frequency of the enhancement-positive cases, which are evaluated by signal intensity ratio, of the affected side, the normal side, and in the normal volunteers, by each segment of the facial nerve. The facial nerve ranging from the geniculate ganglion to the mastoid segment is enhanced not only on the affected side but also on the normal side and in the normal volunteers. However, the internal acoustic meatal segment of the facial nerve is enhanced only on the affected side, which is the major characteristic of Bell's palsy. This suggests that the Bell's palsy lesion may involve the internal acoustic meatal segment of the facial nerve.

Figure 3 shows the results of the signal intensity ratio on the affected side compared with those on the normal side and normal volunteers. The signal intensity ratios in the geniculate ganglion and the tympanic segment were signi-

Y. Koike (✉), H. Tojima, H. Maeyama, and M. Aoyagi
Department of Otolaryngology, Yamagata University School of Medicine, Iida-Nishi, Yamagata, 990-23, Japan

Table 1 Number and frequency of enhanced-positive cases determined by signal intensity ratio

	Bell's palsy		Normal
	Affected side	Normal side	
Internal meatus	20/22 (91%)	0/19 (0%)	0/14 (0%)
Geniculate ganglion	22/22 (100%)	18/19 (95%)	13/14 (93%)
Tympanic segment	22/22 (100%)	16/19 (84%)	9/14 (64%)
Mastoid segment	22/22 (100%)	16/19 (84%)	14/14 (100%)

Fig. 1 Left facial palsy in a 42-year-old man. MR scan was obtained 43 days after onset. The axial contrast enhanced T1-weighted images show intense enhancement of internal acoustic meatal segment (*I*), labyrinthine segment (*L*), geniculate ganglion (*G*), tympanic segment (*T*), and mastoid segment (*M*)

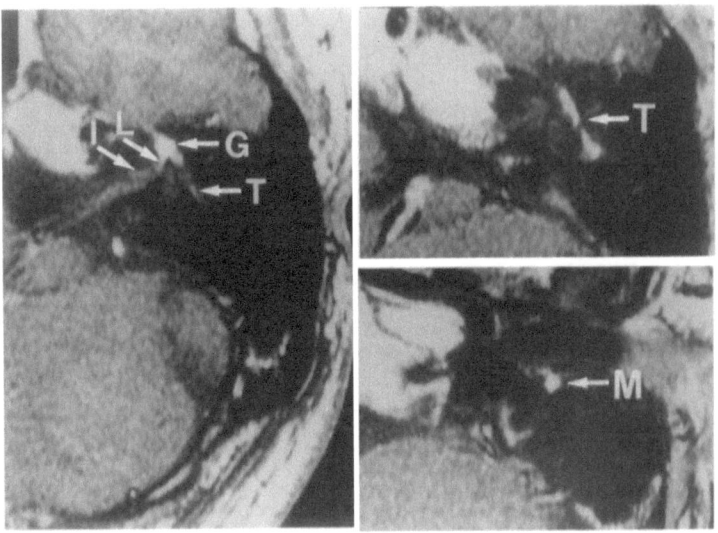

Fig. 2 Same case shown with coronal MR images

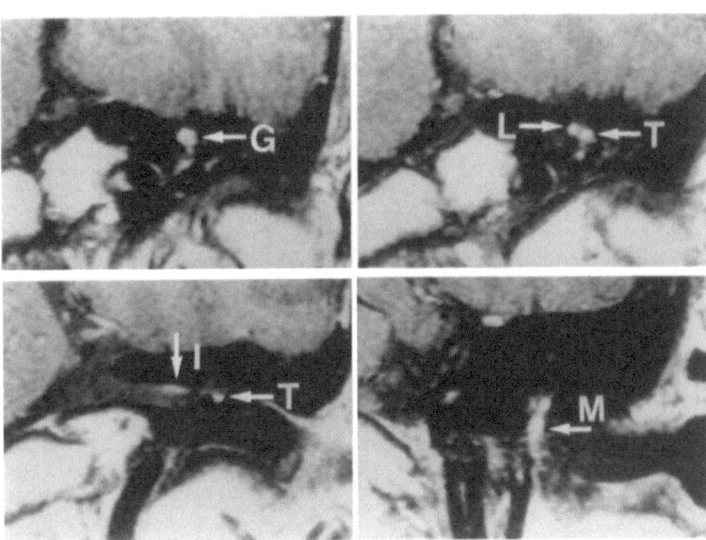

ficantly higher on the affected side than that on the normal side and that in the normal volunteers. The mastoid segment showed a high signal intensity ratio on the affected side, as well as on the normal side and in normal volunteers. The differences between the affected side and other two groups were not significant. Based on these results, it was considered that the geniculate ganglion and the tympanic segment might also provide the chief lesions of Bell's palsy. The results of physiological examinations such as electroneurography and examination of the stapedial reflex were compared with MRI scan results; no relationship was seen.

S348

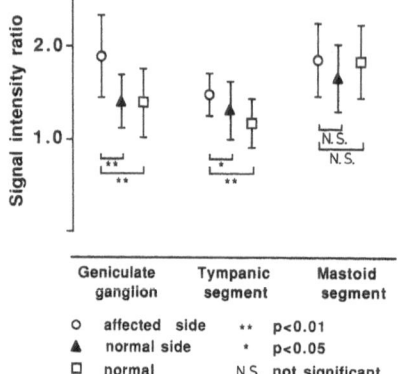

Geniculate ganglion | Tympanic segment | Mastoid segment

○ affected side   ** p<0.01
▲ normal side   * p<0.05
□ normal   N.S. not significant

Fig. 3 Signal intensity ratio results in the affected side compared with the normal side and normal volunteers

Conclusions

1. In a Gd-enhanced MRI of the facial nerve, the signal intensity ratio was a good index for the objective evaluation of contrast enhancement.

2. A characteristic finding was the enhancement of the internal acoustic meatal segment of the facial nerve only on the affected side.
3. The geniculate ganglion, the tympanic segment, and the mastoid segment were enhanced not only on the affected side, but also on the normal side and in normal volunteers. However, the signal intensity ratio of the geniculate ganglion and the tympanic segment was significantly higher on the affected side than on the normal side and the normal volunteers.
4. The severity of facial palsy or the results of physiological examinations bore no relation to the MRI scan results.
5. Based on the above results, a gadolinium-enhanced MRI showed some useful findings in estimating the affected legion of Bell's palsy, whereas it was considered to be of no value for the diagnosis of severity or prognosis.

Reference

1. Daniels DL et al. (1987) Facial nerve enhancement in MR imaging. AJNR 8 : 605–607

Eur Arch Otorhinolaryngology (1994) [Suppl]: S349–S352

Y. Nakao, K. Matsumoto, M. Ochi, and H. Kumagami

Gadolinium-Enhanced Magnetic Resonance Imaging in Experimental Facial Nerve Paralysis

Introduction

Recently, it has been reported that the facial nerve shows enhancement on gadolinium-enhanced magnetic resonance imaging (Gd-MRI) in patients with such conditions as Bell's palsy or traumatic facial nerve paralysis. The site of involvement in Bell's palsy remains unknown, and accurate lesion-site information is useful for surgical planning in cases of facial nerve paralysis. The importance of this technique in detecting the lesion site has been discussed, but the mechanism of facial nerve enhancement is unknown. In the present study, in order to elucidate the correlation between facial nerve enhancement and lesion site, Gd-MRI study was performed in the rabbit.

Methods

Seven rabbits weighing about 2 kg each were used. The rabbits were anesthetized with an intravenous injection of sodium pentobarbital (30 mg/kg body weight). After exposing the facial nerve under an operating microscope, facial nerve paralysis was produced by the following methods: (1) nerve crushing with a hemostat forceps for 20 s at the center of the mastoid portion; (2) ligature with silk in the same portion; and (3) ligature with silk at the stylomastoid foramen in the extratemporal portion. Gd-MRI was performed with the patient under general anesthesia 4–7 days after the nerve damage, and follow-up Gd-MRI studies were conducted 19–51 days later in two rabbits.

Y. Nakao (✉), K. Matsumoto, and H. Kumagami
Department of Otolaryngology, Nagasaki University,
School of Medicine, 7-1, Sakamoto Machi, Nagasaki, 852, Japan

M. Ochi
Department of Radiology, Nagasaki University, Japan

MRI was performed on a 1.5-T superconducting magnet (Signa, GE Medical Systems, Milwaukee). A sagittal T1-weighted spin-echo image was used for localization (Fig. 1). Axial and coronal T1-weighted images through the temporal bones and posterior fossa were obtained. For T1-weighted images, an echo time of 20 ms was used with a repetition time of 400 ms. Slice thickness was 3 mm with an interslice gap of 1.5 mm. Gadolinium-diethylenetriamine-pentaacetic acid (Gd-DTPA) was administered intravenously at a dosage of 0.1 mmol/kg body weight. T1-weighted images were obtained both before and after administration of Gd-DTPA.

To define the anatomy of the rabbit facial nerve, T1-weighted images were obtained from a fresh rabbit cadaver. Prior to MRI, a flexible tube filled with 0.19% Gd-DTPA solution was bonded after removing the facial nerve ranging from the internal auditory canal to the stylomastoid foramen.

Moreover, the facial nerve from the nerve root to the stylomastoid foramen was observed using the technique of fluorescein angiograhy [5]. Seven days after nerve crushing injury with a hemostat forceps at the center of the

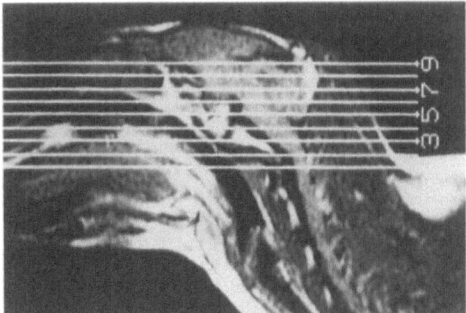

Fig. 1 Sagittal T1-weighted image is used to position subsequent axial sections through the temporal bone and posterior fossa

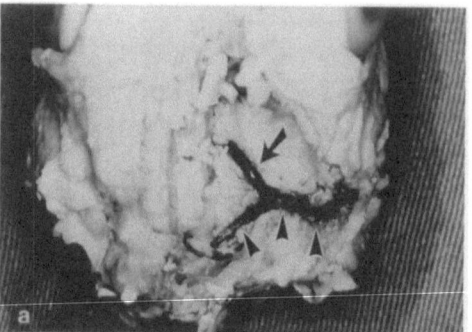

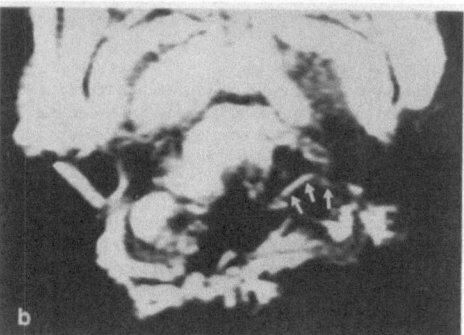

Fig. 2 **a** Rabbit cadaver specimen with attached tube (*arrowheads*) filled with Gd-DTPA solution after removing the facial nerve. The *arrow* points to the major petrosal nerve. **b** T1-weighted axial image shows enhancement (*arrows*) along the tube

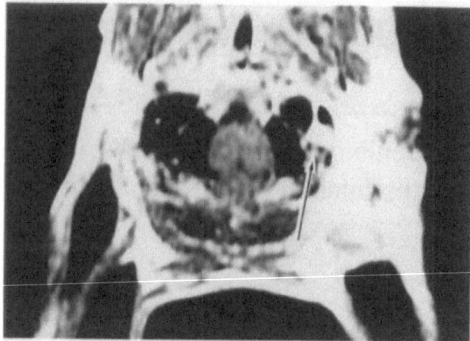

Fig. 3 Animal 3. Gadolinium-enhanced MRI shows enhancement with enlargement (*arrow*) in the geniculate ganglion and the tympanic segment

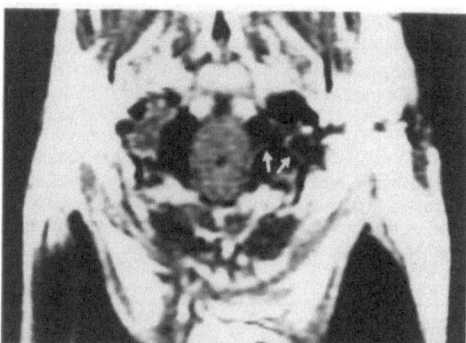

Fig. 4 Animal 5. Gadolinium-enhanced MRI shows enhancement (*arrows*) from the internal auditory canal to the tympanic segment

mastoid portion, as in the MRI study, 1.2–1.3 ml/kg of a fluorescent substance (Fluorecite) was injected intravenously. Fifteen minutes after the injection of Fluorecite, the rabbit was killed by intravenous injection with 5 ml sodium pentobarbital. The facial nerve was exposed by surgical removal of the bony wall, and then observed using a fluorescence eye fundus camera (Kowa RC-M).

Results

Figure 2 shows the rabbit cadaver specimen with attached tube and T1-weighted axial image. Enhancement was observed along the tube.

The Gd-MRI results are summarized in Table 1. On Gd-MRI performed 4–7 days after the nerve damage, five of

the seven animals showed facial nerve enhancement on the paralytic side. In animals 1 through 4 receiving crush injury at the center of the mastoid portion, facial nerve enhancement with enlargement was observed in the geniculate ganglion and the tympanic segment (Fig. 3). The mastoid segment was obscured by soft tissue enhancement. In animal 5 receiving nerve ligature at the center of the mastoid portion, enhancement was observed from the internal auditory canal to the tympanic segments (Fig. 4). In animal 6 and 7 receiving nerve ligature at the stylomastoid foramen, no enhancement of the nerve was seen.

In the follow-up scans in animals 3 and 4, the facial nerve enhancement was diminished in size compared to that in the initial study (Fig. 5).

Figure 6 shows the fluorescence finding in the normal facial nerve. Fluorescence was observed along the entire

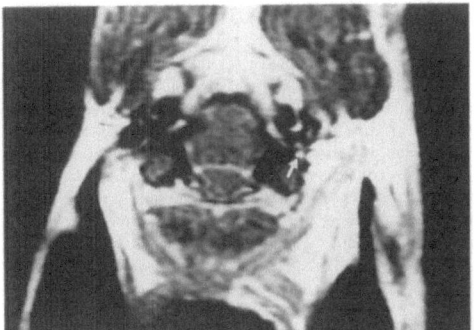

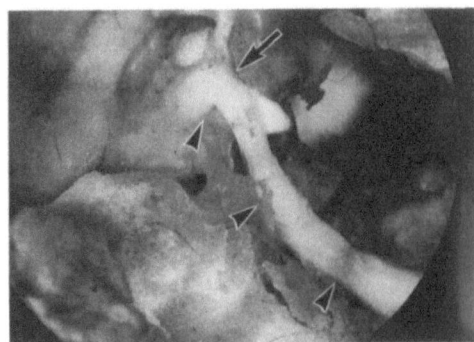

Fig. 5 Animal 4. Follow-up scan performed 51 days later shows enhancement (*arrow*) in the tympanic segment

Fig. 6 Normal facial nerve from the nerve root to the mastoid portion. Fluorescence is visible along the nerve through the distal portion of the internal auditory canal segment (*arrowheads*) but not proximal to this portion. The *arrow* points to the geniculate ganglion

Fig. 7a, b Facial nerve 7 days after crush injury at the mastoid portion. **a** An edematous change (*arrowheads*) is seen proximal to the site of injury. The *arrow* points to the site of injury. *Small arrowheads* indicate the distal side of the facial nerve. **b** Fluorescence is visible at the edematous portion (*arrow*) but not in the distal side including the lesion site

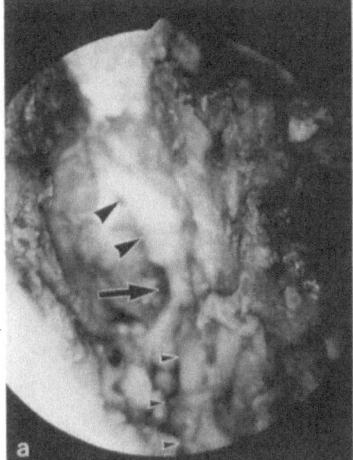

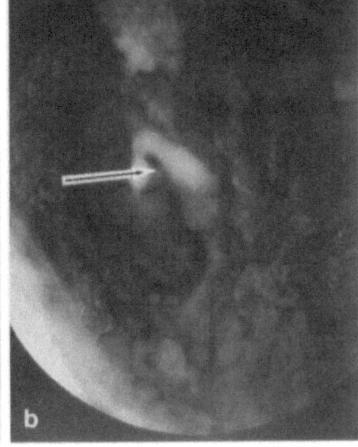

Table 1 Magnetic resonance enhancement characteristics in seven animals with experimental facial nerve paralysis. IAC, internal auditory canal; +, enhancement; −, no enhancement

Animal number	Injury		Days after injury	Enhanced segment of facial nerve		
	Site	Method		IAC	Labyrinthine/ geniculate	Tympanic
1	Mastoid	Crush	4	−	+	+
2	Mastoid	Crush	7	−	+	+
3	Mastoid	Crush	5	−	+	+
			19	−	−	+
			47	−	−	−
4	Mastoid	Crush	7	−	+	+
			51	−	−	+
5	Mastoid	Ligature	4	+	+	+
6	Extratympanic	Ligature	5	−	−	−
7	Extratympanic	Ligature	7	−	−	−

course of the nerve through the distal portion of the internal auditory canal segment, but it was not observed in the region proximal to this portion. In the crushed facial nerve, on the other hand, edematous change was observed proximal to the site of injury as shown in Fig. 7a. Fluorescence was observed at the edematous portion but not in the distal side including the lesion site (Fig. 7b).

Discussion

Gadolinium-DTPA is a paramagnetic agent which decreases the spin lattice relaxation time in tissues where it accumulates, resulting in improved contrast enhancement in T1-weighted images. As Gd-DTPA is distributed almost exclusively in extracellular spaces, its influence is most pronounced in regions with increased extracellular fluid, such as areas of inflammation, tumor, and edema [4]. However, most of the brain is not enhanced, because this agent dose not cross the blood-brain barrier. In the normal facial nerve of the rabbit, intravenous injection of Fluorecite resulted in fluorescence of the entire nerve through the distal portion of the internal auditory canal segment. Such a staining seems to be an important fact in explaining an enhancement along the normal facial nerve in the facial canal [2]. It is considered that Gd-DTPA is also distributed in this portion.

With Fluorecite injected intravenously, the facial nerve stains from the proximal side to the distal side in the intratemporal portion, whereas it stains from the distal side to the proximal side in the extratemporal portion [3]. This flow seems to be responsible for the edematous change proximal to the site of injury in animals damaged at the intratemporal portion. At the surgery of Bell's palsy, swelling of the facial nerve proximal to the site of compression was also confirmed by Fisch et al. [1].

In this study, fluorescence was observed at the edematous portion proximal to the site of injury but not in the distal side including the lesion site. Furthermore, facial nerve enhancement was observed proximal to the site of injury in animals damaged at the mastoid portion. These findings suggest that the facial nerve is enhanced at the edematous portion resulting from nerve damage because of increased extracellular fluid within the nerve.

References

1. Fisch U, Felix H (1983) On the pathogenesis of Bell's palsy. Acta Otolaryngol (Stockh) 95 : 532 – 538
2. Gebriski SS, Talian SA, Niparko JK (1992) Enhancement along the normal facial nerve in the facial canal: MR imaging and anatomic correlation. Radiology 183 : 391 – 394
3. Kumagami H, Nakao Y (1988) Fluorescence findings of the facial nerve at decompression operation. Acta Otolaryngol Suppl (Stockh) 446 : 126 – 131
4. Millen SJ, Daniels DL, Meyer GA (1990) Gadolinium-enhanced magnetic resonance imaging in facial nerve lesions. Otolaryngol Head Neck Surg 102 : 26 – 33
5. Pau HW (1987) Revascularization of fascia after tympanoplastic grafts. Arch Otorhinolaryngol 239 : 7 – 13

Eur Arch Otorhinolaryngology (1994) [Suppl]: S353–S355

J. Kronenberg, C. Fuchs, and E. Bendet

Preoperative Radiologic Assessment of Facial Nerve in Cochlear Implant Surgery

Facial nerve palsy was reported as a complication of cochlear implant surgery at a rate as high as $1\% - 3\%$ [3, 4]. Even though temporary, it may have a profound effect on the patient's well being. Our clinical impression was that the knowledge of the anatomical relationship of the facial nerve to various adjacent structures in the surgical field may help avoid this complication and also influence the decision on which side to implant. Facial recess, the distance from the facial nerve to the external auditory canal, and the distance from the facial nerve to the round window niche were previously measured [1, 2]. However, we believe that these parameters are insufficient in predicting the likelihood of facial nerve palsy in cochlear implant surgery. Of 20 patients operated on in our departmet since 1989, two patients (10%) had temporary facial palsy that resolved spontaneously after 2 weeks in one patient and 6 weeks in the other. In one additional patient (5%), the round window niche could not be reached through the posterior tympanotomy approach and a canal wall-down mastoidectomy had to be performed. We have analyzed the temporal bone anatomy on high-resolution computerized tomograhy (HRCT) of these three patients and supplemented the information with data of the other operated patients and of additional unoperated patients who served as a control group.

Materials and Methods

We used the HRCT at a 20° incline, parallel to the fronto-meatal line. Slice thickness was 1.2 mm and the table

J. Kronenberg (✉) and E. Bendel
Department of Otorhinolaryngology, Sheba Medical Center,
Tel-Hashomer, Israel and Sackler School of Medicine,
University of Tel-Aviv, Tel-Aviv, Israel

C. Fuchs
Department of Statistics, Beverly and Raymond Sackler
Faculty of Exact Sciences, University of Tel-Aviv, Tel-Aviv, Israel

increment was 1 mm. The proposed approach is based on the values of following three measurements (Fig. 1); the length of the line connecting the facial nerve and the round window membrane (L1); the lenth of the perpendicular line between the facial nerve and the posterior wall of the middle ear (L2); and the angle (α) between the two lines. These parameters were measured on both ears of the 20 operated patients examined retrospectively and of 16 other patients examined for various reasons. The 72 examined ears thus formed two groups of ears. The first group included the 20 operated ears and the second one was made up of the 20 unoperated ears of the same patients and of the 32 ears from the uoperated patients. There were 23 males and 13 females; the age ranged from 8 to 72 years with a mean of 44 years. We analyzed the distribution of the three parameters with respect to sex, age, and side. The values of

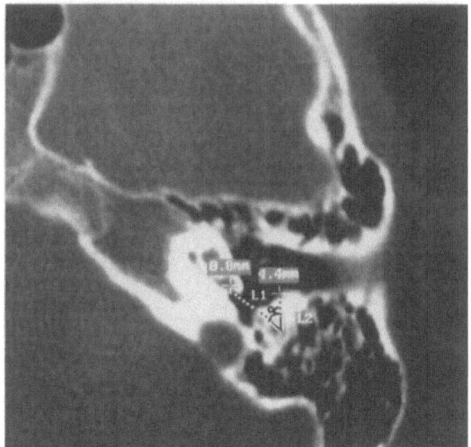

Fig. 1 The HRCT of an operated patient: L1 (4 mm), L2 (8 mm)

S 354

the parameters measured on the two sides of each patient were then compared in a matched pairs analysis. The L1, L2, and α values from the 17 operated ears with no complications were defined as a "reference sample" to which we compared the entire operated group. Shewhart charts [6] and multivariate MP charts [5] were used in the data analysis.

Results

The distance L1 between the round window membrane and the facial nerve in the sample of 72 ears varied from 4.0 to 11.2 mm with a mean of 7.43 (standard deviation 1.56 mm). The length L2 between the facial nerve and the posterior wall of the middle ear ranged from 1.0 to 5.3 mm with a mean of 2.95 (standard deviation of 0.95 mm). The angle α between these two lines varied from 36.2° to 90.0° with a mean of 63.70° (standard deviation of 12.44°). We note that the values of the analyzed parameters vary considerably both among patients as well as between the two sides of the same patient.

No statistically significant differences in the three parameters were found either between males and females or between the left and right sides except for a borderline significant value of 0.06 found for L1 and angle α whose means were smaller on the left side than on the right side. A highly significant positive correlation of the age with the angle α was also noted (p value = 0.0025).

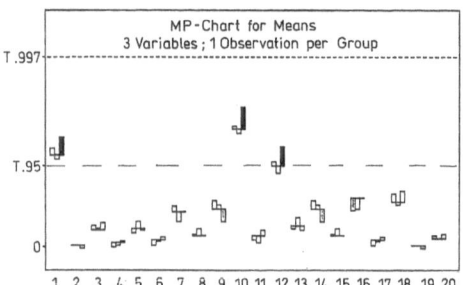

Fig. 3 The multivariate profile chart: *The black bars* correspond to the α measurements of the patients with complications in surgery

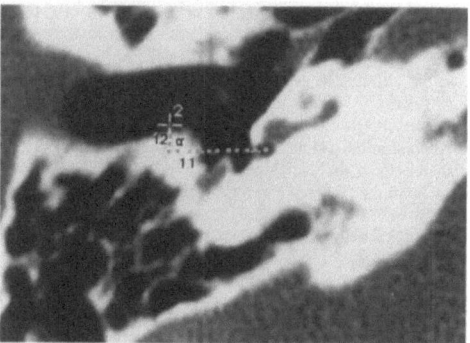

Fig. 4 The HRCT of an operated patient with a wide α angle

The values of the parameters (L1, L2, and α) were plotted on three separate Shewhart charts (Fig. 2). The upper critical level (UCL) and the lower critical levels (LCL) are displayed on the charts by horizontal lines at ± 3 standard deviations around the mean of the "reference sample" formed by the 17 patients without complications, with whom all 20 observations were compared. We can see that for the parameters L1 and L2, none of the observations deviate from the standards. However, the chart for α (Fig. 2c) reveals clearly that patients 10 (with an angle α of 89.0°) and 12 (with α of 89.5°), who had temporary facial palsy, and patient 1 (with α of 90.0°), who required canal wall-down mastoidectomy, had outlying values which reached or exceeded the upper critical level. The multivariate profile (MP) chart (Fig. 3), which displays simultaneously the univariate and the multivariate measures of dispersions, presents an even more conclusive picture. We can see in this figure that the three observations with complications, patients 1, 10, and 12, do indeed deviate

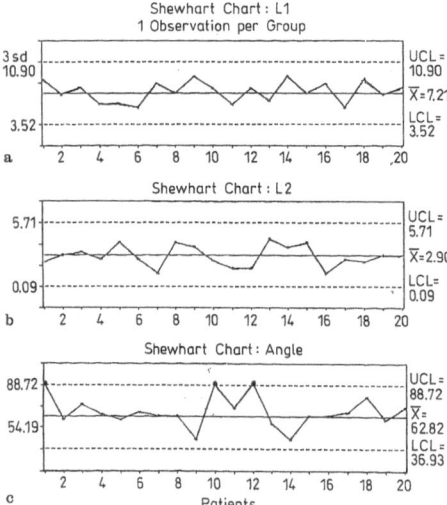

Fig. 2 The Shewart charts for L1 (a), L2 (b), and α (c)

significantly from the "reference sample" exceeding the critical value at a significance level of 0.05. In this chart, the vertical position of each symbol represents the overall deviation of all the parameters from the mean of the "reference sample." Critical values are marked by horizontal lines on the chart. The bars in the symbol correspond to the three variable sequentially. They increase in size and darken as the level of significance of the deviation increases. The bars extend either above or below the base line according to the sign of the deviation. We observe that the third bar in each of those symbols which represents the angle α is large and painted black, thus defining outlying values.

Discussion

The two length measurements and the angle between them can easily be obtained from the patients' HRCTs. From the analysis of the distributions of those parameters we can conclude that there are considerable variations, both among individuals as well as between the two sides of the same person. No significant relationship was detected with respect to sex and side. The L1 and L2 measurements were also not correlated with age. However, the distribution of α with respect to other factors was quite different with a positive correlation both between the angle and age as well as between the angles in the two sides of the same person.

From the point of view of the cochlear implant surgery, the distance L2 appeared to be important for the determination of ease of approach into the middle ear. A small facial recess results in the unavoidable sacrifice of the chorda tympani. The longer the distance L2, the easier is the approach. On the other hand, the distance L1 was found to be of importance only in connection with the angle α between the two lines. The latter was found to be the crucial parameter for this surgical procedure. Angles between 44° and 80° seem to provide an easy and safe access

to the round window niche. An angle wider than 85° (Fig. 4) means that the round window niche is placed far posteriorly in the sinus tympai and can hardly be seen through the opened facial recess, thus posterior angling of the drill is required in order to reach the round window niche. Such a maneuver would endanger the facial nerve by heating it with the revolving drill shaft. In angles near 90°, the round window niche cannot be reached at all through a posterior tympanotomy approach and cochleaotomy or canal wall-down mastoidectomy will be required. The two patients who had facial palsy had angles near to 90° (89.0° and 89.5°, respectively) and the patient in whom a canal wall-down mastoidectomy was done had an angle of 90.0°.

We believe that the simple roentgenological approach outlined above, based on the analysis of the HRCT of the temporal bone, can minimize the likelihood of facial nerve injury.

Acknowledgements The authors wish to express their gratitude to Professor J. Braham for his critical review and to Mrs. C. Halpern for her assistance.

References

1. Balkay T, Dresbach J (1987) Surgical anatomy and radiographic imaging of cochlear implant surgery. Am J Otol 3 : 195 – 200
2. Balkany T et al. (1986) Radiographic imaging of the cochlear implant candidate: preliminary results. Otolaryngol Head Neck Surg 95 : 592 – 597
3. Cohen NL et al. (1988) Medical or surgical complications related to the Nucleus multichannel cochlear implant. Ann Otol Rhinol Laryngol 97 [Suppl 135]: 8 – 13
4. Cohen NL et al. (1987) Problems and complications of cochlear implant surgery. Ann Otol Rhinol Laryngol 96 [Suppl 128]: 5 – 14
5. Fuchs C, Benjamini Y (1989) Multivariate profile charts for SPC. Series in applied statistics 91-01, Department of Statistics, Tel Aviv University
6. Wadsworth MH Jr et al. (1986) Modern methods for quality control and improvement technology. Wiley, New York

Eur Arch Otorhinolaryngology (1994) [Suppl]: S356–S357

POSTERS

M. L. Navarrete, A. Rovira, P. Quesada, and M. García

Gadolinium-Enhanced Magnetic Resonance Imaging in Bell's Palsy

Introduction

The etiopathogenesis of Bell's palsy is not yet well known. The lesion site of facial nerve has been determined as being in the entrance to the internal auditive conduct [1].

Not very long ago, radiological diagnosis in patients with Bell's palsy was only a diagnosis of exclusion.

The evaluation of the temporal bone has changed since the rise of computerized tomography (CT); however, with magnetic resonance (MR), the facial nerve can be seen in a pathological state [2]. Studies using a contrast mean such as gadolinium (Gd) may help to clarify some questions about the pathogenesis of the disease.

The aim of this study was to acquire data that will help us find out about the etiopathogenesis of Bell's palsy using MR with Gd.

Material and Methods

Seven patients in the acute phase of the disease were followed from September to December 1991. Four men and three women between 27 and 63 years old were studied. All patients showed complete facial paralysis at the beginning. Electrophysiological examination by electroneurography (ENoG) at 10 days of evolution established severe paralysis in all cases (ENoG <20%).

A study using MR was performed on days 3–40 of evolution (average, 19 days). All patients were examined under superconductive magnet of 1.5 T (Magneton, Simens, Erlangen, Germany). A cranial coil was used with T1-weighted spin-echo sequences (600/20/3; TR/TE acquisitions). Images of the temporal bone in the axial and coronal sections were obtained, before and after administration of Gd (0.1 mmol/kg). As study parameters a section depth of 3 mm, a distance between sections of 0.1 mm, and a matrix of 256×256 were used. The sequences T1 after contrast were obtained immediately after the administration of Gd. The evaluation of findings by MR was done without knowing clinical findings. To get this evaluation, images of axial and coronal cuts were carefully examined, assessing the presence of contrast along the differents portions of the affected and nonaffected facial nerves.

Results

All patients showed uptake of Gd along more than two portions of facial nerve, i.e., uptake positive to the inflammatory edema. There were several uptake patterns: the labyrinthine and tympanic portions showed uptake in six cases, the geniculate ganglion and the mastoid segment in five cases, and the intracanalicular portion in four cases. In none of these cases did we observe uptake in the nonaffected facial nerve or in other cranial nerves.

Often the affected nerve path was only observed in one of the projections, noting the optimal evaluation of the mastid segment in the axial projection and the intracanalicular one in the coronal projection.

Discussion

The diagnosis of Bell's palsy is based on clinical findings. Clinical and electrophysiological topodiagnosis studies have demonstrated the proximal site lesion in severe facial paralysis [3]. It seems that MR in Bell's palsy is optimal if done during the first 2 weeks of evolution. However, there are studies which conclude identical results performed in the acute phase as in the tardive phase [4].

The first studies demonstrated Gd uptake by the intrapetrous portion of facial nerve in patients diagnosed as

M.L. Navarrete, A. Rovira, P. Quesada, and M. Garcia
Hospital Valle de Hebrón, Universidad Autónoma, Barcelona

having Bell's palsy [5]. Gd spreads preferentially in the extracellular spaces and only gets through the hemato-encephalic barrier (HEB) if this is broken. The uptake mechanism in Bell's palsy is unknown, but it seems related to the hypervascularization of the perineural structures or to HEB disruption [6].

Image evaluation by MR is based on the outline changes of facial nerve and the Gd uptake distribution although this uptake is not specific for Bell's palsy [7].

Until now studies by MR in Bell's palsy have concluded that uptake by the facial nerve is in the majority of cases diffuse, with strangulation of the edematous facial nerve in the fallopian conduct. A diffuse uptake by the facial nerve preferentially from the geniculate ganglion to the mastoid segment has been observed and in a few cases also in the intracanalicular portion [8]. In our series, we observed tympanic and labyrinthine uptake as the most frequent, followed by the geniculate ganglion and mastoid segment. We also observed uptake in the intracanalicular portion in four of the seven cases.

In this series it was found that uptake of all presented Gd occurred in more than one portion, but in some the uptake was not continous, probably because this was secondary to a failure in the cut orientation.

On the other hand, in case 6 hyperintense nodular image was found in the geniculate ganglion site secondary to the flat marrow temporal bone; this could lead to false interpretation if it is not compared with the previous results obtained before contrast administration.

Almost all the studies carried out until now seem to show that there is no correlation between the severity of facial paralysis and the degree of uptake. In the reviewed studies, the authors agree that the results of using MR with Gd would not constitute a proof in Bell's palsy patients [6, 8].

Thus, our study supports our previous work about the benefit of tympanic and labyrinthine facial nerve decompression in patients with maximal paralysis.

References

1. Gantz BJ, Gmür A, Fisch U (1982) Intraoperative evoked electromyography in Bell's palsy. Am J Otolaryngol 3 : 273 – 278
2. Teresi L, Lufkin R, Wortham D et al. (1987) MR imaging of the intratemporal facial nerve by using surface coils. AJR 148 : 589 – 594
3. Yanagihara N, Kitani S, Gyo K (1988) Topodiagnosis of lesions in Bell's palsy. Ann Otol Rhinol Laryngol [Suppl] 97 : 14 – 17
4. Schwaber MK, Larson TC, Zealear DL, Greasy J (1990) Gadolinium enhanced magnetic resonance imaging in Bell's palsy. Laryngoscope 100 : 1264 – 1269
5. Daniels DL, Czervionke L, Pojunas KW et al. (1987) Facial nerve enhancement in MR imaging. AJNR 8 : 605 – 607
6. Millen SJ, Daniels DL, Mayer G (1990) Gadolinium enhanced magnetic resonance imaging in facial nerve lesions. Otolaryngol Head Neck Surg 102 : 26 – 33
7. Millen SJ, Daniels DL, Meyer GA (1989) Gadolinium enhanced magnetic resonance. Laryngoscope 99 : 2257 – 2260
8. Tien R, Dillon WP, Jackler RK (1990) Contrast enhanced MR imaging of the facial nerve in 11 patients with Bell's palsy. AJNR 11 : 735 – 741

Eur Arch Otorhinolaryngology (1994) [Suppl]: S 358 – S 360

A. May, J. Nebe, M. Keidel, R. Verhagen, and H.C. Diener

Hemifacial Spasm Caused by Posterior Inferior Cerebellar Artery Elongation – Diagnostic Value of Angiomagnetic Resonance Imaging

Clinical Picture and Epidemiology

Hemifacial spasm (HFS) is characterized by painless unilateral involuntary contractions (spasm) of the mimic muscles innervated by the seventh cranial nerve. At the beginning of the disease, the contractions usually occur in the orbicularis oculi muscle and later on progress to involve the entire ipsilateral face over several years. Nevertheless, both bilateral occurrence [1] and familial incidence [2] are described in a few cases. HFS occurs with greater incidence on the left facial sice [3], with women being more affected than men (Ratio 2:1).

Tics, focal cortical seizures, blepharospasm, facial myokymia, tardive dyskinesia, and ephaptic excitation after Bell's palsy are easily distinguished by history, course, and clinical symptoms. Additionally, in testing the orbicularis oculi reflex, the finding of synchronous bursts of electromyographic activity in the orbicularis oculi and orbicularis oris muscles is pathognomic for HFS [4].

Pathogenesis

The etiology of HFS is believed to be an irritation of a "parabiotic" site along the course of the facial nerve. The most common cause is a chronic vascular compression of the nerve root by an aberrant or ectatic artery. As revealed during surgery, this is the case with the anterior inferior cerebellar artery (AICA) in 54%, the posterior inferior cerebellar artery (PICA) in 38%, the vertebral artery in 11%, and more than one vessel in 3% of cases [5]. More rarely, the compressing vessel is a vein near the central part of the facial nerve at the point in the pontocerebellar cisterna where the nerve leaves the brain stem.

Compression by larger arterial or arteriovenous malformations (AVM) or by tumors in the cerebellopontine angle (e.g., acoustic neuroma) are also described in the literature [6], as well as idiopathic spasm and those caused by damage of the nucleus due to pontine infarction [7].

A. May, J. Nebe, M. Keidel and H.C. Diener
Department of Neurology, University of Essen, Hufelandstr. 55, 45122 Essen, Germany

R. Verhagen
Department of Radiology, University of Essen, Germany

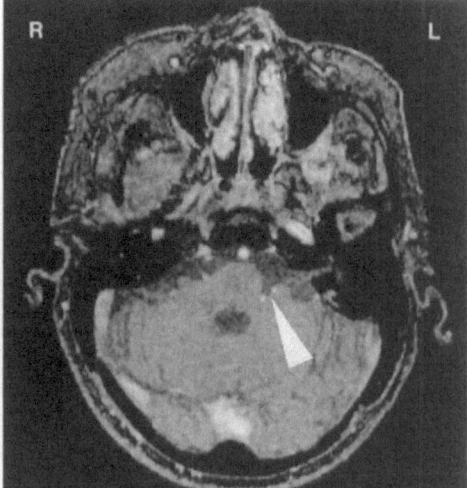

Fig. 1 Magnetic resonance tomogram of steady state free precession (SSFP) sequences: pons, cerebellum, and left facial as well as left vestibulocochlear nerve with neighbouring vascular loop (*arrow*)

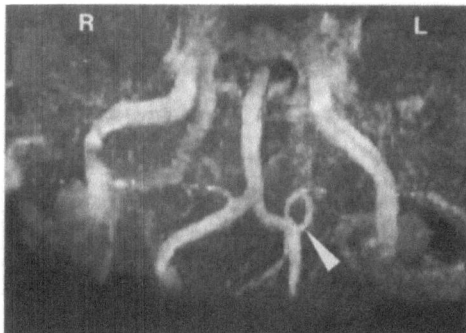

Fig. 2 Reconstruction of the skull base vessels by using magnetic resonance tomogram of steady state free precession (SSFP) sequences: identification of the vascular loop (*arrow*) of the left cerebellopontine angle as a segment of the left posterior inferior cerebellar artery

Radiological Diagnostics

Based on this theory of pathogenesis, before the introduction of magnetic resonance imaging (MRI), computerized tomography (CT) of the posterior fossa, with and without contrast media, was the prevalent screening method to demonstrate vascular compression in HFS. Cerebral angiography is generally reserved for patients without relevant findings in the auxillary examinations or for those with a planned operative microvascular decompression. With contrast medium MRI, it is possible to exclude a symptomatic HFS due to tumors or AVM and to demonstrate facial nerve compression by ectatic or elongated vessels. Just recently, the demonstration of cerebral vessels by MRI angiosequences has become available. Thus it has become possible to identify the arteries demonstrated in the conventional MRI.

To demonstrate the efficiency of angio-MRI in evaluating HFS, we present a case report of a patient with HFS who visited our clinic in November 1991.

Case Report

An otherwise healthy 34-year-old woman had a 2 1/2-year history of left primary HFS. Her symptoms began with painless twitching of the left orbicularis oculi muscle and progressed over the next year to involve the ipsilateral orbicularis oris muscle as well. There was no evidence of a facial palsy either in the previous history, by clinical neurological examination, or by electroneurography. Electromyographic responses following preauricular stimula-

tion of the seventh nerve showed synchronous bursts in the simultaneous recordings of the orbicularis oculi and oris muscles. Cranial CT scans and conventional roentgenograms of the internal acoustic meatus showed no pathological findings. Only with MRI could the etiology be shown to be a compression of the left facial nerve by a vessel in the pontocerebellar angle: MRI scans revealed a vessel located in the direct vacinity of the left facial nerve. The angiosequences of MRI identified the artery as the PICA and demonstrated the close relationship between nerve and artery in the cerebellopontine angle (Figs. 1 and 2).

Therapy

Microsurgical decompression of the facial nerve in the causal therapy. Despite of usually excellent results, there are complications in 3%–10% [8], the most common being a surgical lesion of the eight nerve with resulting hearing loss or deafness.

Alternatively, in short-lasting HFS, a therapeutic trial with carbamazepine (400–1000 mg per day) can be undertaken with the intention of neuron membrane stabilization. In recent years, local injections of botulinum A toxin into the orbicularis oculi muscle have been successfully introduced [9].

Conclusion

We report an example of the efficiency of MRI and angio-MRI in clarifying the etiology of HFS. We conclude that in the diagnosis of HFS, (noninvasive) angio-MRI is not only a supplementary, but rather an alternative technique to cerebral angiography. This holds true especially for those patients in whom other radiological findings are equivocal or in the early diagnosis of HFS when a surgical microvascular decompression is not indicated.

References

1. Holds JB, Anderson RL, Jordan DR, Patrinely JR (1990) Bilateral hemifacial spasm. J Clin Neuro Ophthalmol 10:153–154
2. Carter JB, Patrinely JR, Jankovic J, McCravy J, Boniuk M (1990) Familial hemifacial spasm. Arch Opthalmol 108:249–250
3. Schrader V (1987) Hemispasmus facialis. In: Brandt T, Dichgans J, Diener HC (eds) Therapie und Verlauf neurologischer Erkrankungen. Kohlhammer, Stuttgart, pp 70–71
4. Stöhr M (1987) In: Stöhr M, Bluthardt M (eds) Atlas der klinischen Elektromyographie und Neurographie. Kohlhammer, Stuttgart, p 67
5. Baba T, Matsushima T, Fukui M, Hasuo K, Yasumori K, Masuda K, Kuromatsu C (1988) Relationship between angiographical manifestations and operative findings in 100 cases of hemifacial spasm. No Shinkei Geka 16:1355–1362

6. Janetta PJ (1981) Hemifacial spasm. In: Samii M, Janetta PJ (eds) The cranial nerves. Springer, Berlin Heidelberg New York, pp 484–493
7. Kawamaki M, Sato T, Tochigi S, Ito T (1990) Lacunar pontine infarction with hemifacial spasm as the initial symptom. Stroke 21/8 : 1236
8. Janetta PJ (1986) Microvascular decompression for hemifacial spasm. In: May M (ed) The facial nerve. Thieme, New York, p 126
9. Elston JS (1992) The management of blepharospasm and hemifacial spasm. J Neurol 239 : 5–8

Eur Arch Otorhinolaryngology (1994) [Suppl]: S 361 – S 362

FREE PAPERS AND POSTERS

M. L. Navarrete, J. L. Fernández, P. Quesada, F. Casamitjana, and M. Pellicer

Computerized Tomography Demonstration of Labyrinthine Facial Nerve Decompression Viability by the Transattical Approach

Introduction

At present, total facial nerve decompression is the only therapeutic method to prevent the progression of the facial nerve lesion and its secondary sequelae. This method is also used for other causes of facial paralysis where the nerve lesion is located on the preganglionar facial nerve segment [1 – 6].

There are two surgical approaches to the three facial nerve segments: the combined middle fossa-transmastoid approach and the transattical-transmastoid one. The latter was described by Salaverry in 1974 and modified by us in 1979 [7, 8].

In order to overcome the existing scepticism about the labyrinthine facial nerve approach by this method (published by several authors), we made this confirmatory study by computed tomography (CT) scan in the postoperative period.

Material and Methods

We followed 16 patients with severe Bell's palsy, i. e., with more than 90 % degenerated nerve fibers. All were treated by total facial nerve decompression using the transattical-transmastoid approach. These patients were studied preoperatively by two dimensional CT scan to examine the labyrinthine facial nerve access through the attical cavity.

The postoperative confirmation of the labyrinthine facial nerve decompressin was made by two-dimensional CT scan at 45 – 60 days after surgical treatment.

M. L. Navarrete, J. L. Fernández, P. Quesada, F. Casamitjana, and M. Pellicer
Department of Otorhinolaryngology and Neuroradiology, Autonomous University of Barcelona, Spain

We performed the CT examination in axial projection, using tomographic sections of 1.2 mm every 1.5 mm with ultra-high resolution technique (Elscint 2400). The axial projection in the temporal bone study give the best visualization of the labyrinthine and tympanic facial nerve segments and the best attical area measure. These data are fundamental for estimating the transattical decompression viability.

We used the same method postoperatively to evaluate facial nerve decompression.

Results

In this study the results are only iconographic. On the basis of several tomographic attical sections performed after transattical facial decompression, we can see how the decompression area reached the first facial nerve portion (Figs. 1 – 3), confirming the viability of the labyrinthine facial nerve approach by the transattical approach.

Discussion

In our experience, a minimal attical area exists that theoretically mates the transattical-transmastoid approach viable. By CT scan, this area was evaluated as being 36 mm^2 [9]. In this way ce can evaluate the viability of the transattical approach before surgical treatment and confirm it during the operation. Later, these results are proved by high-resolution CT scan.

We have to point out that when performing the postoperative scan study it is useful to use axial and coronal tomographic sections. This helps a lot in attical radiological evaluation.

Although the efficiency of surgical decompression in Bell's palsy is doubted by some authors, this is the only treatment we can use at present to prevent progression of the facial nerve lesion and the establishment of secondary sequelae in patients who suffer from severe facial paralysis (more than 90% degenerated fibers) [1–5, 7, 10–12].

Nowadays, we have two approach techniques to achieve total facial nerve decompression: the combined middle fossa-transmastoid approach suggested by House in 1961 and the transattical-transmastoid approach proposed by Salaverry in 1974.

The transattical approach is an extralabyrinthine approach which reaches the labyrinthine facial nerve following a straight line beginning in the posterior zygomatic root and going on to the hammer head and semicircular horizontal and superior channels [7, 9]. This approach allows facial nerve decompression from its labyrinthine portion to the stylomastoid for amen. It has advantage of allowing total nerve exploration without performing a craniotomy. In 1979, using the ideas suggested by Bernstein [13], Pulec [3], and Salaverry [8], May developed the transmastoid-extralabyrinthine-subtemporal approach, similar to the transattical approach. He treated 92 cases of peripheral facial pàralysis, stating that the advantages of this technique outweigh the potential risk of middle and internal ear lesions [14]. However, in our experience this risk was not present, because hearing loss secondary to ossicular chain lesion is minimized after our technique, i.e., including the posterior zygomatic rout in the attical drilling and maximal chinning of the external auditory channel and tegumen tympani [7, 12].

The sensorineural hearing loss secondary to drill near the labyrinth can be prevented using serum irrigation at body temperature [12, 15].

However, the transattical approach has the disadvantage of being difficult when the attical cells are poorly developed. This has been observed in a small percentage of cases [10, 12]. This problem can be resolved by two-dimensional preoperative CT examination [9, 10]. In this case, we use a middle fossa approach.

Thus, in our experience concerning the similar results and the different risks involved in the two techniques, we propose the transattical approach as the treatment of choice in cases where a facial nerve decompression is indicated.

References

1. Fisch U (1981) Surgery for Bell's palsy. Arch Otolaryngol 107:1–11
2. Sterkers JM, Sterkers D (1983) Chirurgie du nerf facial. Encycl Méd Chir Paris 20260 A20
3. Pulec JL, (1966) Total decompression of the facial nerve. Laryngoscope 76:1015–1028
4. McCabe BF (1977) Some evidence for the efficacy of decompression of Bell's palsy: immediate motion postoperatively. Laryngoscope 87:2246–2249
5. Graham M, Kariush JM (1989) Total facial nerve decompression for recurrent facial paralysis: an update. Otorhinolaryngol Head Neck Surg. 101/4:442–444
6. May M (1985) Surgical rehabilitation of facial palsy: total approach. In: May M (ed) The facial nerve. Thieme, New York, pp 695–777
7. Quesada P, Lopez D (1984) Tratamiento quirúrgico de la parálisis facial. Ponencia Soc Esp ORL: 271–293
8. Salaverry MA (1974) Transattical approach. A technique variation for total decompression of the facial nerve. Rev Brasil Otorhinol 40:262–264
9. Navarrete ML, Pellicer M, Fernandez JL, Rovira A, Quesada P (1991) Predicción de la viabilidaó del abordaje transattical en la cirugia de decompresión del nervio facial. ORL Dips 3:148–154
10. Quesada P, Navarrete M, Fernandez JM, Gimeno V (1991) Estado actual del tratamiento quirurgico de la paralisis facial idiopática. ORL DIPS 3:138–142
11. Boedts B (1986) Facial nerve surgery. Acta Otorhinolaryngol Belg 40 1:179–186
12. Navarrete ML, Quesada P, Martinez MJ (1988) Indicaciones operatorias en la paralisis facial a frigore. Nervi craniales. Ponencia Soc Lat ORL: 346–350
13. Bernstein L (1961) A surgical approach to the tympanic portion of the facial nerve with methods of preoperative investigation. Ann Otorhinolaryngol 70:194–204
14. May M (1982) Transmastoid total facial nerve exploration for acute facial paralysis. In: Graham MD, House WF (eds) Disorders of the facial nerve. Raven, New York, pp 413–417
15. Navarrete ML, Quesada P (1991) Le traumatisme acoustique dans la chirurgie de decompression transatticale du nerf facial. Cahiers ORL XXVI 2:74–78

Eur Arch Otorhinolaryngology (1994) [Suppl]:S363

ABSTRACTS

M. Yanagida, K. Usihiro, T. Iwaho, C. Ino, Y. Hosada, and T. Kumazawa

Depiction of Affected Facial Nerve with Gd-DTPA Enhanced MRI

We performed enhanced MRI (using Gd-DTPA) in 91 patients with facial palsy to investigate the enhanced portion of the facial nerve.

We made MRI examinations in several stages in 70 patients with Bell's palsy. In many patients examined at an early stage of the disease, enhancement was seen in the central part of the facial nerve in segments of the internal auditory canal and labyrinthine; however, in patients examined in later stages enhancement was mainly observed in the peripheral areas such as horizontal and vertical segments. Even in the cases of repeated MRI (18 cases) for the same patient, the enhanced area tended to shift from the central peripheral areas with the passage of time.

In most patients with Ramsay Hunt syndrome, enhancement was shown in the segment of the internal auditory canal and labyrinth. This observation suggested that histological changes in the internal auditory canal and labyrinthine segment in patients with Ramsay Hunt syndrome were more intense than those in patients with Bell's palsy.

In a case of postoperative facial palsy, enhancement was observed in a vertical segment which had not been injured during surgery. And in a case of intracanalicular facial nerve schwannoma, intense enhancement was shown not only in the tumor itself but also in the labyrinthine, horizontal, and vertical segments. Our follow-up MR studies with Bell's palsy and these two cases indicated that the histological change of increased permeability shifts from the injured point to the peripheral side of the facial nerve with time.

M. Yanagida, K. Usihiro, T. Usihiro, C. Ino, Y. Hosoda, and T. Kumazawa
Department of Otolaryngology, Kansai Medical University Osaka, Japan

Eur Arch Otorhinolaryngology (1994) [Suppl]: S 364

ABSTRACTS

C. Wagner-Manslau and V. Bonkowski

Idiopathic Facial Nerve Palsy (Bell's Palsy): Morphological Changes in MRI

Purpose Indiopathic facial nerve palsy, so-called Bell's palsy, is thought to be a reactivation of herpes simplex virus located in the ganglion geniculi. The peripheral mastoideal part of the facialis nerve is thought to have a reactive edema. Does MRI show pathomorphological changes in virologically and immunologically positive cases?

Method and Material We investigated 24 patients within 24 h of the beginning of Bell's palsy, 3 with chronic palsy of the facial nerve and 1 after restitution of Bell's palsy using the following methods: SE-T2 and prot (TR 2000/ TE 30, 100), SE-T1 (TR 600/TE 30), and i.v. Gd-DTPA (0,1 mmol/kg).

Discussion In agreement with the literature the anatomy of the facialis nerve is easily reproducible. Virological, immunological, and histological studies indicate that the idiopathic facialis nerve palsy is caused by a reactivation of herpes simplex virus. The expected edema is seen in all acute cases as an abnormal enhancement or a prolonged T2 relaxation in the ganglion geniculi or in the mastoideal, labyrinthal, or meatal parts of the facial nerve.

Results

	n	Meatal	Labyrinthal	Ganglion	Meastoidal
Normal anatomy	50	No E	No E	No E	No E
Bell's palsy	24	1+, 3 (+)	8+, 3 (+)	8 T2+, 18 Gd +, 1 (+)	12+, 3 (+)
Chronic facial palsy	3	No E	No E	No E	No E

No E = no enhancement; +, enhancement after i. v. Gd-DTPA; (+), little enhancement; T2+, hyperintense in T2.

C. Wagner-Manslau and V. Bonkowski
Nuklearmedizinische Klinik, TU München, Ismaninger Str. 22,
81675 München, Germany

Eur Arch Otorhinolaryngology (1994) [Suppl]: S365

G. Oberascher and E. Doringer

High-Resolution Computed Tomography Imaging
of the Facial Nerve Canal in Temporal Bone Fractures

Injuries to the facial nerve canal in cases of temporal bone fractures can cause cosmetic and functional deficiencies according to the severity of facial paralysis. In order to obtain information on what imaging plane (axial/coronal) the injured canal can best be demonstrated, an experimental study on the temporal bone of traumatized cadavers was performed. Fractures of all parts of the facial nerve canal were inflicted under microscopic conditions and subjected to analysis. Usin petrosal bones specific of recently deceased patients. The specimens were examined by high-resolution computed tomography (HR-PCT). Varying degrees of sensitivity in the imaging of the different segments could be demonstrated. The following results were btained, from which conclusions could be established: (1) In cases of temporal bone fractures in combination with facial paralysis (immediate or delayed) axial and coronal HR-PCT in 1-mm planes should be performed. (2) The meatal and labyrinthine segment is best seen in the axial plane. (3) The best identification of the mastoidal portion is in the coronal plane. (4) The entire tympanic segment does not permit a satisfactory diagnosis as in the other segments, either in the axial or the coronal plane. (5) It is highly recommended that the labyrinthine segment be divided into proximal, ganglion geniculi, and distal regions.

Imaging of the temporal bone in trauma cases is a very helpful instrument for topodiagnostic identification of facial nerve canal injuries. In combination with clinical and electrophysical testing procedures the appropriate surgical approach can be chosen.

G. Oberascher
Department of Otolaryngology, General Hospital,
Müllner Hauptstr. 48, 5020 Salzburg, Austria

E. Doringer
Department of Radiology, General Hospital,
Müllner Hauptstr. 48, 5020 Salzburg, Austria

Eur Arch Otorhinolaryngology (1994) [Suppl]: S 366

ABSTRACTS

M. Toshima, S. Hashimoto, S. Koike, and T. Takasaka

Facial Palsy Due to Intracranial Vascular Lesion

Of the many disorders which may cause facial nerve palsy, vascular lesions in the cerebellopontine (CP) angle are uncommon. Two cases of such etiologies will be presented and discussed in this paper. The first case was that of a 73-year-old woman. She had suffered from left-sided incomplete facial nerve palsy for 2 months. She was referred to our clinic because therapy had not been effective. MR imaging revealed a mass lesion in the left CP angle adjacent to the left vertebral artery, which was proven to be an aneurysm by angiography. The second case was that of a 15-year-old girl. She was referred to our clinic for further examination and treatment of left-sided incomplete facial nerve palsy. Neurotological examination revealed left hearing loss, horizontal gaze nystagmus to the right, and hypesthesia of her left face. MRI revealed a mass lesion in the left CP angle with signal voids interpreted as hemosiderin deposits. Angiography was normal in that region. These findings suggested cavernous hemangioma in the left CP angle.

M. Toshima, S. Hashimoto, S. Koike, and T. Takasaka
Department of Otolaryngology, Tohoku University School
of Medicine, Sendai 980, Japan

Eur Arch Otorhinolaryngology (1994) [Suppl]: S367

ABSTRACTS

A. Kumar, M. Mafee, and M. Dailey

Imaging in the Differential Diagnosis of Facial Paralysis

Until recently, high-resolution computerized tomography was the imaging study of choice in the evaluation of facial paralysis. The disadvantage of this technique was that it was difficult to image the extracranial and intracranial segments of the nerve. Evidence of pathology in its intratemporal course was inferential, being judged by changes in density of bone surrounding the fallopian canal. Magnetic resonance imaging offers the clinician an advantage in that the whole course of the nerve can be imaged, and contrast enhancement can be used to detect pathology, since normal cranial nerves do not enhance. Can paralysis due to specific pathological disorders be diagnosed using this new technology? To answer this question we studied patients with facial paralyses secondary to multiple sclerosis, chronic granulomas, sarcoidosis, facial neuromas (both traumatic and neoplastic), isolated glomus tumor arising from the facial nerve, Ramsay Hunt syndrome, and cholesteatoma. On the basis of our experience, we conclude that when the information from imaging studies is combined with the clinical and electrophysiological data, an etiologic diagnosis can be achieved.

A. Kumar, M. Mafee, and M. Dailey
Department of Otolaryngology, Head- and Neck Surgery,
University of Illinois at Chicago, Chicago, USA

Eur Arch Otorhinolaryngology (1994) [Suppl]: S 368

J.M. Chen, C. Moll, and U. Fisch

Value of MRI and Intraoperative Frozen Sections in Defining the Extent of Facial Neurinoma

Seven cases of intratemporal facial neurinomas were treated between 1986 and 1991. Preoperative MRI studies and intraoperative frozen sections were used to determine the extent of the neurinoma infiltration. Gadolinium-enhanced MRI was helpful in planning the surgical approach, and in defining the extent of tumor involvement. Frozen sections on the other hand were often misleading, giving frequent false-positive reports of inadequate resection. Ultimately, tumor infiltration, especially in the proximal direction, is best judged by its gross intraoperative appearance under high magnification, with the aid of MRI.

Complete removal was achieved in all seven cases, with excellent functional outcome in those with a sufficiently long follow-up. The difficulty in establishing an intraoperative histologic diagnosis of neurinoma infiltration in the presence of organized neural fibers is emphasized.

J.M. Chen, C. Moll, and U. Fisch
ENT Department, University Hospital, 8091 Zürich, Switzerland

Eur Arch Otorhinolaryngology (1994) [Suppl]:S369

ABSTRACTS

G.-M. Sprinzl and W.F. Thumfart

Topographical Anatomy of the Facial Nerve

Introduction. An understanding of the anatomy of the facial nerve demands a high degree of three-dimensional imagination from ENT surgeons and anatomists. Because of its long intratemporal course as well as its branching in the parotid region, the facial nerve is often impaired by traumatic and tumorous processes. This contribution describes the topographical anatomy of the facial nerve from the surgical viewpoint. Special attention is paid to computerized examination of the (bone) density of the temporal bone.

Method. After removing the roof of the internal auditory meatus with a milling cutter in five temporal bones, the facial nerves were dissected. Five macerated temporal bones were embedded in plastic material and then sawn into parallel sections 1.5 mm in thickness. Radiographs taken from the sections were analyzed with the help of a computerized image analyzing system (Atari, Mockenhaupt, Cologne). These parts of the nerves, lying distal to the stylomastoid foramen, were dissected in a formalin-fixated head.

Results. The dissections presented accurately demonstrate all the peripheral parts of the facial nerve. Maximum density, mostly found in the area of the labyrinth, and minimum density, overall in the region of the tegmen tympani, show weak points in the osseous pattern of the temporal bone. The relationship between the parotid gland and the facial nerve is also presented.

Discussion. This complete description of the most important directional structures such as the internal auditory canal, the vertical crista (Bill's bar), the greater superficial petrosal nerve, the geniculate ganglion, the chorda tympani, the styloid process, and the parotid gland helps orientation in surgical dissection of the temporal bone as well as of the parotid gland area. High-resolution computed tomography today is the most important diagnostic method for the temporal bone. The radiographs of the sections give a better resolution and subsequent geometrical three-dimensional reconstruction.

G.-M. Sprinzl and W.F. Thumfart
Universitätsklinik für Hals-Nasen-Ohrenheilkunde Innsbruck,
Anichstr. 35, 6020 Innsbruck, Austria

Eur Arch Otorhinolaryngology (1994) [Suppl]: S 370

ABSTRACTS

A. L. Kossovoi

X-Ray Symptomatology of the Facial Canal Involvement in Chronic Otitis

Facial nerve is a well-recognized complication of chronic suppurative otitis. Clinical signs of chronic epitympanitis were investigated using the Schüller/Mayer modified Chausse III projection and lateral and anterior posterior tomography in 415 patients.

The facial canal appeared involved in 38 patients, and cholesteatoma developed in 34 of them. Destruction in the tympanic portion was found in 15 cases, the descending one in 18, and both sites in 5. The signs of tympanic portion involvement were observed in Chausse III view as the appearance of tympanic portion lumen with simultaneous thinning of the lower part of horizontal semicircular canal. The signs of descending portion involvement on lateral tomograms were the loss of the canal bony wall on its route through the destruction cavity in the mastoid.

Facial palsy developed in all patients with the tympanic portion lesion and in ten cases with the descending one. On operatin the walls of the fallopian canal proved to be destroyed at the compromised site in all patients.

A. L. Kossovoi
X-ray Department, Institute of Advanced Medical Studies,
St. Petersburg, Russia, 193015

Surgical Techniques

Eur Arch Otorhinolaryngology (1994) [Suppl]:S373–375

T. Kunihiro, T. Matsunaga, and J. Kanzaki

Clinical Investigation of Hypoglossal-Facial Nerve Anastomosis

Introduction

In our previous study of acoustic neuroma patients who had facial nerve paralysis after tumor resection, we reported that, in contrast to the result in those undergoing no reanimation procedures postoperatively, no apparent correlation was seen between the patients' self-estimation and the physician's evaluation of facial movement in those who had undergone hypoglossal-facial nerve anastomosis. In the present study, we have conducted a more systematic investigation about the correlation between these "subjective" and "objective" evaluations. On the basis of our results, we will discuss their clinical implications.

Materials and Methods

This study included 34 patients (male, 18; female, 16). Their ages ranged from 40 to 72 years (mean, 56.4 years). All patients had undergone hypoglossal-facial nerve anastomosis at the Department of Otolaryngology, Keio University Hospital 7 months to 9 years before assessment. Fifteen patients underwent this cross-nerve anastomosis because the facial nerve had been transected during acoustic neuroma removal, and single-stage intracranial reconstruction had not been feasible. Sixteen patients underwent this procedure because of poor restoration of facial function despite anatomical preservation of the facial nerve. In the remaining three patients, it was performed because of no or poor return of facial function despite prior intracranial

reconstruction. Acoustic neuroma removal had also been performed in all patients at the Department of Otolaryngology, Keio University Hospital.

The senior author (TK) interviewed 28 of the patients and evaluated their facial movements according to Yanagihara's three-rating scale [1] and House's grading system [2]. After each interview, TK handed a questionnaire to the patient, which was mailed back to TK after being filled out. Six other patients also responded to the questionnaire, although their facial movement was not assessed. (Their data was included in the analysis of the subjective evaluations only.) The questionnaire included the following two questions among others: (1) "How many points out of 100 would you give your facial movements, in comparison with your 'normal' facial movements prior to your acoustic neuroma operation?" and (2) "How satisfied are you with your present facial movements: a, satisfied; b, fairly satisfied; c, not very satisfied or dissatisfied?" We then analyzed the relationships among these four parameters.

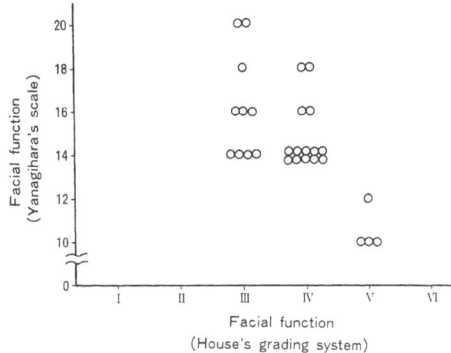

Fig. 1 Relatinship between two objective evaluations (Yanagihara's scale vs. House's grading system)

T. Kunihiro
Department of Otolaryngology, National Yokohama Hospital

T. Matsunaga and J. Kanzaki
Department of Otolaryngology, School of Medicine,
Keio University, 35 Shinanomachi, Shinjuku-ku, Tokyo 160, Japan

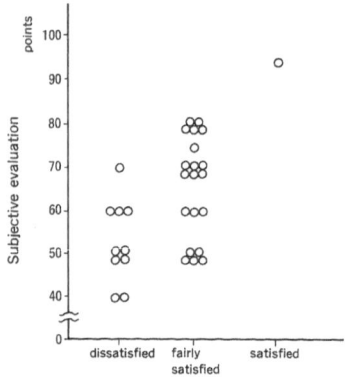

Fig. 2 Relationship between subjective evaluation and overall satisfaction. A significant difference was found in distribution between the groups of "dissatisfied" and "fairly satisfied" ($p < 0.05$)

Results

When evaluated according to House's grading system, facial function was classified as grade III in 10 patients and grade IV in 14 patients, whereas in the remaining 4 patients, it was classified as grade V. According to Yanagihara's scale, on the other hand, all patients fell between 10 and 20 points (mean, 14.7 points). No significant difference was found in distribution between grade III and grade IV ($p = 0.11$), but grade V showed a significantly lower range of distribution than grade III or grade IV ($p < 0.05$) (Fig. 1).

The subjective evaluation scores ranged from 40 to 95 points (mean, 63.0 points). No significant difference was found between the sexes ($p > 0.05$). As regards overall satisfaction, 9 patients answered "satisfied" and 15 patients "fairly satisfied," while the remaining 8 patients answered "not very satisfied" or "dissatisfied." Two patients did not answer this question. There was a positive correlation between the subjective evaluation and overall satisfaction (Fig. 2).

In contrast, no significant correlation was detected between the objective and subjective evaluations ($p > 0.05$) (Fig. 3a, b). Nor was overall satisfaction significantly correlated with the objective evaluations ($p > 0.05$). (Fig. 4a, b).

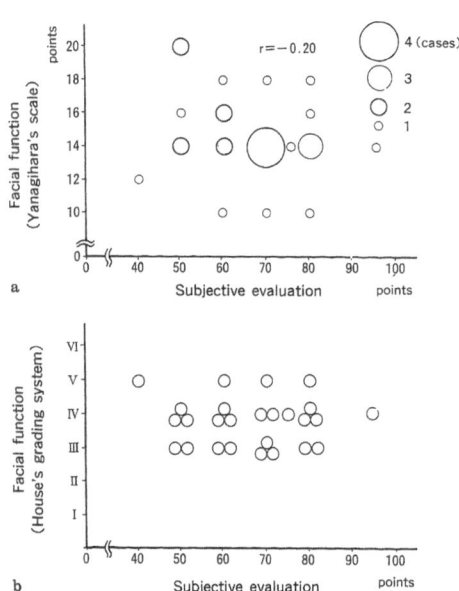

Fig. 3 Relationship between objective and subjective evaluations. **a** Yanagihara's scale vs. subjective evaluation; **b** House's grading system vs. subjective evaluation

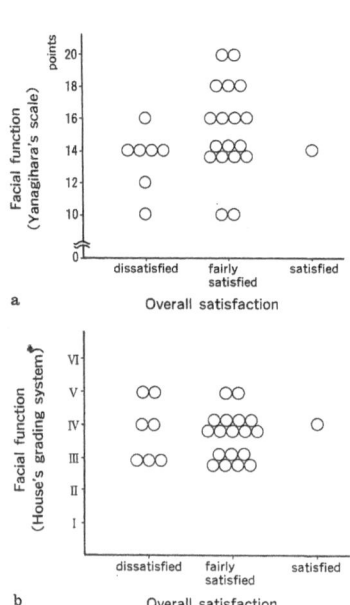

Fig. 4 Relationship between objective evaluation and overall satisfaction. **a** Yanagihara's scale vs. overall satisfaction; **b** House's grading system vs. overall satisfaction.

Discussion

This study substantiated the results of our previous investigations [3, 4]. Although we evaluated the patients' facial movements according to House's grading system in addition to Yanagihara's three-rating scale in this study, no significant correlation was detected between the objective and subjective evaluations in either case.

This seems to be partly explained by the fact that the patients never obtained normal facial movements as a result of hypoglossal-facial nerve anastomosis. All patients suffered from various degrees of sequelae. These included mass movements, hypertonia, blepharoptosis, and hypoglossal nerve paralysis. These sequelae may have negatively affected the patients' overall satisfaction, and thus their subjective evaluation in a way that was unanticipated. In fact, even among patients who did not undergo any facial reanimation procedure, the correlation coefficient between objective and subjective evaluations was only 0.26 in the subgroup of patients whose facial function was 10–20 points [3]. The patients' psychological status may also give a partial explanation. We reported in the previous study [5] that the patients' subjective evaluation was inversely proportional to their score on the Self-Rating Questionnaire for Depression. Pensak et al. [6] pointed out that patients who dealt with their debilities most readily expressed appreciation for the close patient-physician relationship they experienced and that many of these patients noted a high degree of empathy from coworkers and family. In addition, unrealistic expectations of patients before undergoing this cross-nerve procedure may also have lowered subjective evaluation and overall satisfaction in varying degrees.

The results of this study imply the importance of sufficient prior explanation concerning the facial movements that can be expected after hypoglossal-facial nerve anastomosis. Or, a new grading system may be required for evaluating the facial movements of patients who undergo facial nerve reconstruction procedures.

References

1. Yanagihara N (1977) Grading of facial palsy. In: Fisch U (ed) Facial nerve surgery. Aesculapius, Birmingham/USA, pp 533–536
2. House JW (1983) Facial nerve grading systems. Laryngoscope 93:1056–1069
3. Kanzaki J (1990) Surgical treatment of acoustic neuroma (in Japanese) ORL (Tokyo) 33 [Suppl 3]: 380–387
4. Kunihiro T, Kanzaki J, O-Uchi T (1991) Hypoglossal-facial nerve anastomosis – clinical observation. Acta Otolaryngol Suppl (Stockh) 487:80–84
5. Kunihiro T, Kanzaki J, O-Uchi T, Ogawa K, Harada T (1991) Further study of the evaluation methods for the facial function after hypoglossal-facial nerve anastomosis (in Japanese). Otol Jpn 1:71–75
6. Pensak ML, Jackson CG, Glasscock ME III, Gulya AJ (1986) Facial reanimation with the VII–XII anastomosis: analysis of the functional and psychologic results. Otolaryngol Head Neck Surg 94:305–310

Eur Arch Otorhinolaryngology (1994) [Suppl]: S376 – S377

L. Bignardi and C. Aimoni

Salvage Decompression of the Facial Nerve

Introduction

Ischemia and inflammation phenomena, as well as demyelinization of the nervous fibers, play an important role in the multifactorial etiology of the so-called idiopathic facial nerve paralysis (IP), either of viral or immune origin. Conventional therapies, which consist of vasodilatatives, cortisone, and more recently antivirals have not proved effective in changing the natural evolution of facial paralysis. It is widely acknowledged that idiopathic palsy has a favorable evolution in most cases (84% according to Peitersen). It has also been suggested that surgical treatment based on accurate neurophysiological principles be used [2]. It is under discussion whether in cases of late facial paralysis functional recovery can be achieved through surgery, when neither a waiting conduct nor medical therapy has led to a noticeable real recovery of the nervous function.

The aim of our work was to show the results of surgical salvage decompression carried out on eight cases of idiopathic palsy observed at the ENT Clinic of Ferrara in the period 1983 – 1991. The long "lag period" between the onset of palsy and decompression and the satisfactory quality of the results, evaluated with the visual method of Ralli et al. [6], 6 – 8 months after surgery, enabled us to reconsider the real advantages of "delayed" surgical decompression, in the cases of idiopathic paralysis which do not give a response to traditional therapies.

Methods and Materials

We carefully studied eight cases of VII idiopathic paralysis at the ENT Clinic of Ferrara between 1983 and 1992. The patients were 4 females and 4 males aged between 3 and 52

L. Bignardi and C. Aimoni
ENT Clinic, University of Ferrara, Italy

years. Most patients (6/8) complained at the early phase of the idiopathic paralysis of retroauricular pain, radiating into the nape, face, and pharynx. All patients had undergone careful ENT, neurological, and oculistic evaluation, and the following examinations were made: pure-tone audiogram and stapedial reflex test; Schirmer's test; laboratory tests; electromyography (EMG); CT of petrous bones (four out of eight cases): normal; MNR (one case): normal.

Patients with idiopathic paralysis were observed at our clinic after a valuable period of time from the onset of the disease (2 days – 10 months); in this time lapse they underwent cortisone therapy (prednisone) and neurotrophic and vasoactive therapy, and they were observed using a periodical EMG test.

On the basis of Ralli et al.'s proposal on the assessment of mimic muscle functionality (according to House's grading), we expressed the static and dynamic deficiency of the three facial muscle groups (forehead, eye, mouth) as a grading (0–4) relative to their capacity for voluntary contraction.

In three out eight cases the mimic muscles functionality proved to be totally damaged (= 0%); the other five patients showed ranges between 10% and 45%. No real improvement of the mimic muscle functions was observed in the patients after the medical therapy and/or in relation to the long period of presurgical observation, while from the EMG examination we observed a progressive depletion of the nervous regenerative capacity.

In our series of cases the shortest interval between the onset of paralysis and decompression was 10 weeks, the longest 40, with an average of 20 weeks. Three out of eight patients underwent opening of the fallopian canal as far as the geniculate ganglion, after the incus had been removed which had previously been reinserted. In all cases we opened the epineurium right along the tympanic and mastoid segments; facial nerve segments, whose epineurium has been disconnected, were covered with abdominal fat.

The surgical findings were in all cases of perineural edema and in one case there were signs of previous hemorrhage. Together with these vascular changes, evident signs of nervus structure damage were noticed in two patients with the longest waiting times.

The clinical-instrumental evaluation of the functional recovery of the three facial muscle groups was carried out using the visual method of Ralli et al., at the following times: 2 weeks after surgical operation and 2, 6, and 8 months after operation.

The results of the fourth postoperative examination proved to be effective and steady during the subsequent follow-up. At the first postoperative examination carried out 2 weeks after decompression, six out of eight patients had a facial muscle recovery of between 10% and 50%; while two out of eight patients had a recovery of between 55% and 60%. At the second examination carried out 2 months after surgery, four out of the eight patients had achieved a full functional recovery (100%); the other four had a recovery of between 50% and 90%. Six months after the operation eight out of the eight patients obtained a full functional recovery (100%) and this situation remained unchanged at the subsequent follow-up.

Facial nerve decompression, according to the above indicated technique, has not in any case involved complications and relevant sequelae (transmissive or neurosensory hearing loss, tinnitus, cerebral fluid leak, infections). In three out of the eight patients chorda tympani section showed no relevant complications. In three out of the eight patients it was necessary to remove the incus, which had been reinserted in order to open the facial canal as far as the geniculate ganglion.

Conclusion and Discussion

We have already stated that, essentially paralysis generally has a favorable prognosis even without surgery. However, it has to be acknowledged that the recovery of the nervous functions can have better results through facial nerve surgery rather than with any other therapy, in selected cases, when surgery is performed within 5 days from the onset of the paralysis and includes the labyrinthine segment.

It is also true that, at least in Italy we face long-standing inaction, since neurologists have worried about their EMG signs of unfavorable evolution and patients have asked for medical improvement of their condition.

Our experience is relevant to this kind of observation and offers as a solution the resort to a sort of compromise surgery. This compromise is based substantially on the failure of any kind of treatment or therapy and on the requirements of our patients. This compromise refers to surgery which has been limited to the tympanic-mastoid segments of the nerve. This limitation has been brought in with the aim of improving the cost-benefit relationship of surgery, considering that serious sequelae can turn up during labyrinthine tract decompression. This "Italian" solution has led in the observed cases to very satisfactory results and to no relevant sequelae. Apart from any consideration on the spontaneous recovery of facial muscle functions, hardly to be expected with longstanding paralysis, we think that edema and inflammation, which characterize the pathogenesis of idiopathic paralysis and lead to structural compression of the nerve in the narrowest tract of the fallopian canal, can be discharged and drained with decompression distal to the critical site of entrapment. As a result even conditions of the nervous segment which has not been treated can improve and a feedback mechanism can be interrupted.

References

1. Adour KK (1991) Medical management of idiopatic (Bell's) palsy. Otolaryngol Clin North Am 24 (3)
2. Fish U (1991) Surgery for Bell's palsy. Arch Otolaryngol 107
3. Marsh MA, Coker NJ (1991) Surgical decompression of idiopatic facial palsy. Otolaryngol Clin North Am 24 (3)
4. May M, Klein SR (1983) Facial nerve decompression complications. Laryngoscope 93
5. May M, Klein SR, Taylor FH (1985) Idiopathic (Bell's) facial palsy: natural history defies steroid or surgical treatment. Laryngoscope 95
6. Ralli G, Magliulo G, Parisi L (1987) Riflesso stapediale e paralisi di Bell. Sua evoluzione nella prima settimana di malattia. Acta Otorhinol (Ital) 7 : 495 – 500

Eur Arch Otorhinolaryngology (1994) [Suppl]: S 378–S 379

FREE PAPERS AND POSTERS

S. Hashimoto, T. Chiba, M. Toshima, S. Koike, and T. Takasaka

Is Facial Nerve Decompression Surgery Effective?

Introduction

Since steroid therapy has been proven to be effective on facial nerve palsy, many doctors have abandoned facial nerve decompression surgery (FND), and it is usually used only for traumatic facial palsy. However, there are still a few cases which cannot be cured by steroid therapy. With such cases or the cases which were not properly treated, we have used FND in the late period. In this paper, the results of this surgery are reported and its effectiveness is discussed.

Materials

The indication for FND is: (1) there is no sign of recovery after more than 3 months from the onset of palsy and (2) no response is seen in the nerve excitability test (NET) or less than a 10% response with electroneuronography (ENoG), regardless of how the patient was treated initially. During the 3 years of the study, we have operated on eight patients (Table 1) excluding traumatic facial palsy. Of these cases, four were Bell's palsy and another four were Ramsay-Hunt syndrome. Three patients had initially been treated by high-dose steroid therapy (two patients in our clinic and one patient elsewhere), and four patients by conventional dose steroid therapy (initial dose, predonisolone 60 mg or less) elsewhere. Another patient had not been treated at the time of onset because he was a fisherman in the Pacific ocean.

The operation was performed with the patient under general anesthesia using the transmastoid approach. In seven cases, the tympanic and the mastoid segment of the facial nerve was fully exposed and the nerve sheath was opened. In one case, only the mastoid segment was decompressed because the stapedial reflex was positive. In every case, various grades of neural edema were observed and no nerve atrophy was noted.

Table 1 Case summary

Case	Diagnosis	Previous treatment	Score (%)	Op. days
K.O.	Hunt	HDS	10	136
B.S.	Hunt	Steroid	5	116
K.M.	Hunt	None	8	80
H.S.	Bell's	Steroid	5	118
A.M.	Bell's	HDS	20	120
T.T.	Bell's	HDS	15	104
Y.S.	Bell's	Steroid	15	108
E.S.	Hunt	Steroid	10	110

Op. days, days from onset of palsy to operation; HDS, high-dose steroid therapy.

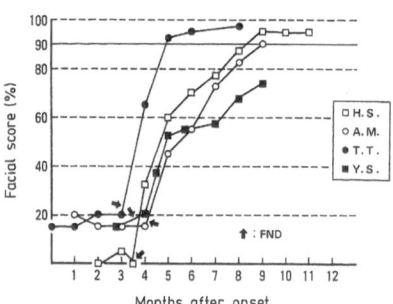

Bell's palsy

t : FND

☐ H.S.
○ A.M.
● T.T.
■ Y.S.

Fig. 1 Course of recovery, Bell's palsy. *Arrows* indicate the time of surgery. Note that every case shows quick recovery within 1 month after surgery. Case Y.S. is still recovering

S. Hashimoto (✉), T. Chiba, M. Toshima, S. Koike, and T. Takasaka
Department of Otolaryngology, Tohoku University School
of Medicine, 1-1 Seiryo-cho, Aoba, Sendai 980, Japan

Hunt's syndrome

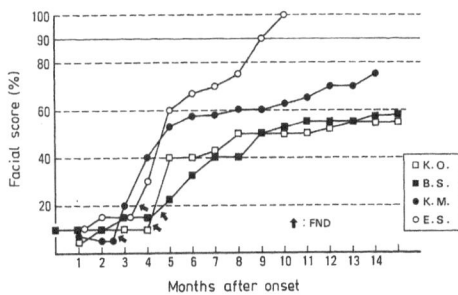

Fig. 2 Course of recovery, Ramsay-Hunt syndrome. *Arrows* indicate the time of surgery

Results

After surgery, all patients started to recover within 1 month and four patients fully recovered with a facial score of 90% or more without obvious synkinesis or contraction (House-Blackmann grade I or II) in 6 months. Two patients of Ramsay-Hunt syndrome showed moderate recovery with a facial score of around 60% (House-Blackmann grade III). The other two patients are still recovering (Figs. 1, 2).

Discussion

Facial nerve decompression surgery (FND) was once a popular and major therapy for idiopathic facial palsy (Bell's palsy). However, since Stennert [3], Adour [1], and others proved its efficacy on Bell's palsy, steroid therapy has become very popular and it is almost certain that steroid therapy should be the first choice. In contrast, FND has become to be applied less frequently. There exists great controversy as to whether or not to operate on the patient with Bell's palsy.

Nevertheless, there are a few patients who show complete denervation of the facial nerve and show no signs of recovery even after high-dose steroid therapy. There are also patients who suffer from severe sequelae after inappropriate therapy such as vitamins or stellate ganglion blocks. We operated on eight such patients after 80–136 days from the onset of palsy. We included the patients who suffered from severe palsy after Ramsay-Hunt syndrome because the main pathology of its facial palsy is also considered to be entrapment neuropathy.

Timing of Surgery

The timing of surgery is also a controversial subject. It has been believed that surgery should be performed in the early period of the disease to prevent the progression of nerve degeneration. After treating 90 patients with Bell's palsy and 9 patients with Ramsay-Hunt syndrome by high-dose steroid therapy in our clinic, only 2 patients failed to recover. All other patients showed signs of recovery within 3 months from the onset of palsy even after severe denervation (no response in NET). Thus, in the early period of palsy, there is a good chance of recovery after steroid therapy. We think that there is no reason to give up the possibility of recovery without surgical intervention and that a patient will show signs of recovery within 3 months if he or she does recover. Therefore, we decided to wait for at least 3 months.

Extent of Decompression

The labyrinthine segment of the facial nerve is considered to be the main site of entrapment neuropathy as described by Fish and Felix [2]. It has also been stated that neural edema usually progresses distally after initial injury of the facial nerve. Thus, in the late period of the disease, neural edema may still exist in the tympanic and mastoid segment. On the other hand, the edema in the labyrinthine segment and geniculate ganglion will disappear earlier because these portions have easy access from the internal auditory meatus of facial hiatus. We think that the main site of entrapment neuropathy in the late period is the tympanic and/or mastoid segment. This is one of the reasons why we use the transmastoid approach instead of the middle fossa approach. Another reason is that this procedure is a safe operation compared with the middle fossa approach, which is more risky and might be life threatening. As the best result is not guaranteed by any type of surgery, one cannot offer a risky procedure. FND by the transmastoid approach does no harm to the nerve as long as the surgery is carefully and well executed without touching the nerve itself during bone work, and is effective as described above.

After surgery, all patients started to recover within 1 month although the timing of surgery varied. This result indicates that this operation initiated the recovery. We conclude that facial nerve decompression surgery is effective and should be used if the initial treatment has failed.

References

1. Adour KK, Hetzler DG (1984) Current medical treatment for facial palsy. Am J Otolaryngol 5:499–502
2. Fish U, Felix H (1983) On the pathogenesis of Bell's palsy. Acta Otolaryngol (Stockh) 95:532–538
3. Stennert E (1979) Bell's palsy – a new concept of treatment. Arch Otorhinolaryngol 225:265–268

Eur Arch Otorhinolaryngology (1994) [Suppl]: S380–S382

FREE PAPERS AND POSTERS

K. Nakamura, S. Murakami, T. Kozawa, and N. Yanagihara

Surgical Treatment of Synkinesis

Introduction

Synkinesis is the most troublesome and common sequela seen in the recovery course of facial nerve palsy. However, no appropriate treatment has been developed so far. We used selective neurectomy on two patients with synkinesis and obtained good results; this technique has often been utilized for hemifacial spasm.

Case 1

The first patient was a 59-year-old female. Six years ago she suffered from left facial palsy and had recovered incompletely in 6 months. She subsequently complained of involuntary contraction of her shoulder during speaking. She also had ptosis and some other synkinesis. Contraction of the platysma while whistling was noted. Before surgery the route of the cervical branch and the marginal mandibular branch was percutaneously mapped, checking the contraction of the lower lip and the platysma with electrostimulation. A skin incision was made along the supposed line on the cervical branch. Three cervical branches could be recognized beneath the platysma and were directly electrostimulated to obtain functional mapping. According to the result it was decided which branch to amputate. A section of the nerve branch was cut off, about 1 cm long at the electrostimulated point. Other synkinesis involving the eye closure was still seen but suspension surgery brought good symmetry. Especially the synkinesis involving the platysma almost disappeared and the mimetic movement seemed to be satisfactory and no recurrence of her complaint was observed for 2 years after surgery (Fig. 1).

Case 2

The second patient was a 75-year-old female. Four years ago she suffered from right facial palsy and achieved incomplete recovery. She subsequently complained of high-grade synkinesis between the orbicularis oris muscle and the orbicularis oculi muscle. When she whistled, her eye was completely closed. Preoperatively the route of the branches was transcutaneously mapped using electrostimulation. Here it is important to find the most peripheral point that the orbicularis oculi and oris muscles are simultaneously contracted. After mapping, nerve block was tried using 1–2 ml 2% lidocaine around the zygomatic branch. The result of this suggested neurectomy had the potential to stop the synkinesis. Surgery was performed in the same way as superficial parotidectomy. The facial nerve was dissected as much as possible. Each branch was functionally investigated by electrostimulation. The branch through which both the orbicularis oculi and oris muscle are simultaneously contracted was selected for neurectomy. Other branches which innervated separately to the orbicularis oculi and oris muscle were preserved as much as possible. Three branches were amputated. Each branch selected was temporarily blocked by placing a piece of cotton soaked with 2% lidocaine. After this procedure the nerve trunk was stimulated to check what effect could be obtained. If the blocking effect was not enough, additional anesthetics were needed. Electrostimulation of each branch was performed in order to confirm the blocking effect. After this procedure, neurectomy was performed and the nerve ends were ligated with silk thread to prevent the start of sprouting. Mimetic movement after surgery appeared to be satisfactory. Complete eye closure followed by whistling was much reduced and the eye and mouth could be moved separately (Fig. 2).

K. Nakamura (✉), S. Murakami, T. Kozawa, and N. Yanagihara
Department of Otolaryngology, Ehime University School
of Medicine, Shigenobu-cho, Onsen-gun, Ehime 791-02, Japan

Fig. 1 Mimetic movement before and after surgery of case 1. Symmetry of the face was recovered with suspension of the left upper eyelid. *Upper*, preoperative; *lower*, postoperative

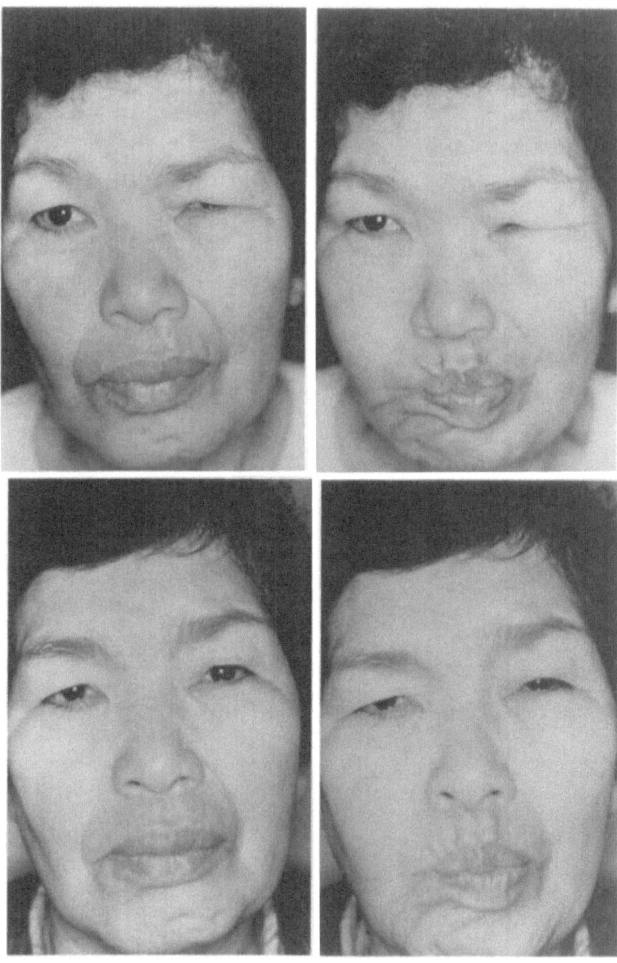

Discussion

The principle of selective neurectomy is to control the hyperkinesis of a muscle by replacing with palsy. Therefore, only for the case in which postoperative palsy is evaluated to be much more comfortable than the preoperative symptoms, neurectomy will be applicable for synkinesis. From this standpoint, neurectomy of the cervical branch is thought to be an effective treatment for synkinesis involving the platysma.

The cause of synkinesis is thought to be misdirection of the nerve fibers of the intratemporal segment. Therefore,

selective neurectomy is not a radical treatment for this pathological change but a treatment just for symptoms. However, this surgery seems to be helpful for the control of severe synkinesis.

When neurectomy is utilized for surgical treatment of synkinesis, the following points are crucial. To find the nerve which causes synkinesis and cut it through completely is essential, but avoiding excessive neurectomy is also important because many patients with synkinesis have incomplete recovery of facial palsy. Intraoperative nerve block using local anesthetics is very useful to estimate the effect of neurectomy and to avoid excessive neurectomy.

Fig. 2 Mimetic movement before and after surgery of case 2. Complete eye closure followed by whistling was much reduced. *Right*, preoperative; *left*, postoperative

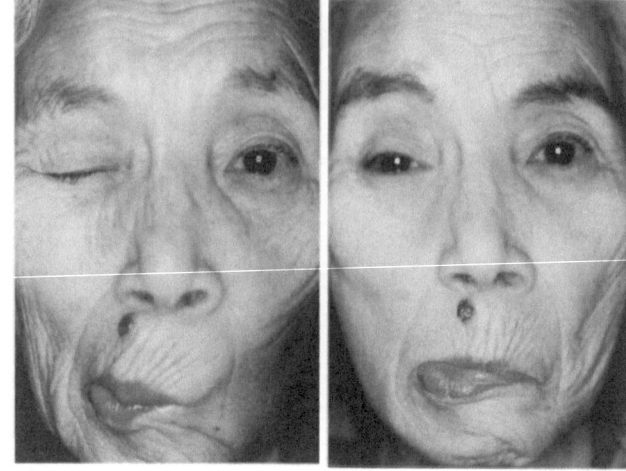

Eur Arch Otorhinolaryngology (1994) [Suppl]:S383–S386

J. B. Anon, S. P. Lipman, W. Thumfart, and D. A. Sibly

Parotidectomy with the Nerve Integrity Monitor II

Introduction

While the technique of parotidectomy is well described in multiple surgical atlases, techniques of monitoring the facial nerve during this surgery have had little emphasis. Probably the most commonly employed method is having the surgical assistant keep a constant view of the face and warn the surgeon of any facial motion. This may be supplemented with stimulation by small, disposable handheld probes or larger battery-operated units. Since 1988 we have been using the Xomed Nerve Integrity Monitor II (NIM II). This device allows the surgeon to continuously monitor the facial muscle electromyographic (EMG) signals via needle electrodes placed within specific muscles of the face. These signals are displayed via waveform on a monitor with an accompanying audible output. With this technique of monitoring the facial nerve, we feel that safer parotidectomy surgery can be performed.

Technique

Following induction of general anesthesia, the patient is prepared and draped in the usual fashion for parotidectomy surgery. We have found that self-adhesive plastic drapes allow full visualization of the entire face beyond the sterile surgical field. A NIM II electrode is shown in Fig. 1. The electrodes are placed in a sterile manner as shown in Fig. 2. The forehead electrode (arrow #1) is the patient ground. There are two active electrodes inserted into the orbicularis oculi muscle (arrow #2) and two active electro-des inserted inferiorly into the region of the orbicularis oris muscle (arrow #3). The lead wires are then fed underneath the drapes and are attached to the NIM II monitoring device, which is off the surgical field. Once these facial electrodes have been positioned, a sixth negative (anode) electrode is inserted into the patient's contralateral shoulder (not shown). This negative electrode creates a return for electric current from the stimulator.

Once all of the electrodes have been properly inserted, the resistance of the electrode system itself need to be established. A maximum resistance of $10\,000\,\Omega$ is desired to eliminate external noise factors. It should also be noted that the NIM II has muting circuitry so that when a cautery device is activated, the monitor will automatically be bypassed until the cauterization current has been deactivated. Following a check of the electrodes, the resting muscle activity is subsequently measured (approximately 30 mV or less). Increases in electrical activity within the muscle will be displayed visually and audibly on the NIM II.

Surgery begins in the usual fashion; Fig. 3 shows a parotid gland exposed. The facial nerve is identified and stimulated by the NIM II handheld probe. This stimulator probe has an adjustable electrical range from 0.05 mA to 3.0 mA. There is insulation up to the very tip of the probe to prevent electrical interference. As the region of the facial nerve is approached, a setting of 1.0 mA is utilized. For direct stimulation of the nerve, a setting of 0.25 mA is used. We never exceed 1.0 mA throughout.

J. B. Anon, S. P. Lipman, W. Thumfart, and D. A. Sibly
Saint Vincent Health Center Laser Ear, Nose and Throat
Surgery of Erie, Peach Street Medical Building, 3580 Peach Street,
Suite 106, Erie, PA 16508 814/864-9994, USA
and University Ear, Nose and Throat Clinic, Innsbruck, Austria

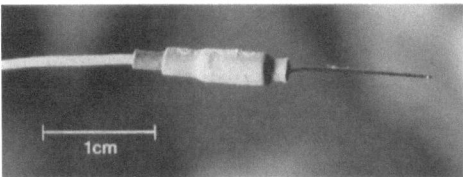

Fig. 1 A Nerve Integrity Monitor (NIM) II electrode

Fig. 2 Placing of electrodes. *1*, Patient ground. *2*, Orbicularis oculi muscle. *3*, Orbicularis oris muscle region (see text for details)

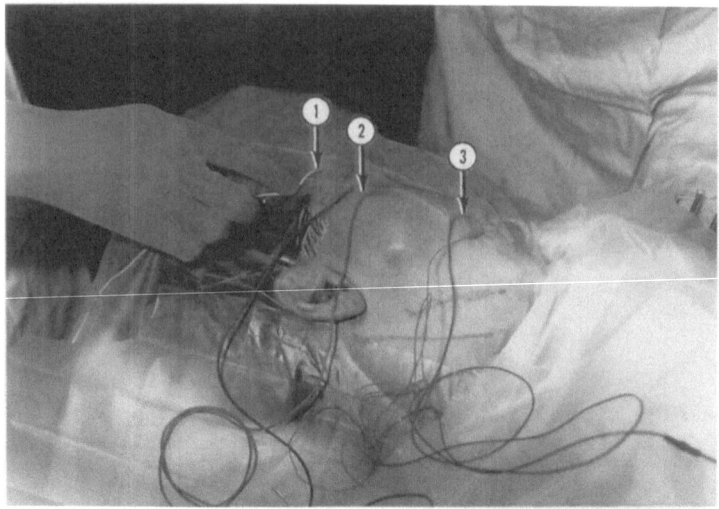

Fig. 3 Parotid gland exposed

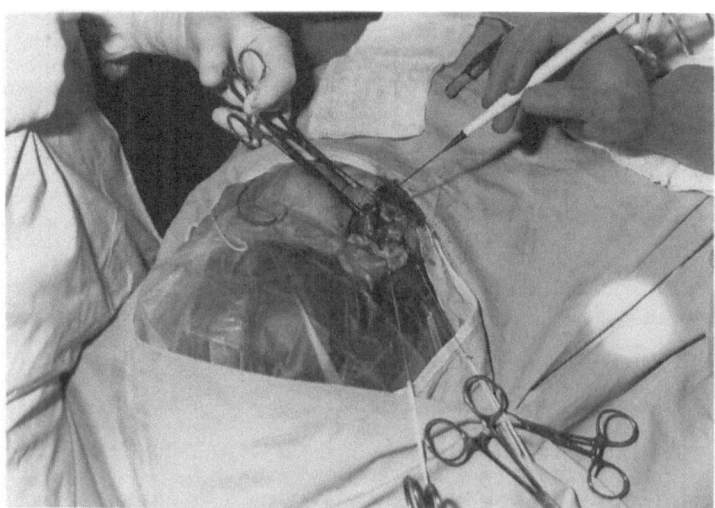

As surgery progresses and the branches of the facial nerve are followed, the NIM II monitor shows ongoing EMG activity. If the nerve is stimulated directly, such as with the probe or a surgical instrument which is dissecting too closely to the nerve, there will be an increase in the EMG activity greater than the aforementioned 30 mV. This change is registered as a sinusoidal waveform as shown in Fig. 4. Artifacts such as two metal instruments touching each other in the surgical field will yield a very sharp waveform with no time duration between the upward and downward peaks. This is demonstrated in Fig. 5. Also, as mentioned earlier, these waveforms are accompanied by

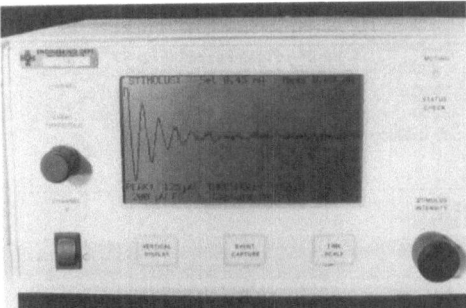

Fig. 4 Increase in electromyographic (EMG) activity (sinusoidal waveform) on direct stimulation of nerve

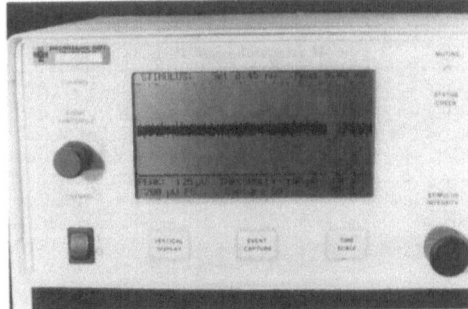

Fig. 6 Traction stimulation

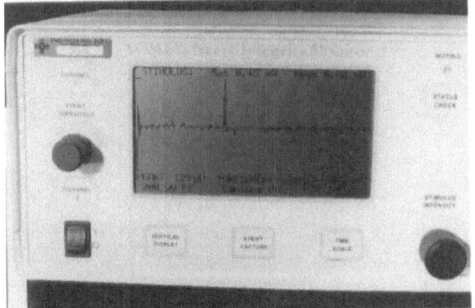

Fig. 5 Sharp waveform produced when two metal instruments touch

somewhat distinctive tones. With experience, the surgeon is able to distinguish some differences in waveform based upon sound alone.

Another advantage of the NIM II is the ability to measure the amount of stretching of the facial nerve. Often during surgery when the nerve is not monitored, the surgeon has the assistant stop retracting the parotid gland in order to let the facial nerve rest. This supposedly prevents the temporary palsy that can occur after parotidectomy by reducing the tension on the facial nerve. (It also has the advantage of allowing the surgeon a moment's respite from the tedious surgical dissection!) The continuous NIM II monitoring of the status of the facial nerve allows the surgeon to know when the nerve is being overstimulated by direct traction. This traction stimulation is shown in Fig. 6, where an abundance of EMG activity is noted across the entire screen. When this occurs, the assistant should relax tension on the nerve and within a short while the EMG activity rapidly declines and the surgery can proceed safely.

Results

To date, we have done approximately 40 parotidectomies using the NIM II monitor. Of these, two patients developed permanent palsy of a branch of the facial nerve. Both of these patients had malignancies that were intimately associated with the nerve and required more aggressive dissection. Two patients, also with malignancies, had facial nerves closely approximated to the tumor; however, the resultant postoperative palsies were temporary.

We are unable to accurately compare the results to our cases prior to using the NIM II monitor as one of the main surgeons (J.B. Anon) began using this monitor immediately after his residency training.

Discussion

We feel the NIM II monitor has added a margin of safety to the surgery which was previously not available. As our experience with this device has grown, there are several key points which need to be emphasized. First, it is important that the technician in charge of the device be very familiar with the equipment. Our technicians are electroencephalogram (EEG) technicians who have had extra training in monitoring techniques. The NIM II has some subtle nuances which require more than just a casual understanding of the instrument. Sometimes when there is confusion as to whether the facial nerve is actually being stimulated or we are simply close to the nerve, our technicians are able to interpret the signal, which clarifies the situation. While the surgeon could position the NIM II so that he can view the waveforms, this is distracting, and we therefore feel that having a separate technician involved is mandatory. A second point we have found is that during surgery, spontaneous EMG signals can be displayed on the screen with no direct stimulation of the nerve. Experience has shown that this actually represents a change in the patient's level of anesthesia from a deeper state to a lighter state. As the patient begins to awaken, muscle motions are picked up by the monitor. Our technicians at this point will notify the anesthesiologist and the patient's anesthesia stage will be deepened. A third interesting finding is that EMG signals can occur during surgery with simple irrigation of the surgical field. Further exploration of this has found that cold saline irrigation leads to nerve irritation and stimulation. This problem can be circumvented by using warm saline.

Conclusion

As the field of otolaryngology grows, surgical safety must continue to be emphasized. The NIM II has been described for otologic procedures [1, 2], but has been somewhat disregarded in other surgical procedures. We have described our technique for using the NIM II during parotid surgery. We currently are using the NIM II for almost all ear surgeries, surgeries involving the submandibular gland, neck node dissections, and during thyroid surgery.

References

1. Leonetti JP, Brackmann DE, Prass RL (1989) Improved preservation of facial nerve function in the infratemporal approach to the skull base. Otolaryngol Head Neck Surg, 101/1 : 74 – 78
2. Niparko JK, Kileny PR, Kemink JL, Lee HM, Graham MD (1989) Neurophysiologic intraoperative monitoring. II. Facial nerve function. Am J Otol 10/1 : 55 – 61

Eur Arch Otorhinolaryngology (1994) [Suppl]: S 387 – S 388

POSTERS

R. Ferreira Bento, E. Resende De Almeida, and A. Miniti

Anastomosis of Intratemporal Facial Nerve with Fibrin Tissue Adhesive

Introduction

Traumatic facial paralysis can be iatrogenic or catastrophic. The iatrogenic lesion can be deliberate or inadvertent. The catastrophic can be form temporal bone fracture, firearm shooting, or cutting lesions of the face.

The facial nerve is present a long way inside a bone canal within the temporal bone, making anastomosis technically difficult owing to limited space. This difficulty is made worse by the presence of cephalorhachidian liquid in some cases and by an even more limited space when the anastomosis has to be carried out on the inner auditory canal, on the posterior cranial fossa, or close to important structures such as the labyrinthine block.

To repair a damaged peripheral nerve there are four basic types of techniques described in the literature: (1) the epineural suture, first described by Hueter in 1873 [1], (2) the tubulization method, first described by Bugner in 1891 [2], (3) the peripheral suture, first described by Langley and Hashinoto in 1917 [3], and (4) fibrin glue in nerve anastomosis stabilization, first described by Young and Medawar in 1940. This adhesive can be obtained as a commercial product or made from homologous blood.

The objective of this paper is to show some practical steps that can be performed for intratemporal facial nerve repair with a easy method and good result by an ear, nose, and throat specialist with microsurgical training just for ear surgery or by a head and neck surgeon.

Principles and Basic Rules of Facial Nerve Anastomosis

There are certain basic rules for repair and treatment of the acquired peripheral nerve anastomosis which have been derived from experience with obtained results. These rules must be observed when the decision regarding treatment is taken; they have direct influence on the final result.

Once the diagnosis of the total or partial facial nerve has been done, based on clinical and electrophysiological signs of Wallerian degeneration, the nerve has to be explored in the least possible time using these principles:

1. For partial lesions, only partial repair is required.
2. Whenever possible, try end-to-end anastomosis, even if it is necessary to reroute the nerve.
3. If item is not possible, homologous graft must be performed; the nerve we prefer is the sural nerve.
4. The anastomosis must be left in a situation without tension for possible withdrawal or mobilization.
5. The repair must be done sooner after the lesion since the time is directly proportional to the result.
6. Regarding the anastomotic stump preparation, they always must be handled taking at least 0.5 cm off the sheath. Distal of each stump. Do not use scissors, but a very sharp scalpel so as to avoid the possibility of stumps being crushed. This cutting must be performed at the last moment before the anastomosis is done.
7. An adequate increase with surgical microscope must always be used so as to carry out the anastomosis with the least nerve trauma possible.
8. Ideal fascicle alignment involves trying to make longitudinal vessels meet or establish a mesoneuroposition; choose the most adequate position in the nerve rotational direction.

R. Ferreira Bento, E. Resende de Almeida, and A. Miniti
Department of Otolaryngology, University of São Paulo
Medical School, Rua Pedroso Alvarenga 1255 cj-22-04531,
São Paulo, Brazil

Advantages and Disadvantages of Anastomosis Stabilization Techniques

Epineural Suture

The advantages of epineural suture are: short execution time; simplicity of execution in relation to the perineural suture; the intraneural content is not manipulated and therefore not iatrogenically hurt; minimum possibility of local foreign body reaction, since intraneural stitches are not used.

The disadvantages are: possibility of an incorrect fascicular alignment; necessity of using several stitches so as to prevent neuroma formation.

Fascicular or Perineural Suture

The advantages of fascicular or perineural sature are: adequate coaptation of fascicle, in spite of it being difficult to decide which distal fascicle corresponds to the proximal one.

The disadvantages are: longer surgery time; greater technical difficulty; greater possibility of foreign body reaction and intraneural fibrosis because of intraneural manipulation; greater iatrogenic trauma possibility; greater need for training in microsurgery techniques.

In some kinds of nerves in which the fascicles are well individualized, this technique is ideal, but in the facial nerve, mainly in its intratemporal portion, this individualization does not occur.

Tubulization

The advantages of tubulization are: least surgery time; technical facility; least possibility of intraneural foreign body reaction.

The disadvantages are: problems in the anastomosis stabilization, since there is no fixation; possibility of local foreign body reaction, since the method does not use homologous material; problems concerning fascicular alignment.

Gluing with Fibrinic Tissue Adhesive

The advantages of gluing with fibrinic tissue adhesive are: least surgical time; greater technical facility; absence of local foreign body reaction; least iatrogenic trauma of the nerve.

The disadvantages are: problems concerning fascicular alignment.

Discussion

As far as the advantages and disadvantages of each method are concerned, we must bear in mind the fact that the intratemporal facial nerve does not have a very precise fascicular differentiation (mainly the most proximal segment) and that there is a big technical difficulty regarding sutures owing to the limited space, the presence of important structures in the neighborhood, and sometimes the presence of cephalorhachidian liquid, all factors which complicate the procedure. In the intratemporal segment of the facial nerve, our experience has led us to use the different anastomosis methods in the following order:

1. We use gluing with tissue adhesive as the method of choice.
2. If gluing is not possible, we use epineural suture.
3. If epineural suture is not possible, we use entubulization with temporal muscle fascia.

We have not used the anastomosis covering with tissue from fascia or perichondrium.

Conclusion

The results obtained with the routine use of this technique by several surgeons with only micro-otological surgery training and without nerve microanastomosis training were excellent, all patients showing clinical and electrophysiological signs of nervous regeneration.

References

1. Bugner VO (1891) Über die Degenerations- und Regenerationsvorgänge an Nerven nach Verletzungen. Beitr Pathol 10:321–331
2. Hueter K (1873) Die allgemeine Chirurgie. Vogel, Leipzig
3. Langley JN, Hashimoto M (1917) On the suture of separate nerve bundles in a nerve trunk and on internal nerve plexus. J Physiol (Lond) 51:318
4. Young JZ, Medawar PB (1940) Fibrin sutures of peripheral nerves. Lancet 2:126–128

Eur Arch Otorhinolaryngology (1994) [Suppl]:S389

ABSTRACTS

J. G. Spector

Treatment of Facial Paralysis in Humans by Neural Methods

Human facial nerve regeneration was compared in three repair systems: autologous neural cable grafts ($N = 56$), direct end-to-end anastomosis ($N = 34$), and VII–XII anastomosis ($N = 26$). The data were analyzed based on the following criteria: facial symmetry and muscle tone at rest, degree of total facial reinnervation, voluntary motion, synkinesis, and electrophysiological testing. Facial tone and symmetry at rest and electrophysiologic tests were similar, while voluntary motion and facial reinnervation were decreased and synkinesis increased in the autologous cable graft repairs and VII–XII anastomosis. Electrophysiologic tests of the innervated muscles failed to distinguish between the three repair methods in successful regenerates. Neural cable grafts and VII–XII anastomosis were associated with more mass movement less fine precise emotive facial movement and more synkinesis. Excellent results, especially cable graft repairs, diminish with time because of continual progressive synkinesis, which may take up to 4 years to develop.

J. G. Spector
Department of Otolaryngology, Head & Neck Surgery, Washington University School of Medicine, St. Louis, Missouri 63110, USA

Eur Arch Otorhinolaryngology (1994) [Suppl]: S 390

ABSTRACTS

B. Toussaint, F. Decroocq, and C. Simon

Facial Reanimation by XII to VII Nerve Anastomosis After Surgery on the VIII Nerve

The results are reported of 18 hypoglossal-to-facial nerve anastomoses after surgery on the acoustic nerve, especially for neurinoma. The restoration of a basic muscle contraction was studied with a delay of more than 9 months. The best results were obtained with a short time difference between tumor extirpation and nerve anastomosis, less than 3 months.

The results show a basic restoration of the contraction in 90% of the cases studied and in 50% of the cases with dynamic muscle contraction, especially in the lower territory. Sometimes spontaneous animation was noted.

Using House and Brackmann's classification, most of the total and complete facial paralysis was 6th degree before surgical anastomosis, and 4th degree 1 year after surgery. Otherwise, the consequences of this anastomosis on tongue function, elocution, and deglutition are minimal and do not cause trouble for the patient. Finally 75% of the patients had a better muscular function when they move the tongue spontaneously.

In conclusion, considering these results and those of many other authors, we think that those XII to VII nerve anastomoses have a specific place in the surgical treatment of facial reanimation after paralysis. The technique has a place between direct suture of the nerve or nerve grafts using branches of the superficial cervical plexus and surgically paliative techniques such as muscle transfers and suspensions.

B. Toussaint, F. Decroocq, and C. Simon
C.H.R.U. 29, avenue du Mal de Lattre de Tassigny, 54000 Nancy, France

Eur Arch Otorhinolaryngology (1994) [Suppl]:S391

G. Schram, V. Gallati, S. Michel, and U. Fisch

Rehabilitation After Hypoglossus-Facial Crossover

The long-term results of 82 patients with hypoglossus-facial crossover are reviewed.

The effect of rehabilitation training on the final result, particular'y in eyelid closure, is emphasized.

G. Schram, V. Gallati, S. Michel, and U. Fisch
ORL Department, University Hospital, Zürich, Switzerland

Eur Arch Otorhinolaryngology (1994) [Suppl]: S 392

ABSTRACTS

I. Schneider, A. Gunkel, E. Stennert, and W. F. Neiss

Development of the Nerve Conduction Velocity After Hypoglossal-Facial Nerve Anastomosis: An Electroneurographic Study

Hypoglossal-facial nerve anastomosis (HFA) is nowadays a common technique for reinnervation of the paralyzed face and an ideal model to study the plasticity of the brain, because functional end results of facial movement can be influenced by mimical training. To further study regeneration of the facial nerve by functional parameters, we measured time and amount of increase of the nerve conduction velocity (NCV) before and after resection and reconstruction of the nerve by a unilateral HFA.

Methods Thirty-six adult female Wistar rats were examined. Before the operation the stimulus-response latencies, the amplitudes, and the nerve conduction velocities (NCV) of the facial nerve were measured. Neuromyographic conductions were carried out at the m. levator labii (MLL) with special bipolar surface electrodes and at the m. orbicularis oculi (MOO) with concentric needle electrodes. Postoperative measurements were performed by exposing the site of anastomosis and directly stimulating the hypoglossal nerve proximal to the anastomosis. In the first 8 weeks electroneurographic measurements were performed at weekly intervals and thereafter at 10, 16 and 20 weeks after surgery.

Results The mean preoperative NCV at the MLL was 26.3 ± 1.3 m/s and at the MOO 22.2 ± 2.3 m/s. As soon as 21 days after nerve suture, first stimulus responses with an NCV of $1-2$ m/s were detected. From this time on, there was a continuous increase of the NCV. Ten weeks after surgery the mean NCV reached 15.4 ± 1.7 m/s (MLL) and 15.1 ± 1.3 m/s (MOO), 58.7% (MLL) and 68.2% (MOO) of the initial value. Twenty weeks after operation there was only a slight further increase to 17.5 ± 1.07 m/s (MLL) and 16.5 ± 2.2 m/s.

These data show that our rat model for performing an HFA and the electromyographic control of regeneration of the nerve and reinnervation of the facial muscle with special minielectrodes works very well. As we expected, the increase in the NCV in the first 10 weeks was very fast and then slowed down, to reach a maximum of 66.7% (MLL) and 74.2% (MOO) of the original value after 20 weeks.

Supported by the Deutsche Forschungsgemeinschaft (Ne 412/1-1).

I. Schneider, A. Gunkel, and E. Stennert
Department of Otorhinolaryngology, University of Cologne,
Joseph-Stelzmann-Str. 9, 50924 Cologne, Germany

W. F. Neiss
Department I of Anatomy, University of Cologne, Cologne, Germany

Eur Arch Otorhinolaryngology (1994) [Suppl]: S393

ABSTRACTS

J. K. Terzis

The "Babysitter" Principle: Experience and Results in 25 Cases

Purpose To present the introduction and our 6-year clinical experience of a new technique for facial reanimation by which ipsilateral "strong" motor donors are used to preserve denervated targets in complete or partial facial palsies until contralateral VII nerve motor fibers take over.

Methods In complete or partial facial palsies, a small segment of the ipsilateral XII nerve was used as a motor donor to rapidly reinnervate selective denervated targets while the contralateral VII nerve fibers are regenerating through cross-facial nerve grafts. In a second stage the distal ends of the cross-facial nerve grafts were coapted with more peripheral branches of the involved facial nerve. The "babysitter" XII nerve serves only to maintain the bulk of the facial muscle while the cross-facial nerves carrying fibers from the contralateral VII nerve function as the "pacemakers." The indications and intricacies of this combined technique are presented in cases of complete and portial facial palsies. If denervation time is over 2 years, one needs to supplement this procedure with local or free vascularized muscle transfers.

Results Twenty-five cases have been performed to date. Follow-up ranges from 3 months to 6 years. Exemplary results are discussed in detail. Contrary to previous reports a rewarding degree of symmetrical coordinated animation was achieved even after prolonged denervation of the (facial muscle up to 2 years). In cases where satisfactory reanimation was not accomplished by the "babysitter" technique, provision of new muscle was carried out at a later date.

Conclusion (1) After 6 months of denervation the facial musculature atrophies, thus cross-facial nerve grafting is not effective. (2) Six years ago, the author introduced a new technique that may restore function to the paralyzed face after up to 2 years of denervation by the combined use of "babysitter" and "pacemaker" nerves. The "babysitters" are cranial motor nerves on the ipsilateral side of the lesion other than the facial nerve and they are used to "quickly" send motor fibers to the denervated facial muscle. The "pacemakers" are always the fibers of the contralateral facial nerve. The combination of the two sources of motor fibers has restored regarding degress of synchronous and coordinated animation to the previously paralyzed face. (3) In late cases of facial paralysis or in cases where adequate reinnervation was not achieved, the author proceeded with the addition of local or free vascularized muscle procedure to complete reanimation of the paralyzed face.

J. K. Terzis
Eastern Virgina Medical School, Microsurgical Research Center –
MRC, 700 Olney Road, Norfolk, VA 23507, USA

Eur Arch Otorhinolaryngology (1994) [Suppl]: S 394

ABSTRACTS

M. L. Cheney, A. E. Petropoulos, and M. J. McKenna

Trigeminal Neoneurotization of the Paralysed Facial Musculature

Many investigators have entertained the concept of facial muscle reinnervation from the trigeminal pathway following facial nerve paralysis. In this paper we present a documented clinical case as well as experimental evidence that trigeminal facial crossover does occur and can be used as a concept to maximize early rehabilitation of the paralyzed face. A case is presented demonstrating unequivocal clinical evidence of trigeminal facial cross-innervation. A 62-year-old white female underwent a left parotidectomy 30 years ago. In December 1990, left facial paralysis developed over 24 h. CT scan revealed a deep lobe parotid tumor. She then underwent a total parotidectomy with sacrifice of the facial nerve at the stylomastid foramen. Ten months later, she spontaneously demonstrated the ability to smile on the left side while chewing. This was documented both photographically and by video and confirmed by EMG testing. We hypothesize that this phenomenon is due to trigeminal facial crossover. Furthermore, other patients who had undergone a temporalis transposition procedure for facial reanimation after facial nerve paralysis also demonstrated facial movement upon mastication, in excess of that which could be attributable to the temporalis transposition alone. We have studied this phenomenon in animal model, in which the temporalis transposition procedure was performed at varying intervals post facial nerve transection. After an appropriate period, the zygomaticus major muscle was injected with a histochemical marker to evaluate the reinnervation process.

M. L. Cheney, E. Petropoulos, and M. J. McKenna
Harvard Medical School, Massachusetts Eye and Ear Infirmary,
Boston, Massachusetts 02114, USA

Eur Arch Otorhinolaryngology (1994) [Suppl]: S 395

ABSTRACTS

J. F. Sanchez-Marle

Surgical Repair of the Facial Nerve at the Base of the Skull: The Mastoid-Parotid Approach

The mastoid-parotid approach involves an otological stage for proper identification of the proximal nerve stump, and a careful high cervicofacial dissection to find the distal portion of the facial nerve. In our experience it represents the best technique to resolve injuries of the VII cranial nerve at the extratemporal base of the skull. We have managed ten cases with this approach. Etiology, surgical indications, systematization, possible alternatives, and our results are presented.

J. F. Sanchez-Marle
Central Army Hospital, Mexico City, Mexico

Eur Arch Otorhinolaryngology (1994) [Suppl]: S 396

ABSTRACTS

K. W. Zhang and Z. T. Shun

Microvascular Decompression by the Retromastoid Approach for Idiopathic Hemifacial Spasm: Experience of 300 Patients

Our experience is reported of 300 patients with idiopathic hemifacial spasm in which microvascular decompression was accomplished by the retromastoid approach between April 1985 and January 1992. The surgical procedure and the advantages of the retromastoid approach are described. Vascular compression of the nerves was noted in all patients at operation. Therefore, we suggest vascular compression is the main cause of idiopathic hemifacial spasm. Two hundred and seventy-seven patients had symptoms which disappeared postoperatively, which gives a 92.3% cure rate. In addition, 7.7% of the patients were not cured; therefore, we suggest the possible existence of other etiologies.

K. W. Zhang and Z. T. Shun
Department of Otoneurosurgery, PLA Air Force Xiang Fan Hospital, 441003 Xiang Fan City, Hu Bei Province, China

Eur Arch Otorhinolaryngology (1994) [Suppl]: S 397

ABSTRACTS

G.M. O'Donoghue

Endoscopic Anatomy of the Facial Nerve and Related Structures

This study describes the endoscopic anatomy of the cerebellopontine angle (CPA) and basal cisterns. Endoscopes were introduced into the basal cisterns and it was found that the neurovascular structures of this angle could be seen in detail. The course of the facial nerve from the pontomedullary junction to the porus can be clearly seen. Endoscopy is likely to complement contemporary micro-surgical procedures. The need for minimally invasive surgery may mandate further study of the application of this type of endoscopy in surgical practice. It is stressed that considerable cadaver experience should be obtained with this technique prior to any application in the operating room.

G.M. O'Donoghue
Department of Neurotology, University Hospital, Nottingham, UK

**Facial Nerve Research:
New Approaches and Results**

Eur Arch Otorhinolaryngology (1994) [Suppl]:S401–S402

E. Senba, T. Saika, and T. Matsunaga

Expression and Regulation of Neuropeptides in Rat Facial Motoneurons

It is well known that axotomy causes a variety of morphological and chemical changes in motoneurons. Enzymes and other substances related to neuronal transmission, such as choline acetyltransferase or nicotinic acetylcholine receptor (α_3 subunit) [3], are decreased in rat facial motoneurons after facial nerve transection. On the other hand, house keeping enzymes are increased in the same situation. Recently it has been demonstrated that motoneurons contain various kinds of neuropeptides, such as calcitonin gene-related peptide (CGRP), cholecystokinin (CCK), or galanin (Gal) [2], although their functional roles are stil obscure. They might play some role in the process of regeneration, because axotomy remarkably enhances the expression of these peptides.

In situ hybridization histochemistry, using synthesized oligonucleotides of 40–60 bases complementary to each mRNA as probes, was employed to study the changes in synthesis of these peptides and other substances in facial motoneurons following axotomy. In control rats, 38%, 55%, and 7% of the facial motoneurons expressed α-CGRP, β-CGRP, and CCK mRNAs, respectively. No Gal mRNA-containing motoneurons were observed in these animals. The levels of mRNA for α-CGRP, CCK, and Gal were increased while the β-CGRP mRNA level was decreased after axotomy. The levels of mRNAs for these peptides returned to the control values by 2–4 weeks after nerve crushing, whereas nerve resection had more prolonged effects.

In addition to neuropeptides, the growth-associated protein GAP-43, a neuron-specific phosphoprotein, is also synthesized in facial motoneurons in response to axotomy. This protein seems to play a role in axonal outgrowth

during neuronal development and regeneration [4]. GAP-43-positive motoneurons could be identified at 1 day after facial nerve crushing or resection. The signal intensity of GAP-43 mRNA increased until 7 days after the insult and then subsequently gradually decreased.

It is also documented that immediate early genes of the jun family, which encodes transcriptional regulators, are activated in axotomized motoneurons [1]. C-*jun* mRNA is only weakly expressed in intact motoneurons. Marked elevation of its level was observed in axotomized motoneurons and the elevated level was maintained for several weeks. In motoneurons of the L4, 5 levels of the spinal cord, an increase of the c-*jun* mRNA level was apparent as early as 6 h after the sciatic nerve transection. This increase was followed by upregulations of α-CGRP and GAP-43 mRNAs, which appeared 1 day after the insult. These findings suggest that Jun protein is one of the transcriptional activators of some peptides or proteins in motoneurons.

The next question is how the transcription of c-*jun* mRNA is activated in injured motoneurons. There are at least two possible mechanisms: (1) Retrograde transport of some factors synthesized by Schwann cells in the degenerating nerves leads to upregulation of c-*jun* mRNA and (2) blockade of axonal flow eliminates suppressive factors which are normally retrogradely transported from the target tissues to suppress the transcription of c-*jun* gene. We examined whether the c-*jun* mRNA level was increased or not when axonal transport was interrupted without causing axonal degeneration. For this purpose, we applied the well-known axonal flow blocker vinblastine. Low doses of vinblastine (50–100 μM) were applied to the sciatic nerves for 15 min and the rats were allowed to survive for 6 days. Vinblastine at low doses (<150 μM) caused no sign of axonal degeneration at the electron microscopic level. This treatment also induced marked enhancement of c-*jun*, α-CGRP, and GAP-43 mRNA levels in motoneurons, suggesting that a blockade of transcriptional repressor from the target tissues plays key roles in the regulation of these genes and controls the regeneration process of injured axons and motoneurons.

E. Senba (✉)
Department of Anatomy and Neurobiology, Wakayama Medical College, 27 Kyuban-cho, Wakayama 640, Japan

T. Saika and T. Matsunaga
Department of Otolaryngology, Osaka University Medical School, Osaka 565, Japan

References

1. Leah JD, Herdegen T, Bravo R (1991) Selective expression of Jun proteins following axotomy and axonal block in peripheral nerves in the rat: evidence for a role in the regeneration process. Brain Res 566:198–207
2. Saika T, Senba E, Noguchi K, Sato M, Kubo T, Matsunaga T, Toh-yama M (1991) Changes in expression of peptides in rat facial motoneurons after facial nerve crushing and resection. Mol Brain Res 11:187–196
3. Senba E, Simmons DM, Wada E, Wada K, Swanson LW (1990) RNA levels of neuronal nicotinic acetylcholine receptor subunits are differentially regualted in axotomized facial motoneurons: an in situ hybridization study. Mol Brain Res 8:349–353
4. Skene JHP (1989) Axonal growth-associated proteins. Annu Rev Neurosci 12:127–156

Eur Arch Otorhinolaryngology (1994) [Suppl]: S403 – S406

FREE PAPERS AND POSTERS

T. Arzberger, E. Ritter, and A. Weindl

Human Facial Nucleus: Choline Acetyltransferase and Calcitonin Gene-Related Peptide*

Introduction

Of the cranial nerves the facial nerve in man is of special interest for two reasons: (1) facial expression forms a "window," through which the inner world, i. e., psychic states such as emotions, are nonverbally communicated to the outer world, (2) the facial nerve is afflicted in a great variety of central and peripheral neurological diseases. Many studies concerning the identification and localization of neuroactive substances have been carried out in the facial nucleus of experimental animals, because perfusion fixation warrants excellent tissue preservation for immunocytochemical studies. However, in the human, to the best of our knowledge, no systematic studies have been reported in the literature. In the framework of a larger study on the distribution in the human brainstem of choline acetyltransferase (ChAT), the biosynthetic enzyme of acetylcholine, and of calcitonin gene-related peptide (CGRP), both present in cranial and spinal motoneurons, we have focused on the facial nerve. To evaluate the distribution of the neurotransmitter acetylcholine and of CGRP, a neuropeptide which exists in two forms in humans (CGRP I and II) differing in three amino acids [14] and rat (CGRP α and β) differing in one amino acid [1], we employed Nissl staining, immunostaining for ChAT or for CGRP I/II, and immuno-double-staining for ChAT and CGRP I/II on sections of the human brainstem containing the facial nucleus.

T. Arzberger, E. Ritter and A. Weindl
Neurologische Klinik der Technischen Universität München, Möhlstr. 28, 81675 München, Germany

* Supported by grants from DFG (We 608/8-3) and BMFT (01 KL 9001)

Material and Methods

Early postmortem human brain specimens were obtained from the Department of Forensic Medicine, Ludwig Maximilian University, Munich. The brainstem was excised, divided into smaller pieces by sections perpendicular to the sagittal axis, and fixed by immersion in 10% formaldehyde in 0.1 M phosphate buffer, pH 7.4. The ages of these control persons (one male, one female) were 60 and 65 years. Death was caused by cardiac arrest. Postmortem time was 4.5 h and 7 h. After a fixation period of several weeks the blocks were washed in TBS (0.02 M Tris; 0.125 M NaCl; pH 7.4) for a couple of days and transferred into 20% sucrose in TBS for cryoprotection until they sank to the bottom. Then 50- to 60-μm sections were cut in a cryostat and stored in 5% sucrose in TBS at -20 °C until use.

Nissl Staining Defrosted sections were washed 3×5 min in TBS, mounted on gelatine-chromalum-coated slides, air-dried, stained in 0.5% cresyl fast violet (Fluka), dehydrated, and embedded in Entellan (Merck).

Immunohistochemistry Pretreatment of Sections Defrosted free floating sections were washed 3×5 min in TBS. To block endogenous peroxidase and to eliminate melanin granules or lipofuscin, sections were pretreated according to Guntern et al. [7] for 20 min in 0.25% $KMnO_4$, washed briefly in distilled water, and immersed in Pal's solution (1% K_2SO_4 in 1% oxalic acid). To expose immunoreactive epitopes in overfixed tissue, sections were treated with 1% $NaOH/0.9\%$ H_2O_2 for 10 min and finally washed 5×5 min in TBS.

Double Staining Sections were incubated successively (a) in a mixture of polyclonal antibodies to both forms of human CGRP (diluted 1 : 1000) of rabbit origin (Peninsula) and of monoclonal antibodies to ChAT (20 μg/ml) of mouse origin (Boehringer) dissolved in TBS additionally

S404

containing 20% normal goat serum, 2% bovine serum albumin (BSA), and 0.5% Triton X (TBS+) overnight at room temperature (RT), (b) in a mixture of goat anti-rabbit IgG (1:100; Sigma) and goat anti-mouse IgG (1:100; Sigma) in TBS+ for 1 h at RT, and (c) in a mixture of rabbit PAP (peroxidase antiperoxidase) complexes (1:100; Sigma) according to Sternberger [15] and mouse APAAP (alkaline phosphatase-antialkaline phosphatase) complexes (1:50; DAKO) according to Cordell et al. [5] in TBS+ for 1 h at RT. Steps (b) and (c) were repeated. Between all steps sections were washed 3×5 min in TBS. To visualize ChAT the sections were incubated for 20 min in 0.1 M Tris pH 8.2 containing 0.2 µg/ml naphthol AS-MX phosphate (substrate), 1 mg/ml fast red salt (chromogen), 20 µl/ml dimethylformamide, and 1 µl/ml 1 M levamisole (blocks endogenous alkaline phosphatase). To visualize CGRP the sections were subsequently incubated for 1 min in 0.1 M Tris pH 7.4 containing 0.015% H_2O_2 (substrate) and 1 mg/ml diaminobenzidine (DAB; chromogen). Finally, sections were mounted on gelatine-chromalum-coated slides and embedded in a water-soluble medium containing glycerol (Sigma).

Single Staining *CGRP.* The same procedure as described for double staining was applied omitting the reaction of APAAP.

ChAT A similar procedure as described for double staining was applied replacing the solution of step (c) with a solution of monoclonal mouse PAP complexes (Sigma) diluted 1:100 in TBS+. Consequently the final enzymatic reaction was in Tris/DAB/H_2O_2 (se above) for 1 min. Mounted single-standed sections were dehydrated and embedded in Entellan (Merck).

Results

On Nissl-stained sections the facial nucleus was grouped in several divisions. According to Olszewski and Baxter [11], a dorsal, intermediate, medial, ventral, ventromedial, and ventrolateral subnucleus could be discerned. Single staining with PAP for ChAT (Fig. 1) revealed that ChAT neurons represent the vast majority of Nissl-stained

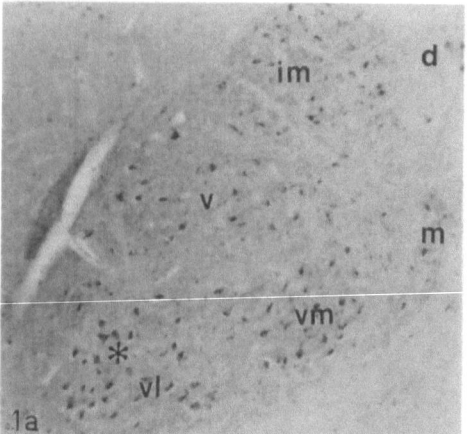
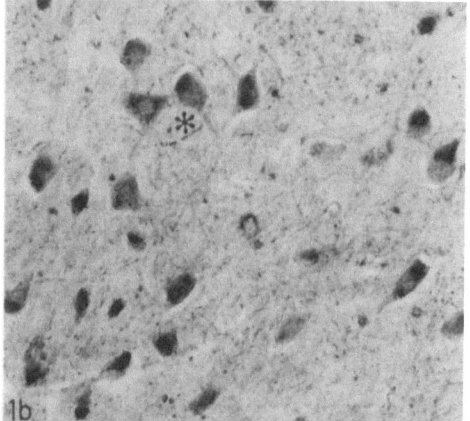
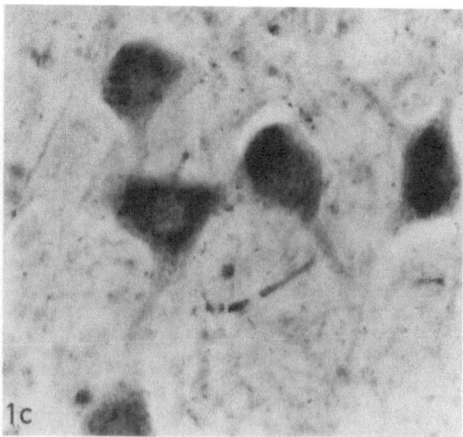

Figs. 1–3 Human facial nucleus. Frontal sections. PAP reaction for ChAT (Fig. 1) and CGRP (Fig. 2), and double staining for ChAT (APAAP) and CGRP (PAP) (Fig. 3). The facial nucleus can be subdivided into sveral groups of neurons: dorsal (*d*), intermediate (*im*), medial (*m*), ventral (*v*), ventromedial (*vm*), and ventrolateral (*vl*) group. The vast majority of neurons of the facial nucleus contain ChAT (Fig. 1) and CGRP (Fig. 2). Both markers are colocalized in the same neurons (Fig. 3). Figs. 1a, 2a, 3a, ×30; Figs. 1b, 2b, 3b, ×120; Figs. 1c, 2c, 3c, ×300; • indicates areas of subsequently enlarged details

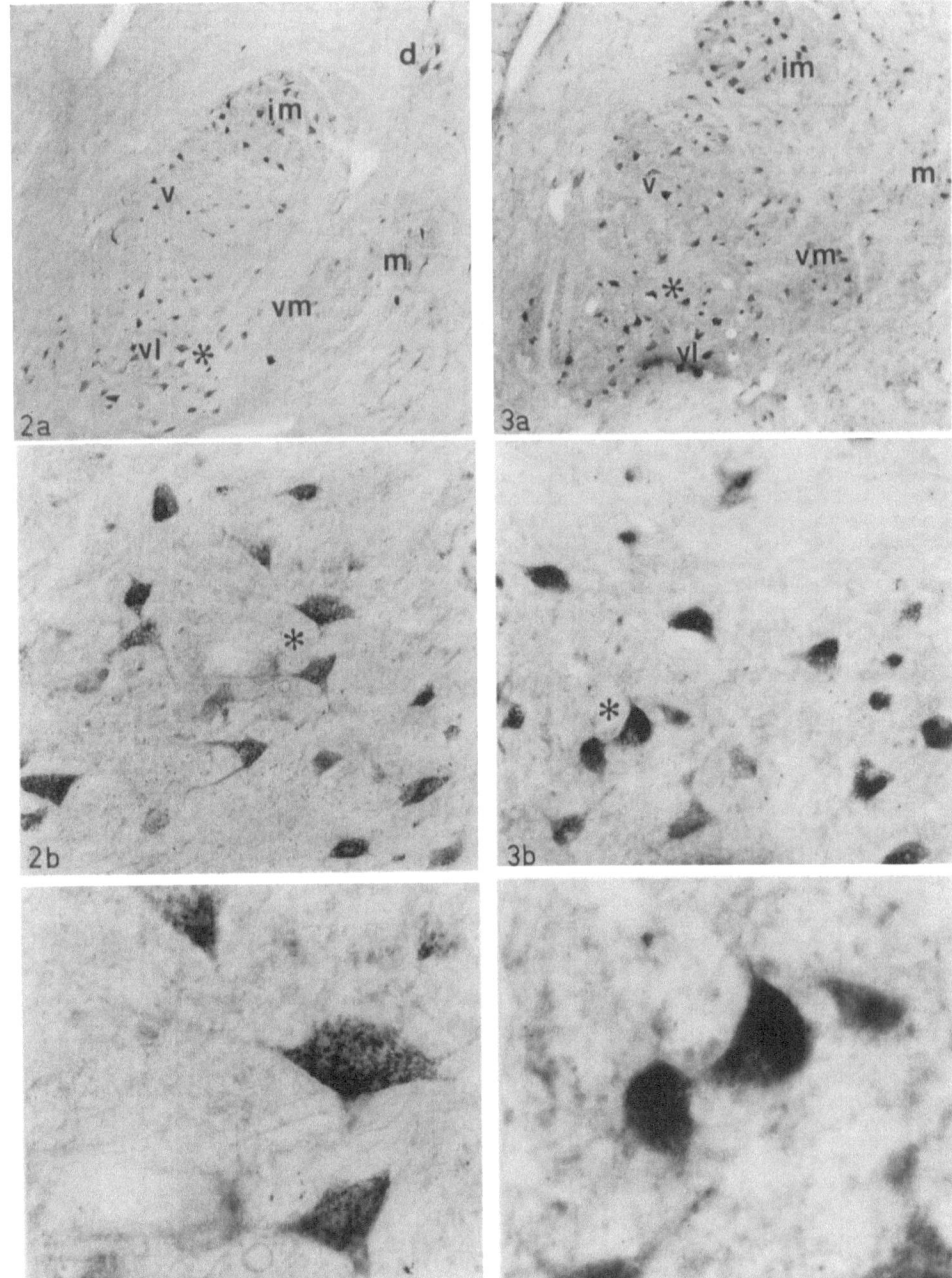

neurons. Single staining for CGRP (Fig. 2) revealed that the majority of neurons in all subnuclei display CGRP immunoreactivity (CGRP-IR). CGRP was present in a granular distribution within the neuronal perikarya (Fig. 2b, c). The application of the double staining method for ChAT and CGRP on the same section (Fig. 3) revealed that CGRP-IR was present in nearly all ChAT immunoreactive neurons. While ChAT was marked by a more diffusely distributed red staining, CGRP-IR was distributed within Nissl substance-like brown-stained granules. On double-stained sections only rarely was a cell found which appeared to have only ChAT- or only CGRP-IR. The intensity of ChAT-IR appeared higher in the intermediate and ventral subnucleus, whereas the CGRP-IR appeared to be more intense in all other subnuclei.

Discussion

Batten et al. [3] found colocalization of CGRP more in medial than in lateral portions of the facial nucleus of rat and cat. Takami et al. [17] using single staining on adjacent sections found CGRP in 80% of rat facial ChAT neurons. Using double staining we have found a colocalization of ChAT- and CGRP-IR in the vast majority of neurons of all subnuclei of the human facial nerve. The granular distribution represents CGRP-IR in Golgi bodies and secretory vesicles [4]. While it is well established that acetylcholine is the transmitter of facial motoneurons at the neuromuscular junction, the function of CGRP in cholinergic motoneurons is not yet clearly understood. Several hypotheses have been put forward concerning the role of CGRP, which has been reported to regulate the synthesis of nicotinic acetylcholine receptors [6, 10]. In facial motoneurons CGRP and its mRNA are increased after axotomy [2, 8, 16] and may mediate reactive hypertrophy of astrocytes and proliferation of microglial cells [9]. Saika et al. [13] showed that this increased mRNA encodes α-CGRP, while mRNA for β-CGRP is decreased after axotomy, suggesting that only α-CGRP has a trophic function, whereas β-CGRP may work as a neurotransmitter. In the transected sciatic nerve, CGRP mediates axonal-endoneurial cell interaction during peripheral nerve regeneration [12]. In transected nerves CGRP may act on connective tissue to facilitate nerve outgrowth and appears to have an antisprouting effect [12]. It is noteworthy that in the human facial nucleus, which from clinical experience is seen to have a good capacity for regeneration, CGRP is abundantly present in cholinergic facial motoneurons.

References

1. Amara S, Arriza J, Leff S, Swanson L, Evans R, Rosenfeld M (1985) Expression in brain of a messenger RNA encoding a novel neuropeptide homologous to calcitonin gene-related peptide. Sciene 229 : 1094 – 1097
2. Arvidsson U, Johnson H, Piehl F, Cullheim S, Hökfelt T, Risling M, Terenius L, Ulfhake B (1990) Peripheral nerve section induces increased levels of calcitonin gene-related peptide (CGRP)-like immunoreactivity in axotomized motoneurons. Exp Brain Res 79 : 212 – 216
3. Batten T, Appenteng K, Saha S (1988) Visualisation of CGRP and ChAT-like immunoreactivity in identified trigeminal neurones by combined peroxidase and alkaline phosphatase enzymatic reactions. Brain Res 447 : 314 – 324
4. Caldero J, Casanovas A, Sorribas A, Esquerda J (1992) Calcitonin gene-related peptide in rat spinal cord motoneurons: subcellular distribution and changes induced by axotomy. Neuroscience 48 : 449 – 461
5. Cordell J, Falini B, Erber W, Ghosh A, Abdulaziz Z, MacDonald S, Pulford K, Stein H, Mason D (1984) Immunoenzymatic labeling of monoclonal antibodies using immune complexes of alkaline phosphatase and monoclonal anti-alkaline phosphatase (APAAP complexes). J Histochem Cytochem 32(2) : 219 – 229
6. Fontane B, Klarsfeld A, Hökfelt T, Changeux J (1989) Calcitonin gene-related peptide, a peptide present in spinal cord motoneurons, increases the number of acetylcholine receptors in primary cultures of chick embryo myotubes. Neurosci Lett 71 : 39 – 63
7. Guntern R, Vallet P, Bouras C, Constantinidis J (1989) An improved immunohistostaining procedure for peptides in human brain. Experientia 45 : 159 – 161
8. Haas C, Streit W, Kreutzberg G (1990) Rat facial motoneurons express increased levels of calcitonin gene-related peptide mRNA in response to axotomy. J Neurosci Res 27 : 270 – 275
9. Lazar P, Reddington M, Streit W, Raivich G, Kreutzberg G (1991) The action of calcitonin gene-related peptide on astrocyte morphology and cyclic AMP accumulation in astrocyte cultures from neonatal rat brain. Neurosci Lett 130 : 99 – 102
10. New H, Mudge A (1986) Calcitonin gene-related peptide regulates muscle acetylcholine receptor synthesis. Nature 323 : 809 – 811
11. Olszewski J, Baxter D (1953) Cytoarchitecture of the human brain stem. Karger, Basel
12. Raivich G, Dumoulin F, Streit W, Kreutzberg G (1992) Calcitonin gene-related peptide (CGRP) in the regenerating rat sciatic nerve. Restor Neurol Neurosci 4 : 107 – 115
13. Saika T, Senba E, Noguchi K, Sato M, Kubo T, Matsunaga T, Tohyama M (1991) Changes in expression of peptide in rat facial motoneurons after facial nerve crushing and resection. Mol Brain Res 11 : 187 – 196
14. Steenbergh P, Höppener J, Zandberg J, Lips C, Jansz H (1985) A second human calcitonin/CGRP gene. FEBS Lett 183 : 403 – 407
15. Sternberger L (1986) Immunocytochemistry, 3rd edn. Churchill Livingstone, New York
16. Streit W, Dumoulin F, Raivich G, Kreutzberg G (1989) Calcitonin gene-related peptide increases in rat facial motoneurons after peripheral nerve transection. Neurosci Lett 101 : 143 – 148
17. Takami K, Kawai Y, Shiosaka S, Girgis L, Hillyard C, Macintyre I, Emson P, Tohyama M (1985) Immunohistochemical evidence for the coexistence of calcitonin gene-related peptide- and choline acetyltransferase-like immunoreactivity in neurons of the rat hypoglossal facial and ambiguus nuclei. Brain Res 328 : 386 – 389

Eur Arch Otorhinolaryngology (1994) [Suppl]: S407–S409

M. J. Bernardo, P. Ablanedo, C. Suarez, M. Alvarez-Uria, and J. L. Llorente

Nerve Growth Factor: Morphological and Morphometric Findings on Facial Nerve Regeneration in the Rabbit

Introduction

Nerve growth factor (NGF) is indispensable for the correct functioning of the sympathetic and sensorial autonomic nervous system, with multiple effects and potential clinical applications, specifically in Alzheimer's disease [2]. We are not aware of a specific active trophic factor on the motor system, analogous to the NGF, which would correspond to a muscle-derived protein [5, 6]. The "target-derived" trophism is an aspect of the autonomic system which is still under discussion. At the present time, it is believed that the NGF is synthesized by glial cells, astrcytes, and laminine [7]. The aim of this study is tu use the facial nerve, which is a mixed nerve, like the sciatic nerve and the trigeminal nerve [1], and to evaluate the possible effect of NGF on all its fibers.

Material and Methods

Four New Zealand albino rabbits weighing 1 – 1.7 kg were used. All the animals received a sharp transection of the third portion of the facial nerves. In the right section 1000 ng 2.5 S-NGF (Bethesda Res. Lab.) was instillated, surrounding the nerve with Gelfoam soaked with NGF. On the left side the nerve section was instillated with 0.5 ml sali-

M.J. Bernardo (✉), C. Suarez, and J.L. Llorente
Department of Otolaryngology, Hospital Central Universitario de Oviedo, Asturias, Spain

P. Ablanedo
Department of Pathology, Hospital Central Universitario de Oviedo, Asturias, Spain

M. Alvarez-Uria
Department of Cellular Biology, Hospital Central Universitario de Oviedo, Asturias, Spain

ne serum. The animals were put to death after 80 days and the right and left facial nerves submitted for study.

All animals were perfused with a solution of glutaraldehyde, dehydrated, and embedded in Epon 812 and the nerves were fixed in osmium tetroxide. Blocks were stained with uranyl acetate and lead citrate.

Thin sections were examined with a Siemens Elmistrop 102 electron microscope. Photographs taken from semithin sections were studied morphometrically by an automatic image analysis system (Kontron Videoplan DRCD). The parameters evaluated were number and diameter of the nerve fibers, which were later submitted for statistical analysis. For each specimen, one or more sectons which were distal and proximal to the site of the nerve transection were studied.

Results

Light Microscopy

All the right and left facial nerves in the area proximal to the section showed no alterations (Fig. 1A), except in the areas near the section neuroma where endo- and perineural fibrosis was observed. In the distal area and beyond the neuroma, the nerve was seen to have a thick circular and interfascicular perineurum. We noted a marked intraneural vascular network and absence of intraneural free spaces, predominance of myelinic thin and medium size fibers, and isolated groups of amyelinic fibers. This configuration persisted until the exit of the nerve through the stylomastoid foramen. No differences were found between the right and left nerves in any of the animals (Fig. 1B, C).

Electron Microscopy

In the areas proximal to the section the myelinic fibers were more abundant than the amyelinic ones, which were

Fig. 1A–C Semifine section. Toluidine blue, ×750. A Control section of the facial nerve at the level of the geniculate ganglion. B Distal portion of the right facial nerve 2 months after transection, with NGF application. C Distal part of the left facial nerve 2 months after transection without NGF

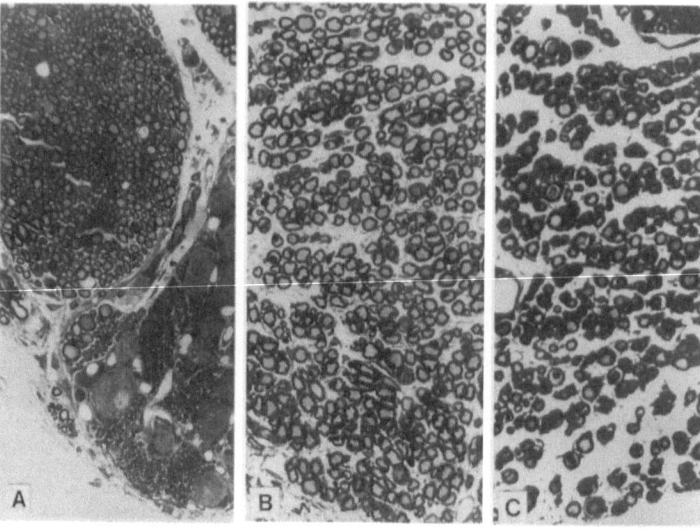

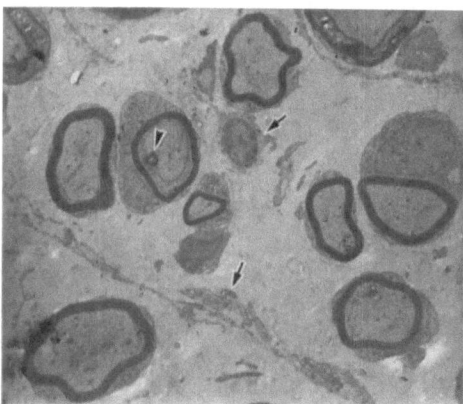

Fig. 2 Remyelinated axon intraxonal myelinic bodies (*arrow*). Fibroblast prolongatin (*arrow*), EM, ×3000

In the distal areas the myelinic fibers were smaller and consisted of fine sheaths with normal axonal organization and isolated laminar aggregates representing myelinic deposits. These deposits were also seen in the Schwann cells, which had prominent mitochondria and dense electron bodies which corresponded to lipoid deposits. There was no difference between the right and left sides in the elements which made up the nerve.

Morphometry

The histogram of the proximal portion of the facial nerves had a unimodal curve similar to the normal facial nerve, with an average diameter of myelinic fibers of 5.16 μm. The highest number of these fibers ranged between 4 and 8 μm, the greatest frequency of fibers being between 5 and 7 μm. There were no differences between the two sides. The histograms of the distal portion of the nerves lost this unimodal configuration with fibers of all sizes being found, and small myelinic fibers were seen to predominate. This showed that regeneration was not complete.

surrounded by the cytoplasm of the Schwann cells, which had abundant organelles and finger-like prolongations without phagocytic deposits. They were myelin sheaths which surrounded the axons formed by neurotubes and neurofilaments. In the interstitial area there existed collagen fibers, which we found at varying concentrations, among which fibroblast prolongations were observed (Fig. 2).

Statistical Analysis

The mean diameter of fibers was submitted for statistical analysis. Variance analysis sowed that the substance factor (NGF versus saline serum) was not a factor of heterogeneity and did not influence the disparity of the groups. In contrast, the zone factor (distal versus proximal) did prove to be a factor of heterogeneity. With a level of confidence of 95%, the NGF did not influence the average diameter of myelinated fibers 60 days after the transection of the facial nerve.

Discussion

The section of the sciatic nerve acts in Wallerian degeneration just as a real trophic factor in the perisectional region [3]. The behavor of the Schwann cells after the transection of the mixed peripheral nerve [4] justified the local application of NGF in the section. However, we have not found positive effects of NGF when faced with a substance lacking in trophic properties such as saline serum.

References

1. Davies AM (1990) NGF synthesis and NGF receptor expression in the embryonic mouse trigeminal system. J Physiol (Paris) 84: 100–103
2. Hefti F, Schneider LS (1991) Nerve growth factor and Alzheimer's disease. Clin Neuropharmacol 14 [Suppl 1]: 562–576
3. Poduslo JF (1985) Regulation of myelinatin Schwann cell transition from a myelin-maintaining state to a quiescent state after permanent nerve transection. J Neurochem 44: 388–400
4. Schawab ME, Thoenen H (1985) Nerve growth factor. Its action modes. J Neurosci 5: 2415–2423
5. Seckel BR (1990) Enhancement of peripheral nerve regeneration. Muscle Nerve 13: 785–800
6. Slack JR, Hopkins WG, Pockett S (1983) Evidence for a motor nerve growth factor. Muscle Nerve 6: 243–252
7. Varon S, Adler R (1981) Trophic and specifying factors directed to neuronal cells. Adv Cell Neurobiol 2: 115–163

Eur Arch Otorhinolaryngology (1994) [Suppl]: S410–S412

K. Matsumoto. Y. Nakao, and H. Kumagami

Observation of Motoneurons After Recovery from Experimental Facial Nerve Paralysis

Introduction

In Bell's palsy and in Ramsay Hunt's syndrome, sequelae such as synkinesis, facial spasm, or contracture occur during recovery from facial nerve palsy. The mechanism of these sequelae has not yet been sufficiently clarified. The misdirection of regenerating nerve fibers at the site of injury may result in synkinesis. However, other possible mechanisms of synkinesis, including rearrangement of synaptic vesicles in the facial nucleus, have been suggested [1]. In the present study, the alteration of motoneurons in the brainstem after recovery from experimental facial nerve paralysis was examined by the retrograde horseradish peroxidase (HRP) technique in rabbits.

Methods

Six rabbits weighing about 2 kg each were used for the facial nerve damage test group. Under general anesthesia, the intratemporal portion of the facial nerve ranging from the stapedial muscle to the stylomastoid foramen was exposed under an operating microscope, and then crushed with a hemostat forceps for 20 s at the center of the vertical portion. Three months after the nerve injury, the return of motor function was evaluated by testing the corneal reflex. Six months after the nerve injury. 10 μl of 50% HRP (TOYOBO) solution was injected into the zygomatic muscle on the recovered side using a microliter syringe. Great care was taken to avoid unintentional spilling of the solution. After a survival time of 48 h, the animals were anesthetized and fixed by intracardiac perfusion with 2.5% glutaraldehyde in 0.2 mol phosphate buffer (pH, 7.2). The brainstem was then removed and cut serially into 100-μm-

K. Matsumoto (✉), Y. Nakao, and H. Kumagami
Department of Otolaryngology, Nagasaki University,
School of Medicine, 7-1, Sakamoto Machi, Nagasaki, 852, Japan

thick pieces in a transverse plane on a freezing microtome. Staining for peroxidase activity was carried out by the diaminobenzidine (DAB) method. For the control study, 13 rabbits were used. The zygomaticus, orbicularis oculi, orbicularis oris, and masseter muscles were exposed under the operating microscope, and then injected with the same volume of HRP. Similarly, after exposing the extratemporal portion of the facial nerve trunk, the nerve was transected and the proximal stump immediately put into a plastic capsule filled with HRP solution. The following procedure for the control group was the same as that described for the recovery case.

Results

The rabbits showed drop ear immediately after the nerve damage. Touching the cornea caused no blink on the

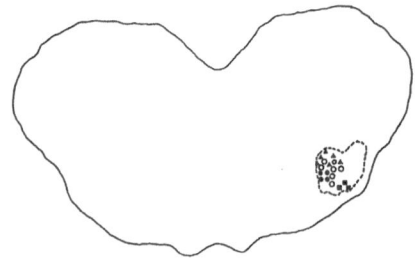

▲ Orbicularis Oculi
■ Orbicularis Oris
● Zygomaticus
○ Zygomaticus (recovered)

Fig. 1 Drawing of transverse section showing HRP-labeled facial neurons in the control and recovered animals

Table 1 Number and location of labeled neurons following injection of HRP into the facial nerve or masseter muscle in the control animals

Animal number	Injection site	Labeled cells		Other site labeled in brainstem
		Number	Location	
1	Facial nerve	575	Medulla/ventral	None
2	Facial nerve	1190	Medulla/ventral	None
3	Facial nerve	1562	Medulla/ventral	None
4	Masseter	56	Pons/dorsal	None
5	Masseter	63	Pons/dorsal	None
6	Masseter	116	Pons/dorsal	None

Table 2 Number and location of labeled neurons following injection of HRP into the facial muscles in the control and recovered animals

Animal number	Synkinetic movement	Injection site	Labeled cells		Other site labeled in brainstem
			Number	Location in facial nucleus	
Control animal					
7	–	Orbicularis oculi	23	Dorsomedial	None
8	–	Orbicularis oculi	24	Dorsomedial	None
9	–	Zygomaticus	16	Ventromedial	None
10	–	Zygomaticus	25	Ventromedial	None
11	–	Zygomaticus	35	Ventromedial	None
12	–	Orbicularis oris	11	Ventrolateral	None
13	–	Orbicularis oris	20	Ventrolateral	None
Recovered animal					
1	–	Zygomaticus	20	Medial	None
2	+	Zygomaticus	20	Medial	Nuclei reticularis
3	+	Zygomaticus	26	Medial	Nuclei reticularis
4	+	Zygomaticus	29	Medial	Nuclei reticularis
5	+	Zygomaticus	29	Medial	Nuclei reticularis
6	+	Zygomaticus	30	Medial	Nuclei reticularis

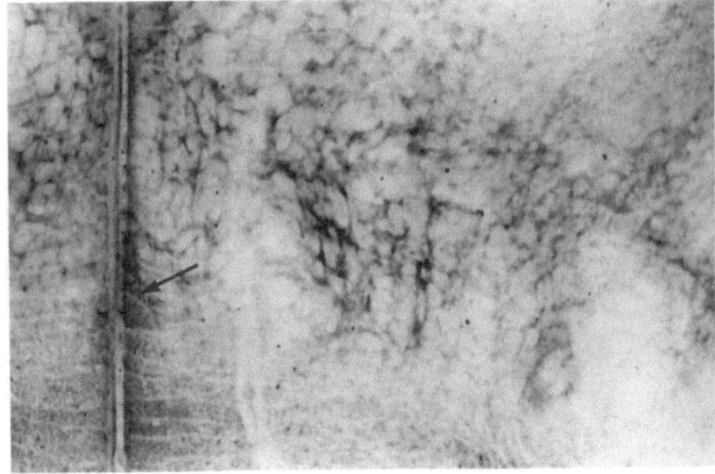

Fig. 2 Photomicrograph of transverse section of HRP-labeled cells in the brainstem from an animal which observed synkinetic movement (←: raphe)

damaged side. Three months later, however, the animals were able to raise their auricles and to produce blinking. In addition, in five of the six animals, synkinetic movement of the auricle was observed only on the damaged side simultaneously with the eye blink. Table 1 summarizes the results in the control animals following injection into facial nerve or the masseter muscle. The facial nucleus was distributed in the ventral protion of the medulla. The labeled neurons of the masseter muscle were distributed in the dorsal portion of the pons. Table 2 summarizes the results in the control and recovered animals following injection into facial muscles. Labeled neurons of the orbicularis oculi muscle were located in the dorsomedial portion of the facial nucleus, while labeled neurons of the zygomatic muscle and the orbicularis oris muscle were located in the ventromedial and ventrolateral portion respectively of the facial nucleus. The motoneurons supplying the facial muscles in the control rabbit were somatotopically organized, and there were no labeled neurons in other nuclei in the brainstem. On the other hand, in recovered animals labeled neurons innervating the zygomatic muscle were located

not only in the ventromedial portion but also partially in the dorsomedial portion where there were labeled neurons innervating the orbicularis oculi muscle in control animals (Fig. 1). There was no significant difference in the size or number of labeled neurons compared to control animals.

Furthermore, in animals observed with synkinetic movement, multipolar neurons of various sizes were labeled bilaterally in the reticular formation from the pons to the medulla (Figs. 2, 3). These neurons contained granules of HRP which were brown in color but paler than those in the facial nucleus.

Discussion

Our finding that the somatotopic organization of the facial nucleus was obscure in the recovered animals is similar to that reported previously in rats [5]. This is thought to be due to the fact that regenerating axons are misdirected at the site of injury. The brainstem afferent fiber system to the facial nucleus was examined in the cat following the injection of cholera toxin as a retrograde tracer into the facial nucleus [2]. Labeled neurons were observed bilaterally in the nuclei reticularis of both the pons and medulla. Therefore, the labeled neurons found bilateraly from the pons to the medulla in the present study are considered to be premotor neurons to the facial nucleus. The lower brainstem reticular formation can control a variety of spontaneous and reflex facial movements [4]. The pontine reticular formation area described as a pontine blink premotor area plays a role in blink reflex [3]. It seems that the premotor neurons labeled in this study may also have a role in muscle movements after recovery from facial nerve paralysis.

Acknowledgements Animal experiments were carried out in the Animal Center of Nagasaki University.

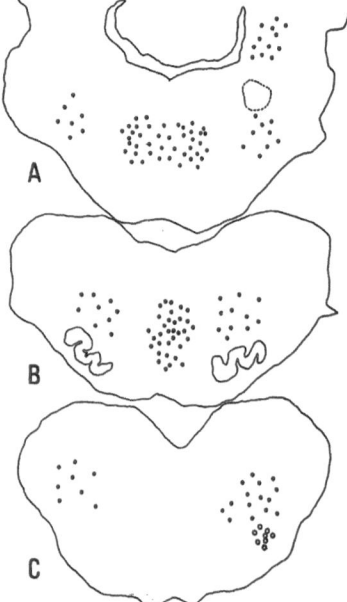

Fig. 3A–C Drawing of transverse sections from the three different levels of the brainstem in animals which observed synkinetic movement. **A** level of trigeminal motor nucleus; **B** level of superior olivary nucleus; **C** level of facial nucleus

References

1. Crumley RL (1979) Mechanisms of synkinesis. Laryngoscope 89 : 1847–1854
2. Fort P, Sakai K, Luppi PH, Salvert D, Jouvet M (1989) Monoaminergic, peptidergic, and cholinergic afferents to the cat facial nucleus as evidenced by double immunostaining method with unconjugated cholera toxin as a retrograde tracer. J Comp Neurol 283 : 285–302
3. Holstage G, Tan J, Han JV, Graveland A (1986) Anatomical observations on the afferent projections to the retractor bulbi motoneuronal cell group and other pathways possibly related to the blink reflex in the cat. Brain Res 374 : 321–334
4. Sherrington CS (1917) Reflexes elicitable in the cat from pinna, vibrissae and jaws. J Physiol 51 : 401–431
5. Thomander L (1984) Reorganization of the facial motor nucleus after peripheral nerve regeneration. Acta Otolaryngol (Stockh) 97 : 619–626

Eur Arch Otorhinolaryngology (1994) [Suppl]: S413–S415

K. Ishii and N. Takeuchi

Extracellular Matrix Arrangements of Rat Facial Nerve

Introduction

The nonneural elements of the peripheral nerve trunk are three different kinds of connective tissue sheath; epineurium, perineurium, and endoneurium. They play a role in protecting the nerve against stretching and compressive forces. The perineurium also forms a permeability barrier. The aim of this study is to observe the three-dimensional architecture of the connective tissue of rat facial nerve, and investigate the components.

Material and Methods

Electron Microscopy

Normal adult rats were perfused through the left ventricle with Karnovsky's solution. For the SEM study specimens were fixed in the same fixative, immersed in 70% ethanol for 2 days, freeze-cracked and stored in 10% aqueous solution of NaOH for 5 days [1], rinsed in distilled water, treated with 2% tannic acid solution and fixed in 2% OsO_4, dehydrated and transferred to isoamyl acetate, critical-point dried, and observed under the scanning electron microscope. For the TEM study, facial nerves were fixed in 2.5% glutaraldehyde plus 1% tannic acid, post fixed in 1% OsO_4, dehydrated, and embedded in Epon. Ultrathin sections were observed under the transmission electron microscope.

Immunomorphology

Specimens were frozen in liquid nitrogen and embedded in tissue-Tek medium without fixation. Cryostat sections

K. Ishii (✉) and N. Takeuchi
Department of Otorhinolaryngology, Faculty of Medicine,
University of Tokyo, 7-3-1 Hongo, Bunkyo-ku, Tokyo 113, Japan

were incubated with first antibody (collagen type I, III, V, VI, fibronectin, laminin). After washing in PBS, the sections were incubated with FITC-labeled goat IgE-rabbit antibody. They were examined by immunofluorescent microscopy.

Results

Electron Microscopy

There was no great difference in findings between the SEM and TEM studies regarding the extratemporal segment and distal portion of the intratemporal segment of the facial nerve.

Epineurium In the distal portion, the epineurium was composed of a thick bundle of collagen fibrils as seen by the TEM study. The cell digestion method with 10% NaOH removed the cellular elements. In the SEM survey the thick bundle of collagen fibers in the epineurium were seen in a flat tape-like shape and ran a wavy and oblique course.

Perineurium In the TEM stdy, the perineurium of the distal portion was composed of four to seven layers of perineural cells which were invested by basal laminae. There were collagen fibrils of a smaller diameter than those in the epineurium. The SEM study revealed that the collagen component of the perineurium consisted of sheets of a network of thin collagen bundles. In the proximal portion, rat facial nerve lost the rigid structure of the epineurium and perineurium, and there were only the periostium and a thin network of fibroblasts and collagen fibrils between the bone of the facial canal and the endoneurium.

Endoneurium Under TEM observation, in the distal portion the endoneurium consisted of collagen bundles and

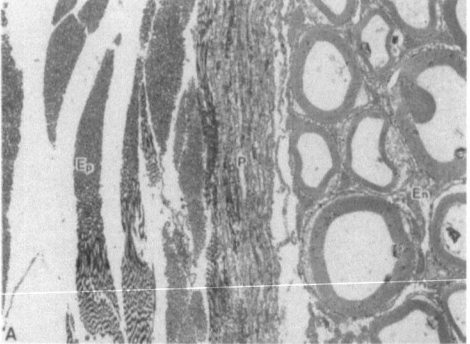

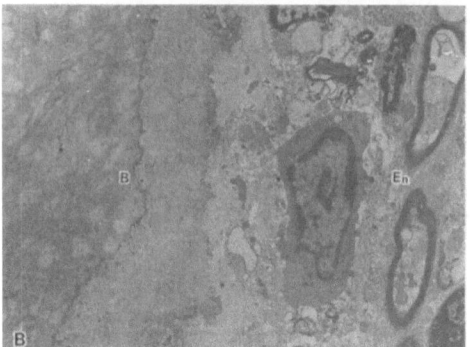

Fig. 1A, B Intratemporal segment of the rat facial nerve. **A** Distal portion. Epineurium (*Ep*), perineurium (*P*), endoneurium (*En*), ×3000. **B** Proximal portion. Interspace between the endoneurium (*En*) and bone (*B*)

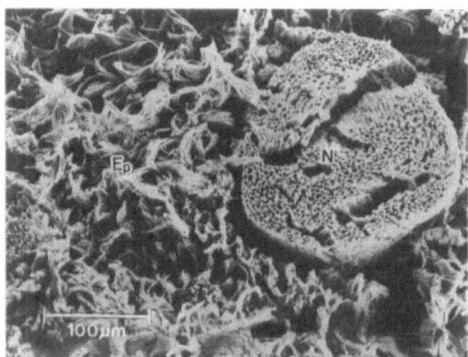

Fig. 2 Distal portion of the intratemporal segment digested with NaOH. Nerve trunk (*N*), epineurium (*Ep*), ×500

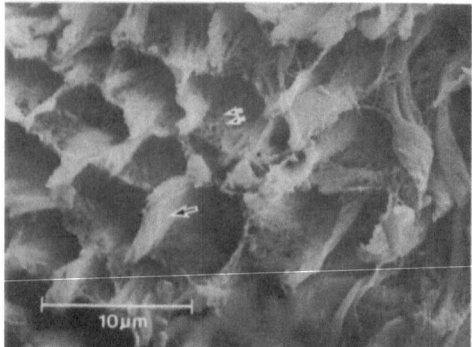

Fig. 3 Endoneurium in the distal portion of the intratemoral segment digested with NaOH. Thick collagen bundle (*arrow*) and delicate meshwork of thin collagen fibrils (*double arrow*), ×6300

fine collagen fibrils beneath the basal laminae of the Schwann cell. After NaOH treatment, the endoneurium showed numerous cylindrical tubes within which individual nerve fibers ran. These cylindrical tubes were composed of two layers of collagen fibrils, thick collagen bundles ran longitudinally along the nerve fibers in the outer layer, and the inner layer was composed of delicate meshworks of thin collagen fibrils. In the proximal portion of the facial nerve from the half of the horizontal segment, the two-layer structure of collagen fibrils was absent with only individual collagen fibrils running straight or in a slight oblique direction (Figs. 1 – 3).

Immunomorphology

Epineurium The epineurium was stained with anti-type I and III collagen and anti-fibronectin antibody. But no type V collagen and laminin stainning was noted.

Perineurium Type III and V collagen, laminin, and fibronectin stainings were present but type I collagen was not present.

Endoneurium Type I, III, V, and VI collagen, laminin, and fibronectin were codistributed. The expression of these antibodies in the endoneurium was as strong in the proximal portion as in the distal portion of the facial nerve (Fig. 4).

Fig. 4A–D Immunofluorescent microscopic demonstration of matrix components of the facial nerve. **A** Extratemporal segment, fibronectin, ×50. **B** Extratemporal segment, collagen type V, ×100. **C** Extratemporal segment, collagen tye I, ×50. **D** Proximal portion of the intratemporal segment, laminin, ×50

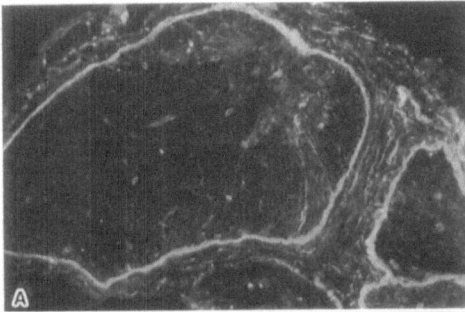

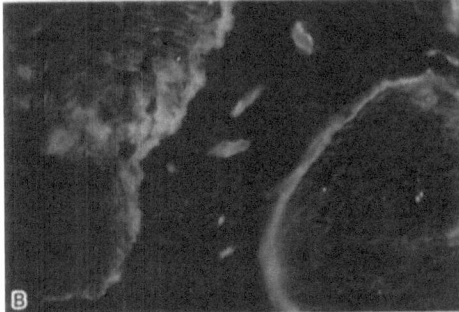

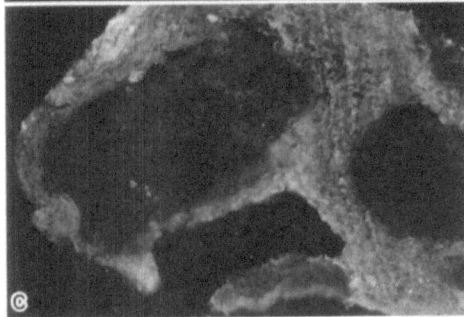

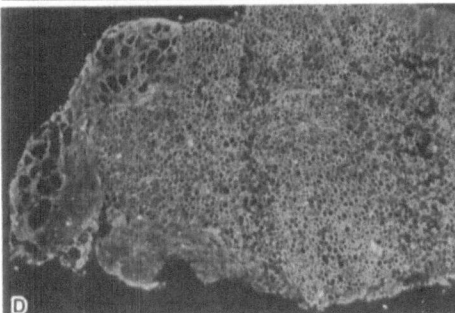

Discussion

Recently, Ohtani [1] introduced a cell-digestion method with NaOH treatment, and Ushiki and Ide [2] demonstrated a fine three-dimensional structure of the rat sciatic nerve with this method. On the other hand, the course of the facial nerve is very different from other peripheral nerves (sciatic nerve, etc.) because it runs in a bony canal of the temporal bone. The thick collagen bundles of the epineurium of the peripheral nerves which run in the soft tissue may play a role in protecting the nerve against longitudinal stretching forces, but the fact that the facial nerve has the same epineurial structure in the vertical segment, where it is rarely loaded with compressive or stretching forces, is very interesting. The lacework of collagen bundles in the perineurium may contribute to the resistance against the expanding force and to the maintenance of intrafascicular pressure (Ushiki 1990). The perineurium also forms a permeability barrier. Therefore, in the presence of facial nerve edema, in the vertical segment the perineurium may strongly related to the mechanism of facial nerve palsy, but in the proximal portion in which the facial nerve lost epineurium and perineurium, the mechanism may be the same as in the vertical segment. Ushiki et al. demonstrated two layers of collagen fibrils in the endoneurium of the rat sciatic nerve. They supposed that the longitudinally oriented collagen fibrils may play a role in resisting the stretching force along the nerve fibers, and the inner fine collagen meshworks may serve to protect the nerve fibers against compressive forces. However, the perineurium and endoneurium also changed their matrix structure to scarcely separated collagen fibrils running in the mid-horizontal segment. Therefore, the facial nerve of the proximal portion may be much weaker against the forces and invasion of toxic substances or inflammation from outside than that of the distal portion.

Generally, type I and III collagen exist in elastic tissues such as skin and blood vessel walls. They may form the stress resistance property of epineurium and endoneurium. Type V collagen and laminin are often associated with basement membrane. They may be distributed in the basement membrane of the Schwann cells in the endoneurium and that of the perineurial cells in the perineurium. Fibronectin existed in all connective tissue, and may act as a contact-mediator of connective tissue in nerve.

References

1. Ohtani O (1987) Three-dimensionnal organization of the connective tissue fibers of the human pancreas. A scanning electron microscopic study of NaOH treated tissue. Arch Histol Jpn 50 : 557–566
2. Ushiki T, Ide C (1990) Three dimensional organization of the collagen fibrils in the rat sciatic nerve as revealed by transmission and scanning electron microscope. Cell Tissue Res 260 : 175–184

Eur Arch Otorhinolaryngology (1994) [Suppl]: S416 – S417

J. A. M. Murray, R. Mountain, and M. Willins

Best Method for Facial Nerve Anastomosis

Introduction

The facial nerve is divided or sacrificed and grafted in a significant number of patients with a parotid malignancy. Rehabilitation of the face is of paramount importance to the patient and it is essential that efforts are made to restore facial nerve continuity if at all possible. The best of the traditional four methods of facial nerve anastomosis, viz. absorbable sutures, non-absorbable sutures, glue or wrapping have never previously been evaluated as a whole. It was regarded as unethical and impossible to perform a randomised controlled trial using human patients for this study due to the infinite number of variables which have to be considered so an experiment using the facial nerve of the rat was designed.

Methods and Materials

Live healthy Sprague-Dawley rats of 6 – 8 weeks old of between 200 and 300 g were used. The rats were anaesthetised without any neuromuscular blocking agent. The facial nerve was aproached by a longitudinal linear incision across the cheek and the nerve was found easily as it exited from the parotid gland. The nerve was dissected free of underlying muscles. A Digitimer Ltd. isolator stimulator model DS2 was used as a source of electrical energy. Two hooked electrodes lifted the nerve just clear of the underlying muscles. The voltage was increased until there

was a minimal movement of the rat's snout. The voltage was then increased again until maximum movement was noted. A small pin stuck in the animal's snout accentuated any movement to make recognition easier. Summation was avoided by resting between impulses. The nerve was then either used as a control or sectioned and re-anastomosed. The end result was photographed using a fixed system to allow an immediate and late postoperative comparison. The animal was allowed to recover and re-anaesthetised 70 days later. The nerve was redissected, the anastomotic site photographed and a minimal and maximal nerve twitch voltage noted. The animal was then sacrificed and the nerve examined histologically. The anastomotic agents used were $2 \times 10/0$ absorbable sutures (Vicryl-Ethicon), $2 \times 10/0$ non-absorbable sutures (Ethilon-Ethicon), Tisseel tissue glue and a thin collagen film wrap. All the experiments were randomised and blind. The histological sections were viewed through a compound microscope (Jemaned, Karl Zeiss, Jena) connected to a video, 3 semi-automated image analysis system (Analytical Measuring Systems Ltd, Pampisford, Cambridge). Distribution histograms of myelinated nerve fibre diameters were compiled from the sections using a Magiscan M2a automated image analysis system (Joye-Loebl Ltd, Gateshead, Cleveland, UK). Artefact rejection was set to eliminate fibres in the 0.75 range of the function $(4 \pi A)$ over $p \ sq$ where $\pi = 3.14286$, $A =$ cross sectional ara of the axon in square microns and $p =$ perimeter (microns). This effectively excludes fibres not cut in transverse section and those showing excessive crenation due to poor fixation. Fibre size distributions were compared using Ogival (accummulated frequency curves).

J. A. M. Murray (✉) and R. Mountain
Otolaryngology Unit, Lauriston Building, The Royal Infirmary, Edinburgh EH3 9EN, U. K.

M. Willins
Ethicon Laboratories, Bankhead Avenue, Edinburgh, U. K.

Results

The experiments were arranged as follows. Five rats compared Ethilon with a control, five rats compared Vicryl with a control, five rats compared Tisseel with a control and five rats compared the collagen wrap with a control. Twenty rats compared Ethilon with Vicryl and 20 rats compared glue and the collagen wrap. Ten further rats were used to test any deleterious effect on the intact nerve of the substances used.

Photography There was no significant difference in the size of the transverse diameter with the nerves comparing pre- and postoperative states and between any of the anastomotic agents used. A qualitative assessment was made at the time of the anastomosis and at postmortem and agan no significant difference was found, either comparing pre- and postoperative states and any of the anastomotic agents.

Electrophysiology Overall no superior method was found at either the minimal nerve stimulatin or maximum nerve stimulation levels. In such a large volume of numbers, a few spurious statistically significant results emerged. The occasional result of significance in a mass of data must be regarded with common sense and not held as a success of an experiment if no other data support it.

Histology Both approximal and distal nerve sections were studied and again no significant difference between any of the groups was found.

Discussion

The buccal division of the rat facial nerve is an excellent nerve to use as an animal model. There may be some criti-cisms levelled at using rats and the translation of any work from rats to human facial nerves but, nevertheless, the animal model is valid to a limited extent. This experiment shows that the material used, i.e. absorbable, non-absorbable, a collagen tube and a plasma glue are inert to the nerve and allow natural healing of a divided facial nerve with minimal influence from the materials themselves. This would certainly suggest that the discussion over exactly what material should be used on the grounds of interference with axon regrowth should now be discounted and more attention paid to the practical details of the site of the nerve section. It is suggested that if the site allows the nerves to lie together without movement, e.g. within the temporal bone, then probably glue or a tube would be appropriate, particularly as this area may be difficult to suture, whereas in the extratemporal portion of the facial nerve, where there is potential for more movement of the face, a suture material may be appropriate. There appears to be no difference in the end result of the different types of repair to the facial nerve itself.

Reference

1. Murray JAM (1992) ChM thesis, University of Edinburgh

Eur Arch Otorhinolaryngology (1994) [Suppl]:S418–S419

FREE PAPERS AND POSTERS

T. Takeda, S. Takeda, K. Kozakura, and H. Saito

An Animal Model of Ischemic Facial Palsy

Introduction

Although the pathogenesis of idiopathic facial palsy still remains to be settled, ischemia of the facial nerve is thought to be one of the most likely etiological factors. The intratemporal portion of the facial nerve receives blood supply from three major sources; that is, the internal auditory artery, the petrosal branch of the middle meningeal artery, and the stylomastid artery [1]. Of these arteries, the petrosal branch of the middle meningeal artery, the so-called petrosal artery, provides the main arterial supply to the geniculate ganglion, where the vascularity is much richer than elsewhere in the course of the facial nerve. Therefore, this artery seems to be a key to the solution of the pathogenesis of idiopathic facial palsy. In the preset study, we studied influences of interruption of the petrosal artery on the facial nerve.

Materials and Methods

Animals used were 50 guinea pigs in the present study. These animals were divided into two groups for the following two experiments: Experiment No. 1, in which we measured blood flow in the facial nerve at the geniculate ganglion using laser Doppler flowmetry in ten guinea pigs, and studied the effects of interruption of the petrosal artery on the blood flow in the facial nerve. In Experiment No. 2, we investigated the motor function and histological changes of the facial nerve within 3 days after interruption

T. Takeda (✉), S. Takeda, K. Kozakura, and H. Saito
Department of Otolaryngology, Kochi Medical School, Kohasu, Oko-cho Nankoku, Kochi, 783, Japan

of the petrosal artery in 40 animals. The motor function was estimated by blink reflex and an antidromic evoked facial nerve response. The degree of facial palsy was graded by blink reflex (+3, complete loss of reflex; +2, unable to close eye completely; +1, delayed reflex; 0, normal). Antidromic facial nerve responses were recorded from the geniculate ganglion, according to a method described by Tashima K et al. [2]. Animals were put to death 3 days after the interruption and histological changes were examined light microscopically. The interruption of the petrosal artery was carried out by transection of this artery in the attic.

Results

Experiment No. 1

Interruption of the petrosal artery resulted in almost complete ischemia of the facial nerve at the geniculate ganglion, but interruption of the stylomastoid artery caused no change in blood flow in the facial nerve.

Experiment No. 2

Interruption of the petrosal artery produced facial palsy within 3 days after the interruption in 29 of 40 guinea pigs (72.5%). As to grade of facial palsy, grade +3 was found in 9 animals, grade +2 in 5 animals, and grade +1 in 15 animals. In cases with inomplete palsy (grade +1 or +2), weakness of blink reflex was observed during 2–3 days after the operation. But in cases with complete palsy (grade +3), loss of blink reflex appeared as early as 1 day after the interruption. Antidromic facial nerve response were relatively well evoked in cases with incomplete palsy. But no antidromic facial nerve response was evoked, or waves, generated proximal to the recording site, reduced or disappeared in animals with complete palsy. Characteristic histological changes of the facial nerve were nerve swelling. The facial canal was occupied by the swollen facial nerve. This swelling was most marked at geniculte level and was evident in the tympaic and mastoid segments. It was most severe in cases with complete palsy. Swelling was also noted in cases without facial palsy, although to a less striking degree. This swelling of the facial nerve was mainly caused by swelling of the individual nerve fibers. The myelin sheaths were elongated and made thinner by swelling axons and were less stained with Luxor fast blue stain compared to those of the control side. A clustering of nerve fibers of varying size was noted.

Discussion

Ischemia of the facial nerve is thought to be one of the most likely etiological factors in idiopathic facial palsy. The blood supply in the facial nerve has been studied morphologically in considerable detail. However, we have little information on its hemodynamics. The present study using a laser Doppler flowmeter revealed that the blood flow in the geniculate ganglion of the facial nerve comes not from the stylomastid artery but mainly from the petrosal artery. Thus, interruption of the petrosal artery resulted in a marked decrease in facial nerve blood flow at the geniculate ganglion. Indeed this ischemic change caused facial palsy within 3 days in 72.5% of the guinea pigs. Antidromically evoked facial nerve responses and histological findings suggested that facial palsy was caused by nerve conduction block due to edema of the nerve distal to the geniculate ganglion.

Recently, a target lesion site in idiopathic facial palsy has been thought to be the central portion around the geniculate ganglion. This experimentally induced facial palsy is similar to idiopathic facial palsy in humans with respect to a lesion site. Therefore, this animal model would provide us with a new tool to evaluate the pathogenesis of facial palsy.

References

1. Blunt MJ (1954) The blood supply of the facial nerve. J Anat 88 : 520 – 526
2. Tashima K, Takeda T, Saito H et al. (1990) Antidromically evoked facial nerve responses in guinea pigs: a basis for clinical applications in patients with facial palsy. Eur Arch Otorhinolaryngol 247: 151 – 155

Eur Arch Otorhinolaryngology (1994) [Suppl] : S 420 – S 421

S. Kitani and N. Yanagihara

Experimental Studies on Antidromic Evoked Potential of the Facial Nerve

Introduction

A method of recording antidromic evoked potential (AEP) of the facial nerve is supposed to have advantages over conventional tests, such as evoked electromyography (eEMG), electroneuronography, and nerve excitation test, in predicting the prognosis of facial palsy in its early stage. However, a comparison of these tests has not yet been studied. The aim of this paper is to investigate the diagnostic value of AEP in predicting the prognosis of facial palsy in comparison with that of eEMG in animal models.

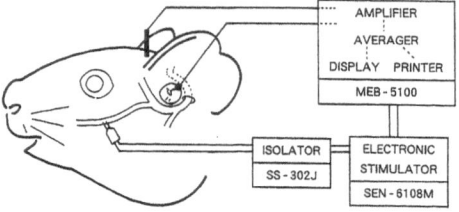

Fig. 1 Experimental setup

Materials and Methods

The experiments were conducted on 57 normal guinea pigs. Following intraperitoneal anesthesia using pentobarbital sodium (30 – 50 mg/kg), the intratemporal segment of the facial nerve was exposed by the superior approach under the operating microscope. In order to produce experimental facial nerve paralysis, the nerve trunk was clamped just peripheral to the geniculate ganglion using a needle holder designed for microvascular surgery (compressed group, $n = 50$). The superior labial branch of the facial nerve was exposed and then stimulated directly by a pair of bipolar electrodes each separated by 1 mm. Figure 1 shows the experimental setup. A square wave electrical pulse, 10 μs in duration and 20 – 40 V in amplitude, were repeatedly applied at 0.5 s intervals. For recording of AEP,

S. Kitani (✉)
Department of Otolaryngology, Yawatahama City Hospital,
1-638 Ohira, Yawatahama, Ehime, 794, Japan

N. Yanagihara
Department of Otolaryngology, Ehime University, Ehime, Japan

two active electrodes were placed on the posterosuperior aspect of the external ear canal and on the nerve trunk just below the stylomastoid foramen, respectively. The inactive electrode was placed on the parietal scalp, and the earth was placed on the back of the neck. Averaging of 64 or 124 trials was performed with MEB-5100 (Nihon Koden). While recording the AEP, the eEMG from the orbicularis oris muscle was simultaneously registered with bipolar needle electrodes. The AEP and eEMG were registered from the 2nd to the 20th day after compression. In the control group ($n = 7$), the facial nerve was exposed at the geniculate ganglion but not clamped. The AEP and eEMG were recorded between the 2nd and the 18th day.

Results

Table 1 summarizes the results of the experiments. Both AEP and eEMG were clearly identified on the 2nd day. On the 3rd day, AEP was unelicited in all animals except one in which a small response was recorded through the electrode at the stylomastoid foramen. In contrast, eEMG was recorded in four of the eight animals. On the 4th day, AEP was unobtainable in any of the three animals, while the eEMG was recorded in one of the three animals. At this

Table 1 Results of the experiments

Day after compression			2	3	4	5~7	8~10	13~16	19~20
No. of evoked	AEP	EAC	2	0	0	0	1	5	6
		SMF	2	1	0	0	1	10	6
	eEMG		2	4	1	0	0	4	4
No. of total experimented animals			2	8	3	8	7	14	8

AEP, antidromic evoked potential; eEMG, evoked electromyography; EAC, external auditory canal; SMF, stylomastoid foramen

early stage, of the animals from which the eEMG was not obtained, no AEP was registered.

From the 5th to the 7th day, neither AEP nor eEMG were obtained from any of the eight animals. On the 8th to the 10th day, AEP was evoked in one of the seven animals while eEMG was not. On the 13th to the 16th day, AEP was evoked from the stylomastoid foramen in 10 of the 14 animals. In contrast, eEMG was registered from only 4 of the 14 animals. On the 19th to the 20th day, AEP was obtained in six of the eight animals while the eEMG was obtained in four animals.

In the control group, AEP was obtained at any time tested between the 2nd and the 18th day.

Discussion

The advantages of AEP are due to its ability to directly detect the pathological condition of the involved site. Following damage to the nerve, Wallerian degeneration occurs and spreads centrally and distally. There are two main possibilities to explain the progress of physiologial degeneration: (1) degeneration takes place simultaneously along the entire length of the fiber, (2) degeneration follows a centrifugal course. According to the former, both AEP and eEMG should be involved at the same time. Instead, our results tend to support the latter, due to the disappearance of AEP before that of eEMG. Thus, the results indicate that AEP correlates better than eEMG to the condition of facial nerve lesion. These results of the present experimental study are thought be useful in interpreting of AEP recorded from the patient with acute intratemporal facial nerve paralysis. We attempted to record AEP in 12 patients with facial palsy at various time after the onset. However, AEP was observed only in two patients. In one of the patients, AEP was recorded on the 3rd diseased day. In the other patient, AEP was recorded on the 38th diseased day soon after the palsy disappeared. The AEP can be recorded in human subjects with facial palsy, but more investigation is needed to know its clinical value.

Eur Arch Otorhinolaryngology (1994) [Suppl]: S 422

POSTERS

B. Csillik, E. Knyihár-Csillik, E. Kukla-Dobi, I. Tajti, A. Czigner, and G. W. Kreutzberg

Function-Dependent Expression of Calcitonin Gene-Related Peptide in Neuromuscular Junctions of Facial Muscles

Motor end plates of various mammalian and amphibian muscles express calcitonin gene-related peptide (CGRP). It has been assumed (Fontaine et al. 1986) that CGRP in the neuromuscular junctions is involved in the regulation of the synthesis of the alpha-subunit of the nicotinic acetylcholine receptor. However, motor end plates in the facial muscles, innervated by the facial nerve, fail to exert any CGRP immunoreactivity. We sought to solve this controversy by immobilization of related muscles by injecting bupivacaine (Marcain) twice daily into the tissue space between the masseter and buccinator muscles of the rat. Bupivacaine is known to block action potentials in nerve and muscle as well as the action of acetylcholine at the neuromuscular junction, thereby paralyzing the muscle. We found slight immunoreactivity of motor end plate CGRP after 4 days' continuous bupivacaine treatment; after 10 days the reaction was comparable to that seen in strongly reacting muscles (e. g., flexor digitorum brevis). It is concluded that immobilization of the muscles induces an accumulation of CGRP in the normally negative motor end plates, strongly supporting the hypothesis on the regulatory role of CGRP upon the acetylcholine receptor.

References

Fontaine B, Klarsfeld A, Hökfelt T, Changeux J-P (1986) Calcitonin gene-related peptide, a peptide present in spinal motoneurons, increases the number of acetylcholine receptors. Neurosci Lett 71:59

B. Csillik (✉)
Harvard University, Medical Education Center, The Holmes Society, 260 Longwood Avenue, Boston, MA 02115, USA

E. Knyihár-Csillik, E. Kukla-Dobi, I. Tajti, A. Czigner, and G. W. Kreutzberg
Department of Anatomy, Albert-Szent-Györgyi Medical University, H-6701 Szeged, Hungary

Eur Arch Otorhinolaryngology (1994) [Suppl]: S 423 – S 424

POSTERS

N. Kanoh, T. Kumoi, T. Minatogawa, T. Kobayashi, T. Okada, and H. Seguchi

Ultracytological Localization of K⁺-Dependent, p-Nitrophenylphosphatase Activity in Cat Facial Nerve

Introduction

The transport of Na and K ions across the plasma membrane of the neuron seems to be a prerequisite for the conductance of nerve impulses. The localization of Na-K ATPase activity in the sciatic nerve, among other peripheral nerves, has been previously reported by several authors. However, little is known as to the localization of Na-K ATPase activity in the facial nerve.

The present study was designed to investigate the localization of ouabain-sensitive, K⁺-dependent p-nitrophenylphosphatase (K-NPPase) activity, the second dephosphorylative property of the Na-K ATPase complex, in the horizontal portion of the cat facial nerve, using the new method proposed by Kobayashi et al. [1].

Materials and Methods

Preparation of Tissues

Intratemporal facial nerves were obtained from normál cats weighing 2.8 – 4.0 kg. Under ketamine hydrochloride anesthesia, the animals were perfused via the heart with a fixatime containing 2% paraformaldehyde and 0.05% glutaraldehyde in 0.1 M cacodylate buffer, pH 7.4, for 10 min. The facial nerve was removed from the temporal bone and further fixed in the same fixative for 1 h at 0 – 4°C.

Cytochemical Procedure

Materials were cut into sections 40 µm thick with a Microslicer. The tissue slices were rinsed with 50 mM Tricine buffer, pH 7.5, for 15 min and incubated in a medium reported by Kobayashi et al. [1]. Observation was performed with a JEM-100S electron microscope.

As controls, tissue samples were incubated in substrate-free medium, in medium containing 10 mM ouabain, and in medium in which K⁺ had been replaced with Na⁺.

Results and Discussion

K-NPPase activity revealed the fine granular reaction product on the cytoplasmic side of the plasma membrane of Schwann cells and axons (Fig. 1). In the node of Ranvier,

N. Kanoh (✉), T. Kumoi, T. Minatogawa, and H. Seguchi
Department of Otolaryngology, Hyogo College of Medicine, 1-1, Mukogawa-cho, Nishinomiya, 663 Hyogo, Japan

T. Kobayashi and T. Okada
Department of Anatomy and Cell Biology, Kochi Medical School, Kohasu, Okoh-cho, Nankoku, Kochi 783, Japan

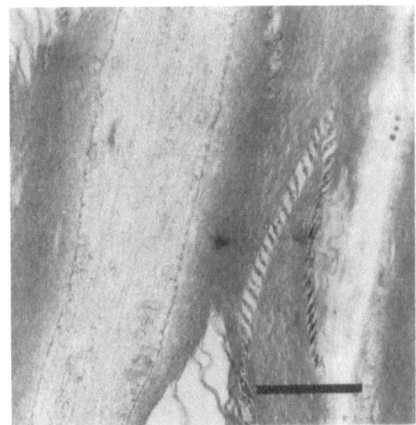

Fig. 1 Ouabain-sensitive, K⁺-dependent p-nitrophenylphosphatase (K-NPPase) activity in a longitudinal section of axon of facial nerve. *Bar,* 1 µm

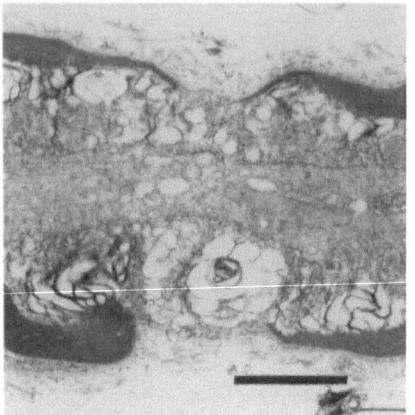

Fig. 2 A node of Ranvier. *Bar* = 1 μm

reaction product was observed when tissues were incubated in substrate-free medium.

To our knowledge, this is the first report on the cytochemical localization of Na-K ATPase activity in the horizontal portion of the cat facial nerve.

When compared with the histo- and cytochemical data on the sciatic nerve provided by other researchers, the results seem controversial. One of the main reasons could be the different methodological approach. However, in previous immunocytochemical studies of the sciatic nerve, Na-K ATPase activity was reported to be localized at the nodal axolemma, astrocytic foot processes, and the paranodal regions of the Schwann cells, including nodal microvilli, which coincides with the findings reported in this paper. Thus there seems to be no significant difference between the localization of Na-K ATPase in the sciatic and the facial nerve.

From the clinical point of view, this fundamental study on the localization of Na-K ATPase activity in the facial nerve is expected to become an important fact to be taken into consideration for the elucidation of the cause of idiopathic facial palsy (Bell's palsy).

the reaction product was localized not only on the nodal portion, but also on the paranodal and internodal portions of the axolemma and on the microtubules in the axon cylinder. Enzyme activity was also localized in the cytoplasmic side of the plasma membrane of the terminal paranodal loop of Schwann cells (Fig. 2). In controls, formation of reaction product was almost completely inhibited when 10 mM ouabain was included in the medium. No

Reference

1. Kobayashi T, Okada T, Seguchi H (1987) Cerium-based cytochemical method for detection of ouabain-sensitive, potassium-dependent, p-nitrophenylphosphatase activity at physiological pH. J Histochem Cytochem 35 : 601 – 611

Eur Arch Otorhinolaryngology (1994) [Suppl]: S425 – S427

POSTERS

S. Murakami and N. Yanagihara

Degeneration and Regeneration of Neuromuscular Junction in Guinea Pig Mimic Muscle – A Scanning Electron Microscopic Study

Introduction

Morphological changes in the neuromuscular junction (NMJ) postsynaptic membrane at the motor end plate have been studied with light and transmission electron microscope during experimental denervation and reinnervation. However, only a few studies have been demonstrated in mimic muscle and these have failed to reveal the overall morphological changes in the MNJ. The purpose of this study is to clarify the three-dimension morphological changes in NMJ after facial nerve section and suture in guinea pig by use of scanning electron microscope (SEM).

Materials and Methods

The orbicularis oculi muscle of adult guinea pigs weighing 300 – 400 g were used. In the denervated experiment, the extratemporal facial nerve trunk was resected 3 mm in length. The muscle was removed for 1 – 4 weeks and processed for SEM examination. In the reinnervation experiment, immediate perineural nerve suture was performed with 10.0 monofilament nylon under operating microscope immediately after nerve section. The muscle was examined 5 – 11 weeks after nerve suture.

The excised muscle was fixed in 3% glutaraldehyde for 3 h and postfixed in 2% osmium tetroxide. After osmication, the specimen was rinsed in distilled water and then treated with 8N-HCl for 30 min at 60°C to remove the intramuscular connective tissue components [1]. The specimen was dehydrated through a graded series of ethanol and immersed in isoamyl acetate. After drying by the critical point method and a sputter coating with platinum, the specimen was examined in a Hitachi S-500-SEM.

Results and Comments

NMJ consisted of terminal axon covered with Schwann cell and subneural apparatus (SNA) in the muscle fiber. Normal SNA was characterized by deep and clearly outlined labyrinthine primary synaptic clefts (Fig. 1A, large arrow) and numerous narrow slits openings of the junctional folds (secondary synaptic clefts; Fig. 1A, small arrow) in the primary synaptic clefts. During the first 2 weeks after nerve section, primary synaptic clefts became shallower. The junctional folds gradually decreased in number and became wider and shorter (Fig. 1B). After week 3, muscle fiber became atrophied and primary synaptic clefts elevated and with an irregular surface. Junctional folds decreased in number (Fig. 1C). At week 4, the SNA could still be recognized as an irregular elevation, but the number of discernible SNA had remarkably decreased in this week (Fig. 1D).

In the early stage of reinnervation, primary synaptic clefts were small and sarcoplasmic ridges obscure. The junctional folds appeared to be shallow, short slit-like openings (Fig. 2A, B). After week 7, the primary synaptic clefts became large and increased their depth, though they were less regular in shape than those in normal muscle. Junctional folds gradually increased in number and depth (Fig. 1C). At week 9, some SNA regenerated and acquired normal structural organization (Fig. 1D).

The sequence of events during reinnervation seems to be in the reverse order to denervation processes. The denervation and reinnervation stages of the SNA varied considerably among muscle fibers. This was because the speed of denervation and reinnervation depends mostly on the size of nerve fiber; both are faster in large nerve fibers than in small ones.

S. Murakami and N. Yanagihara
Department of Otolaryngology, Ehime University School
of Medicine, Shigenobu-chou Onsen-gun, Ehime, 791-02 Japan

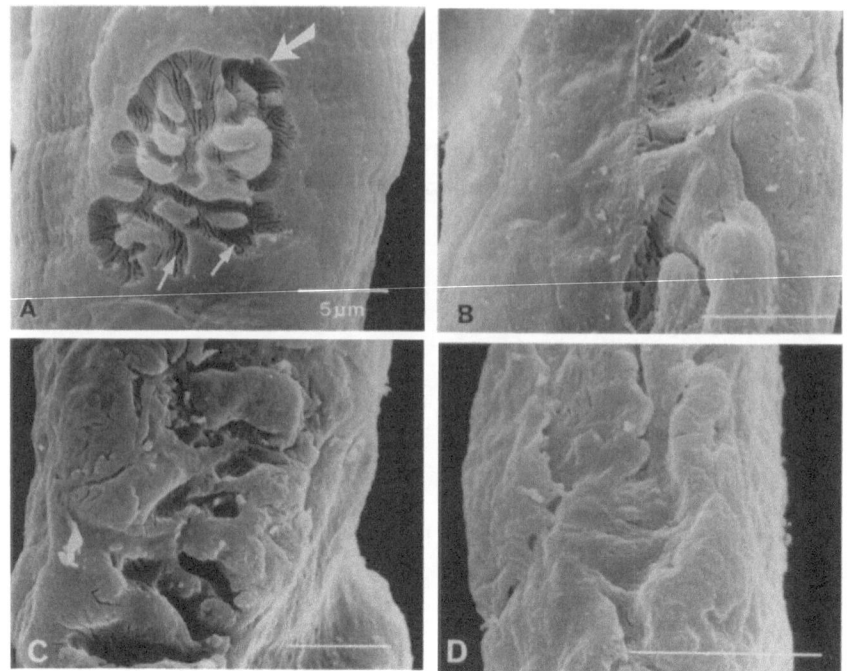

Fig. 1A–D Degeneration process of neuromuscular junction (NMS). **A** Intact NMJ; *large arrow,* primary synaptic cleft; *small arrows,* secondary synaptic clefts. **B, C, D** Weeks 2, 3 and 4, respectively, after nerve section. *Bar,* 5 μm

Reference

1. Desaki J, Uehara Y (1981) The overall morphology of neuromuscular junctions as revealed by scanning electron microscopy. J Neurocytol 10:101–110

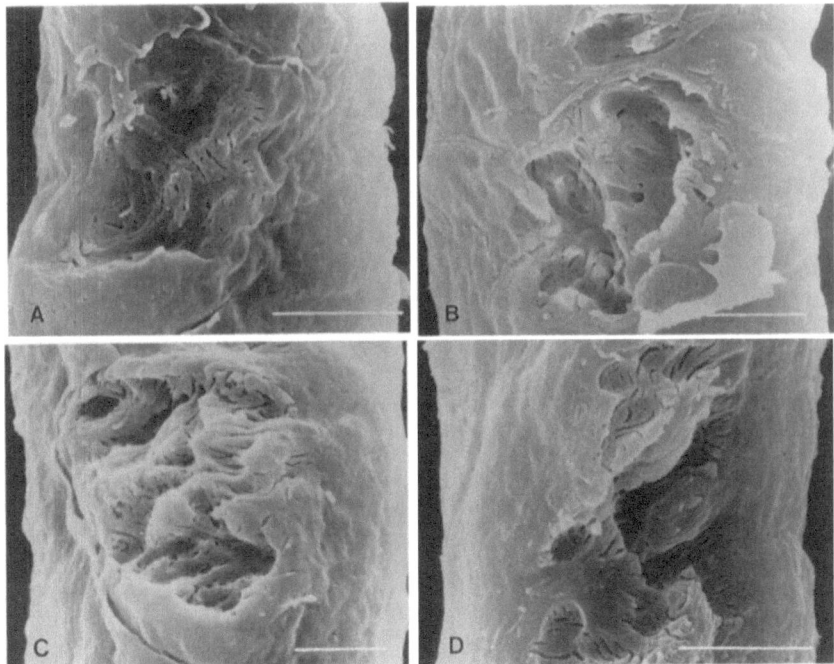

Fig. 2A–D Regeneration process of neuromuscular junction at weeks 5 (**A**), 6 (**B**), 7 (**C**), and 9 (**D**) after nerve suture. *Bar*, 5 μm

Eur Arch Otorhinolaryngology (1994) [Suppl]: S428–S429

POSTERS

P. Ablanedo, M. J. Bernardo, C. Suarez, M. Alvarez-Uria, and J. L. Llorente

Nerve Growth Factor: Optic and Ultrastructural Findings on Facial Nerve Degeneration in the Rabbit

Introduction

After the discovery by Hamburger [3] and Levi-Montalcini [5] of the nerve growth factor (NGF), other neurotrophic factors such as brain-derived neurotrophic factor (BDNF) and cilliary neurotrophic factor (CNTR) [6] were found. At present we do not know whether a specific trophic factor exists that acts on motor fibers. On the other hand, the effect of the NGF on sensory fibers is known. Therefore, we used this factor locally on the transected area of a mixed nerve, such as the facial nerve, evaluating its possible action during the degeneration period.

Material and Methods

For this study we used seven male white New Zealand rabbits, weighing a average of 1 kg. The third portion of the intrapetrous facial nerve was approached and a complete transection of the nerve, before the exit of the chorda timpani, was carried out. On the right side at the section point 1000 ng 2.5 S-NGF (Betseda Research Labaratory was instilled localy, overing the nerves with gel foam sponges soaked in NGF. On the left side the same technique was applied and at the section point 0.5 ml saline serum was instilled. The animals were killed in sequence after 24 h and 2, 3, 5, and 19 days after surgery. An intracardial per-

M. J. Bernado (✉), C. Suarez, and J. L. Llorente
Department of Otolaryngology, Hospital Central Universitario de Asturias, c/Pedro Masaveu 25, 33007, Oviedo, Asturias, Spain

P. Ablanedo
Department of Pathology, Hospital Central Universitario de Asturias, c/Pedro Masaveu 25, 33007, Oviedo, Asturias, Spain

M. Alvarez-Uria
Department of Cellular Biology, Hospital Central Universitario de Asturias, c/Pedro Masaveu 25, 33007, Oviedo, Asturias, Spain

fusion with glutaraldehyde was performed and the right and left facial nerves from each animal were extracted for histologial study.

Results

Under light microscopy the proximal areas of all the nerves appeared to be normal, with the exception of a small segment close to the section which displayed characteristics similar to those of the regenerated distal areas.

After 24 h intact myelinic fibers appeared, alternating with others which were degenerated, fragmentation of the myelin sheath, axonal vacuolization, and intra-axonal occupation.

In the area distal to the section after 2 days, the early degenerative changes were more noticeable, with disarrangement and demyelinization of the fibers and loss of the intraneural structure. Three days after the section, myelinic fibers which were not yet degenerated alternated with clearly degenerated fibers. These nondegenerated myelinated fibers were no longer observed after the fifth or sixth day after the section, a time at which the degeneration of the distal nerve was complete. Axons were demyelinated, the myelin being fragmented and endoneurally situated. Globular axonal forms were also seen and the perineurum was preserved. After 19 days, marked perisectional fibrosis was observed as well as axonal sprouts thus the nerve appeared to be regenerating.

Distal to the section, the nerve configuration was similar to a nonmanipulated nerve, made up of fibers of medium and small size and scarce areas with degenerated fibers showing vacuolization and increase in interneural fibrosis. No differences were found between the left and right nerves at this time.

Ultrastructurally, 24 h after the section, the distal zones were already seen to show early signs of degeneration. Myelin deposits were observed intraxonally or in the cytoplasm of the Schwann cells, and degeneration among the fibers was not uniform (Fig. 1). At this time some fibers

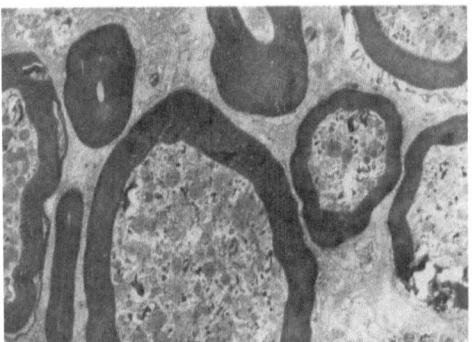

Fig. 1 Distal area near section 24 h after nerve transection. Electron micrograph showing myelinic degenerated fibers. Vacuolization and multivesicular bodies in Schwann cells and from the axon

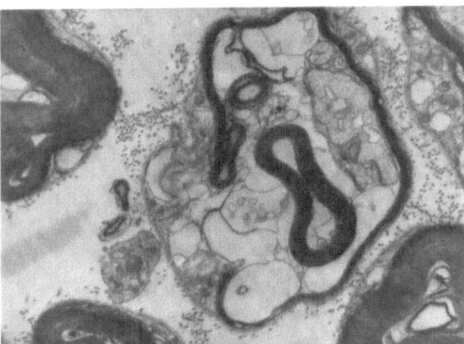

Fig. 2 Distal area 3 days later than in Fig. 1. Numerous dense bodies and myelin-like intra-axon. Partial conservation of myelin

showed complete axon-myelin degeneration with laminar multivesicular and myelin-like bodies and the disappearence of the organelles from the Schwann cells and from the axons. After 3 days, a clear degeneration appeared with axon-myelin disruption (Fig. 2) and concentric laminar

bodies and some nondegenerated fibers still remaining. Small amounts of collagen were seen in the interstitial area as well as remnants of free myelin. Five to six days after the section, the degeneration of the axon and the myelin was complete, with vacuolization and large dilations affecting all the fibers. After 19 days we observed predominance of the myelinated fibers with irregular and stellate forms. Only a few amyelinic fibers and endoneural capillaries and little collagen were seen. The whole sequential study showed no valuable ultrastrucdural differences between the right and left nerves in the distal areas. The proximal areas showed no degeneration except in the perisectional region.

Discussion

The ligature of the sciatic nerve [2] and its transection [4] produce an increase in NGF and mRNA-NGF, respectively, on both sides of the transection in the first steps of regeneration, showing that the non-neuronal cells which surround the nerve fibers can produce or convey it; for this reason the local application of NGF would have a positive effect on the first stages of regeneration. In our series using NGF versus saline serum locally, we found no modification of one substance compared to the other in this phase.

References

1. Barde Y, Edgar D et al. (1982) Purification of a new neurotrophic factor from mammalian brain. EMBO J 1 : 549 – 553
2. Fitzgeral M, Wall PD (1985) Nerve growth factor counteracts the neurophysiological and neurochemical effects of chronic sciatic nerve section. Brain Res 332 : 131 – 141
3. Hamburger VJ (1934) The effects of wing bud extirpation on the development of the central nervous system in chick embryos. J Exp Zool 68 : 449 – 494
4. Heumann R et al. (1987) Changes of NGF synthesis in nonneural cells in response to sciatic nerve transection. J Cell Biol 104 : 1623 – 1631
5. Levi-Montalcini R (1966) The NGF: its mode of action on sensory and sympathetic nerve cells. Harvey Lect 60 : 217 – 219
6. Manthorpe M, Varon S (1985) Regulation of neuronal survival and neuritic growth in the avian cilliary ganglion. In: Guroff G (ed) Growth and maturation factors, vol 3. Wiley, New York

Eur Arch Otorhinolaryngology (1994) [Suppl] : S 430

POSTERS

O. Guntinas-Lichius, E. Stennert, and W. F. Neiss

Stereological Estimation of the Volume and Neuron Number of the Facial and Hypoglossal Nucleus of the Rat*

Recently developed stereological methods allow an unbiased and efficient estimation of structural quantities. In order to study the effect of an operation at the facial and hypoglossal nucleus on the volume, neuron number, and neuron density in the nuclei of origin, we investigated these parameters in the normal untreated facial and hypoglossal nucleus using two stereological methods: Cavalieri's principle and the fractionator.

Material and Methods Fifty-six female Wistar rats (BOR:WISW) were fixed by perfusion, the brainstems were embedded in paraffin, and 6-μm sections through facial and hypoglossal nucleus were Nissl-stained. The volume was estimated by Cavalieri's principle using ten equidistant sections per nucleus and the neuron number was counted by the fractionator using five equidistant pairs of adjacent sections as physical disectors. The neuron density was calculated from neuron number and volume of the nucleus.

As the ranges show, there was a large interindividual variation between animals, although all rats were taken from the same closed SPF colony. A right vs. left side analysis indicated no systematic side asymmetry, the intraindividual side asymmetry was negligible, and a linear regression left vs. right side of all parameters showed that a big (small) left nucleus was always highly correlated to a big (small) right nucleus ($r = 0.63 - 0.93$; $P = 0.001$).

The neuron density was nearly twice as high in the hypoglossal as in the facial nucleus. A craniocaudal analysis of the sections through the nuclei showed that the neuron density was nearly homogeneous in all parts of the facial and hypoglossal nucleus.

Results

Facial nucleus	Mean ± SD in %	Range
Volume	$0.83 \text{ mm}^3 \pm 12\%$	$0.4 - 1.0 \text{ mm}^3$
Neuron number	$3835 \pm 14\%$	$2518 - 5085$
Neuron density	$4621 \text{ mm}^{-3} \pm 18\%$	$3300 - 7537 \text{ mm}^{-3}$
Hypoglossal nucleus	Mean ± SD in %	Range
Volume	$0.29 \text{ mm}^3 \pm 13\%$	$0.22 - 0.41 \text{ mm}^3$
Neuron number	$2487 \pm 14\%$	$1728 - 3312$
Neuron density	$8576 \text{ mm}^{-3} \pm 17\%$	$5807 - 13400 \text{ mm}^{-3}$

O. Guntinas-Lichius (✉), E. Stennert, and W. F. Neiss
Department I of Anatomy and Department of Otolaryngology, University of Cologne, Joseph-Stelzmann-Str. 9, 50924 Cologne, Germany

* Supported by the Deutsche Forschungsgemeinschaft (Ne 412/1-1).

Eur Arch Otorhinolaryngology (1994) [Suppl]: S431

POSTERS

T. Evgenjeva

Effects of Motor Neuron Disorders on Feeding Behavior of Sturgeons, Inhabiting the Volga River

The locomotion and feeding behavior of sturgeons (*Acipencer guldenstadti*) was studied and facial muscles and olfactory barbels were examined using light and scanning electron microscopy. The barbels of the surgeon serve to provide a sense of smell in the search for food. In 18 (8 male, 10 female) sturgeons aged 8–19 years with clinical characteristics of skeletal muscle pathology caused by ecological pollution, the contraction and innervation of the facial muscle and barbels were examined. The results indicated degenerative changes in muscle associated with destruction of myofibrils. It was found that the innervation of the barbels was disturbed and the ability to search for food impaired. The movements of the barbels were much slower than those in healthy fish.

Thus the myofibrillar apparatus of the facial muscle was found to be in a pathological state compared to normal skeletal muscles and provides an interesting model for the investigation of various environmental factors. The state of the muscle function can therefore be monitored by barbel activity.

T. Evgenjeva
Institute of Evolutionary Animal Morphology and Ecology, Moscow, GUS, Lenenski, pr. 33, B-71

Eur Arch Otorhinolaryngology (1994) [Suppl]:S432–S433

Y. Kawasaki, H. Aruga, S. Ogino, K. Hashimoto, K. Yamanishi, and T. Matsunaga

Detection of Varicella Zoster Virus DNA by Polymerase Chain Reaction in Clinical Samples from Patients with Hunt's Syndrome

Introduction

It is well known that Hunt's syndrome is caused by the reactivation of varicella zoster virus (VZV), and as viral isolation from vesicle fluid is very difficult due to the high lability of the virus, usually laboratory diagnosis is carried out by serological testing. For direct immunofluorescence, well-prepared cellular smears are necessary. Diagnosis by antibody detection is not possible in the early days of disease and is complicated by cross-reactions to herpes simplex virus.

The polymerase chain reaction (PCR) is a novel technique that amplifies a specific sequence of DNA in vitro efficiently and rapidly using synthetic oligonucleotide primers in a series of denaturation, reannealing, and extension steps with heat-stable Taq polymerase [4]. In this study, we established a system of PCR for VZV and used it to detect VZV DNA in clinical samples from patients with Hunt's syndrome.

Materials and Methods

For certification of the specificity of the PCR in this system, DNA from cells infected with five human herpesvirus – VZV, cytomegalovirus (CMV), human herpesvirus 6 (HHV-6), and herpes simplex virus types 1 (HSV-1) and 2 (HSV-2) – were extracted, purified, and used as templates in the PCR.

Y. Kawasaki (✉), H. Aruga, S. Ogina, and T. Matsunaga
Department of Otolaryngology, Osaka University Medical School, Osaka, 553, Japan

K. Hashimoto
Japan Clinical Assay Laboratories Ltd.

K. Yamanishi
Department of Virology, Research Instititute for Microbial Diseases, Osaka University

For determination of the sensitivity of the PCR, a sample of cloned VZV DNA was amplified with primers of glycoprotein I (gpI).

As clinical samples, three vesicles' fluid, 12 crusts of skin lesions, and a swab of palatal ulcer from 13 Hunt's syndrome patients were collected.

Samples collected from patients were added to PCR buffer with nonionic detergents and proteinase K and were homogenized until no pieces were visible. These samples were incubated at 55 °C for at least 1 h and at 95 °C for 10 min to inactivate the proteinase. A total of 25 μl of this lysate was used for PCR reaction.

DNA was amplified in a total volume of 100 μl reaction mixture consisting of 50 mM KCl, 10 mM Tris-HCl (pH 8.3), 1.5 mM MgCl$_2$, 0.01% gelatin, deoxynucleotide triphosphate mixture (dATP, dGTP, dCTP and dTTP at a final concentration of 200 μM), and 2.5 U Taq DNA polymerase. The sequences of the two oligomers, which were regions of gpI, were synthesized and used as primers. A total of 30 cycles of the amplification reaction were carried out in a DNA thermal cycler. Annealing was performed at 60 °C for 2 min, extension at 72 °C for 5 min, and denaturation at 90 °C for 1 min [2].

The amplified product was detected by agarose gel electrophoresis and stained with ethidium bromide. For Southern blot analysis, separated DNA fragments were transferred and denatured. Hybridization procedure and immunological detection was carried out according to the standard protocols of Lion [3] and Kessler [1].

Results

Specificity and sensitivitiy of the Polymerase Chain Reaction

The specificity of the PCR was evaluated by using four other human herpesviruses (CMV, HHV-6, HSV-1, HSV-2). No band of the expected 677-bp size was detectable

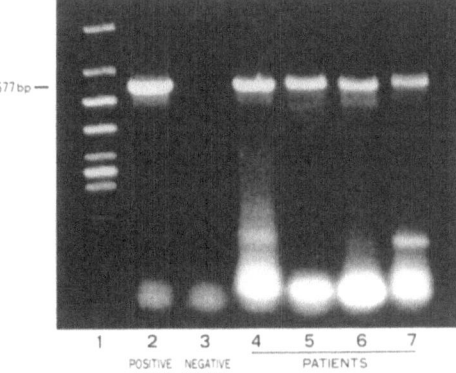

677 bp —

1   2   3   4   5   6   7
POSITIVE NEGATIVE   PATIENTS
CONTROL CONTROL

Fig. 1 Detection of varicella zoster virus (VZV) DNA by polymerase chain reaction (PCR) in clinical samples by direct gel electrophoresis.
Lane 1, molecular weight standards. *Lane 2,* positive VZV DA control. *Lane 3,* reaction mixture alone.
Lanes 4–7, crusts of skin lesions and swab of palatal ulcer from patients. VZV DNA from all clinical samples were detected by direct gel electrophoresis

after amplification of these viruses. For determination of sensitivity of the PCR in this study, a sample of cloned VZV DNA was amplified. VZV DNA fragments were detected in an agarose gel by ethidium bromide staining at a level of 5×10^3 copies; 5×10^2 copies of VZV DNA were detected by Southern blot analysis.

Detection of Varicella Zoster Virus DNA

Sixteen clinical samples were collected from 13 patients diagnosed clinically as having Hunt's syndrome, and VZV DNA in these samples was examined by PCR. All clinical samples were detected by direct gel electrophoresis and Southern blot analysis (Fig. 1).

Discussion

In this study, VZV DNA was detected in all vesicles, crusts, and in a swab of palatal ulcer by direct gel electrophoresis, and specificity was proved by Southern blot analysis. As described in the introduction, virus isolation from patients with VZV infection is difficult even from vesicles because of the lability of the virus. In the case of patients with Hunt's syndrome, clinical diagnosis is not difficult according to symptoms, but virological or serological diagnosis is often difficult and complicated. In some cases, seroconversion is not detected, and because vesicles observed in patients with Hunt's syndrome are generally small and are often replaced with crusts at the time of consultation, isolation of the virus is almost impossible. In contrast, this PCR method does not require the presence of live or intact infectious virus. Very small amounts of DNA or partially degenerated DNA of VZV can also be detected. Moreover, it is of interest that VZV DNA was detected even in patients who were treated with systemic or local acyclovir therapy. These experiments demonstrated that this PCR method was useful for detecting VZV in clinical samples from patients with Hunt's syndrome.

References

1. Kessler C (1991) The DIG technology – a survey on the concept and realization of a novel bioanalytical indicator system. Mol Cell Probes 5 : 161 – 205
2. Kido S, Ozaki T, Asada H, Higashi K, Kondo K, Hayakawa Y, Morishima T, Takahashi M, Yamanishi K (1991) Detection of varicella-zoster virus (VZV) DNA in clinical samples from patients with VZV by the polymerase chain reaction. J Clin Microbiol 29 : 76 – 79
3. Lion T, Hass OA (1990) Nonradioactive labeling of probe with digoxigenin by polymerase chain reaction. Anal Biochem 188 : 335 – 337
4. Saiki RK, Scharf S, Faloona F, Mullis KB, Horn GT, Erlich HA, Arnheim N (1985) Enzymatic amplificaton of β-globin genomic sequences and restriction site analysis for diagnosis of sickle cell anemia. Science 230 : 1350 – 1354

Eur Arch Otorhinolaryngology (1994) [Suppl]: S434

ABSTRACTS

W. F. Neiss, O. Guntinas-Lichius, A. Gunkel, D. N. Angelov, and E. Stennert

Stereological Evaluation of Neuronal Plasticity in Rat Brainstem After Hypoglossal-Facial Anastomosis*

Using stereological methods for the estimation of neuronal cell number, neuronal packing density, and the volume of brain regions, we have investigated the quantitative structural changes that take place in the facial and hypoglossal nucleus of the rat brainstem following surgery of the peripheral nerves.

Material and Methods. In 249 rats either a HFA was performed microsurgically or a facial-facial or hypoglossal-hypoglossal anastomosis or both nerves were transected and 10 mm of the distal portion removed. Four to 112 days postoperation (dpo) all rats were fixed by perfusion and stereological evaluation was performed in 6-μm paraffin serial sections after Nissl staining (compare Guntinas Lichius et al., this symposium).

Results. Axotomy of the facial or hypoglossal nerve without nerve suture, i. e., axotomy of the facial nerve during HFA or resection of both peripheral nerves, causes loss of motoneurons and shrinkage of the facial or hypoglossal nucleus. This degeneration seems to start as early as 14–28 dpo, is evident at 42 dpo, and further progresses until at last 112 dpo, at which date – in comparison to the untreated contralateral side of the brainstem – 30%–40%

of all motoneurons have disappeared in the facial or hypoglossal nucleus. In parallel to the reduction in the number of motoneurons, the degenerating facial or hypoglossal nucleus also loses 30%–40% of its volume. The packing density of the motoneurons remains, however, constant in both nuclei during degeneration.

Following axotomy with nerve suture i. e., suture of the hypoglossal nerve in HFA or hypoglossal-hypoglossal anastomosis and suture of the facial nerve in facial-facial anastomosis, there is regeneration of the peripheral nerve and of its nucleus of origin. During this regeneration neither loss of nerve cells nor shrinkage of the facial or hypoglossal nucleus could be detected in our material.

Facial or hypoglossal regeneration after simple re-anastomosis shows the same reaction pattern over the same time course, whereas hypoglossal regeneration after HFA differs during the acute phase of neurite outgrowth (14–42 dpo) in that HFA seems to stimulate the cellular reactions in the regenerating hypoglossal nucleus more intensely.

Conclusion. Microsurgical suture of the cut facial or hypoglossal nerve in rats serves to maintain the central neuronal structures of these nerves completely.

W. F. Neiss, O. Guntinas-Lichius, A. Gunkel, D. N. Angelov, and E. Stennert
Department I for Anatomy and Department of Otolaryngology, University of Cologne, Joseph-Stelzmann-Str. 9, 50924 Cologne, Germany

* Supported by the Deutsche Forschungsgemeinschaft (Ne 412/1-1) and the Humboldt-Stiftung (Angelov).

Eur Arch Otorhinolaryngology (1994) [Suppl]: S435

ABSTRACTS

M. V. Kozlova, V. U. Kalentchuk, and N. G. Slepko

Role of Opioid Peptides and Substance P in the Regeneration of CNS and PNS Nervous Tissue

Cultures of PNS, CNS, and glioma C_6 are very convenient models for testing the biologial activity of factors in neural regeneration. According to our studies opioid peptides (OP) [endogenous, but also synthetic analogues (substance P, SP)] change not only the intensity of neurite outgrowth, but also survival and adhesion properties of PNS and CNS neurons. This type of peptide activity was measured in dissociated culture of rat spinal cord by aggregation assay. It was found that the aggregation during peptide action was increased on average 1.6- to 1.7-fold compared to controls, thus altering cell adhesion and increasing survival of neurons and glial cells. We obtained data on increased survival of PNS neurons CNS in culture many years ago. OP and SP change ot only survival, neurite outgrowth and neuron adhesion, but also the properties of PNS and CNS glial cells. The rate of migration of Schwann cells and spinal cord astrocytes increased under the effect of OP and SP, altering their adhesion and survival. It was shown on glioma C_6 cells that proliferation activity, DNA synthesis, and degree of differentiation (GS, CNP, GPDH activity) altered with OP and SP action; GPDH activity of Schwann cells and oligodendroeytes increased; the number of cells labeled with the astrocyte marker (GFAP) increased in the presence of OP in the growth medium.

Thus, our findings and the literature to date suggest that OP and SP may play a role in the development and regeneration of neurons and glial cells of PNS and CNS tissue.

These results were the basis for the treatment in clinical practice of ALS and MS [by the dalargin analogue of (Leu)-enkephalin]. These peptides, especially dalargin, can be used for regeneration in the case of facial nerve injury.

M. V. Kozlova, V. U. Kalentchuk, and N. G. Slepko
Institute of Experimental Cardiology of the Research,
Cardiology Center, Moscow, CIS

Eur Arch Otorhinolaryngology (1994) [Suppl]: S436

ABSTRACTS

D. N. Angelov, A. Gunkel, O. Guntinas-Lichius, E. Stennert, and W. F. Neiss

Reinnervation of Rat Vibrissae After Hypoglossal-Facial Anastomosis: A Horseradish-Peroxidase Study *

The movement of whiskers in rat is solely controled by motoneurons of the facial nerve. Hence the musculature of the whiskerpad is a good model to study the time course of mimic reinnervation after hypoglossal-facial-anastomosis (HFA) in this animal. We have investigated this question morphologically (for physiological data see: Schneider et al., this symposium), counting the number of motoneurons that were labeled by retrograde transport of horseradish peroxidase (HRP) injected into the whiskerpad at different postoperative survival times. These results were compared with the normal number of HRP-labeled facial motoneurons (HRP applied into the whiskerpad of the nonoperated contralateral side).

Material and Methods In 42 rats an HFA was performed, and 48 h before sacrifice 2 mg HRP (type VI-A, Sigma, no. P-6782) in 0.2 ml distilled water was administered into both whiskerpads. At intervals of 14, 18, 21, 28, 42, 56, and 112 days postoperation (dpo) the rats were fixed by perfusion and HRP activity revealed in 50-μm vibratome sections of the brainstem.

Results Injection of HRP into the normal whiskerpad of the untreated contralateral side labeled 1278 ± 97 (mean ± SD, $n = 42$) motoneurons, all of which were localized in the lateral facial subnucleus. After HFA no cells were labeled up to 21 dpo. The first HRP-labeled motoneurons coul be detected in the hypoglossal nucleus at 28 dpo, at which day 46 ± 21 (mean ± SD, $n = 6$) labeled nerve cells were counted. Gradually this number increased to 565 ± 63 at 42 dpo, 1096 ± 52 at 56 dpo, and 1172 ± 32 at 112 dpo. Surprisingly, HRP-marked neurons were also observed scattered throughout the whole facial nucleus of the operated side. Their numbers amounted to 268 ± 35 (mean ± SD, $n = 6$) at 42 dpo, 700 ± 107 at 56 dpo, and 797 ± 85 at 112 dpo.

Conclusions (1) HFA effected the regeneration and outgrowth of hypoglossal neurons into a facial domain. (2) The crosscut proximal stump of the facial nerve spontaneously regenerated into its original peripheral despite HFA.

D. N. Angelov, A. Gunkel, O. Guntinas-Lichius, E. Stennert, and W. F. Neiss
Institut I für Anatomie and Hals-, Nasen- und Ohrenklinik der Universität zu Köln, Cologne, Germany

* Supported by the Humboldt-Stiftung (Angelov) and the Deutsche Forschungsgemeinschaft (Ne 412/1-1).

Eur Arch Otorhinolaryngology (1994) [Suppl]: S437

ABSTRACTS

M. Papaxanthos, J. Koenig, A. Guilhaume, V. Darrouzet, D. Portmann, J.M. Aran, and J.P. Bébéar

Biomaterials Used in Nerve Regeneration Chambers as Substrata for Spinal Cord Neurons Cultured In Vitro

Despite marked advancements in microsurgical techniques, the prognosis for complete functional recovery after peripheral nerve transection and resutrue in man is poor. Various biomaterials have been used in nerve regeneration chambers. However, their in vitro properties in relation with the cell to substratum (biomaterials) adhesion of neurite growth cones have rarely been studied. Spinal cord neurons cultured in vitro are shown to respond differently to the various biomaterials used as substrata. The authors emphasize the importance of studying biomaterials as substrata in the same condition as those used in vivo.

M. Papaxanthos, J. Koenig, A. Guilhaume, V. Darrouzet,
D. Portmann, J.M. Aran, and J.P. Bébéar
Clinique Universitaire ORL, INSERM Unité 229, Bordeaux, France

Eur Arch Otorhinolaryngology (1994) [Suppl]: S 438

M. Papaxanthos, J. Koenig, J. Dupont, A. Guilhaume, J.M. Aran, and J.P. Bébéar

Fibrin Sealant (Tissucol) as a Substratum for Spinal Cord Neurons Cultured In Vitro

Many in vivo studies have shown the technical advantages of fibrin sealant in the facial nerve anastomosis. The results of this use outweigh those achieved with microsurgical suture. Fibrin sealant is used as a substratum for spinal cord neurons cultured in vitro. The authors emphasize the importance of the respective concentrations of its componets and proposals for its optimal use are made.

Without changing its adhesive qualities so appreciated by neurosurgeons, we propose modifications so as to transform the universal Tissucol into specific Neurocol.

M. Papaxanthos, J. Koenig, J. Dupont, A. Guilhaume, J.M. Aran, and J.P. Bébéar
Clinique Universitaire ORL, INSERM Unité 229, Bordeaux, France

Eur Arch Otorhinolaryngology (1994) [Suppl]:S439

ABSTRACTS

J. G. Spector and P. Lee

Facial Nerve Regeneration Through Semipermeable Porous Chambers

Peripheral nerve regeneration, over a 10-mm transectional gap, was determined in 70 rabbit buccal divisions of the facial nerve using two entubational systems (semipermeable porous and impermeable silicone chambers) and three naturally occurring media (serum, blood, saline) during a 5-week period. The number of myelinated axonal regenerates at the midchamber and 2 mm into the distal transected neural stump were counted in each group and compared to normative pooled myelinated axonal counts in nine normal rabbit buccal divisions of the facial nerve. Semipermeable porous chambers had an overall greater regeneration success rate (75% vs. 42.8%) and regained, on average, a higher number of myelinated axons (51.4% vs. 26.1%) than silicone chamber regenerates. Semipermeable porous chambers containing serum or blood had significantly higher regeneration success, myelinated axonal couts, and percentages of neural innervation of the distal transected neural stump. Both entubational systems produced similar axonal counts with intraluminal saline. The highest overall success rate (93.7%) and average number of myelinated axons per chamber (3072) were achieved in porous chambers filled with serum. The greatest variability in myelinated axonal counts (0–3266 axons) and percentage distal stump innervation (5.5%–98.1%) was seen in silicone chambers filled with saline. The percentage myelinated axons from the midchamber that innervated the distal stump was greater in porous chambers with blood (73%) and serum (54%) than in silicone saline chambers (43%). On average, the distal stumps from porous chambers filled with serum (47%) and blood (33.5%) regained a higher percentage of normal myelinated axonal counts than silicone-saline chambers (12.5%). The implications of these results is that both the construction of the entubational chamber and the intraluminal medium have a significant influence on neurite regeneration. Semipermeable porous chambers with intraluminal serum have a strong neurite-promoting potential in peripheral neural regeneration of rabbit facial nerves.

J. G. Spector and P. Lee
Department of Otolaryngology, Head & Neck Surgery, St. Louis, Missouri 63110, USA

Eur Arch Otorhinolaryngology (1994) [Suppl]: S 440

ABSTRACTS

J.G. Spector, P. Lee, A. Derby, G. Frierdich, G.R. Neises, and D.G. Roufa

Comparison of Rabbit Facial Nerve Regeneration in Nerve Growth Factor-Containing Silastic Tubes to Autologous Cable Grafts

Previous reports suggest that nerve growth factor (NGF) enhanced significantly nerve regeneration in rabbit facial nerves (Chen et al.). We compared facial nerve regeneration in silastic tubes prefilled with NGF or cytochrome C (Cyt. C, control) to autologous neural grafts. A 10-mm silastic tube prefilled with a solution of either NGF or Cyt. C in saline was implanted to bridge an 8-mm neural gap in the buccal division of the rabbit facial nerve. At 3 weeks there was a more mature neural organization, greater fascicular organization, and more proliferative neovascularization in NGF-treated regenerates. At 3 and 5 weeks computer-assisted morphometric examination at the midtube revealed no significant difference in the number of myelinated or unmyelinated axons in NGF or Cyt. C treated implants. However, at 5 weeks, NGF regenerates, when compared to their respective preoperative controls, had a greater percentage of myelinated axons (46% vs 18%). For cable graft repair an 8-mm autologous segment of the buccal nerve was removed, rotated 180°, and sutured to bridge the neural gap. The number of myelinated axon regenerates in the autologous nerve graft at 5 weeks were significantly greater than those growing through the silastic tubes. However, in the neural graft the majority of the axons were found in the extrafascicular connective tissue (66%). The majority of these myelinated fibers did not find their way into the distal neural stump. Implanted NGF containing silastic tubes of 15 mm length (13 mm neural gaps) for 7 weeks failed to show a neural regenerate and the PC12 tissue assay and anti-NGF antibody demonstrated no NGF activity in the intrasilastic tube serum. We conclude that NGF improves facial nerve regeneration over an 8-mm neural gap. NGF effects over longer distances need further clarification. In neural graft repairs intrafascicular regenerates are the major axons reinnervating the distal transacted nerve segment. The number of myelinated axons innervating the distal stump in NGF-filled silastic tubes and autologous nerve grafts are similar. Thus neural grafts may not be superior to entubational repairs.

J.G. Spector, P. Lee, A. Derby, G. Frierdich, G.R. Neises, and D.G. Roufa
Department of Otolaryngology, Head & Neck Surgery, Washington University School of Medicine, St. Louis, Missouri 63110, USA

Eur Arch Otorhinolaryngology (1994) [Suppl]: S441

ABSTRACTS

J. C. Dort, M. Wolfensberger, and H. Felix

Carbon Dioxide Laser Repair of the Facial Nerve: An Experimental Study in the Rat

The facial nerve is often injured by trauma, infection, or during the course of tumor resection. Many techniques of nerve anastomosis have been described with the current standard nerve repair using the microscope and monofilament suture. The purpose of this study was to evaluate the CO_2 surgical laser as a tool for facial nerve anastomosis. Following preliminary electrical measurements, 36 nerves were anastomosed using either laser or conventional monofilament suture. Laser anastomosis had neither beneficial nor detrimental effects on nerve regeneration. This method of anastomosis may be advantageous when surgical access is limited. In addition, this study found that the use of CO_2 laser as a dissecting or vaporizing tool in proximity to intact facial nerves results in degenerative changes.

J. C. Dort
Department of Surgery University of Calgary, Rm 193, 3330 Hospital Dr. Nih, Calgary, Alberta, Canada T2N 4N1

M. Wolfensberger and H. Felix
Department of Otolaryngology of the University of Zürich, Zürich, Switzerland

Eur Arch Otorhinolaryngology (1994) [Suppl]:S442

ABSTRACTS

Y. Hosomi, M. Kinishi, H. Hosomi, and M. Amatsu

A New Animal Model of Facial Nerve Palsy Using a Freezing Method

The etiology of Bell's palsy is still unknown. It is generally accepted that the edema and the ischemia in the fallopian canal are the major pathogenic factors of Bell's palsy. From this standpoint, few animal models have been established. A new animal model of facial nerve palsy caused by freezing is reported. Mongoian gerbils were used. The middle ear space was frozen microscopically with dimethylether liquid propane gas, after myringotomy. The onset of palsy was confirmed by the loss of both blink and movement of the whiskers. Facial movement was evaluated, and the evoked EMG was recorded 1, 3, and 5 weeks later after the onset of facial palsy. Temporal bones were sectioned and subjected to histopathological study.

Out of 50 animals thus frozen, 47 (94%) had complete facial palsy. This animal model of facial nerve palsy is characterized by the high occurrence of palsy in the temporal bone without direct manipulation of the nerve. In most animals, facial movements recovered completely within 5 weeks. The amplitude of the evoked EMG was not found 1 week after onset. Three and 5 weeks after onset, the evoked EMG was seen although the amplitudes were less than those of the nonaffected side.

In the pathological study, the empty endoneural spaces were observed 1 week after onset and decreased 3 and 5 weeks after onset, though empty spaces were still seen.

Y. Hosomi, M. Kinishi, H. Hosomi, and M. Amatsu
Department of Otolaryngology, Head and Neck Surgery,
Kobe University, School of Medicine, Kobe, Japan

Immunology

Eur Arch Otorhinolaryngology (1994) [Suppl]: S445–S446

M. Mañós-Pujol, J. Nogués, A. Ros, M. Dicenta, M. Mestre, and E. Buendía

Etiopathogenesis of Bell's Palsy: An Immune-Mediated Theory

The findings reported in a series of works related to the nature of Bell's palsy suggest that immune alterations play an important role in the etiopathogenesis of Bell's palsy [1]. Humoral immunity alterations have been reported during the acute phase of Bell's palsy, suggesting an inflammatory reaction triggered by a viral infection [1–3]. Herpes viruses have been proposed as Bell's palsy triggers because their infections present epidemiological [4–6] and clinical similaritis [6–8]; furthermore herpes viruses have been reported in the ganglia of some cranial nerves [9–10].

Cellular immune disorders similar to those found in autoimmune demyelinating and viral diseases have also been reported in Bell's palsy patients [11–14]. The pathologial studies performed in Bell's palsy patients described in inflammatory reaction with lymphocytic infiltrates [15–16]. Evidence of isochrome polyneuropathy and demyelinating pheomena have been described in cranial and peripheral nerves [17–19] in patients with Bell's palsy.

These series of works therefore support an immune-mediated mechanism triggered by a viral infection in the pathogenesis of Bell's palsy [20]. As the real etiopathogenic mechanism is still unknown, we suggest that a viral infection triggers the facial paralysis according to the following events: the antigenic determinants of the nerve cells and myelin are modified during viral replication within the ganglionar nerve cells. Then, a T-lymphocyte-mediated immune response is triggered against the modified nerve cells, producing an immunomediated segmentary horizon-tal demyelination expressed clinically as facial paralysis. Once this phenomena is controlled remyelination begins and the facial paralysis clinically improves.

As the immune response is genitically controlled, a individual susceptibility is present in Bell's palsy associated with class II (DR linked gene) antigens [13, 21, 22]. Our conclusion is that Bell's palsy is an acute demyelinating disease, triggered by a viral infection, that produces an immune-mediated segmentary demyelination in a genetically predetermined population.

References

1. Mañós-Pujol M et al. (1990) Lymphoproliferative response to facial nerve extracts in patients with Bell's palsy. Preliminary report. In: Castro D (ed) The facial nerve. Kugler and Ghedini, Amstelveen, pp 339–343
2. Jonsson L et al. (1990) The cellular and humoral response in Bell's palsy. In: Castro D (ed) The facial nerve. Kugler and Ghedini, Amstelveen, pp 215–220
3. Diamante VG (1990) Some aspects of Bell's palsy; pathogenesis. In: Castro D (ed) The facial nerve. Kugler and Ghedini, Amstelveen, pp 311–313
4. McCormick DP (1972) Herpes simplex virus as a cause of Bell's palsy. Lancet 1, 937–939
5. Adour KK (1976) Cranial polyneuritis and Bell's palsy. Arch Otolaryngol 102 : 262–264
6. Adour KK et al. (1978) The true nature of Bell's palsy: an analysis of 1000 consecutive cases. Laryngoscope 88 : 787–801
7. Djupesland G et al. (1977) Acute peripheral facial palsy: part of a cranial polyneuropathy? Arch Otolaryngol 103 : 641–644
8. Valhne A et al. (1981) Bell's palsy and herpes simplex virus. Arch Otolaryngol 107 : 79–81
9. Baringer JR et al. (1973) Recovery of herpes simplex virus from human trigeminal ganglion. N Engl J Med 81 : 648–650
10. Mulkens PSJ et al. (1980) Acute facial paralysis: a virological study. Clin Otolaryngol 5 : 303–309
11. Aviel et al. (1983) Peripheral blood T and B subpopulations in Bell's palsy. Ann Otol Rhinol Laryngol 92:137–141
12. Mañós-Pujol M et al. (1985) T-lymphocyte subpopulations in Bell's palsy. In: Portmann M (ed) Facial nerve. Masson, New York, pp 197–202
13. Bumm P et al. (1990) The results of immunological regulation and immunogenetics in Bell's palsy. In: Castro D (ed) The facial nerve. Kugler and Ghedini, Amstelveen, pp 211–214

M. Mañós-Pujol, J. Nogués, A. Ros, and M. Dicenta,
Department of ORL, Ciutat Sanitaria i,
Universitaria de Bellvitge, Barcelony, Spain

M. Mestre and E. Buendía
Department of Immunology, Ciutat Sanitaria i,
Universitaria de Bellvitge, Barcelony, Spain

14. Jonsson L et al (1988) Depression of T cels in Bell's palsy. Ann Otol Rhinol Laryngol 97 : 138 – 143
15. Reddy JB et al. (1966) Histopathology of Bell's palsy. Eye Ear Nose Throat Monthly 45 : 62 – 65
16. Proctor G et al. (1976) The pathology of Bell's palsy.Trans Am Acad Ophthalmol Otolaryngol 82 : 70 – 79
17. Adour KK et al. (1980) Herpes simplex polyganglionitis. Otolaryngol HNS 88 : 270 – 274
18. Odkvist L et al. (1982) Evidence of polyneuropathy in Bell's palsy. In: Graham MD, House WF (eds) Disorders of the facial nerve. Raven, New York, pp 303 – 305
19. Thomander L et al. (1990) Magnetic resonance imaging in patients with Bell's palsy. In: Castro D (ed) The facial nerve. Kugler and Ghedini, Amstelveen, pp 195 – 197
20. Adour KK et al. (1991) Medical management of idiopathic (Bell's) palsy. Otolaryngol Clin North Am 24 (3): 663 – 673
21. Gorodezky C et al. (1990) HLA ad T-cell subpopulations in Bell's facial paralysis. In: Castro D (ed) The facial nerve. Kugler and Ghedini, Amstelveen, pp 315 – 317
22. Shibahara T et al. (1990) A possible association of HLA with Bell's palsy as an etiologial genetic factor. In: Castro D (ed) The facial nerve. Kugler and Ghedini, Amstelveen pp 323 – 325

Eur Arch Otorhinolaryngology (1994) [Suppl]: S447–S448

FREE PAPERS AND POSTERS

P. Bumm and G. Schlimok

T-Lymphocyte Subpopulations and HLA-DR Antigens in Patients with Bell's Palsy, Hearing Loss, Neuronitis Vestibularis, and Ménière's Disease

Numerous and various immunological tests have been made in the last few years for researching and diagnosing immunological diseases of the labyrinth. In spite of the different possibilities for immunological testing, Veldmann [8] is right in talking of the diagnostic dilemma of recognizing supposed immuno-otological diseases. This is also true to the same degree for the facial nerve.

In this study some days after onset of the paralysis different lymphocyte tests were made in peripheral blood in order to analyze the general, systematic immune system in various otological diseases and peripheral facial paralysis. On one hand, it involves recognizing immunoregulation, in which the T-helper lymphocytes (CD4)/T-suppressor lymphocyte (CD8) ratio is determined. On the other hand, it involves a testing method to measure immunogenetics by HLA-DR typing. The first results were reported at the 6th International Symposium on the Facial Nerve in Rio de Janeiro [3]. The results with a large number of patients have become so stabilized that a new report should be made.

In this article no further details concerning the findings in HLA-DR typing will be given. The typing was more difficult due to the cortisone treatment of Bell's palsy. Only HLA-DR3 and HLA-DR4 were studied. No relative increase of risk was found for both antigens in muscle palsy. A simplified, hypothetical scheme for immunoregulation is: The macrophage produce interleukin. (1) This causes the proliferation of CD4 helper cells, which leads to an activation of CD8 suppressor cells by interleukin. (2) B cells, which produce antibodies, are activated by CD4 helper cells and are impeded by CD8 suppressor cells. The CD4/CD8 ratio was determined by an immunofluorescence method.

Figure 1 shows the findings of immunoregulation in various otoneurological diseases. The CD4-helper/CD8-suppressor cell ratio is indicated on the ordinate. The normal values of the method can be found in the boxes. The "KO" stands for a control group of 51 healthy persons, as shown on the x-axis.

A pathological CD4/CD8 quotient appears in 57% of cases of Meniere's disease, 48% of neuronitis vestibularis, and 39% of Bell's palsy. These findings of Bell's palsy confirm the measurements of Manos-Pujol et al. [6], who reported for the first time about changes in lymphocyte subpopulation. Although other researchers were not able to confirm these findings, our findings confirm his results.

Figure 2 presents the immunoregulation CD4/CD8 in various acute hearing losses. A healthy control group "KO" is indicated on the x-axis, followed by a group of 52 patients with sudden hearing loss, who demonstrated a pathological quotient in about 50%. Eight patients had hearing loss due to otobasal fractures, nine had tinnitus and

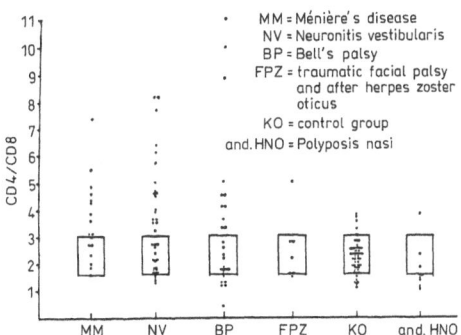

Fig. 1 CD4/CD8 quotients in various otoneurological diseases and in a control group (*KO*) of 51 healthy persons. The normal values are given *in the boxes*

P. Bumm and G. Schlimok
ENT Clinic and Department of Hematology, Zentralklinikum,
Stenglinstrasse, 86156 Augsburg, Germany

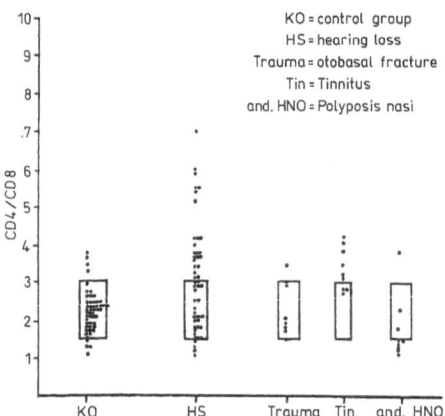

Fig. 2 CD4/CD8 quotient in various acute hearing losses and in a control group (*KO*) of healthy persons. The normal values are given *in the boxes*

decrease of suppressor cells. The calculation of the absolute lymphoyte count results in the fact that the decrease of the total T lymphocytes is due to a suppression of both lymphocyte subpopulations. The evaluation indicates that the immunological imbalance is due to a greater percentage decrease of CD8 cells and not to an increase of CD4 helper cells.

The decrease of suppressor cells is the essential immunopathological finding of this study. The possible hypothesis is that through the decreased suppressor cells the control of plasma cells is reduced, the so-called "forbidden clons" become active. These "forbidden clons" may then produce autoantibodies against the facial nerve.

According to today's immunological knowledge, the immunological imbalance described here is most likely consistent with an autoimmune disease. It is interesting to note that the immunological imbalance described here has a great similarity to findings in multiple sclerosis, as described by Reinharz et al. [7] and Bach et al. [2].

another nine patients had different non-otoneurological ENT diseases. It is also interesting to note here that there is only an imbalance in CD4/CD8 quotient in inner ear diseases of unknown genesis [4]. This finding favors a causative immunological origin. A change in the quotient CD4/CD8 appears only in facial paralysis of unknown origin, such as Bell's palsy, but not in facial paralysis of known origin such as traumatic facial paralysis and in the healthy control group. A normal quotient was also found in herpes zoster oticus paralysis [3]. It seem possible, however, that virus infections can have a triggering effect, resulting in a malfunction of the immunosystem.

Djupesland et al. [5] speak of a cranial polyneuropathy. Adour [1] established that Bell's palsy involves an acute, benign, cranial polyneuritis. The findings of this study support the hypothesis of ADOUR, because the same immunological imbalance was found in various cranial nerve diseases such as sudden hearing loss, vestibular lesion, and Bell's palsy.

The main question is whether the immunological imbalance CD4/CD8 is due to an increase of helper cells or a

References

1. Adour K (1985) Bell's palsy as viral-cranial polyganglionitis. In: Portmann M (ed) Proceedings of the 5th international symposium on the facial nerve Bordeaus. Masson, New York, pp 233–236
2. Bach MA, Phan-Dinh-Tuy F, Bach JF et al. (1980) Deficit of suppressor T cells in active multiple sclerosis. Lancet 303 (3): 1221–1223
3. Bumm P, Schlimok G (1988) The results of immunological regulation and immunogenetics in Bell's palsy. In: Castro D (ed) The facial nerve. Proceedings of the 6th international symposium on the facial nerve, Rio de Janeiro. Kugler and Ghedini, Amsterdam, pp 319–321
4. Bumm P, Muller, EC, Grimm-Müller, U, Schlimok G (1991) T-lymphocyte subpopulations and HLA-DR antigens in patients with hearing loss, neuronitis vestibularis, Meniere's disase and Bell's palsy. Laryngol Rhinol Otol 70:260–266
5. Djupesland G, Miklos D, Stien R et al. (1977) Acute peripheral facial palsy. Arch Otolaryngol 103:641–644
6. Manos-Pujol M, Buendia E, Mestre M et al. (1985) T-lymphocyte subpopulations in Bell's palsy. In: Portmann M (ed) Proceedings of the 5th international symposium on the facial nerve. Masson, New York, pp 197–202
7. Reinherz EL, Weiner HL, Hauser SL et al. (1980) Loss of suppressor T-cells ina active multiple sclerosis. N Engl J Med 303:125–129
8. Veldmann JE (1986) Cochlear and retrocochlear immune-mediated inner ear disorders. Pathogenetic mechanisms and diagnostic tools. Ann Otol Rhinol Laryngol 95:535–540

Eur Arch Otorhinolaryngology (1994) [Suppl]: S449–S451

A. Formenti, M. Galli, G. Termine, M. Corbellino, and N. Massetto

Electrophysiologic Pattern and T-Cell Subsets in Bell's Palsy

Introduction

The etiology of Bell's palsy (BP) is as yet undefined. Among the candidates are various infectious agents and in particular viruses ubiquitous in distribution and with persistence and/or latency sites in nervous cells as herpes virus [1–3]. Besides alterations in the humoral arm of the immune system, with an increase of circulating immune complexes [4], signs of activation in the cellular compartment are described [5–8]. These findings may be indirect clues directing us towards an infectious agent. Nevertheless autoimmune phenomena have also been suspected, such as in sudden hearing loss and in other inner ear disturbances [9]. The natural history of Bell's palsy is on the other hand quite protean, suggesting a variety of pathogenetic events, all leading ultimately to nerve damage but with different outcomes. Immunologic alterations observed at onset and during BP show a relevant degree of variability that evidently emerge when large case files are considered. In our research we investigated a possible correlation between evoked SR and ENoG that gives clues to the outcome and degree of nerve impairment [10], and the determination of lymphocyte subsets. The aim of this study was to consider whether such an approach could allow us to identify subcategories of BPs, differing on the basis of prognosis and laboratory findings.

Material and Methods

The study was performed at the ENT Department, Fatebenefratelli Hospital, Milan, from 1989 to 1991. We investigated a consecutive series of 86 (53 male, 33 female) patients who came into our observation within 10 days from the onset of BP and without prior treatment. Subjects harboring metabolic disturbances were excluded as were those with underlying neurologic or neoplastic diseases. Patients with herpes zoster oticus, intravenous drug users, alcoholics, cases of Melkersson-Rosenthal syndrome, and HIV-1 positive individuals were similarly excluded. CD4-positive and CD8-positive lymphocyte subsets were determined from whole blood by cytofluorimetric analysis (Orhto spectrum III-Ortho/Diagnostics, Raritan NJ) at the time of first observation. SR was recorded using an Amplaid 720 impedance meter. ENoG was performed by Nicolet Compact Four. Both tests were carried out every 5 days in the first 3 weeks from onset of BP. The worst electrophysiologic data recorded during the observation period were chosen. The time needed for facial recovery almost up to House degree II was take into account. All the patients received 6-methyl prednisolone, 40 mg (daily) i.m., with progressive reduction to zero over the following 7 days. Statistical analysis was performed with X^2, Student's t test, and the test for linear trends, when appropriate.

A. Formenti (✉) and G. Termine
ENT Department, Fatebenefratelli Hospital, Milan, Italy

M. Galli and M. Corbellino
Clinic of Infectious Diseases, University of Milan, Italy

N. Massetto
Department of Neurology, S. Paolo Hospital, Milan, Italy

Results

The percentage of patients with BP over 45 years was higher, even if not significantly so, in women (63.6 vs. 41.5%; $X^2 = 3.14$; $p > 0.05$). A relative increase of white blood cell, total lymphocyte, and T lymphocyte counts was confirmed. In particular, 37.2% of cases showed white cell counts $> 104/mm^3$, 31.4% total lymphocyte counts $> 3 \times 103/mm^3$, 30.2% CD8 lymphocyte counts $> 900/mm^3$, 24.4% CD4+/CD8+ cell ratios > 2.2, and 15.1%

S 450

Tab. 1 Nervous fiber impairment measured by ENoG and Stapedial reflex in 86 cases of Bell's palsy

% of impairment	N	%
0–25	26	30.2
26–50	10	11.6
51–75	21	24.4
76–100	29	33.8
Stapedial reflex		
Positive	20	24.4
Negative	66	75.6

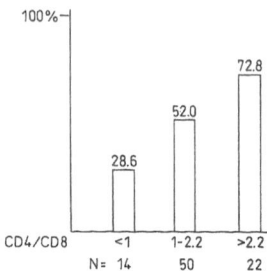

Fig. 1 Nervous fiber impairment > 50% and absence of stapedial reflex on BP patients grouped by CD4/CD8 ratio. $p < 0.01$ (test for linear trend)

CD4+/CD8+ cell ratios <1. Patients older than 45 years showed a higher percentage of CD4+/CD8+ ratios >2.2 (37.2% vs. 13.9% in patients under 45; $p<0.05$). The results of the ENoG determinations are reported in Table 1. In the majority of patients (58.2%), nervous fiber impairment was higher than 50%. Age significantly influenced the degree of compression, with more than 50% of impairment in 53.6% of the subjects aging more than 45 yars and 34.9% in those younger ($p<0.01$). The stapedial reflex was absent in 75.6% of cases. When the patients were grouped by CD4/CD8 ratio, the percentage of subjects with nervous fiber impairment >50% and compromised stapedial reflex was significantly different in the three groups ($p<0.01$, test for linear trend) (Fig. 1). Patients with ratios >2.2 had significantly longer periods of recovery (42 ± 16.5 versus 19.4 ± 9.5 and 15 ± 4.9 days in the other two groups; $p<0.001$). The shortest recovery time was observed in subjects with ratios <1. The difference between this group and the patients with ratios ranging from 1 to 2.2 was significant ($p<0.05$). The recovery time was also influenced by age (27.8 ± 17.1 days in subjects aged more than 45 years vs. 17.1 ± 5.4 in younger patients, $p<0.01$).

Discussion

Our data confirm a relative frequence of immunological abnormalities in Bell's palsy. Age influenced either the degree of nerve compression or the time of recovery and, as expected, the percentage of high CD4/CD8 ratios among the studied population. Nevertheless, the prevalence of increased CD4/CD8 ratios seems to be unusually high, when compared to the age-adjusted standards of our laboratory. In a previous study this phenomenon was responsible for the lack of a statistically significant difference, due to a high standard deviation between BPs and age- and sex-matched healthy controls (8). Thus, we suggest the existence of a BP subgroup showing a panel of distinctive features represented by age over 45, high degree of nerve impairment, longer time of recovery, and elevated CD4/CD8 cell ratio. This observation might be the basis for future studies on the mechanisms implicated in facial nerve damage in these cases. Presently the available data do not permit further comment. Similar findings have been reported in cases of sensorineural hearing loss by Yoo et al. [11] and by ourselves [12]. The high frequency of elevated CD4/CD8 ratios was interpreted as an expression of autoreactivity [11]. A second subset of BP patients is represented by individuals with shortened time of recovery, lower degree of nerve impairment, and CD4/CD8 ratios lower than 1, not significantly influenced by age. This pattern resembles one which could be expected in an acute (viral?) disease. Nevertheless no analogy was found between this group and the data previously reported in Ramsay Hunt syndrome (8), in which we observed higher CD4/CD8 ratios. Herper zoster oticus is, however, a manifestation more frequently observed in the elderly and due to a reactivation of a virus in steady state. VZV (in the case of herpes sine herpete) and HSV have been indicated as a possible cause of BP (1, 3). In our opinion these viruses might be involved in the pathogenesis of BP without necessarily inducing detectable alterations in peripheral T-cell subsets. In fact, a relevant number of BP patients did not show any significant immunological abnormality. The etiopathogenesis of BP remains to be clarified. The identification of subgroups such as the ones evidenced in this paper might be a useful tool for further investigations.

References

1. Adour KK, Byl FM, Nilsinger RL (1978) The true nature of Bell's palsy: analysis of 1000 consecutive patients. Laryngoscope 88: 787–901
2. Clark JR, Carlson RD, Sasaki CT, Steere AC (1985) Facial paralysis in Lyme disease. Laryngoscope 95: 1341–1345
3. Fleury H, Chilotti P, Bonnici JF, De Pasquier P, Portmann D, Bebear JP, Portmann M (1990) IgM against herpes viruses in Bell's palsy. In: Castro D (ed) The facial nerve. Proceedings of the 6th international symposium. Kugler and Ghedini, Amsterdam, pp 221–223

4. Formenti A, Galli M, Cocchini F (1985) Circulating immune complexes in idiopathic facial palsy. In: Portman M (ed) The facial nerve. Proceedings of the 5th international symposium. Masson, New York, pp 236–239

5. Maños Pujol M Buendia E, Mestra M (1985) T-lymphocyte subpopulations in Bell's palsy. In: Portmann M (ed) The facial nerve. Proceedings of the 5th international symposium. Masson, New York, pp 197–202

6. Maños Pujol M, Buendia E, Mestra M (1987) Cellular immune abnormalities in patients with recurrent Bell's palsy. Clin Otolaryngol 12 : 283–287

7. Maños Pujol M, Sierra A, Buendia E, Mestre M, Maños Gonzalbo M (1990) Lymphoproliferative response to facial nerve extracts in patients with Bell's palsy. In: Castro D (ed) The facial nerve . Proceedings of the 6th international symposium. Kugler and Ghedini, Amsterdam, pp 339–342

8. Formenti A, Galli M, Massetto N et al. (1990) Immunological aspects of Bell's palsy. In: Castro D (ed) The facial nerve. Proceedings of the 6th international symposium. Kugler and Ghedini, Amsterdam, pp 211–214

9. Mc Cabe BF (1979) Autoimmune sensorineural hearing loss. Ann Otol Rhinol Laryngol 88 : 585–589

10. Kimura Y, Tojina H, Inamura H (1990) Stapedial reflex in patients with Bell's palsy: comparison of SR with electroneurography. In: Castro D (ed) The facial nerve. Proceedings of the 6th international symposium. Kugler and Ghedini, Amsterdam, pp 369–372

11. Yoo TJ, Floyd R, Ishibe T, Shea JJ, Bowman C (1985) Immunologic testing of certain ear diseases. Am J Otol 6 : 96–100

12. Ponzi S, Galli M, Formenti A, Castellani C (1988) T cell subsets in sudden hearing loss. Proceedings of the 1st European congress of otolaryngology, Paris

Eur Arch Otorhinolaryngology (1994) [Suppl]: S452–S453

FREE PAPERS AND POSTERS

V. Bonkowsky, K. Deusch, and E. Moschovakis, C. Wagner-Manslau, and R. Kau

Immunological Findings in Bell's Palsy

Introduction

Despite the many theories formulated in the last several decades, the etiology of Bell's palsy is still unknown. Histologic findings of Liston and Kleid [5] in one patient, who died 1 week after the onset of a complete facial palsy of a ruptured abdominal aneurysm, showed that the entire nerve was infiltrated by inflammatory cells suggesting a viral neuritis. Clinical and experimental studies also support an infectious-immunologial etiology [2, 4, 7]. The aim of the present study was to investigate the humoral and cellular immune response in patients with Bell's palsy.

Patients and Methods

Seventy-six patients with Bell's palsy were studied. The patients were between 4 and 79 years of age (mean age, 36 years). All patients were examined and followed up by the same physician.

Humoral Immune Response

Virus-specific IgG and IgM antibodies against herpes simplex virus type 1 (HSV-1) and varicella zoster virus (VZV) were determined by ELISA in all of the patients during the acute phase on days 1–10 (mean day 5). The soluble interleukin-2 receptor (sIL-2R) was determined in the serum of 20 patients by an enzyme immunoassay (EIA, Immunotech) within 2 days after the onset of facial palsy. The

V. Bonkowsky (✉)
HNO-Universitätsklinik Regensburg, Franz-Josef-Strauß-Allee 11, 93042 Regensburg, Germany

K. Deusch, E. Moschovakis, C. Wagner-Manslau, and R. Kau
ENT Department, Klinikum Rechts der Isar, TU München, Germany

results were compared with a sex- and age-matched control group with no herpes labialis in the history ($n = 20$). Moreover the results of IgG and IgM antibodies against HSV-1 in patients with Bell's palsy were compared with the antibody titer against HSV-1 in patients with herpes labialis ($n = 20$).

Cellular Immune Response

The lymphoproliferative response against human facial nerve antigen was observed in 14 patients. Two facial nerves were obtained by immediate autopsy from one patient who died of myocardial infarct. The intratemporal parts of the facial nerves were prepared according to the method described by Manos-Pujol [6], but without separation in different portions. Then a lymphocyte transformation test (LTT) was performed by using the prepared human facial nerve as antigen. The response was measured by ^{3}H-thymidine incorporation to DNA in a β-counter. The stimulation index (SI) was expressed in counts per minute experimental/control. A positive reaction was defined at values > 3. The detailed procedure of the LTT is described elsewhere [3].

Results

Humoral immune Response

1. IgM antibodies against HSV-1 or VZV could be found in 16% of patients.
2. An increased IgG antibody titer against HSV-1 or VZV could be found in 59%, but this raised titer was not diagnostic of an acute infection or reactivation.
3. A comparison of HSV-1 antibody titers between patients with Bell's palsy and patients with herpes labialis showed nearly identical antibody titers in both diseases (Table 1).

Table 1 Comparison of HSV-1 antibody titers in Bell's palsy ($n = 76$) and herpes labialis ($n = 20$)

	Bell's palsy	Herpes labialis
IgM positive	6 (7.5%)	1 (5%)
IgG > 1 : 5120	39 (51.5%)	17 (85%)
IgG man value	1 : 15800	1 : 12500

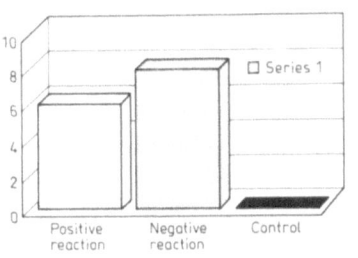

Fig. 1 Increased stimulation index vs. human facial nerve antigen in the lymphocyte transformation test in patients with Bell's palsy

The median serum level of soluble interleukin 2 receptor was elevated in the acute phase of Bell's palsy (153 pM +/ -48 pM) compared with a control group (51 pM +/ -32 pM).

Cellular Immune Response

In 6 of 14 patients (42%) a lymphoproliferative response (positive reaction) to human facial nerve antigen was observed (Fig. 1).

Discussion

The results of this study demonstrate that in 16% of Bell's palsy patients an acute infection or reactivation of HSV or VZV was evident (IgM positive). Similiar results were reported by Adour [2], Djupesland [4], and Mertens [7]. Of course this temporal coincidence of an acute HSV-1 infection with Bell's palsy is no proof of the etiological role of this virus. In addition to this temporal coincidence further factors must support the assumed viral etiology. Comparison of the elevated IgG antibodies in Bell's palsy – a supposed reactivation of HSV-1 – to the IgG antibodies in herpes labialis – a sure reactivation of HSV-1 – showed that the titer was about the same in both diseases. These serological findings are well compatible with the hypothesis that the reactivation of HSV-1 plays an important role in the pathogenesis of Bell's palsy. The observation of a lymphoproliferative response to human facial nerve antigen suggests that the lymphocytes of patients with Bell's palsy were sensitized against certain components of the facial nerve. According to the results of Abramsky et al. [1], this component could be the peripheral nerve P1L basic protein. The data of these study suggest that in many cases of Bell's palsy an immunological process is triggered by a reactivation of herpes simplex type 1 virus.

References

1. Abramsky O, Webb C, Teitelbaum D, Arnon R (1975) Celular immune response to peripheral nerve basic protein in idiopathic facial paralysis (Bell's palsy). J Neurol Sci 26 : 13 – 20
2. Adour KK (1985) Bell's palsy as a viral cranial polyganglionitis. In: Portmann M (ed) The facial nerve. Masson, Paris, pp 233 – 236
3. Berger P, Koja S, Rogowski M, Vollrath M (1989) Der Lympho-zytentransformationstest zum Nachweis einer immunologischen Innenohrschwerhörigkeit. HNO 37 : 153 – 157
4. Djupesland G, Bordal P, Johannsen TA (1976) Viral infection as a cause of acute facial palsy. Arch Otolarynol 102 : 403 – 407
5. Liston SL, Kleid S (1989) Histopathology of Bell's palsy. Laryngoscope 99 : 23 – 26
6. Manos-Pujol M, Sierra A, Buendia M, Manos Gonzalbo M (1990) Lymphoproliferative response to facial nerve extracts in patients with Bell's palsy. Preliminary report. In: Castro D (ed) The facial nerve. Kugler and Ghedini, Amsterdam, pp 339 – 342
7. Mertens T, Thomas J-P, Zippel C, Eggers H-J (1982) Peripheral facial palsy and viral infections – findings and problems. Med Microbiol Immunol 171 : 77 – 83

Eur Arch Otorhinolaryngology (1994) [Suppl]: S454 – S455

A. Formenti, M. Galli, G. Termine, A. Lupo, M. Corbellino, and N. Massetto

Prevalence of *Borrelia burgdorferi* Antibodies in Bell's Palsy in a Metropolitan Area of Northern Italy

Introduction

Borrelia burgdorferi is the causative agent of Lyme disease, a multiphasic disorder affecting the skin, heart, joint, muscle, and nervous systems [1]. Meningitis, cranial neuritis, and radiculoneuritis represent the clinical spectrum of neurological manifestations of Lyme disease [2]. Several reports from central and northern Europe indicate that Bell's palsy (BP) may be caused by *B. burgdorferi* [3 – 5], giving a possible explanation for a consistent proportion of BP cases. The aim of this paper is to evaluate the prevalence of *B. burgdorferi* related cases in a consecutive series of BP observed in subjects living in a metropolitan area of northern Italy.

Methods

The study was performed at the ENT Department, Fatebenefratelli Hospital, Milan, from 1988 to 1991 on a consecutive series of 104 patients with BP. Subjects with underlying metabolic, neurologic, and neoplastic diseases, intravenous drug users, alcoholics, HIV-1-positive patients, and patients with Ramsay Hunt or Melkersson-Rosenthal syndrome were excluded from the study. Anti-*B. burgdorferi* antibodies were sought for by commercially available IFA for IgG and IgM antibodies and by ELISA, from sera drawn at the first observation and 15 days later; 85 age- and sex-matched patients with laryngeal nonneo-

plastic diseases, observed as outpatients in the same period of time, served as controls.

Results

Significant titers of anti-*B. burgdorferi* IgG and IgM antibodies were present only in 1 out of 104 patients with BP (0.9%) while all the controls tested negative. The positive patient was a 46-year-old male, living in an urban environment and working as a clerk. No history of tick bites or other anamnestic evidence of exposure to *B. burgdorferi* infection was reported, except occasional jogging in open fields. The patient tested repeatedly negative for VDRL and TPHA. The serum anti-*B. burgdorferi* IgG titer was 1:160 and 1:320 15 days later. The ELISA-IgG determinations were positive during all the observation period. At the onset of facial palsy the patient had elevated CD8+ T lymphocytes (1782/mm^3), reduced CD4+ cells (369/mm^3), and an inverted ratio (0.2). The recovery time was long (3 months) despite antibiotic therapy, started 8 days after the onset of facial palsy.

Discussion

Since the discovery and isolation of *B. burgdorferi*, Lyme borreliosis has been increasingly recognized worldwide. *B. burgdorferi* has been isolated also in several domestic animals, such as dogs, horses, and cattle. Spirochetes identical or strictly similar to *B. burgdorferi* have been isolated in various ticks other than the *Ixodes* genus [1]. Currently available data suggest that the prevalence in the healthy population ranges from 2% to 10% in healthy blood donors and reaches about 45% in forestry workers [6]. It is probable, however, that strong differences attributable to environmental factors might exist in different geographic areas. According to our knowledge, no information is

A. Formenti (✉) and G. Termine
ENT Department, Fatebenefratelli Hospital, Milan, Italy

M. Galli, A. Lupo and M. Corbellino
Clinic of Infectious Diseases, University of Milan, Italy

N. Massetto
Department of Neurology, S. Paolo Hospital, Milan, Italy

available as to the seroprevalence of *B. burgdorferi* in the Milan area. Our serosurvey evidences an extremely low prevalence also in a selected population of patients suffering from a condition, such as BP, that resulted in other studies frequently associated with B. burgdorferi infection [3–5].

IFA methods prepared from whole *Borrelia* cells and ELISA techniques relying on sonicated whole cell preparations may have problems of cross-reactivity and sensitivity. Nevertheless patients with early disseminated manifestations of Lyme disease, such as meningoradiculoneuritis, test positive in 80% – 98% of cases [6]. In conclusion, *B. burgdorferi* seems to be only an occasional cause of facial palsy in Milan. Different paths are to be followed in order to find the principal causes of BP in urban settings.

References

1. Burgdorfer W (1991) Lyme Borreliosis: ten years after discovery of the etiologic agent, B. Burgdorferi. Infection 19:257–262
2. Pachmer AR, Steere AC (1985) The triad of neurologic manifestations of Lyme disease: meningitis, cranial neuritis and radiculoneuritis. Neurology 35:47–53
3. Clark JR, Carlson RD, Sasaki CT, Steere AC (1985) Facial paralysis in Lyme disease. Laryngoscope 95:1341–1345
4. Jonsson L, Stiernstedt G, Carlson J, Strömberg A, Sjöberg O, Larsson A (1990) Tick-borne Borrelia infection in Bell's palsy: a serological and cerebrospinal fluid study. In: Castro D (ed) The facial nerve. Proceedings of the 6th international symposium. Kugler and Ghedini, Amsterdam, p 199
5. Hanner P (1990) The relationship of Borrelia antibody titers to CSF alterations in Bell's palsy. In: Castro D (ed) The facial nerve. Proceedings of the 6th international symposium. Kugler and Ghedini, Amsterdam, pp 327–328
6. Stanek G (1991) Laboratory diagnosis and seroepidemiology of Lyme borreliosis. Infection 19:263–267

Eur Arch Otorhinolaryngology (1994) [Suppl]: S456–S458

FREE PAPERS AND POSTERS

M. Ikeda, M. Kawabata, M. Kuga, H. Nakazato, H. Tomita, and K. Kawano

Anti-*Borrelia burgdorferi* Antibodies in Sera of Patients with Facial Paralysis

Introduction

Borrelia burgdorferi is a pathogenic spirochete which causes Lyme disease mediated by members of the Ixodidae, as discovered in 1982 [1]. Lyme disease is a complex multisystem disorder. Many cases of this disease were found and reported for the first time in Lyme, Connecticut, United States in the latter half of the 1970s [2]. There are reports, particularly from Europe, maintaining that *B. burgdorferi*, which is the pathogenic spirochete of Lyme disease, is involved in causing Bell's palsy [3–5]. Cases have also been described in Japan where ECM occurred after a tick bite and the patients were serologically diagnosed as having Lyme disease [6]. It is important therefore to examine the relation between Bell's palsy and *B. burgdorferi* in Japan. In the present study, the authors focused on patients residing in or near Toky whose main complaints were associated with facial paralysis.

Subjects and Methods

Studies were conducted on 98 patients with acute peripheral facial paralysis who visited the ENT Clinic of Nihon University Itabashi Hospital, during the 1-year period from July 1990 to June 1991. The 98 patients consisted of 68 cases with Bell's palsy, 20 cases with Ramsay Hunt syndrome or zoster sine herpete, and 10 cases with

M. Ikeda (✉), M. Kuga, H. Nakazato, and H. Tomita
Department of Otolaryngology, Nihon University School
of Medicine, 30-1 Oyaguchi, Itabashi-ku, Tokyo 173, Japan

M. Kawabata and K. Kawano
Department of Clinical Pathology, Nihon University School
of Medicine, 30-1 Oyaguchi, Itabashi-ku, Tokyo 173, Japan

recurrent or bilateral facial paralysis. The breakdown by sex was 62 males and 36 females. In none of the 98 patients were abnormal symptoms observed in other organs which could be clearly identified with the clinical spectrum of Lyme disease. Nor were there any cases with other spirochete infections such as syphilis.

Two kinds of antigen were employed for detecting anti-*B. burgdorferi* antibodies in the sera. One was the antigen referred to hereafter as Wh-antigen, which was prepared from extracts of sonicated whole *B. burgdorferi* spirochetes. The other antigen, referred to hereafter as F-antigen, was from a commercially available kit (DAKOPATTS Co.). The F-antigen was a flagellum protein (flagellin fraction) antigen of 41 kilodaltons (kDa) from *B. burgdorferi*.

The indirect enzyme-linked immunosorbent assay (ELISA) was adopted to determine the serum IgG and IgM antibodies against these two antigens. The ELISA involving the Wh-Antigen, as a criterion for judging positivity, at which 95% of 150 healthy Japanese controls proved negative was designated as the specific cutoff level. As regards the antibodies to the F-antigen, the OD values adopted for judging positivity were based on the judgment critera of the kit.

Results

Table 1 summarizes the positivity ratios for IgG and IgM antibodies reacting with the Wh-antigen and F-antigen. A comparison between Bell's palsy and the patients with varicella zoster virus infection revealed that, with the exception of when IgG antibody was examined, more cases of a positive reaction for antibodies were observed in Bell's palsy. The difference was statistically significant ($p < 0.05$). In the study using F-antigen, three (4.4%) of the Bell's palsy patients displayed a positive reaction for IgG or IgM antibody, while one (5.0%) with varicella zoster virus infection demonstrated positivity. All cases which reacted positively to F-antigen also reacted positively to Wh-antigen. The

Table 1 Detection rates of anti-*Borrelia burgdorferi* antibodies in patients with facial paralysis

	Wh-antigen			F-antigen		
	IgG Ab	IgM Ab	IgG/M Ab	IgG Ab	IgM Ab	IgG/M Ab
Bell's palsy (68 cases)	13 (19.1%)	13 (19.1%)*	22 (32.4%)*	2 (2.9%)	1 (1.5%)	3 (4.4%)
Ramsay Hunt syndrome/ zoster sine herpete (20 cases)	2 (10.0%)	0	2 (10.0%)	1 (5.0%)	0	1 (5.0%)
Recurrent/ bilateral paralysis (10 cases)	0	1 (10.0%)	1 (10.0%)	0	0	0
Total (98 cases)	15 (15.3%)	14 (14.3%)	25 (25.5%)	3 (3.1%)	1 (1.0%)	4 (4.1%)

*$p < 0.05$.

Table 2 Detection rates of anti-*Borrelia burgdorferi* antibodies by ELISA employing sonicated whole spirochete antigen in patients with Bell's palsy in relation to season of onset

	April to September	October to March
IgG Ab positive cases	6 (17.1%) *	7 (21.2%)
IgM Ab positive cases	3 (8.6%) *	10 (30.3%)
IgG and/or IgM Ab positive cases	7 (20.0%)	15 (45.5%)

*$p < 0.05$.

next stage of the present investigation was to examine the seasonal occurrence ratio of facial paralysis among the cases with Bell's palsy in which antibodies reacted positively to Wh-antigen (Table 2). This is attributable to the fact that the occurrence of facial paralysis increased to a statitical significant ($p < 0.05$) extent from fall to winter (October to March).

The authors conducted clinical observations on the occurrence of facial paralysis among patients with Bell's palsy whose anti-*B. burgdorferi* antibody reacted positively to Wh-antigen. The positivity among females was significantly high ($p < 0.05$). Comparative studies were also carried out by age, ratio of complete paralysis, results of nerve excitability tests (NET), results of topographical diagnosis of facial nerve paralysis, and ratio of complete recovery. The findings revealed no statistically significant differences between antibody-positive and antibody-negative cases.

Discussion

The present results revealed a major differece between the positivity ratio for Wh-antigen and that for F-antigen in the patients with Bell's palsy. Since the Wh-antigen is a sonicated whole *Borrelia* spirochete antigen, whereas the F-antigen is a 41-kDa protein antigen, it is assumed that the specificities of the two are different [7]. At present, the authors cannot accurately explain the high positive ratio for Wh-antigen in the cases of Bell's palsy. However, there is one finding from the clinical examinations. This is the fact that none of the patients showing a positive reaction had any past experience of tick bite or ECM, or any clinical history suggestive of Lyme disease. It is also important that the positivity ratio for F-antigen did not clearly rise in the patients studied in the present study. When these are taken into account, we cannot simply conclude that the cases displaying a positive reaction to the Wh-antigen in the present study can be diagnosed as the infection with B. *burgdorferi* or as Lyme disease. It is more logial to presume that, although the cause remains unclear, the high positivity ratio for Wh-antigen observed in the cases of Bell's palsy is a result of nonspecific reactions caused to cross-reactions to *B. burgdorferi*.

Analysis by season of the frequency of occurrence of positive reactions to Wh-antige among the patients with Bell's palsy revealed that the ratio rises to a statistically significant extent from October to March. This suggests that factors triggering nonspecific reactions may be present during the seasons from fall to winter. The results of the present study also raised the possibility that the factor in question could be some type of microorganism which shows cross-reactions with sonicated whole pirochete antigen of *B. burgdorferi*. Further studies along these lines could provide valuable information for elucidating the cause of Bell's palsy.

References

1. Burgdorferi W, Barbour AG, Hayes SF, Benach JL, Grunwaldt E, Davis JP (1982) Lyme disease: a tick-borne spirochetosis? Science 216:1317–1319

2. Steere AC, Malawista SE, Snydman DR et al. (1977) Lyme arthritis: an epidemic of oligoarticular arthritis in children and adults in three Connecticut communities. Arthritis Rheum 20: 7–17
3. Jonnson L, Stiernstedt G, Thomander L (1987) Tick-borne *Borrelia* infection in patients with Bell's palsy. Arch Otolaryngol Head Neck Surg 113:303–306
4. Olsson I, Engervall K, Asbrink E, Carlsson-Nordlander B, Hovmark A (1988) Tick-borne borreliosis and facial palsy. Acta Otolrayngol (Stockh) 105:100–107
5. Bjerkhoel A, Carlsson M, Ohlsson J (1989) Peripheral facial palsy caused by the *Borrelia* spirochete. Acta Otolaryngol (Stockh) 108:424–430
6. Kawabata M, Baba S, Iguchi K, Yamaguti N, Russel H (1987) Lime disease in Japan and its possible incriminated tick vector. *Ixodes persulcatus*. J Infect Dis 156:854
7. Grodzicki RL, Steere A (1988) Comparison of immunoblotting and indirect enzyme-linked immunosorbent assay using different antigen preparations for diagnosing early Lyme disease. J Infect Dis 157:790–797

Eur Arch Otorhinolaryngology (1994) [Suppl]: S459 – S462

POSTERS

D. Lopez Aguado, J. Rivero, M. E. Campos, B. Perez, P. Evora, R. Gutierrez, and L. Diaz-Flores

Macrophages and Schwann Cells in Myelin Disintegration

Introduction

In a severely injured neural trunk, degenerative changes are produced in the distal segment (Wallerian degeneration) creating an appropiate environment for axonal regeneration. Degradation and digestion of the myelin cover are among these degenerative phenomena.

Even if the role of Schwann cells in the disintegration and elimination of myelin is not questioned [1 – 3], the action of the migrating macrophages in Wallerian degeneration is by no means clear. Different authors have postulated some interrelationships between the macrophagic cells and Schwann cells in the myelin elimination process [4 – 7], but the origin of these phagocytes has long been debated.

Olsson et al. [8] and Asbury [9] concluded that a part of the macrophagic population in degenerating nerves is presumably of hematogenous origin. The macrophages probably migrate into the nerve through the endothelium of the endoneural vessels. This process is facilitated by means of the release of histamine and serotonin from the endoneural mast cells, increasing the capillary permeability, which aids the passage of the macrophages through the vessel wall [9].

In the present work, the role of macrophages is studied, with particular attention being paid to the participation of the perineural postcapillary venules.

Material and Methods

After interrupting axonal continuity, distal segments of facial nerves were studied by means of histological procedures in adult Sprague-Dawley rat ($n = 30$; average weight, 300 g. Macrophages and Schwann cells were recognized by their ultrastructural characteristics and by their expression of lysozyme, alpha-1-antitrypsin (AAT), alpha-1-antichymotrypsin (AACT), and S-100 protein. To label the monocyte/macrophages that cross the postcapillary venule walls and to follow them in the lesional area, before neural injury 0.1 cc histamine diphosphate (Sigma Chemical Co., St Louis Mo; H-7375) at 1 mg/ml in saline was injected into the epineurium. Monastral blue (MB) (3% suspension); Sigma Chemical Co.; M-3764) was administered intravenously (saphenous vein) at 0.1 cc/100 g body weight.

Results and Discussion

In the early stages of the experiment, most of the cells with the capacity of degrading myelin were Schwann cells (Fig. 1). However, the macrophages rapidly predominated (Fig. 2), while the Schwann cells detached from the residual myelin and underwent mitosis, forming Schwann cell columns.

In cases in which MB was used, the marker was restricted to the cytoplasm of pericytes and endothelial cells of the perineural postcapillary venules and to the macrophages that occur in the space between pericytes and endothelium. Later, the presence of MB was similar, except that some macrophages with MB were in the interstitium (Fig. 3). Finally, MB was observed in numerous cells which degraded myelin (Fig. 4).

Our morphological results agree with those of most of the authors who referred to the interrelationships in the myelin removal function of Schwann cells and macrophagic cells [1, 3 – 7].

D. Lopez-Aguado, J. Rivero, M. E. Campos, B. Perez, P. Evora, R. Gutierrez, and L. Diaz-Flores
Department of ORL and Pathology, Hospital Universitario de Canarias, Facultad des Medicina, Universidad de La Laguna, Tenerife, Canary Islands, Spain

Fig. 1 Schwann cell with numerous myelin laminar bodies in the cytoplasm. ×25000

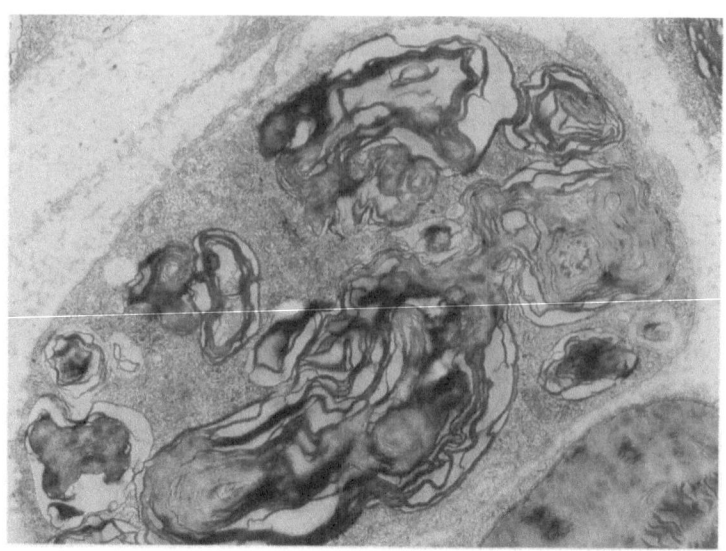

Fig. 2 Macrophages with numerous lysosomes containing myelin debris. ×25000

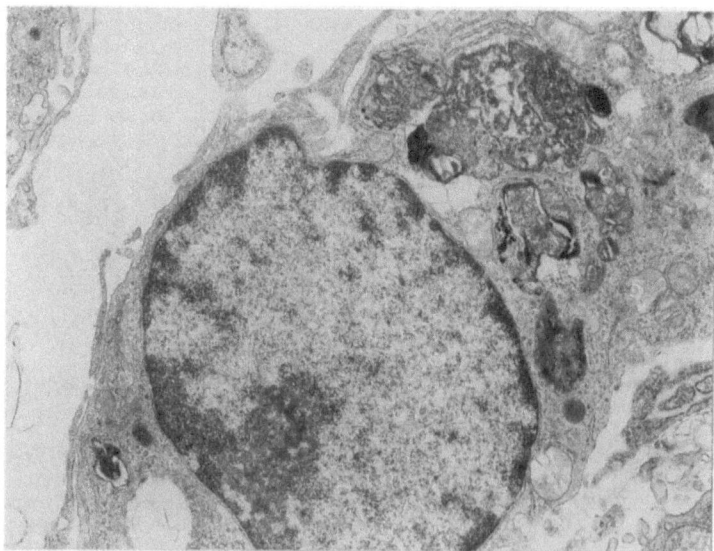

The administration of the marker MB was based on the principle of selective histamine-induced postcapillary venular labeling and on its capacity to be incorporated by macrophages crossing the venular wall.

The results of the present work with the use of MB suggest that most of the macrophages reaching the injured area cross the walls of the postcapillary venules, confirming the studies of Olsson et al. [8, 9] and Asbury [6]. Furthermore, our observations allow us to attribute an important role to the postcapillary venules of the epineurium. This also explains why Ciges et al. [4] did not observe macrophages when ischemia of the facial nerve was produced by isolation from the surrounding tissues using a Teflon tube.

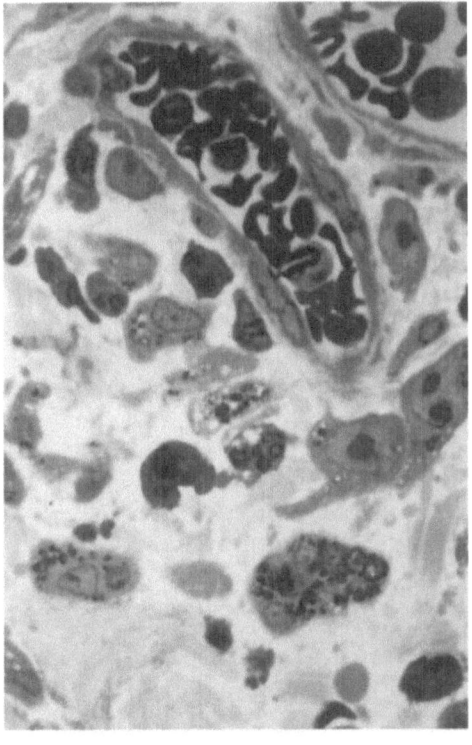

Fig. 3 Macrophage labeling with monastral blue (MB) lie in the interstitium. Toluidine blue, ×50

Fig. 4 Macrophage labeling with monostral blue (MB) and with myelin laminar bodies in the cytoplasm. Toluidine blue, ×100

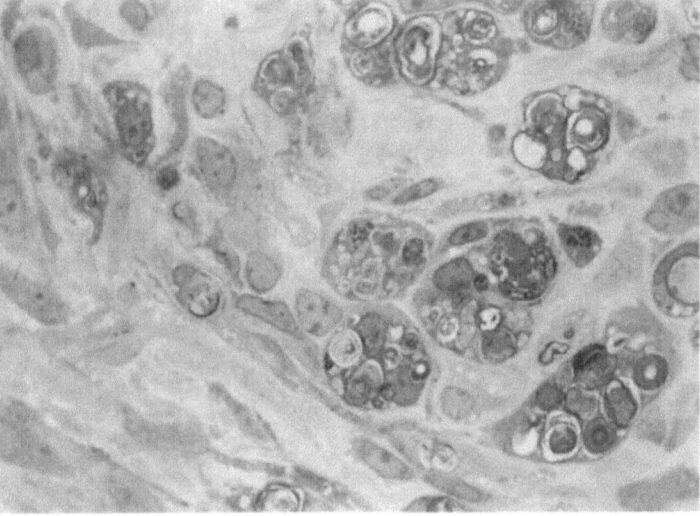

References

1. Berner A, Torvik A, Stenwig AE (1973) Origin of macrophages in traumatic lesions and Wallerian degeneration in peripheral nerve. Acta Neuropathol (Berl) 25 : 228–236
2. Blumke S, Niedorf HR (1966) Electron microscope studies of Schwann cells during the Wallerian degeneration with special reference to the cytoplasmic. Acta Neuropathol (Berl) 6 : 46–53
3. Craviotom H (1969) Wallerian degeneration: ultrastructural and histochemical studies. Bull Los Ang Neurol Soc 34 : 233–341
4. Ciges M, Diaz Flores L, and Lopez Aguada D (1981) Degeneration and regeneration processes in experimental facial nerve paralysis. Acta Otolaryngol (Stokh) 91 : 487–498
5. Lopez Aguado D, Diaz Flores L, Gayoso M, and Ballesteros JM (1979) Comportamiento de las celulas de Schwann en la compresion experimental del nervio facial. Morf Nor Patol [A] 3 : 551–568
6. Asbury AK (1970) The histogenesis of phagocytes during Wallerian degeneration. Proceedings of the VIth International Congress on Neuropathology. Masson, Paris, p 666
7. Williams PL, and Hall SM (1971) Chronic Wallerian degeneration – an in vivo and ultrastructural study. J Anat 109 : 487–498
8. Olsson Y, and Sjostrand J (1969) Origin of macrophages in Wallerian degeneration of peripheral nerves demonstrated autoradiographically. Exp Neurol 23:102–114
9. Olsson Y, and Sjostrand J (1969) Proliferation of mast cells in peripheral nerves during Wallerian degeneration. A radioautographic study. Acta Neuropathol (Berl). 13 : 111–123

Eur Arch Otorhinolaryngology (1994) [Suppl]: S 463

P. Hanner, B. Kaijser, and S. Edström

Incidence of Peripheral Facial Palsy in Patients with Antibodies Against Lyme Borreliosis

Introduction Tick-borne lyme borreliosis is a multi-system malady. Cutaneous alterations are seen in the early stage of the disease and erythema migrans (EM) is an early manifestation followed by the secondary stage of joint, cardial, and neurologic involvements. This may be followed by a tertiary stage of the disease with acrodermatitis atrophicans (ACA) and late musculoskeletal and neurological affections. Facial palsy is a common cranial neuropathy in borreliosis. This study aimed to evaluate the extent to which peripheral facial palsy may be caused by borreliosis in different stages of the disease and over several years.

Methods Seventy-one patients with acute peripheral facial palsy during 1986 and 148 patients from the 1989–1991 period were studied with respect to underlying *borrelia* infection. IgG antibodies were determined using an indirect immunofluorescence method in the acute and convalescent periods. One hundred ad fifty healthy subjects served as controls.

Results During 1986, 23% of the patients had serological evidence of *borrelia* infection. The corresponding values for 1989, 1990, and 1991 were 16%, 10%, and 20%, respectively. The majority of the seropositive patients had no history of previous tick bite or EM. Several patients also had vertigo or hearing loss and three patients demonstrated ACA, referring to the late, tertiary stage of the disease. There were no seasonal variations.

Conclusion Although the first clinical manifestations of Lyme borreliosis are well known and respond well to chemotherapy, facial palsy caused by borreliosis is still a common condition.

P. Hanner, B. Kaijser, and S. Edström
ENT-clinic and Department of Clin Bacteriology,
Sahlgren's Hospital, Göteborg, Sweden

Blood Supply

Eur Arch Otorhinolaryngology (1994) [Suppl]: S467–S468

A. Schadel, H. Theilen, and E. Seifert

Reaction of the Vasa Nervorum of the Facial Nerve During Stimulation with Neurotransmitters

The local blood flow of a tissue depends on the pressure difference in the respective vessel system. In approximate terms, the flow of fluid in an arterial vascular system can be described by the Hagen-Poiseuille law based on the laminar flow of a homogeneous fluid in a rigid tube with wettable walls. The flow-time volume prevailing in a vessel is accordingly proportional to the fourth power of the radius. Regulation of local blood flow is therefore very much more effective when increase of the pressure difference.

The width of the individual vessels is initially determined by the smooth muscle cells present in the vessel walls. Their tonus is under nervous, humoral, and hormonal control as well as being regulated by local metabolic mechanisms. Therefore we examined noradrenaline, acetylcholine, histamine, pH, and adenosine levels.

Our animal experiments were carried out using barbiturate anesthesia with 25 mg sodium pentobarbital/kg body weight. The following parameters were taken into consideration to ensure reproducible experimental conditions:

- Blood pressure and pulse were recorded intraarterially by means of a Seldinger catheter implanted into the contralateral common carotid artery.
- The core temperature of the body was measured rectally in order to be able to detect hypothermia of the experimental animals in good time. Moreover, a heating lamp was used to ensure an adequate temperature for the experimental animals.
- The exposed facial nerve dries out very quickly at least at the surface. Additional alteration of the acid-base equilibrum with reactive vasodilation is to be expected owing to the diffusion of carbon dioxide. In order to

prevent these effects, the area of surgery was overlaid with paraffin oil heated to body temperature after exposure of the facial nerve.
- Using a micropipette and a micromanipulator, the agents to be tested were applied in the form of a deposit into the epineurium of the facial nerve about 5 mm distal to the stylomastoid foramen. The vessel to be investigated was photographed via an automatic photography system over 15 and 30 min after application and the alteration in the vessel diameter was determined. Each measurement was carried out three times and the mean value was taken as the final measurement (by analogy to the procedure of Kuschinsky and Wahl)
- The evaluation was carried out using the image-splitting method. This image-splitting method was tested for its reproducibility by Wahl and Kuschinsky in 1973. Since then, it has been regarded as the standard method for investigations of vascular reaction in neurophysiology.
- The investigations were carried out first of all under physiological conditions, i.e., with an unchanged blood supply to the facial nerve via the stylomastoid artery, the middle meningeal artery, and the anterior-inferior cerebellar artery. Moreover, investigations were carried out after ligature or severance of the stylomastoid artery and after elimination of the terminal branches of the middle meningeal artery. For this purpose, the facial nerve was exposed over the entire fallopian canal into the cerebellopontine angle and raised out of its bony canal with a surgical tenaculum. During this dissection, the small arteriles which traverse to the epineurium of the facial nerve as terminal branches of the middle meningeal artery are destroyed and are no longer available for the further blood supply. The ligation of the anterior inferior cerbellar artery is carried out after the additional performance of partial craniotomy.

After ligature of the stylomastoid artery, the effects described above (contraction and dilation of the resistance vessels) have been demonstrated to be almost unchanged.

A. Schadel and E. Seifert
ENT-Department, Klinikum Mannheim, University of Heidelberg, Mannheim, Germany

H. Theilen
Physiological Institut I, University of Heidelberg, Germany

Only the ligation of the blood supply via the stylomastoid artery and then also the terminal branches of the middle meningeal artery showed markedly reduced reactivity to the agents applied. The reactivity of the facial nerve vaso vasorum is almost completely abolished after ligation of the blood supply via the three afferent dystems of the stylomastoid artery, the terminal branches of the middle meningeal artery, and the anterior inferior cerebellar artery. The remaining blood supply of the facial nerve is evidently still sufficient to ensure undisturbed function. At this point, we there fore refer to our paper read at the meeting of the Politzer Society in Maastricht in June 1991.

The reduced reactivity of the facial nerve vessels to agents after ligation of the blood supply via the three main vascular systems can be explained by dilatation of the blood vessels. A contraction (induced, e. g., by locally applied noradrenaline) would probably bring the facial nerve to the confines of the blood supply which can still be tolerated. However, a further vasodilatation (e. g., by local application of acetylcholine) is clearly possible only to a very limited extent owing to the transmural tissue pressure. On the one hand, the blood vessels supplying the facial nerve evidently have a pronounced autoregulatory mechanism such as is known, for example, from the brain vessels of the cat. On the other hand, the facial nerve reaches the capacity limits of its remaining vascularization after ligation of the blood supply via the individual vessel systems. We are unable to decide to what extent this analysis can be extrapolated to *Homo sapiens*. It is entirely possible that the facial nerve of *Homo sapiens* reaches its limits at an earlier stage.

References

1. Kuschinsky, Wahl
2. Wahl, Kuschinsky (1973)

Eur Arch Otorhinolaryngology (1994) [Suppl]: S469–S470

FREE PAPERS AND POSTERS

F. Satomi, H. Iritani, K. Date, T. Minatogawa, Y. Nishimura, and T. Kumoi

Morphological Changes in Ischemic Facial Nerve Paralysis

Introduction

The etiology of idiopathic facial nerve paralysis is still obscure. Two major concepts are reported in the literature, ischemia of the nerve within the temporal bone, and viral infection of the facial nerve. In the present paper, the morphological changes of the paralyzed facial nerve, atraumatically induced by selective vascular embolization [2], are reported.

Materials and Methods

Healthy adult cats weighing more than 2.5 kg were anesthetized with ketamine HCl, and selective embolization of the internal maxillary and posterior auricular artery was performed with 2.5 ml 1% Avitene (microfibrillar collagen). The loss of the blink or corneal reflex was used to confirm the onset of paralysis. Cats were put to death 1, 7, 14, and 28 days (groups 1 to 4) after the establishment of ischemic facial nerve paralysis. Groups 1 and 2 contained three experimental animals, and Groups 3 and 4 contained four animals. After perfusion with 2% glutaraldehyde, the horizontal segment of the facial nerve was excised, fixed with 2% osmium tetraoxide, embedded in Epon, and sliced into sections 1 μm in thickness. The numbers of myelinated fibers (MF)/mm^2 were counted, and the largest diameter of each fiber was also measured with a computer imaging system (IBAS, Kontron Co., Munich, Germany). The teasing fibers technique was employed for one animal each in groups 1 and 2. The facial nerve of the nonparalyzed side was taken as control.

F. Satomi, H. Iritani, K. Date, T. Minatogawa, Y. Nishimura, and T. Kumoi
Department of Otolaryngology, Hyogo College of Medicine, 1-1, Mukogawa-cho, Nishinomiya, 663 Japan

Results

1. Group 1 (1 day after the establishment of total facial nerve paralysis).
   Scattered degenerated MFs were observed, predominantly found in the central area, most of them belonging to the larger myelinated fiber group. The number of myelinated fibers/mm^2 and the largest diameter did not differ from those in normal specimens (normal, 3535/mm^2, group 1, 3846/mm^2).
2. Group 2 (1 week after establishment of complete facial nerve paralysis).
   The number of MFs was 2539/mm^2.
3. Group 3 (2 weeks after extablishment of complete facial nerve paralysis).
   In two of four animals, the axons of degenerated MFs were already resorbed, but a few normal fibers were spared from Wallerian degeneration in the peripheral zone, and there were many macrophages performing phagocytosis of degenerated myelin debris. In one of four animals, a few swollen fibers were interspersed among the normal MFs. In one animal of group 3, normal-shaped regenerated nerve fibers were observed in about three-fourths of the area in the transversely sectioned plane. This animal had already recovered from facial paralysis, while the other three animals still exhibited paralysis.
4. Group 4 (put to death 4 weeks after establishment of facial nerve paralysis).
   In this group, all four animals showed regenerated nerve fibers, which were small in size, and coated with a thin myelin sheath. One animal in this group showed two crescent-shaped areas of regenerated nerve fibers with normal appearance. Three of four animals had incomplete recovery of facial nerve paralysis on examination before death. The number of regenerated MFs was 8234/mm^2, and the transverse diameter of regenerated fibers was 3–6 μm.
5. Findings of the teased fibers method.

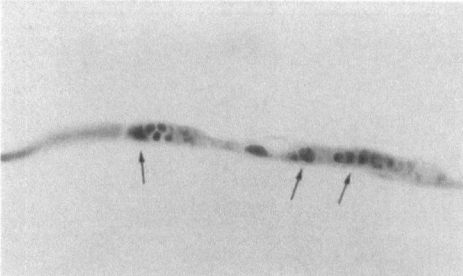

Fig. 1 Teased fiber preparation 1 day after establishment of facial nerve paralysis demonstrating a mixture of myelin ovoids and balls (*arrows*)

The teased fibers examination performed 1 day and 1 week after embolization revealed abnormal myelin thickness within internodes forming myelin ovoids and balls (Fig. 1).

Discussion

Peripheral nerves are extremely well-vascularized structures with elaborate vascular plexuses within and between all structural layers; however, the facial nerve in the temporal bone is different from other nerves in that it is surrounded by a bony canal. Unlike the central nervous system, the peripheral nervous system is relatively resistant to ischemia and is able to survive considerable periods of anoxia with rapid recovery of function, but ischemic neuropathy has proved difficult to study experimentally. Parry and Brown injected arachidonic acid into the femoral artery of normal rats and established an animal model of ischemic tibial nerve palsy [3], and Iritani in 1989 [2] presented an animal model of ischemic facial nerve paralysis in which the main blood supply to the nerve was selectively embolized. In Parry and Brown's observation, 1 day after arachidonate injection microscopic study of sections taken from the distal portion of the posterior tibial nerve revealed early signs of necrosis of neural elements, and 4 days after injection there was more advanced destruction of the endoneural structures. Seven days after arachidonate injection the intramyelinic edema had largely subsided.

The degree of facial nerve damage atraumatically induced by selective vascular embolization of the main blood supply to the nerve was variable. The pathological findings observed at 2 and 4 weeks after establishment of complete facial nerve paralysis were different. Pathological changes were observed on light microscopy 1 day after embolization; however, the area of definite degeneration of fibers was not clearly demonstrated until 14 days after embolization. Absorption of the myelin sheath debris by macrophages was observed in specimens 14 days and 28 days after embolization, and regeneration of fibers was observed 28 days after embolization, although facial nerve function was not yet fully recovered. Examination of single teased fibers 1 day and 1 week after embolization confirmed that the degeneration process [1] had commenced immediately after embolization, as also demonstrated by light microscopic observation.

References

1. Dyck P et al. (1984) Pathologic alterations of the peripheral nervous system of humans. In: Dyck P et al. (eds) Peripheral neuropathy. Saunders, Philadelphia, pp 760–870
2. Iritani H et al. (1989) An animal model for ischemic facial nerve paralysis with a selective embolization. Ear Res Jpn 20:195–196
3. Parry GJ, Brown MJ (1981) Arachidonate-induced experimental nerve infarction. J Neurol Sci 50:123–133

Eur Arch Otorhinolaryngology (1994) [Suppl]: S471–S472

H. Omori, M. Ikeda, N. Kukimoto, H. Kawamoto, A. Ikui, and H. Tomita

Activation of Intravascular Coagulation in Bell's Palsy

Introduction

Although the causes of Bell's palsy are still unknown, it is more or less the unanimous view that ischemic hypothesis and viral hypothesis constitute the main factors. With regard to ischemia, it has been believed that such factors as embolism which occur in vasa nervorum distributing to the facial nerve, or as vasospasm which is induced by dysfunction of the autonomic nervous system, cause ischemia. When considering embolism, it is easily understood that the coagulation functions of individuals are involved in such an abnormality. However, very few studies have so far been made on the functional state of coagulation in patients with facial paralysis. We made a study on the condition of coagulation functions in the acute phase of Bell's palsy based on the clinical examination centering on the thrombin-antithrombin III complex (TAT), and plasmin-α_2 plasmin inhibitor complex (PIC), which have recently attracted much attention as indexes of hypercoagulability. Relationships between the coagulation and the fibrinolytic systems, TAT and PIC, are shown in Fig. 1.

Fig. 1 Relationships between the coagulation and fibrinolytic systems, and TAT and PIC

H. Omori, M. Ikeda (✉), M. Kukimoto, H. Kawamoto, A. Ikui, and H. Tomita
Department of Otolaryngology, Nihon University School of Medicine, 30-1 Oyaguchi, Itabashi-ku, Tokyo 173, Japan

Subjects and Methods

The subjects were 78 patients with Bell's palsy who visited the ENT clinic of Nihon Univerrsity Itabashi Hospital in 1990 and 1991. They visited our clinic within 2 weeks ot the onset of paralysis and had no history of being treated with steroids. Normal subjects were 110 normal adults (70 males and 40 females) for TAT, and 40 normal adults (21 males and 19 females) for PIC. Counts of blood corpuscles, bleeding time, PT, APTT, antithrombin III, FDP, TAT, and PIC were examined. The Standard value of TAT was below 3.0 ng/ml and that of PIC was below 0.8 µg/ml. The values of TAT and PIC obtained from all of the normal subjects were within these standared values. No significant differences between sex and age were recognized in TAT or PIC in normal subjects.

Results

The test results of all the cases were within the normal range for bleeding time, PT, APTT, AT III, and FDP. Cases exceeding normal values were observed for TAT and PIC. Abnormal TAT values in Bell's palsy group were observed in 20 out of 79 patients (25.3%) and a statistically significant difference ($p < 0.01$) was observed versus normal subjects (Table 1). Abnormal PIC values in Bell's palsy were observed in 11 patients (13.9%), and the difference from normal subjects was statistically significant ($p < 0.05$) (Table 2).

Table 1 Detection of TAT abnormality in Bell's palsy cases

		Detection of abnormality
Bell's palsy	(79 cases)	20 cases (25.3%)*
Control	(110 cases)	0 case (0%)*

*$p < 0.0001$.

Table 2 Detection of PIC abnormality in Bell's palsy cases

		Detection of abnormality
Bell's palsy	(79 cases)	11 cases (13.9%)*
Control	(40 cases)	0 case (0%)*

*$p < 0.05$.

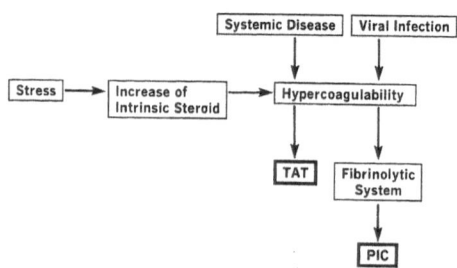

Fig. 2 Hypothesis of the activation of intravascular coagulation in Bell's palsy

It was in three cases that abnormally increased values were observed both for TAT and PIC. Ten out of the 20 patients that indicated abnormal values of TAT were reexamined in their convalescent phases. The results demonstrated that the values were reduced to normal for eight patients, and the values for the remaining two patients were also found to have decreased remarkably. As to PIC, we were able to reexamine two patients. One patient was observed to be within the normal range and the other was found to have a remarkable reduction.

Discussion

Thrombosis is a common phenomenon of disorders causing obstruction of the blood vessel. In this study we evaluated the conditions of coagulation in the acute phase of Bell's palsy. The results indicated that, in Bell's palsy cases, although no abnormal changes were observed in the bleeding time, PT, or APTT, significant abnormalities were observed not only in TAT utilized for early diagnosis of DIC as an index of prethrombotic state but also in PIC, which is believed to be the direct proof of occurrence of thrombus. Moreover, among the cases that exhibited high values in TAT, all of the 10 patients who were reexamined in the convalescent phases showed marked improvement. These findings suggest the possible existence of a factor which causes hypercoagulability and accelerates thrombosis in the acute phase of some patients with Bell's palsy.

It has been recognized that TAT shows high values in such infectious disease as sepsis, various kinds of thrombosis, malignant diseases, pregnancy, tissue injuries, and hepatic dysfunction. On the other hand, PIC has been observed to show high values in thrombosis and hepatic dysfunction. Among the patients with Bell's palsy examined in this study, 20 patients were found also to be suffering from hypertension or diabetes as a systemic disease. Out of those 20 patients, 6 (30%) showed an increase in TAT and 4 (20%) indicated an increse in PIC. It might be possible to assume that these systemic diseases constitute one of the risk factors which could induce the prethrombotic state in Bell's palsy cases.

On other hand, we assume that the increase of intrinsic steroids due to mental or physical stress is important as a cause of the prethrombotic state observed in cases with Bell's palsy showing no abnormality such as systemic diseases or severe infectious disease. Stress has been beieved for a long time to be one of the causative factors of facial paralysis, and it is known that stress causes an increase in intrinsic steroids through ACTH. As thrombosis is also well known as an important side effect of steroids, it might be possible that an increase in intrinsic steroids caused by stress could induce prethrombotic state in Bell's palsy. A hypothesis of the activation of intravascular coagulation in Bell's palsy cases is shown in Fig. 2.

Eur Arch Otorhinolaryngology (1994) [Suppl] : S473 – S474

S. Hegemann, L. Klimek, B. Korves, J. Lamprecht, and S. Wolf

Retinal Videofluorescence-Angiographic Findings in Bell's Palsy

Introduction

Different theories about the etiology of Bell's palsy are discussed. Impaired blood supply to the facial nerve is, by many authors, considered to be the primary cause of the paralysis. It causes nerve swelling and subsequent self-strangulation in its bony canal, leading to the well-known vicious circle first described by Hilger in 1949 [1]. Other diseases such as sudden hearing loss or vestibular neuropathy seem to have a very similar etiology. Indications for generalized microangiopathic alterations leading to impaired blood supply to the nerve were found by various investigators. However, these data are controversial. Methods for microinvasive, direct measurement of facial nerve blood supply might solve this diagnostic problem. Although accurate and standardized methods are in experimental use for animal studies, clinical application in humans seems impossible in the foreseeable future. On the other hand, one can easily observe the retinal vessels in vivo down to the diameter of precapillaries by fundoscopic examination. Retinal blood flow can be measured exactly by means of videofluorescence-angiography. Microangiopathic changes are thus identified with high sensitivity [2, 4]. We postulated that, if impaired blood supply to the facial nerve were due to generalized alterations, we should be able to find those alterations in the retinal vessels as well. Normal retinal blood supply would make a generalized microangiopathy very unlikely.

S. Hegemann, L. Klimek, B. Korves, and J. Lamprecht
Department of Otorhinolaryngology and Plastic Head and Neck Surgery, RWTH University Hospital, 52057 Aachen (Aix la chapelle), Germany

S. Wolf
Department of Ophtalmology and Plastic Head and Neck Surgery, RWTH University Hospital, 52057 Aachen (Aix la chapelle), Germany

Material and Method

At Aachen university hospital a special video analyzing system has been developed allowing quantitative measurement of retinal blood flow. A scanning laser ophthalmoscope with an adapted videosystem is used for fundoscopic examination and digital recording. For videofluorescence-angiography 50 ml/kg body weight of a 10 % fluorescein sodium solution is rapidly injected into the cubital vein, and a videotime generator is started simultaneously.

Fluorescein flow into the retinal vessels is registered from the initial influx to the late venous phase. After a pause of 2–3 min, recording of the fundus is resumed. Optical density measurements can be performed on the video recordings by means of the picture analyzing system in order to determine the circulation parameters of the retina: the arm retina time (ART) and the arteriovenous passage time (AVP).

The ART is the time needed from the bolus injection into the cubital vein to the first appearance of fluorescein in a retinal artery. It allows a very rough estimation of the

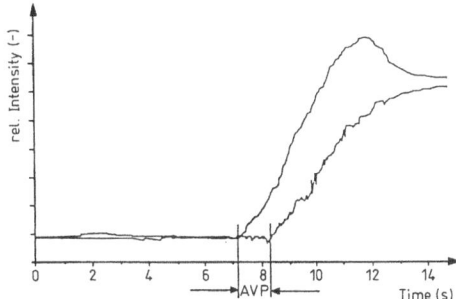

Fig. 1 Characteristic dye dilution curves for measuring the arteriovenous passage time (AVP). (From [4])

S474

macrocirculatory situation. Only gross pathological alterations like marked stenosis of the carotid artery lead to a significantly prolonged ART. The mean normal value is 11.2±3.3 s; values of more than 22 s are considered pathologic.

The AVP is by definition the time between the first appearance of the dye in a retinal artery and in the corresponding vein. If the dilution curves of an artery and its corresponding vein are shown graphically in the same diagram, the distance between the initial points of the rising curves is the AVP (Fig. 1). The mean normal value is 1.45±0.4 s; more than 2.3 s is considered pathologic. The AVP is the shortest circulation time of the indicator through a corresponding area of microcirculation. It is thus a very sensitive indicator for microcirculatory disturbances in the retinal vessels.

Patients

In our prospective study we examined 32 patients suffering from mononeuropathy of cranial nerves. Eleven patients with complete or incomplete Bell's palsy, 17 patients with sudden hearing loss, and 4 with vestibular neuropathy were included in the study. Patients already treated with rheologically active substances prior to videoangiography were excluded. Other exclusion criteria were arterial hypertension of more than 160 over 100 mmHg, diabetes mellitus, allergy to dye, glaucoma, and pregnancy. About 50% of all patients had to be excluded because of previous rheological treatment. Five suffered from diabetes mellitus, one from hypertension, and one from glaucoma. We have seen no patients with allergy to dye or pregnancy.

Results

All patients with Bell's palsy had a normal arm retina time, indicating that there were no major macrocirculatory problems. The mean ART of 11.5±3.1 s was not significantly different from the normal mean. The arteriovenous passage time was normal in 10 of 11 patients. One had a pathologically prolonged AVP of 2.5 s. The mean AVP of the whole group was 1.6±0.4 s. With the one pathological value excluded it was 1.52±0.4 s. Both figures are not significantly different from the normal mean AVP. The patient with the prolonged AVP was a 34-year-old man without any known underlying disease. Blood pressure, hemoglobin, and hematocrit were within the normal range. There was no reason for the prolonged AVP detectable. The 21 patients with sudden hearing loss and vestibular neuropathy all had normal ART and AVP values. The mean values for both parameters were not significantly different from the normal mean. Table 1 summarizes the results. In summary, our results show no pathological ART values. One of 11 cases of Bell's palsy showed indications of a

Table 1. Results of videofluorescence-angiography

	Mean AVP	Mean ART
Normal mean value	1.45±0.4 s	11.2±3.3 s
Pathological value	>2.3 s	>22 s
Bell's palsy (n=11)	1.61±0.4 s	11.5±3.1 s
SHL and VN	1.72±0.4 s	12.2±5.0 s

SHL, sudden hearing loss; VN, vestibular neuropathy

microcirculatory disturbance that could not be exactly identified. In all other cases normal circulation parameters were measured.

Discussion

The method of videoangiography is routinely used in ophthalmology. Its reliability and sensitivity in detecting microcirculatory disturbances has been proven. While blood supply for the inner ear and facial nerve stems mainly from the vertebral artery and the medial meningeal artery, retinal vessels belong to the internal carotid artery system. Nevertheless there seems to be no major difference between these arteries in respect to involvement in microangiopathy. Therefore we consider the retinal vessels to be reasonably comparable to the vessels of the inner ear. We found a pathological AVP value in one case. Except for the AVP, all other blood flow parameters were normal. A mistake in the measuring or analyzing system was excluded by revision of the videorecording. The pathological value of the prolonged AVP for the one patient is unclear, but it has definitely no importance for the explanation of the etiology in the majority of cases. We conclude that generalized microcirculatory disturbances may in some cases cause Bell's palsy, but cannot be detected in the majority of cases. For sudden hearing loss and vestibular neuropathy the same arguments are valid. Bell's palsy seems to be due to local rather than generalized pathology. The final cause remains undiscovered and the facial palsy remains idiopathic.

References

1. Hilger JA (1949) The nature of Bell's palsy. Laryngoscope 59:228–235
2. Reim M, Wolf S (1989) Videofluoreszenzangiographie zur Untersuchung der Hämodynamik des Auges. Fortschr Ophthalmol 86:744–750
3. Stennert E (1980) New concepts in treatment of Bell's palsy. Paper on the 4th international symposium on facial nerve surgery, 2–5 Sept 1980, Los Angeles
4. Wolf S, Jung F, Kiesewetter H, Körber N, Reim M (1989) Video fluorescein angiography: method and clinical application. Graefes Arch Clin Exp Ophthalmol 227:145–151

Eur Arch Otorhinolaryngology (1994) [Suppl]:S475

ABSTRACTS

E. Seifert, A. Schadel and H. Theilen

Evaluation of Total and Perfused Blood Vessels in the Facial Nerve

The theory of primary and/or secondary ischemia leading to the vicious circle postulated by Hilger has become generally accepted. In further animal experimental studies we examined the capillary network of the facial nerve of rabbits. We used, e. g., the method of plastination inaugurated by von Hagens and found a longitudinal and transverse network of capillaries supplying the nerve. The generally accepted theory is that only 25% of all capillaries are perfused in time. However, the normal capillary perfusion of the facial nerve and the amount of in vivo perfused capillaries are still unknown. In awake normocapnic rats we determined the density of the total and perfused capillary network of the facial nerve. The density of perfused capillaries was measured by two intravenous markers (fluorescein isothiocyanate globulin and Evans blue), the density of morphologically existing capillaries was determined according to an immunohistochemical fluorescence method which marked the capillary wall constituent fibronectin. The antibody which attaches to the capillary wall can be made visible by immunofluorescence and peroxidase technique. Comparison of perfused and morphologically existing capillary counts showed very high congruence when fluorescent results were compared. The identity of the perfused and morphologically existing capillary network could be confirmed by a double-staining technique. First, the perfused capillaries were marked by intraveneous application of Evans blue and second the existing capillaries were relocated in the same measuring field by the fibronectin technique. This double-staining technique resulted in identical capillary counts in 92% of all cases. We have to conclude that all existing capillaries are perfused and there is no capillary reserve in the facial nerve like the capillary network of the brain.

E. Seifert, A. Schadel and H. Theilen
ENT Department, Clinic of Mannheim, Mannheim, Germany

Viral Involvement

Eur Arch Otorhinolaryngology (1994) [Suppl]:S479–S481

P.S.J.Z. Mulkens and F.P. Schröder

Virus Isolation Study of the Human Ganglion Geniculi (Nerve VII)

Since Sir Charles Bell, 150 years ago, Bell's palsy (BP) still remains an idiopathic disease. This long history explains why BP turned out to be one of the most controversial entities in otological medicine regarding not only the treatment but also the etiopathogenesis. So it is most obvious that many etiological and pathogenic hypotheses have been presented over the past decades. From the various hypotheses like the vascular, the immunological, and the hereditary, the viral one is widely accepted. Because of the high neurotropism and the frequent association with infection in the face and the head, the focus has been in particular on the herpes simplex virus type I (HSV1) as a possible pathogen. Reviewing the literature the many publications on the subject of the relationship between BP and HSV1 can be divided into clinical and experimental studies (Table 1).

Table 1 Studies of the relationship between Bell's palsy and herpes simplex virus

Clinical
    Serological
    Histological
    Virus isolation

Experimental
    HSV1 inoculation in the stylomastoidal foramen in rabbits
    HSV1 injection close to the facial nerve in guinea pigs
    HSV1 retrograde transneuronal transport in mice
    HSV1 recovery in human trigeminal ganglia (nerve V)
    HSV1 recovery in human geniculate ganglia (nerve VII)

P.S.J.Z. Mulkens
Wilhelmina Hospital Assen, The Netherlands

F.P. Schröder
Regional Public Health Laboratory, Groningen and Drenthe, The Netherlands

Clinical serological research has been published by many authors, e.g., by Adour [2] as one of the initial researchers in this direction. Yet there has not been produced significant serological evidence of an HSV1 infection in Bell's palsy patients. Also our own serological study in 124 patients could not provide any sign for HSV1 pathology [11]. In the rare cases – which enabled Proctor [14], O'Donoghue [13], and more recently Liston [10] to carry out a clinical histological postmortem examination of a BP facial nerve – signs of infection have been demonstrated, possibly of viral origin. However, virus isolation examination has not been performed in these BP patient nerves.

At the end of the period in which we treated BP patients with decompression surgery, specimens of an epineurium fragment obtained after splitting the nerve sheath were excised for virus isolation. In one case out of six the culture proved to be HSV1 positive [11]. It is quite impossible now to continue this kind of research since decompression surgery has been abandoned as a beneficial treatment.

Coming to the experimental section, Kumagami presented in 1972 [8] in an animal experimental model the capability of HSV1 to induce facial paralysis in rabbits by inoculating the stylomastoidal foramen with HSV1. However, in our animal experimental model HSV1 injection in guinea pigs close to the surgically exposed facial nerve just inferior to the stylomastoidal foramen did not induce facial paralysis although there was serological evidence for an HSV1 infection [12]. Ishii [7] in a guinea pig model was also not able to induce a facial paralysis, though the peripherally inoculated HSV1 antigens did reach the facial nerve via the petrosal nerve with inflammatory cell response, hemorrhages, degeneration, and necrosis even in trigeminal ganglia and pons. So he suggested a higher resistance of guinea pigs to HSV1.

The above-mentioned capability of HSV1 to migrate centrally by retrograde transneuronal transport has been established in mice by Thomander [15], who demonstrated an invasion by HSV1 from the tongue to the facial complex. Moreover, the use of HSV1 as a transneuronal tracer by Ugolini [16] confirms how easily the HSV1 can reach its neuronal pathways in mice.

In a human experimental model the establishment of latent HSV in trigeminal ganglia by Baringer [3] strongly supported the HSV1 etiology hypothesis in explaining BP. Dealing with this hypothetical etiopathogenesis of an occasional reactivation of latent HSV1 settled in neural tissue, the question rises if HSV1, which might produce a viral neuritis, can be detected in the facial ganglion of non-BP patients. That is why we decided to perform a virus isolation study from the human geniculate ganglion in the facial nerve.

Materials and Methods

Removal of the Geniculate Ganglion In total, 19 geniculate ganglia were removed in sterile fashion from unselected cadavers undergoing autopsy less than 24 h after death. After resection of the temporal bone an endaural approach was used for the microscopic removal of the eardrum and the ossicular chain. Just above the oval window we removed the lateral bony wall and opened the horizontal part of the facial canal with exposure of the nerve. Following the nerve up to the first knee we resected the ganglion (Fig. 1) and sent it in for virus isolation to the Regional Public Halth Laboratory Groningen and Drenthe. For conservation the so-called gly medium was used.

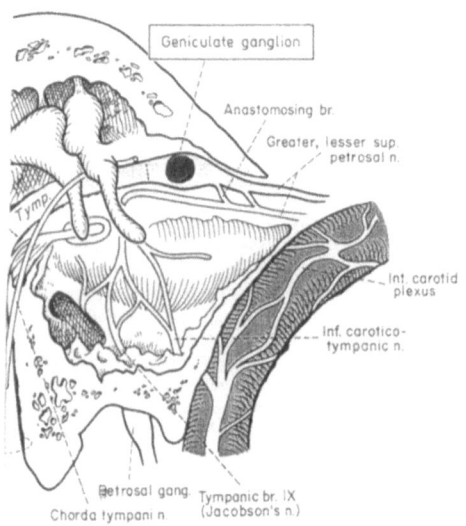

Fig. 1 Resection of the geniculate ganglion

In the period November 1982 until May 1983, 14 temporal bones were resected, immediately deep-freeze stores (-70 °C), and referred to our ENT Dept. within 3 days. These 14 bones were resected at random at the Dept. of Pathology from the University Hospital, Groningen. No case reports were available. From September 1991 up to March 1992 five temporal bones were taken from the Dept. of Pathology in the Wilhelmina Hospital, Assen. These specimens were directly referred to our ENT Department for immediate removal of the ganglia. The available case reports mentioned various causes of death such as apoplexia and cardiac arrests. The average age of the four women and one man was 53.6 years (from 33 to 87 years).

Virus Isolation Procedure The neural tissues were sent to the laboratory in viral transport medium. They were minced and 0.3 ml of the tissue suspension in culture medium was explanted on diploid human embryonic lung fibroblasts. To the medium of these cocultivated cultures 20 μM of the demethylating agent 5-azacytidine was added, according to a poster presentation of Stephanopoulos et al. (Reactivation of herpes simplex virus from latently infected guinea pig neural tissue with 5-azacytidine. D.E. Stephanopoulos, M.G. Myers, J.C. Kappes and D.I. Bernstein. Children's Hospital Research Foundation and J.N. Gamble Inst. Med. Res., Cincinatti, Ohio) at the 11th International Herpesvirus Workshop, Leeds, 1986. Cultures were treated with drug for 3 days, then refed with drug-free medium and observed for CPE for 14 days.

In addition, four shell vial cultures were inoculated each with 0.2 ml tissue suspension. To these cultures 35 μM 5-azacytidine was added after centrifugation at 1000 g for 30 min. After 1 day, immunofluorescence with anti-HSV 1/2 FITC-labeled monoclonal antibodies (Kallestad) was performed on the first coverslip, and in the case of a negative result immunofluorescence was repeated after 7 days on the second coverslip. A second pair of coverslips was used for examination for varicella zoster virus (VZV). In this case indirect immunofluorescence was performed with anti-VZV-monoclonal antibodies (Whittaker bioproducts) and FITC-labeled rabbit-anti-mouse conjugate (Dakopatts).

Results

From all the 19 ganglia it was not possible to isolate a latent HSV1 or any other virus. All the cultures proved to be negative.

Discussion

Accepting viral reinfection as the most likely hypothesis in explaining the etiopathogenesis of Bell's palsy, the attempt to estabish latent HSV1 in the geniculte ganglion is very attractive in supporting this theory, which, however, our results do not. In analysing this situation there are two ways of interpreting these results.

Firstly, we cannot exclude the possibility of a false-negative result. Perhaps the period of 24 h after death, within which we obtained the temporal bones, has been too long. Baringer used a 12-h period and Lewis [9] established that the rate of recovery of HSV1 from trigeminal ganglia is affected by the time elapsed after death: spontaneous reactivation of HSV1 can be maximized when ganglia are obtained within 12 h after death compared with the results after 13–24 h. Secondly, we may consider the possibility of a real lack of latent HSV1 in the geniculate ganglion. In that case we are still able to fit the mentioned transneuronal transfer capability of HSV1 with a supposed migration of HSV1 from the ganglion Gasseri (nerve V) via the petrosal nerve to the facial nerve. Moreover, Davis [4] has demonstrated that HSV1 induced from outside was a high capability to infect especially the geniculate ganglion. According to our negative results an additional study of Ishii [6] may fit because of his finding in his animal experimental model that HSV1 antigen settled more easily in the Gasseri ganglion than in the geniculate ganglion.

Another option has been put forward by Diamante [5] who, reviewing the literature, suggested a mixture of viral reinfection and auto-immunological reactions whereby anti-virus-myelin antibodies, having demyelinating potentials, induce both peripheral and central lesions within the facial nerve and other nuclei belonging to the brainstem. A demyelinating disorder which is comparative with Guillain-Barré syndrome, as well as with systemic lupus erythematosus, is the classical autoimmune disease. This also fits with Adour's [1] report of herpes simples polyganglionitis accompanying Bell's palsy with all the various symptoms of different cranial nerve disorders as well as with the findings of demyelinization in the cited histopathologic studies. Summarizing the discussed results, these might in any case encourage an answer as to whether the HSV1 reinfection hypothesis might be valid. In our opinion, however, the key can be given only by the unique occasion of a fresh Bell's palsy autopsy. A mere histopathologic study, as has already been performed several times, is not sufficient. In such a case an extensive virological study of the whole nerve including the geniculate ganglion is absolutely imperative.

Acknowledgements The authors are grateful to R. v. d. Weg MD and J. v. Buchem MD (Wilhelmina Hospital Assen, Dept. of pathology) for referring the temporal bones of the patients. Our gratitude is also due to Mr. G. Klaucke for his technical assistance and J.D. Bleeker MD for a critical review of the manuscript.

References

1. Adour KK (1976) Cranial polyneuritis and Bell's palsy. Arch Otolaryngol 102:262–264
2. Adour KK, Bell DN, Hilsinger RL (1975) Herpes simplex virus in idiopathic facial paralysis (Bell's palsy). JAMA 233: 527–530
3. Baringer JR, Swoveland P (1973) Recovery of herpes simplex virus from human trigeminal ganglion. N Engl J Med 288: 648–650
4. Davis LE (1981) Experimental viral infections of the facial nerve and geniculate ganglion. Ann Neurol 9: 120–125
5. Diamante VG (1988) Some aspects of Bell's palsy: pathogenesis. In: Castro D (ed) Facial nerve. Kugler and Ghedini, Amsterdam, pp 311–313
6. Ishii K, Kurata T, Sata T, Hao MV, Nomura Y (1988) An animal model of type I herpes simplex virus infection of facial nerve. Acta Otolaryngol Suppl (Stockh) 446: 157–164
7. Ishii K, Nomura Y, Sata T, Kurata T (1990) An animal model of type 1 herpes simplex virus infection of the facial nerve. In: Castro D (ed) Facial nerve. Kugler and Ghedini, Amsterdam, pp 87–90
8. Kumagami H (1972) Experimental facial nerve paralysis. Arch Otolaryngol 95: 305–312
9. Lewis ME, Warren KG, Jefrrey VM, Shnitka TK (1982) Factors affecting recovery of latent herpes simplex virus from human trigeminal ganglia. Can J Microbiol 28: 123–129
10. Liston SL, Kleid MS (1989) Histopathology of Bell's palsy. Laryngoscope 99: 23–26
11. Mulkens PSJZ, Bleeker JD, Schröder FP (1980) Acute facial paralysis: a virological study. Clin Otolaryngol 5: 303–310
12. Mulkens PSJZ, Bleeker JD, Schröder FP, Schirm J, Welling S, Segenhout JM (1985) Bell's palsy: a viral disease? An experimental study. In: Portmann M (ed) Facial nerve. Masson, New York, pp 227–230
13. O'Donoghue GM, Michaels L (1985) Histopathological aspects of Bell's palsy. In: Portmann M (ed) Facial nerve. Masson, New York, pp 248–252
14. Proctor B, Corgill DA, Proud G (1976) The pathology of Bell's palsy. Trans Acad Ophtalmol Otol 82:70–80
15. Thomander L, Aldskogius H, Kristensson K, Vahlne A, Thomas E (1988) Invasion of cranial nerves and brain stem by herpes simplex virus inoculated into the mouse tongue. Ann Otol Laryngol 97:554–558
16. Ugolini G, Kuypers HGJM, Strick PL (1989) Transneural transfer of herpes virus from peripheral nerves to cortex and brainstem. Science 243:89–91

Eur Arch Otorhinolaryngology (1994) [Suppl]: S482 – S486

FREE PAPERS AND POSTERS

H. Honda and A. Takahashi

Virus-Associated Demyelination in the Pathogenesis of Bell's Palsy

Introduction

Idiopathic peripheral facial palsy (Bell's palsy) is a common neuropathy that results from an intrinsic lesion of the seventh cranial nerve. To date, many hypotheses have been presented to explain the etiology of this disorder [1, 2]. However, since the prognosis of facial paralysis is generally good and postmortem studies are quite rare [3], it is difficult to establish the true pathologic nature of Bell's palsy. Even the site along the facial nerve of the lesion is still uncertain.

In an attempt to evaluate the possible pathomechanism of virus-associated demyelination in the development of facial nerve paralysis, we examined the activity of the myelin-associated enzyme 2', 3'-cyclic nucleotide 3'-phosphohydrolase (CNP) [4] in the CSF and the virus serology in patients with Bell's palsy.

Patients and Methods

Patients We examined 164 patients with acute "idiopathic" peripheral facial palsy. Diagnosis of Bell's palsy was made according to Taverner's diagnostic criteria [1]. This study included 75 male and 89 female patients, who ranged from 1 to 89 years of age (average age, 44.2 years); in 80 patients Bell's palsy was right-sided and 9 patients (5.5%) were experiencing a recurrence of the palsy. The majority of the patients had come to our clinic within 7 days of the onset of facial paralysis. At the time of the first visit, peripheral blood was taken for routine laboratory tests, namely, erythrocyte sedimentation rate (ESR), white blood cell count, C-reactive protein (CRP), and cold hemagglutinin (CH) titer.

Virus Serology Serum samples were collected at the time of the first visit and 2 – 5 weeks later. Serum was tested for complement-fixing (CF) antibodies against herpes simplex (HSV), varicella zoster (VZV), mumps, and Coxsackie A9 viruses, and indirect immunofluorescence was carried out to detect IgG antibodies against the capsid antigens of Epstein-Barr virus (EBV). CF antibodies and the antibodies against EBV were considered to be positive at titers of greater than $1:4$ and $1:40$, respectively.

Examination of Cerebrospinal Fluid (CSF) Samples of CSF were obtained from 91 patients within 7 days of the onset of facial paralysis. Cell counts and glucose levels were determined, and total protein was assayed by the method of Lowry et al. [5]. Levels of immunoglobulins (Ig) G, A, and M in CSF were estimated by laser nephelometry.

Assay for 2', 3'-Cyclic Nucleotide 3'-Phosphohydrolase (CNP) Activity in CSF Immediately after sampling, an aliquot of CSF was centrifuged at 1500 rpm and the supernatant was stored at $-80\,°C$ until use. The CNP activity was estimated by the NADP-cycling method as described elsewhere [6]. The activity of the enzyme was expressed as nanomoles per hour per milliliter CSF.

Table 1 Prodromes observed in 124 out of 164 patients with Bell's palsy

Symptoms	No. of cases (%)	Preceding interval days (mean)
Otalgia, retroauricular pain	43 (26.2)	1 – 19 (4.1)
Headache, nuchal stiffness	42 (25.6)	1 – 15 (2.8)
Fever, sore throat, rhinorrhea	32 (19.5)	1 – 21 (5.8)
Nausea	4 (2.4)	2 – 7 (4.0)
Diarrhea	3 (1.8)	5, 7, 15 (9.0)

H. Honda (✉) and A. Takahashi
Department of Neurology, Nagoya University School of Medicine, 65, Tsurumai-cho, Showa-ku, Nagoya, 466 Japan

Table 2 Results of routine laboratory tests in patients with Bell's palsy

Laboratory test	Range			No. of cases with abnormal value (%)	
	No. of cases observed				
Erythrocyte sedimentation rate (mm/h)	≤20	20–40	40≤		
(n = 148) (normal ≤20)[a]	98	39	11	50	(33.8)
White blood cell count (×10³/μl)	≤8.0	8.1–12.0	12.1≤		
(n = 159) (3.5 ≤ normal ≤8.0)	113	37	9	46	(28.9)
C-reactie protein (mg/dl)	≤0.4	0.4≤			
(n = 148) (normal ≤0.4)	122	26		26	(17.6)
cold hemagglutinin titer	≤×32	×64	×128≤		
(n = 148) (normal ≤×32)	129	9	10	19	(12.8)

[a] Normal value was determined according to the data obtained from 76 healthy subjects: 39 males and 37 females who randed in age from 18 to 60 years (average age, 36.9 years).

Table 3 Virus-specific antibody titer in the serum from patients with Bell's palsy

Antibody titer (CF)[a]	≤×4	×8	×16	×32	×64	×128≤
Herpes simplex virus (n = 148)	21[b]	10	75	28	13	1
Varicella zoster virus (n = 148)	142	3	3	0	0	0
Mumps virus (n = 119)	98	7	11	3	0	0
Coxsackie A9 virus (n = 119)	88	8	19	3	1	0
VCA-IgG antibody titer (IF)[c]	≤×40	×80	×160	×320	×640	×1280≤
Epstein-Barr virus (n = 115)	22	31	36	15	11	0

[a] Titer of complement-fixing antibodies.
[b] Number of cases observed. Serum samples were obtained from the patients at the time of the first visit.
[c] Titer of IgG antibodies against the capsid antigen assayed by an indirect immunofluorescence method.

Results

Prodome Early symptoms followed by facial paralysis were seen in 124 of 164 patients, as summarized in Table 1. About one-half of the patients had ipsilateral otalgia and retroauricular pain, and/or occipital headache and nuchal stiffness. Symptoms suggestive of upper respiratory tract infection were not infrequent (19.5%).

Routine Laboratory Findings (Table 2) Erythrocyte sedimentation rate was elevated in 50 (34%) of 148 patients. Leukocytosis was found in 46 (29%) of 159 patients. Serum CRP was positive in 26 (18%) of 148 patients. Thus, at least one-third of the patients had increased ESR, leukocytosis, and/or elevated CRP, which indicated

the presence of an inflammatory reaction. In addition, 19 (13%) of 148 patients had elevated CH titers. Nine patients showed significant changes in CH titers, but none of them had antibodies against *Mycoplasma pneumoniae*.

Virus Antibody Titers Of the 148 patients with Bell's palsy, 127 (86%) had CF antibodies against HSV, and 6 (4%) had CF antibodies against VZV at the time of the first visit (Table 3). Antibodies against mumps and Coxsackie A9 viruses were positive in 21 (18%) and 31 (26%) of 119 patients, respectively. Of the 115 samples of patients' serum examined, 93 (81%) contained IgG antibodies against EBV (Table 3). On subsequent examination, 2–5 weeks after the first

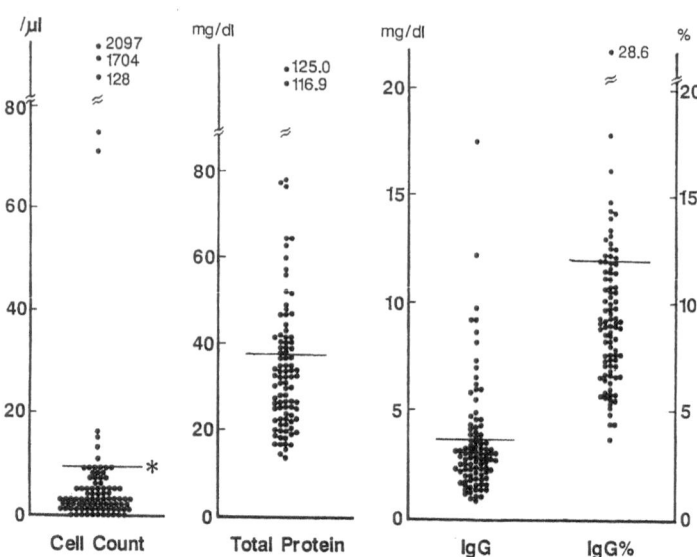

Fig. 1 Cerebrospinal fluid (CSF) findings in 91 patients with Bell's palsy. Samples of CSF were collected at the time of the first visit or within 7 days of the onset of facial paralysis. *Bar* indicated the value of the mean + 2SD in 21 control subjects who had no evidence of organic disorders of the nervous system

sampling, four of 112 patients showed three or fourfold changes in titers of HSV antibodies and one of 86 patients had a fourfold change in the titer of mumps virus antibodies, whereas titers of antibodies against VZV, Coxsackie A9 Virus and EBV remained unchanged in all cases examined.

CSF Findings. Figure 1 shows the results of the examinations of CSF from 91 patients with Bell's palsy. Of 91 patients, nine (10%) had CSF pleocytosis (more than 10 cells/μl), mostly of mononuclear cells, and 30 patients (33%) had elevated protein levels of greater than 37.6 mg/dl (the mean + 2SD value for controls). Among the cases with an increase in CSF protein, pleocytosis was present in only four cases. A total of 28 patients (31%) had elevated levels of IgG of greater than 3.4 mg/dl (the mean + 2SD value for controls) and 15 patients (16%) had an increase in IgG% of more than 12%. Eight patients had elevated levels of IgA, which ranged from 1.0 to 2.3 mg/dl, but the IgM content was below 1 mg/dl in all the cases examined.

The time course of chances in CSF protein content was examined in 14 patients. In five patients the levels of protein in the CSF tended to increase for 3–6 weeks after the onset of the disease and three patients showed a prolonged elevation of protein levels, with values consistently above 50 mg/dl. By contrast, the marked pleocytosis (more than 100 cells/μl) that had been observed in three patients at the first sampling was replaced by a normal cell count within 2–6 weeks.

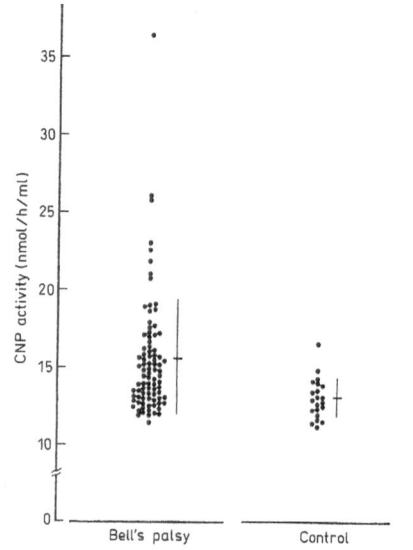

Fig. 2 2′,3′-Cyclic nucleotide 3′-phosphohydrolase (CNP) activity in the CSF. CNP activity was estimated by NADP cycling method (6). CSF samples were obtained from 91 patients with Bell's palsy and 21 control subjects. The enzyme activity was 15.5 ± 3.8 nmol/hr per milliliter (mean ± SD) in the patient group, and was significantly higher than that (13.2 ± 1.3 nmol/h per milliliter) in the control. (Student's *t* test, $p < 0.01$)

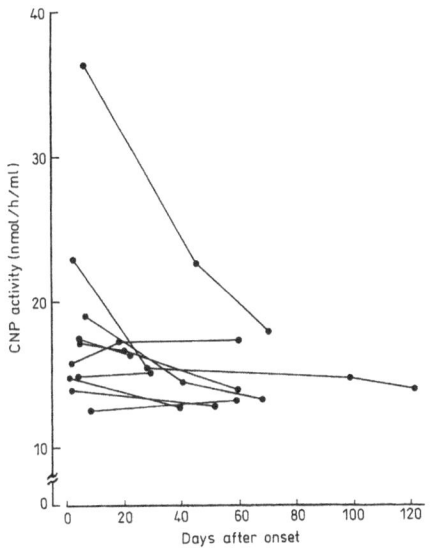

Fig. 3 Th time course of changes in the activity of 2′,3′-cyclic nucleotide 3′-phosphohydrolase in the CSF from ten patients with Bell's palsy

CNP Activity in CSF There was a significant elevation in CNP activity in the patient group (15.5 ± 3.8 nmol/h per milliliter) as compared with that in the control (13.2 ± 1.3 nmol/h per milliliter) (Student's t test, $p < 0.01$) (Fig. 2). At the first sampling, 29 patients (32%) had elevated enzyme activities of greater than the value of the mean + 2SD for the controls (15.8 nmol/h per milliliter). The time course of changes in CNP activity was examined in ten patients at 2–10 weeks after the onset of facial paralysis. Seven showed a decrease and three showed a slight increase in the CNP activity (Fig. 3).

The CNP activity was statistically correlatd with both the total protein ($r = 0.353$, $p < 0.01$) and levels of IgG ($r = 0.259$, $p < 0.05$) in the CSF. An analysis of the correlation between the titer of HSV antibodies and CNP activity revealed that the patients who were positive for the antibodies had higher CNP activity than those who were negative (Table 4). The four patients who showed significant changes with time in the titer of HSV antibodies also had elevated CNP activity, whereas a patient with a recent mumps virus infection, as indicated by changes in antibody titers, did not. Furthermore, the patients who were positive for HSV antibodies tended to have a high incidence of abnormal CSF findings (Table 4). By contrast, there was no significant relationship between the serum antibody titers against VZV, EBV, mumps virus, Coxsackie A9 virus, and the CSF findings, including CNP activity.

Table 4 Relationship between titer of serum HSV antibodies and CSF findings

	No. of cases	Age (years)	CSF findings				
			Cell count (/μl)	Total protein (mg/dl)	IgG (mg/dl)	IgG%	CNP activity (nmol/h/ml)
Controls[a]	21	41.9 ±16.2[b]	3.1 ±2.9	24.8 ±6.4	2.0 ±0.7	8.0 ±2.0	13.2 ±1.3
Patients	91	45.5 ±17.6	47.8 ±29.2	36.1 ±19.1**	3.5 ±2.6**	9.4 ±3.5	15.5 ±3.8**
HSV antibody titer (CF)							
≤×4	17	32.2 ±17.7	3.4 ±2.6	31.1 ±13.3	2.7 ±1.4	8.4 ±2.2	13.8 ±1.9
×8, ×16	53	48.0 ±15.3	75.7 ±50.4	37.5 ±18.9**	3.7 ±2.4**	9.7 ±3.4	15.6 ±3.1***
×32, ×64≤	21	49.9 ±18.6	15.6 ±7.3	36.3 ±23.4*	3.7 ±3.6*	9.7 ±3.2*	16.6 ±5.8**

[a] Controls consisted of 12 males and 9 females who ranged in age from 21 to 71 years (average, 41.9 years), and who had no evidence of organic disorders of the nervous system.
[b] Values are expressed as the mean ± SD.
*, **, *** Statistical significance (Student's t test) at $p < 0.05$, $p < 0.01$ $p < 0.001$ as compared with controls, respectively.

Discussion

The present study demonstrated that Bell's palsy is frequently accompanied by an inflammatory reaction, abnormal CSF findings, and elevated CNP activity in the CSF. Furthermore, the resutls of virus serology suggest that these pathologic changes may be associated with HSV infection or reactivation.

Symptoms suggestive of upper respiratory tract infection were often followed by facial paralysis, and nearly half of the patients had hematological and/or serologial evidence of an inflammatory reaction. Thus, it seems likely that inflamatory changes are frequently involved in the early phases of facial paralysis.

There have been few reports of CSF findings associated with Bell's palsy [7, 8]. The present study demonstrated that a relatively high incidence of CSF abnormalities accompanied facial paralysis, such as increased levels of total protein (30 cases) and IgG (28 cases), and occasional pleocytosis (9 cases) in 91 patients with Bell's palsy. These CSF findings indicate that intrathecal inflammatory or immunological changes occur in a large fraction of patients with Bell's palsy.

It is of interest that these CSF findings are quite similar to those observed in cases of acute inflammatory demyelinating polyneuropathy [9]. In this regard, some investigators [10, 11] have suggested that acute peripheral facial palsy is part of a polyneuropathy. These observations raise the possibility that Bell's palsy may involve a pathomechanism(s) similar to that responsible for Guillain-Barré syndrome or acute polyneuropathy in which inflammatory demyelination leads to nerve injury.

We attempted to examine whether a demyelinating process occurs during the development of facial paralysis. The significant elevation of CNP activity suggests that, at least in some cases of Bell's palsy, the breakdown of myelin does occur, since CNP has been found as a myelin-associated enzyme and elevated CNP activity is thought to be a marker of demyelination [4, 12].

From the changes in virus-specific antibody titers, facial paralysis appeared to be associated with a recent viral infection in only a few patients, namely, infection with HSV in four cases and with mumps virus in one case. These findings suggest the rare association of a primary viral infection with the onset of facial paralysis. However, several lines of evidence suggest that Bell's palsy may be caused by infection or reactivation of viruses, in particular HSV [13, 14], and it has been demonstrated that, in cases of herpes virus infection, the antibody titers only occasionally fluctuate before, during, or after the recrudescence of the infection [15–17]. Therefore, even if a direct connection between the antibodies and the clinical condition remains to be established, it seems possible that high titers of HSV antibodies found in the serum of patients with Bell's palsy are compatible with recurrent or reactivated infection with HSV. Our observation of an association between the antibodies against HSV, but not against EBV, and CSF abnormalities including elevated CNP activity in patients with Bell's palsy supports this hypothesis.

References

1. Taverner D (1955) Bell's palsy: a clinical and elctromyographic study. Brain 78 : 209–228
2. Zulch KJ (1970) "Idiopathic" facial paralysis. In: Vinken PJ, Bruyn GW (eds) Handbook of clinical neurology, vol VIII. North-Holland, Amsterdam, pp 241–302
3. Proctor B, Corgill DA, Proud G (1976) The pathology of Bell's palsy. Trans Am Acad Ophthalmol Otol 82 : 70–80
4. Banik NL, Mauldin LB, Hogan EL (1979) Activity of 2′,3′-cyclic nucleotide 3′-phophohydrolase in human cerebrospinal fluid. Ann Neurol 5 : 539–541
5. Lowry OH, Rosebrough NJ, Farr AL, Randall RJ (1951) Protein measurement with the Folin-phenol reagent. J Biol Chem 193 : 265–275
6. Weissbarth S, Marker HS, Lehrer GM, Schneider S, Bornstein MB (1980) A sensitive fluorometric assay for 2′,3′-cyclic nucleotide 3′-phosphohydrolase. J Neurochem 35 : 503–505
7. Djupesland G, Berdal P, Johannssen TA, Degré M, Stien R, Skrede S (1976) Viral infection as a cause of acute peripheral facial palsy. Arch Otolaryngol 102 : 221–227
8. Park HW, Watkins AL (1949) Facial paralyses: analyses of 500 cases. Arch Phys Med 30 : 749–761
9. Link H (1973) Immunoglobulin abnormalities in the Guillain-Barré syndrome. J Neurol Sci 18 : 11–13
10. Djupesland G, Degré M, Stien R, Skrede S (1977) Acute peripheral facial palsy: part of a cranial polyneuropathy? Arch Otolaryngol 103 : 641–644
11. Sandstedt P, Hyden D, Ödkvist L (1981) Bell's palsy: part of a polyneuropathy? Acta Neurol Scand 64 : 66–73
12. Sprinkle TJ, Mckhann GM (1978) Activity of 2′,3′-cyclic nucleotide 3′-phosphodiesterase in cerebrospinal fluid of patients with demyelinating disorders. Neurosci Lett 7 : 203–206
13. Adour KK, Bell DN, Hilsinger RL (1975) Herpes simplex virus in idiopathic facial paralysis (Bell's palsy). JAMA 233 : 527–530
14. Davis LE (1981) Experimental virus infections of the facial nerve and geniculate ganglion. Ann Neurol 9 : 120–125
15. Hadar T, Tovi F, Sidi J, Sarov B, Sarov I (1983) Specific IgG and IgA antibodies to herpes simplex virus and varicella zoster virus in acute peripheral facial palsy patients. J Med Virol 12 : 237–245
16. Cesario TC, Poland JD, Wulff H, Chin TDY, Wenner HA (1969) Six years experience with herpes simplex virus in children's home. Am J Wpidemiol 90 : 416–422
17. Nahmias AJ, Roizman B (1973) Infection with herpes-simplex viruses 1 and 2. N Engl J Med 289 : 719–725

Eur Arch Otorhinolaryngology (1994) [Suppl]:S487–S488

S. Murakami, T. Sugita, Y. Hirata, N. Yanagihara, and J. Desaki

Histopathology of Facial Nerve Neuritis Caused by Herpes Simplex Virus Infection in Mice

Introduction

Many researchers have attempted to make animal models of facial palsy by inoculating herpes simplex virus (HSV). but without direct injection of HSV into the facial nerve, this has not been successful. In the present study, we succeeded in making an animal model of transient facial nerve palsy by inoculating herpes simplex virus (HSV) into the auricle of mice. The facial nerve histopathology of this animal model was examined.

Materials and Methods

For this study 15 animals were used; 10 animals developed transient facial palsy and 5 animals did not show facial palsy in the course of virus infection. In six out of ten paralyzed animals, bilateral facial nerves were obtained during paralysis and in the other four animals they were obtained after recovery of the paralysis. In five unparalyzed animals the facial nerves were dissected out the 10th day after inoculation. The specimens were examined under the light and electron microscopes. For the light microscope, hematoxylin-eosin staining and toluidine blue staining were used.

Results and Comments

In the paralyzed animals, severe nerve edema was observed in the affected facial nerve compared with the unaf-

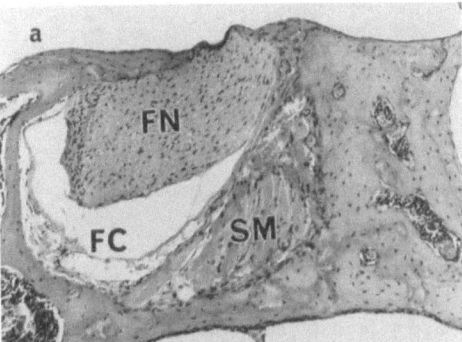

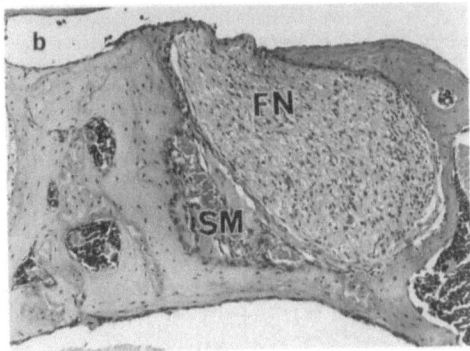

Fig. 1a, b Bilateral facial nerve obtained 2 days after the onset. **a** Unaffected side; **b** affected side; *FN*, facial nerve; *FC*, fallopian canal; *SM*, stapedius nerve

S. Murakami, T. Sugita, Y. Hirata, and N. Yanagihara
Department ot Otolaryngology, Ehime University School
of Medicine, Shigenobu-chou, Onsen-gun, Ehime 791-02 Japan

J. Desaki
Department ot Anatomy, Ehime University School of Medicine,
Shigenobu-chou, Onsen-gun, Ehime 791-02 Japan

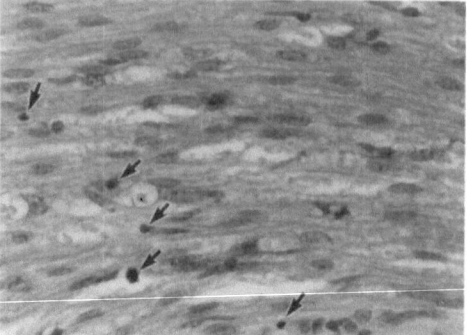

Fig. 2 Infiltration of inflammatory cell (*arrows*)

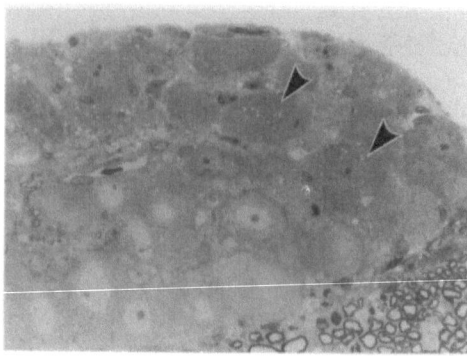

Fig. 4 Vacuolar change in geniculate ganglion (*arrows*)

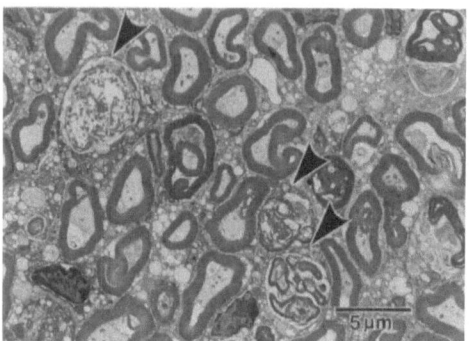

Fig. 3 Degeneration of nerve fibers (*arrows*)

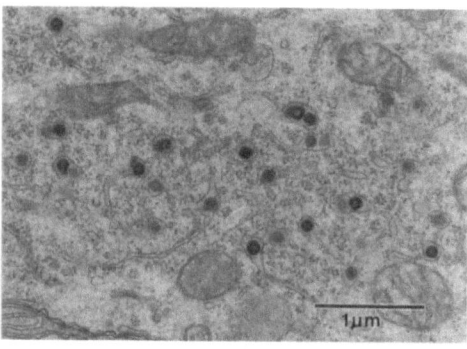

Fig. 5 HSV particles in cytoplasm

fected nerve. In normal facial nerve, there was enough space between the facial nerve and the fallopian canal (Fig. 1a). But no space could be seen in the affected facial nerve (Fig. 1b). This edema disappeared soon after the recovery of facial nerve function. The infiltration of inflammatory cells was seen in the entire length of the affected facial nerve (Fig.2). This change was more prominent in the proximal portion than in the distal portion of the geniculate ganglion. The degeneration of myelin and axon (Fig. 3) were also recognized as being more severe in the proximal part than in the distal part of the geniculate ganglion. In the geniculate ganglion, some of ganglion cells showed vacuolar changes (Fig. 4). Virus particles of HSV were also detected in the geniculate ganglion cells. They were found particularly in the rough endoplasmic reticulum in the cytoplasm. These virus particles were uniform and their size was about 100 nm (Fig. 5).

There have been relatively few reports on the histopathology of Bell's palsy. Some of these reports emphasized edema, inflammatory cell infiltration, nerve degene-

ration, and hemorrhage, suggesting vital neuritis [1–4]. In our animal model, similar changes such as edema, inflammatory cell infiltration, and nerve degeneration were observed. Bell's palsy is an idiopathic facial palsy and viral infection will not be the only etiology. But our study confirmed HSV has enough potential for the pathogenesis of facial palsy and suggested HSV was one of the causes of Bell's palsy.

References

1. Flower EP (1963) The pathogenic findings in a case of facial paralysis. Trans Am Acad Ophthalmol Otolaryngol 67:187–197
2. Proctor B, Corgill DA, Proud G (1976) The pathology of Bell's palsy. Trans Am Acad Ophthalmol Otolaryngol 82:70–80
3. Reddy J, Lui J, Balshi S et al. (1966) Histopathology of Bell's palsy. Eye Ear Nose Throat Monthly 45:62–66
4. Stephen LL, Stephen MK (1989) Histopathology of Bell's palsy. Laryngoscope 99:23–26

Eur Arch Otorhinolaryngology (1994) [Suppl]: S489–S490

J.L. Llorente Pendás, C. Suarez Nieto, M. Oña Gutierrez, A. Martinez, and S. Melon Garcia

Herpes Simplex Virus and Experimental Facial Paralysis

Introduction

Bell's palsy still remains an idioptahic disease. It was the purpose of this study to provoke facial paralysis in rabbits instilled with herpes simplex virus type 1 (HSV-1), to find evidence supporting the etiopathogenic viral theory.

Material and Methods

A total of 48 male white New Zealand rabbits were used. Strain FP-16 of HSV-1 was inoculated into the kidney cels of hamster (BHK-21) with an average dilution of 10^{-4}. Following anesthesia, we proceeded as follows:

- Prior to inoculation and before the death of the animal, oral swabs for viral culture were taken, and peripheral blood for determination of antibodies against the HSV-1 was extracted.
- A quantitiy of 2 ml inoculum was instilled in the mouth or injected into the anterior lateral two-thirds of the tongue or into the perineurum of the facial nerve at its exit at the stylomastoid foramen (Fig. 1). The control rabbits were killed after the injection of a virus transport medium without any handling of the rabbits.

The motor activity of the facial nerve was clinically controlled in the rabbits every 2nd day. Following inoculation a group of rabbits was killed after 1 week, termed the "short technique" (ST), and the other group after 3 weeks, termed the "long technique" (LT). After the death of the

J.L. Llorente Pendás (✉) and C. Suarez Nieto
Department of ENT, Hospital Central de Asturias,
c/Celestino Villamil s/n, 33006 Oviedo, Asturias, Spain

M. Oña Gutierrez, A. Martinez, and S. Melon Garcia
Department of Microbiology, Hospital Central de Asturias,
c/Celestino Villamil s/n, 33006 Oviedo, Asturias, Spain

Material and methods

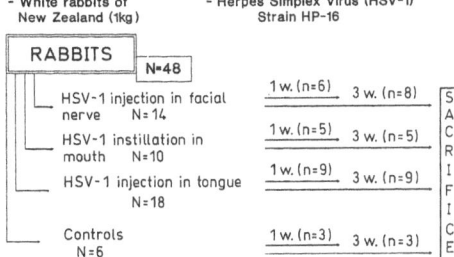

Fig. 1 Distribution of the rabbits

animal, a fragment of the ipsilateral medulla was extracted, and then macerated. Another sample consisted of the macerate of the facial nerve from its exit from the medulla as far as the stylomastoid foramen including the geniculate ganglion (fn/gg). Each sample was submitted to:

1. Block staining by direct immunofluorescence with monoclonal antibodies (Microtrak) against the HSV-1/HSV-2.
2. Culture of the macerates in human fibroblast (MCR-5).
3. Fragmets of the macerates were observed under the electron microscope (EM).
4. The DNA was extracted from a fragment of each sample [4]. Electrophoresis with 10 µl of the dissolved DNA was carried out in a horizontal gel in the Davis type system [4]. Once we had identified the samples containing DNA (although not necessarily viral) this was transferred, in the Manifold apparatus, to nylon membranes for hybridization. The probe used (SNAP by Dupont) was labeled with an alkaline phosphatase enzyme, which linked with the timidine bases. In posi-

tive cases, when precise substrates were added, the enzyme reacted with them, giving a purple coloring after 30 min. The quantity of homologous DNA fixed in the filter was proportional to the intensity of color generated.

5. Detection of human anti-HSV-1 was carried out by means of indirect immunofluorescence on the blood of the animals.

Results

The follow-up of the animals showed no facial paralysis in any of the cases and no animal had vestibular disturbances or secondary neurological effects. The viral cultures in the oral swabs were all negative. The serological study before and after inoculation showed, except in the control rabbits, seroconversion in 100% of the cases. The cultures of the macerates, just as the indirect immunofluorescence in the samples, were found to be negative. The positive results in the EM with the LT and in the sample of 12 fn/gg cases were positive (54.5%), whereas in the ST only 2 cases were positive (10%) ($p<0.001$). With the LT and in the medulla sample, 14 cases were positive (63.6%) and there were no cases with the ST (0%) ($p<0.001$). The samples of fn/gg and those of the medulla were found to be positive in 14 cases (33.3%) and negative in 28 (66.6%) ($p<0.05$). The evaluation of the different administration routes of the inoculum, for the sample of fn/gg, showed no significant differences.

The positive results in hybridization of the 42 rabbits in the sample of the fn/gg were positive with the ST in 6 cases out of 20 (30%) and with the LT none of the 22 cases (0%) ($p<0.05$). In the sample of the medulla, the hybridization with the ST was positive in 12 out of the 20 cases (60%) and with the LT none of the 22 cases (0%) ($p<0.001$). With the ST there existed a greater percentage of positive cases in the hybridizations of the samples from the medulla (12/18) (66.6%) compared with those of the fn/gg (6/17) (35.3%) ($p<0.05$). Taking into account the administration route, the differences in the sample were not significant.

Discussion

In this study, as other authors have found, with the exception of Kumagami [3], we were unable to bring about experimental facial paralysis with similar animal models. The negative cultures suggest that the viral genomes detected by hybridization techniques belong to a virus in the latent phase. We believe that the negativity of the cultures is due to the fact that the rabbits have a very strong immunologi-

cal response against the virus, as shown by 100% seroconversions. This fact would justify the establishment of latency between 48 and 96 h [6].

In EM the LT animals have 65% (26/40) of positive results, whereas those of the ST only have 5% (2/40) ($p<0.01$). The particles found could be virions in a replication state, blocked virions, or remains of viral structures whose DNA has already integrated. Related to the explanation of why there is a very significant difference in the samples comparing ST and LT we can suppose that the virus in its noninfectious form reached the medulla, but due to lack of time did not complete its replication cycle.

With hybridization techniques viral genomes can be detected, although they have lost their morphological appearance and are even found integrated in the genome of the host cell. The majority of the HSV-1 genome is present, between 30% (1) and 50% (5), of the brains of the infected rats in acute and silent forms [5], although the number of viral DNA copies per cell was very low (0.5 to 1 copy per infected cell) [1, 5]. In our series the percentage of positive cases in hybridization with the ST was 30% (6/20) in the sample of fn/gg, and 60% (12/22) in the sample from the medulla and in no case of the LT. There is no doubt that, just as in EM, this percentage could be increased with a larger amount of tissue in the samples. The interpretation of why in the LT we detected no viral genome in any of the cases would correlate with that published by Efstathiou et al. [2], who reported that in the acute or recent infection phase in mice the union segment and the terminal segment of the HSV can be detected, but 1 month after infection the terminal fragment of the viral genome is no longer detected, unless restriction enzymes are used and upon carrying out Southern Blot. Only in this way was a titer of 0.05–0.1 copies/cell found, much smaller than that reported in the medulla of mice killed after 6 days, where between 22 and 178 copies/cell were found [1].

References

1. Cabrera CV, Wohlenberg CH, Openshaw H, Rey-Mendez M, Puga A, Notkins AL (1980) Herpes simplex virus DNA sequences in the CNS of latently infected mice. Nature 288:288–290
2. Efstathiou S, Minson AC, Field HJ, Anderson JR, Wildy P (1986) Detection of herpes simplex virus-specific DNA sequences in latently infected mice and in humans. J Virol 57 (2):446–455
3. Kumagami H (1972) Experimental facial nerve paralysis. Arch Otolaryngol 95:305–312
4. Maniatis T, Fritsch EF, Sambrook (1982) Molecular cloning. A laboratory manual. Cold Spring Harbor Laboratory Manual, Cold Spring Harbor Laboratory
5. Rock DL, Fraser NW (1983) Detection of HSV-1 genome in central nervous system of latently infected mice. Nature 302:523–525
6. Sekizawa T, Openshaw H, Wohlenberg C, Notkins AL (1980) Latency of Herpes Simplex Virus in absence of neutralizing antibody: model for reactivation. Science 210 (28):1026–1028

Eur Arch Otorhinolaryngology (1994) [Suppl]: S491–S492

FREE PAPERS AND POSTERS

H. Inamura, M. Aoyagi, H. Tojima, H. Maeyama, and Y. Koike

Recent Treatment of Ramsay Hunt Syndrome

Introduction

The cure rate for Bell's palsy has improved thanks to recent advances in conservative therapy [1, 2]. For the treatment of Ramsay Hunt syndrome (Hunt's syndrome), antiviral agents and steroids are generally administered, but the prognosis for Hunt's syndrome is less satisfactory than for Bell's palsy. In recent years, high-dose steroid and antiviral agents, such as acyclovir, have been used for the treatment of severe Hunt's syndrome in our clinic. In the present study, the effects of antiviral agents and of high-dose steroid administration in the treatment of Hunt's syndrome are discussed.

Subjects and Method

The subjects were 113 patients with Hunt's syndrome treated conservatively at our clinic since 1983. They consisted of 51 patients treated by the modified Stennert's method with administration of acyclovir (acyclovir combination group), 23 patients treated by modified Stennert's method alone (Stennert's method group), and 39 patients treated by our conventional method (conventional method group). The degree of paralysis was evaluated by a 40-point grading system. All of the patients visited our clinic within the 7th day of onset, and the initial score for facial movement was less than 20 points in all patients. Final recovery was classified as cured in cases where the facial movement score exceeded 36 points without sequelae.

The basic protocol of the modified Stennert's method and acyclovir administration is shown in Table 1. In the acyclovir combination group, acyclovir was administered three times a day every 8 h for 7 days, in addition to the modified Stennert's method. The differences between these three treatment methods are shown in Table 2. The marked differences between these groups were the use or non-use of acyclovir, and the initial and total dosage of prednisolone. The minimum electroneurography (ENoG) values within 2 weeks of onset, which is closely related to the prognosis, were compared among the three groups.

Table 1 Intravenous infusion (Ramsay Hunt syndrome)	Days of treatment	Hydroxyethyl starch (ml/day)		20% Mannitol (ml/day)	Prednisolone (mg/day)	Pentoxifylline (oral) (mg/day)	Acyclovir (mg/day)
	Inpatient						
	1	1000	+	100/16 h	200	300	750
	2	1000	+	100/16 h	200	300	750
	3	1000	+	100/16 h	150	300	750
	4	500	+	50/8 h	150	300	750
	5	500	+	50/8 h	100	300	750
	6	500	+	50/8 h	100	300	750
	7	500	+	50/8 h	75	300	750
	8	500	+	50/8 h	50	300	
	9	500	+	50/8 h	40	300	
	10	500	+	50/8 h	20	300	

H. Inamura (✉), M. Aoyagi, H. Tojima, H. Maeyama, and Y. Koike
Department of Otolaryngology, Yamagata University School
of Medicine, Iida-Nishi, Yamagata, 990-23 Japan

Table 2 Differences between three treatment methods for Ramsay Hunt syndrome

	Acyclovir combination group	Stennert's method group	Conventional method group
Hydroxyethyl starch (low molecular dextran)	1000 ml	1000 ml	1000 ml
Prednisolone (initial dose)	200 mg	200 mg	60 mg
Pentoxifylline	300 mg/day (oral)	300 mg/day (oral)	300 mg/day (oral)
Acyclovir	750 mg/day during 7 days	(−)	(−)

Table 3 Ramsay Hunt syndrome

Treatment	No. of cases	Cured (n)	Cure rate (%)
Stennert's method			
Acyclovir (+)	51	32	62.7
Acyclovir (−)	23	15	65.2
Conventional method	39	14	35.9

* ND; ** $p < 0.01$.

Ramsay Hunt syndrome

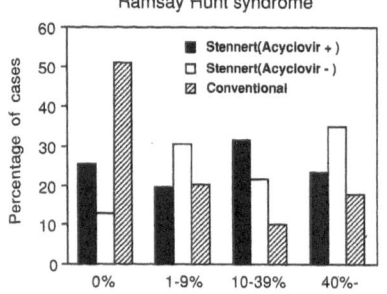

Fig. 1 Distribution of minimum ENoG value in each treatment group. The number of patients with an ENoG of 0% was relatively small in the acyclovir combination group and the Stennert's method group

Results

The cure rate was 62.7% (32/51) in the acyclovir combination group and 64.2% (15/23) with Stennert's method

alone. There was no significant difference between the two groups. On the other hand, the cure rate was 35.9% (14/39) in the conventional method group, showing a significant difference from the other two groups ($p < 0.01$) (Table 3). Therapeutic effects during the same period for Bell's palsy were 97.7% with the modified Stennert's method. Thus, the results of treatment for Hunt's syndrome were less satisfactory than those for treatment of Bell's palsy. Comparing the minimum ENoG level in Hunt's syndrome, while more than half of the cases in the conventional method group showed an ENoG of 0%, or complete denervation was observed, the number of patients with an ENoG of 0% was relatively small in the acyclovir combination group and the Stennert's method group. However, there were no significant differences in ENoG level between the acyclovir-administered or nonadministered groups (Fig. 1).

Discussion

Recently, administration of antiviral agents had been generally practiced in the treatment of Hunt's syndrome, and the usefulness of acyclovir has been reported [3], but the clinical experience is still not sufficient for comparative study. Results obtained in the present study were as follows:

1. The prognosis in Hunt's syndrome was not related to the administration of acyclovir, although the cure rate for Hunt's syndrome improved by the modified Stennert's method, as in Bell's palsy.
2. The reason for the less satisfactory prognosis of Hunt's syndrome, compared with that for Bell's palsy, seemed to be more rapid progression of Wallerian degeneration in spite of the treatment with high-dose steroid.

Acyclovir stimulates healing of auricular herpes and prevents aggravation of viral infection due to steroid administration, so that administration of acyclovir is still desirable in the treatment of Hunt's syndrome. The results of treatment for Hunt's syndrome are still not satisfactory, and further improvement is required.

References

1. Stennert E (1982) New concept in the treatment of Bell's palsy. In: Malcolm D, House G, Heuse WF (eds) Disorders of the facial nerve. Raven, New York, pp 313–318
2. Koike Y, Inamura H et al. (1990) Effects of the administration of the high dose steroids in Bell's palsy – clinical and experimental study. Otorhinolaryngol Head Neck Surg, pp 647–653
3. Dickins JRE, Smith T et al. (1990) Herpes zoster oticus: treatment with intravenous acyclovir. In: Castro D (ed) The facial nerve. Kugler and Ghedini, Amstelveen, pp 113–116

Eur Arch Otorhinolaryngology (1994) [Suppl]:S493–S494

FREE PAPERS AND POSTERS

V. Darrouzet, F. Gharbi, C. de Bonfils, C. Rognon, and J. P. Bebear

Herpes Zoster of the Geniculate Ganglion: Therapeutic Concepts

Introduction

The usual severity of herpes zoster of the genigulate ganglion, or the Ramsay-Hunt syndrome, justifies a certain therapeutic agressiveness. Between 1986 and 1993, we treate 208 acute peripheral facial palsies, 37 of which were Ramsay-Hunt syndromes. Our goal was to carry out a retrospective prognostic analysis according to the time before patient management and the treatments used: acyclovir (ACV) associated with corticotherapy, corticotherapy alone, and decompressive surgery. Only patients with clear clinical syndrome associated with facial palsy and eruption of the concha were analyzed.

Material and Methods

Thirty-seven cases of Ramsay-Hunt syndrome were studied. Twenty patients were seen early before the 3rd week of evolution of their palsy and 17 cases afterwards. This 3-week time period is important since it seems to represent the evolution time of the nerve lesions in the cases of zosterian impairment [6]. All the patients suffered from massive facial palsy: 32 cases of grade V–VI and 5 cases of grade III–IV. In the 20 patients of the first group, 10 patients treated by ACV (ACV+ group) could be distinguished. Seven were given 30 mg/kg ACV for 10 days and three for 7 days. In all cases, the patients were given an adjuvant corticotherapy of 1 mg/kg methylprednisolone and a vasodilator treatment with monitoring of the hepatic and renal functions. Ten patients seen early were not able to benefit from the ACV (ACV- group). The second group included 17 patients seen late and treated with an associa-

tion of corticoids and vasodilators. In the case of unfavorable clinical and electrophysiological evolution at the end of 3 weeks, a decision was made for surgical treatment. This involved decompressing the three portions of the facial nerve with a geniculectomy. Five patients in the ACV-group were concerned and 13 out of the 17 patients seen late.

Results

In addition to the facial palsy, eight patients (22%) suffered from impairment by VZV of the VIIIth cranial pair, in the form of a painful hyperacousia, tinnitus, and deafness with impairment of the high frequencies. This proportion was identical to that found in the literature [9]. In addition, two patients presented impairmetn of the Vth with an endobuccal eruption. Facial prognosis was studied in three subgroups:

- In ACV+ patients, evolution was very favorable in the ten cases with recovery of a normal facial function: seven grade I and three grade II using the House scale.
- In the ACV- group, two patients evolved favorably. Five required a surgical approach (Table 1).
- In the group of 17 patients seen late, 16 evolved unfavorably and 13 were operatedon. The surgical treatment only made it possible to obtain a normal facial function for eight patients (grade I and II). Seven patients had substantial sequelae and six suffered from severe facial palsy (Table 2).

Discussion

When prescribed early, parenterally, in sufficient doses, the high effcetiveness of ACV is confirmed. It transforms the severe prognosis attributed to these facial palsies and related to the size of the lesions of denervation generated by VZV (44% against 14% according to Kansaki [6]). Other

V. Darrouzet, F. Gharbi, C. De Bonfils, C. Rognon, and J.P. Bebear
ENT Department, Pellegrin Hospital, Place Amélie Raba-Léon, 33076 Bordeaux Cedex, France

Table 1 Global prognosis ($N = 37$)

	With ACV $N = 10$ <21 days	Without ACV	
		$N = 10$ <21 days	$N = 17$ >21 days
Favorable	10	2	1
Unfavorable	0	8	16
Surgery	0	5	13

Table 2 Results at 12 months

Grade (House)	ACV+	ACV−	
	$N = 10$ <21 days	$N = 10$ <21 days	$N = 17$ >21 days
I	7	2	2
II	3	4	6
III–IV	0	4	7
V–VI	0	0	2

teams encountered equivalent effectiveness by using the same therapeutic pattern [2] (Table 3). Prescribed at 15 mg/kg per day, ACV seems less effective [4, 8]. The following aspects appear to be decisive factors in the effectiveness of ACV: the earliness of the treatment (all our patients were treated before the 15th day), patients under 70 years of age, and the absence of any cochleovestibular impairment of extension to other territories.

These results somewhat modified our attitude towards facial palsies by VZV, which in the past we tended to ope-

Table 3 Herpes zosters of the geniculate ganglion

ACV	Inamura [4] ($n = 9$) 15 mg/kg 7 days	Dickins [2] ($n = 7$) 30 mg/kg 7 days	Uri [8] ($n = 5$) 15 mg/kg 5–7 days	Bebear [1] ($n = 10$) 30 mg/kg 7–10 days
Results grade I (n)	5	4	1	7
Results grade II (n)	3	1	3	3
Results grade III–IV (n)	1	2	1	0
Results grade V–VI (n)	0	0	0	0

rate on earlier than others, depending on their severity. Currently, if the patient is seen early, before the 3rd week of evolution of the palsy, we give preference to a medical treatment centered on ACV and steroids. If the clinical and electrophysiological evolution proves to be unfavorable (a situation we have yet to encounter), we choose, as for the patients see late, decompressive surgial therapy through the pathway of the middle fossa, the general condition of the patient permitting. If this is not the case and if the hearing is of poor quality, a transmastoidal pathway is then chosen.

Conclusion

This study confirms the high effectiveness of ACV in the Ramsay-Hunt syndrome. Administered early, it stabilizes the lesions of the VIIth nerve, avoids extension towards the VIIIth nerve and other territories and proves to be rapidly effective on otalgia, tinnitus, and vertigo and seems to decrease the frequency of residual pain. The absence of visceral toxicity shown and the progress in serological diagnoses of viral infections make it possible to widen its indications to facial palsies of viral appearance for which it is known that almost 20% are concomitant to asymptomatic herpetic infection [1]. A study is currently ongoing.

References

1. Fleury HJA, Chilotti P, Bonnicci JF, Dupasquier P, Portmann D, Bebear JP, Portmann M (1990) IgM against herpes virus in Bell's palsy. In: Castro D, Facial nerve. Kugler and Ghedini, Amsterdam
2. Dickins JRE, Smith JT, Graham SS (1988) Herpes zoster oticus: treatment with intravenous acyclovir. Laryngoscope 98 : 776–779
3. Fujiwara Y, Yanagihara N, Kurata T (1990) Middle ear – mucosa in Ramsay-Hunt syndrome. Ann Otol Rhinol Laryngol 99 : 359–362
4. Inamura H, Aoyagi M, Tojima H (1988) Effects of acyclovir in Ramsay-Hunt syndrome. Acta Otolaryngol Suppl (Stockh) 446 : 111–113
5. Jackson CG, Johnson GD, Myams VJ, Poe DS (1990) Pathologic findings in the labyrinthine segment of the facial nerve in a case of facial paralysis. Ann Otol Rhinol Laryngol 99 : 327–329
6. Kanzari J (1988) Electrodiagnosis findings in the early stages of Bell's palsy and Ramsay-Hunt syndrome. Acta Otolaryngol Suppl (Stockh) 446 : 42–46
7. Morton P, Thomson AN (1989) Oral acyclovir in the treatment of herpes zoster in general practive. NZ Med J 102 : 93–95
8. Uri N, Greenberg E, Meyer W, Kitzes-Cohen R (1992) Herpes zoster oticus: treatment with acyclovir. Ann Otol Rhinol Laryngol 101 : 161–162
9. Wayman DM, Pham HN, Byl FM, Adour KK (1990) Audiological manifestations of Ramsay-Hunt syndrome. J Laryngol Otol 104 : 104–108

Eur Arch Otorhinolaryngology (1994) [Suppl]: S495–S497

POSTERS

M. L. Navarrete, P. Quesada, V. Gimeno, A. Garcia, and M. Garcia

Acyclovir Versus Steroids in the Treatment of Bell's Palsy

Introduction

Bell's palsy is the most common form of all facial paralyses with a peripheral cause [1]. In spite of this, at present we do not have any specific treatment at our disposal, since the etiopathogenesis of the disease has not been sufficiently proven. Most authors support its immunovirological origin, which implies the reactivation of a latent virus as a leading agent of cross-immunological chain reactions between the facial nerve and the viral antigens [5]. Until now, a number of empirical treatments have been implemented. Findings which demonstrated an inflammatory reaction on a local and systemic level, immunity changes at a peripheral level, and the phenomena of nervous demyelination gave rise to steroidal therapy [6, 7]. Nevertheless, these results have been much disputed. That is why, based on the rising protagonism of the herpes simplex-1 virus in this pathology, serological studies carried out by various authors, the isolation of this virus in specimens of the epineural tissue in a patient with Bell's palsy, and our own experience in this field, we decided to start a treatment with acyclovir for this type of patient beginning in November 1988 [10, 11]. This therapy has not been mentioned in the literature before, except for the treatment of otic zoster [3].

Material and Methods

A total of 151 patients with Bell's palsy were studied. Of these, 100 were studied randomly from a group of 498 cases, gathered between 1983 and 1989, which had been

M. L. Navarrete (✉), P. Quesada, V. Gimeno, A. Garcia,
and M. Garcia
Department of Otorhinolaryngology, Autonomous University
of Barcelona, Spain

treated by steroids. The remaining 51 cases were also selected at random from a group of 121 cases gathered between 1989 and 1990 that had been treated by acyclovir. The steroidal treatment was carried out with prednisone, with an oral dose of 1 mg/kg per day and with decreasing doses every 3 days. The treatment with acyclovir was done with an oral dose of 800 mg/day for 10 days. All the cases had been evaluated previously at the onset of the paralysis, 10 days later, and 1, 3, 6, 9, and 12 months later by otorhinolaryngological and facial exploration. The final clinical assessment was performed at the end of the facial palsy recovery by means of the House and Brackmann scale.

The statistical analysis used to compare the improvement of the patients treated by steroids versus acyclovir was carried out through using the chi-squared test of dependency of improvement on the type of treatment, as well as a differential test of the proportions of patients with or without sequelae for a variable z in both studied groups.

Results

By comparing the progression data at the end of recovery in both groups of patients according to the House and Brackmann scale and by means of a differential test of proportions of the patients who recover without sequelae versus those who recover with more or less important sequelae, we found in the group which received the steroid treatment the same proportion of cases with or without sequelae for $z = 0.7023$ $(0.20 < p < 0.50)$. We reached the same conclusion for the group of patients treated with acyclovir for $z = 0.5630$ $(0.50 < p < 1)$.

In this way, the theory previously sustained according to which most Bell's palsies progressed without any sequelae is refuted.

In addition, we analyzed the likely dependency of the progression of those patients on the kind of treatment received and we observed using the chi-squared test that the progression of patients in independent of the type of treatment received, be it steroids or acyclovir $(0.90 < p < 1)$.

Discussion

The most supported etiopathogenic theory of Bell's palsy, for want of an etiological confirmation, is the immunovirological one. Cross-phenomena of immunological reactions are suspected to exist on the facial nerve as contrasted with viral antigens due to the reactivation of the virus in the geniculate ganglion [5]. Specifically, the herpes simplex virus type 1 is implicated as a leading agent of these phenomena by means of a serological demonstration [11] and pathological nerve studies [10]. These phenomena lead to the degeneration and demyelination of the facial nerve [6, 7]. The presence of immunological chain reactions and zones of demyelination have encouraged the use of steroids as the preferred treatment for Bell's palsy. The results of this therapy have been assessed by various authors with rather different results.

At present, some authors support the steroidal treatment in general [15] and others only when the palsy is extremely serious [18]. Nevertheless, other authors have found no differences [13] even with high doses of steroids used during short periods of time. After reviewing 92 articles on the subject, one author asserted that treatment with steroids would continue to be contraversial since the assessment of results is difficult to carry out in the same way by all. Also in all series, the same control guidelines were not used nor the same doses of steroids. In the same way, the therapy cannot always start early [2].

According to this, the steroidal treatment would treat the effect once the supposed original immunovirological phenomenon began. We deem it important to carry out a special treatment on the source of the disease. In this way we could compare our experience with steroidal therapy versus antiviral drugs, since we cannot compare the steroidal treatment with previous empirical treatments for lack of any file prior to 1983.

At present, acyclovir is the most useful antiviral treatment. It possesses a high therapeutic rate and has few side effects, though it does not eliminate latent viruses. This drug has been used in the treatment of herpes zoster by intravenous administration, which is why most of the bibliographic references deal with this subject. The results are considered good in the otic zone [3] with acyclovir applied by intravenous administration. The same is true for the references on the treatment of lesions produced by the herpes zoster treated orally with acyclovir [9]. Differences are not observed between oral and intravenous administrations in lesions by herpes zoster virus [12].

In relation to the treatment of Bell's palsy with acyclovir, there are few references and intravenous administration is always used. Moreover, results are good [4, 14].

We started using acyclovir orally due to the over crowding of health care services we suffer and the lack of criteria of maximal seriousness for these patients during their first visit. We thought that intravenous therapy was an excessive approach, basing our view on the demonstration of the equal efficiency the two types of administration.

We thought that treatment with acyclovir would inhibit the progression of the lesion produced by the herpes simplex virus on the facial nerve. However, in accordance with our criteria, we did not find any significant statistical difference in relation to the cases which had been treated with steroids.

Thus the progress of these patients dues not seem to be affected by whether steroids or acyclovir is used. The only significant factor which seems to influence the progression of Bell's palsy is the initial degree of seriousness of the nervous lesion, the exact nature of which remains unknown.

In the light of our results, we conclude that most patients do not recover without any sequelae, but that there are similar percentage of recovery with or without sequelae. What really, influences recovery is the degree of seriousness.

The lack of improvement in clinical results by using acyclovir can be explained by the same reasoning: no matter how early we start a treatment, we always treat the effects of the disease, but not its causes. What will happen in the future? Maybe an answer to this question has to do with the feasibility of a vaccine for the herpes simplex virus type 1.

References

1. Adour KK, Bell DN, Hilsinger RL (1975) Herpes simplex virus in idiopathic facial paralysis (Bell's palsy). Jama 233:527–530
2. Al Husain A, Jamal GA, Hilmi AM (1986) Steroids therapy in Bell's palsy. Int J Clin Pharmacol Ther Toxicol 24/8:430–432
3. Dickins JR, Smith JT, Graham SS (1988) Herpes zoster oticus: treatment with intravenous acyclovir. Laryngoscope 98/7:776–779
4. Hase K, Shiraishi M, Hasumi K, Kamiyama Y, Sugita R (1986) The effect of acyclovir on fresh Bell's palsy. Facial N Res Jpn 6:31–34
5. Hughes GB, Barna BP, Kinney SE, Goren H, Sweeney PJ, Valenzuela R, Calabrese LH, Tucker HM (1986) Immune reactivity in Bell's palsy. Otolaryngol Head Neck Ther 95:586–588
6. Liston SL, Kleid MS (1989) Histopathology of Bell's palsy. Laryngoscope 99:23–26
7. Matsumoto Y, Petterson MJ, Pulec JL, Yanagihara N (1988) Facial nerve biopsy for etiologic clarification of Bell's palsy. Ann Otol Rhinol Laryngol 97 [Suppl 13]:22–27
8. May M, Klein SR, Taylor PH (1985) Idiopathic (Bell's) facial palsy: natural history defies steroid or surgical treatment. Laryngoscope 95:406–409
9. Mckendrick MW, McGill J, White JE, Wood MJ (1986) Oral acyclovir in acute herpes zoster. BMJ 293:1529–1532
10. Mulkens PS (1980) Acute facial paralysis: a virological study. Clin Otolaryngol Engl 5:303–310

11. Nakamura K, Yanagihara N (1988) Neutralization antibody to herpes simplex virus type I in Bell's palsy. Ann Otol Rhinol Laryngol 97 [Suppl 137]:18–21

12. Peterslund NA. Esmann V, Ipsen J, Christensen KD, Petersen CM (1984) Oral and intravenous acyclovir are equally effective in herpes zoster. Antimicrob Chemother 14:185–189

13. Prescott CAJ (1988) Idiopathic facial nerve palsy (the effect of treatment with steroids). Laryngol Otol 102:403–407

14. Shiraishi M, Hase R, Kamiyama Y (1987) The effect of acyclovir on Bell's palsy. Facial N Res Jpn 7:199–202

15. Stankiewicz JA (1983) Steroids and idiopathic facial paralysis. Otolaryngol Head Neck Surg 991:672–677

Eur Arch Otorhinolaryngology (1994) [Suppl]: S 498 – S 500

L. J. Schot, P. P. Devriese, R. J. Hadderingh, P. Portegies, and R. H. Enting

Facial Palsy and Human Immunodeficiency Virus Infection

Introduction

Infection with the human immunodeficiency virus (HIV) can cause a wide range of complaints in the field of ear, nose, and throat medicine [7].

A facial paralysis may be the first sign of infection with the virus, or it may occur in the course of the illness. More than 70% of patients who are HIV positive develop neurological complications [6]; in 14% – 27% of cases, these take the form of a peripheral neuropathy [6, 8, 12]. In only 1% – 4% of cases is a cranial nerve alone affected [12, 8].

In Western Europe and North America, only a handful of cases of peripheral facial paralysis in conjunction with HIV infection have been described [3, 4, 8, 9, 11 – 14]. Series of 12 – 16 patients in Central Africa have been described. In more than 90% of these cases, peripheral facial paralysis was the first sign of HIV infection [1, 2].

Between 1986 and April, 1992, 17 patients with a unilateral peripheral facial paralysis in combination with HIV-positive serology were seen at the Academic Medical Center in Amsterdam.

Patients

The 17 patients were all men, with an average age of 35 years (range 24 – 42 years). All of them were seropositive with HIV when the peripheral unilateral facial paralysis occurred. In three of these patients, this paralysis was the first visible sign of HIV infection. In patient 1, the paralysis was caused by an infection with *Aspergillus niger* after

L. J. Schot (✉), P. P. Devriese, R. J. Hadderingh, P. Portegies, and R. H. Enting
Departments of Otorhinolaryngology, Facial Research and Neurology, Academic Medical Centre, Meibergdreef 9, 1105 AZ Amsterdam, The Netherlands

a radical ear operation; patient 2 had had a molar filled in the week before the onset of the paralysis. In patient 3, the clinical picture and the results of tests on the cerebrospinal fluid (CSF) were consistent with an infection with *Treponema pallidum*. Patients 4 – 17 showed the clinical picture of Bell's palsy. Ear, nose, and throat examination revealed no indications of any other causes of the facial paralysis, such as otitis media, varicella zoster, cranial trauma, or tumor of the glandula parotis. In five cases, tests on the CSF indicated aseptic meningitis, in one case they suggested Lues II, and in one case no abnormalities at all. The loss of facial function became total in five of the patients.

Nerve excitability was measured during the paralysis in 12 patients. In all these cases, the nerve retained excitability on both sides. For patient 1, treatment consisted of revision of the radical mastoid cavity with removal of the affected part of the facial nerve and intravenous administration of amfotericine B at a dose of 0.5 mg per kg of body weight for 4 weeks. Patient 3 was given penicillin-G intravenously at a dose of 24 000 000 U per day for 14 days.

Prednisone was prescribed in four cases, at a dose of 60 mg for 4 days, followed by 11 days in which the dose was reduced daily by 5 mg. For three patients there was insufficient follow-up. In patient 1, the total loss of facial function remained, as was to be expected. The other 13 patients showed complete or virtually complete recovery (with slight synkinesis). Table 1 summarizes details of patients and recovery.

Discussion

Age and sex in our group is consistent with the general prevalence of acquired immunodeficiency syndrome (AIDS) in the Netherlands [10]. Patients with HIV infection have an increased chance of developing a (peripheral) facial paralysis, both through their increased chance of neurological complications in general and through their increased

Table 1 Patients and findings

Patient no.	Age	CDC classification	CSF	Paresis-paralysis	Nerve excitability	Prednisone	Follow-up (weeks)	Recovery (Bordeaux classification)
1	42	IV-D	–	Paralysis	–	–	> 52	IV
2	41	II	–	Paralysis	Normal	–	> 52	II
3	29	II	Lues	Paresis	–	–	17	I
4	39	IV-A	–	Paralysis	–	–	13	II
5	33	II	–	Paralysis	Normal	–	4	I
6	39	?	–	Paresis	–	–	2/7	?
7	38	II	Aseptic meningitis	Paralysis	Normal	+	> 52	II
8	32	II	–	Paresis	Normal	–	> 52	I
9	35	III	–	Paralysis	Normal	+	40	II
10	26	IV-C-2	Normal	Paralysis	Normal	–	2	?
11	39	III	–	Paresis	Normal	–	> 52	II
12	41	II	–	Paresis	Normal	+	> 52	I
13	27	II	Aseptic meningitis	Paresis	Normal	–	2	?
14	34	II	Aseptic meningitis	Paresis	Normal	–	> 52	I
15	24	III	Aseptic meningitis	Paresis	Normal	–	> 52	I
16	27	II	Aseptic meningitis	Paresis	–	–	7	I
17	36	IV-C-2	–	Paresis	Normal	–	5	I

CSF, cerebrospinal fluid; CDC, centers for disease control and prevention

chance of contracting infections which may cause facial paralysis, such as herpes zoster. In our series, there were two cases where an infection was involved; patient 1 had an infected radical cavity, and patient 3 had Lues. It is possible that the facial paralysis in patient 2 was brought on by the stress of the dental tratment. In the literature, only two series have been described, both in Central Africa [1, 2], of peripheral facial paralysis with an HIV-positive serology which are comparable in scope to ours, whereas in Western Europe and the USA only isolated cases have been described [3, 4, 8, 9, 11 – 14]. No satisfactory explanation can be given for this, but it seems unlikely that there is a higher incidence of peripheral facial paralysis in the Netherlands than elsewhere.

As has been described elsewhere in the literature, we saw cases in our group of patients where the facial paralysis was the first sign of HIV infection [2, 3, 4, 14]. This means that it is important, in cases of facial paralysis, to consider HIV infection as part of the differential diagnosis. Also in accordance with what had been described in the literature, our group of patients were mostly still in the asymptomatic stage or with only enlarged lymph nodes (CDC classification II and III) [1, 2, 11]. It was also in accordance with the literature that the test on the CSF gave mainly an indication of aseptic meningitis [8, 11, 12]. These abnormal results are found in about 50% of HIV-positive patients with no neurological loss of function, so the value of this finding is not yet clear [6].

In HIV-positive patients with a facial paralysis, examination of the CSF is advisable in order to exclude neurolues or opportunistic infections (such as meningitis tuberculosa, cryptococcal meningitis).

The course of the paralysis in our group was no different from that in patients with Bell's palsy [5].

Remarkably enough, the nerve excitability remained normal; this is in contrast to reports in the literature, which show nerve degeneration in a high percentage of cases with a peripheral europathy resulting from HIV infection [9].

Conclusion

It appears advisable with any patient with a peripheral facial paralysis to consider whether the patient is in a high-risk group for HIV infection.

Where there is facial paralysis and an HIV-positive serology, it is advisable to perform a lumbar puncture to exclude the possibility of neurolues or opportunistic infection. It is especially important with this group of patients to bear in mind the possibility of secondary infections if treatment with prednisone is one of the options.

References

1. Belec L, Georges AJ, Bouree P, Schuller E, Vuillecard E, Di Costanzo B, Martin PMV (1991) Peripheral facial nerve palsy related to HIV infection: relationship with the immunological status and the HIV staging in Central Africa, Centr Afr J Med 37/3 : 88 – 93
2. Belec L, Georges AJ, Vuillecard E, Galin M, Martin PMV (1988) Peripheral facial paralysis indicating HIV infection. Lancet ii : 1421 – 1422
3. Brown MM, Thompson A, Goh BT, Forster GE, Swash M (1988) Bell's palsy and HIV infection. J Neurol Neurosurg Psychiatry 51 : 425 – 426
4. Chilla R, Booken G, Rasche H (1987) Bellsche Parese als Erstsymptom einer HIV-Infektion. Laryngol Rhinol Otol 66 : 629 – 630

5. Devriese PP, Schumacher T, Scheide A, Jongh de RH, Hout-kooper JM (1990) Incidence, prognosis and recovery of Bell's palsy. A survey of about 1000 patients (1974–1983) Clin Otolaryngol 15:15–27
6. Gans J de, Portegies P (1989) Neurological complications of infection with human immunodeficiency virus type 1. Clin Neurol Neurosurg 91:199–219
7. Hadderingh RJ, Tange RA, Danner SA, Eeftinck Schattenkerk JKM (1987) Otorhinolaryngological findings in AIDS patients; a study of 63 cases. Arch Otorhinolaryngol 244:11–14
8. Levy RM, Bredesen DE, Rosenblum ML (1985) Neurological manifestations of the acquired immunodeficiency syndrome: experience at USCF and review of the literature. J Neurosurg 62:475–495
9. Miller RG, Parry GJ, Pfaeffl W, Lang W, Lippert R, Kiprov D (1988) The spectrum of peripheral neuropathy associated with ARC and AIDS. Muscle Nerve 11:857–863
10. Postema CA, Bilert-Mooiman MAJ (1990) AIDS (1982–1989) Ned. Tijdschr Geneeskd 134/44:2148–2150
11. Schielke E, Pfister HW, Einhaupl KM (1989) Peripheral facial nerve palsy associated with HIV infection. Lancet i:553–554
12. Snider WD, Simpson DM, Nielsen S, Gold JWM, Metroka CE, Posner JB (1983) Neurological complicatins of acquired immune deficiency syndrome: analysis of 50 patients. Ann Neurol 14/4:403–418
13. Uldry PA, Regli F (1988) Multinévrite des nerfs craniens et syndrome d'immunodéficience acquise: 5 cas. Rev Neurol 144/10:586–589
14. Wechsler AF, Ho DD (1989) Bilateral Bell's palsy at the time of HIV seroconversion. Neurology 39:747–748

Eur Arch Otorhinolaryngology (1994) [Suppl]:S 501

A. Ramos, A. del Cañizo, I. de Miguel, A.M. Martin, and F.J. Molina

Antibody Response Against the Epstein-Barr Virus in Acute Idiopathic Facial Palsy

The purpose of this study was to determine the correlation between the specific antibody titers against Epstein-Barr virus and the acute phase of idiopathic facial palsy. Specific antibody responses against Epstein-Barr virus, viral capside antigen (VCA), and early antigen (EA) were evulated in 65 patients with facial palsy and 65 healthy adults studied in our Department over an 18-months period. An enzyme-linked immunosorbent assay (ELISA) was used for detection of immunoglobulin G and M (IgG, IgM) antibodies to VCA. We also used an indirect immunofluorescence test for detection of EA antibodies. All the patients were evulated in order to define the neurological and clinical findings. The two groups (patients/healthy) differed with respect to the serological findings. The anti-VCA and anti-EA titers were higher in patients with facial palsy than those of healthy adults ($p < 0.01$). Of patientswith facial palsy, 23.97% showed positive serological findings against Epstein-Barr virus antigens, suggesting that serology against Epstein-Barr virus antigens represents a useful marker relative to the etiology of facial palsy.

A. Ramos (✉), A. del Gañizo, I. de Miquel, A.M. Martin, and F.J. Molina
Hospital Insular G.C.; Clinical Hospital of Salamanca, Las Palmas, Spain

Eur Arch Otorhinolaryngology (1994) [Suppl]:S 502

R.C. Deka

Lower Brainstem Changes in Herpes Oticus with Facial Palsy

Fifteen patientswith facial palsy (five herpes zoster and ten idiopathic) were subjected to auditory brainstem evoked response (ABR) to evaluate the possible brainstem changes in terms of interpeak latency for wave I–III and wave III–V in response to a 60- or 80-dB SL stimulus within the 1st week of the onset. The idiopathic group consisted of ten patients (mean age, 31.8 years) and the herpes zoster group consisted of five patients (mean age, 32.2 years). The right side was affected more (seven idiopathic and four herpes). The herpes group only exhibited hearing loss as a symptom in two patients on audiometry including another patient; three showed mild to moderate loss (40–55 dB). Two patients who showed no hearing loss and two others with 50–55 dB loss (i.e., four patients) showed prolongation of wave I–III IPL only when compared to normative values, i.e., more than normative mean plus 2 SD, suggesting involvement of the 8th nerve and lower brainstem. On the other hand, Bell's palsy (idiopathic) patients showed normal values (I–III = 1.99 ms; III–V = 1.82 ms). Hence herpes zoster not only affects the facial nerve and cochlea, it also affects the brainstem especially the nerve and the pons.

R.C. Deka
Department of ENT, All India Institute of Medical Sciences,
New Delhi, 110029, India

Eur Arch Otorhinolaryngology (1994) [Suppl]: S 503

ABSTRACTS

T. Sugita, S. Murakami, Y. Hirata, Y. Fujiwara, and N. Yanagihara

Facial Nerve Paralysis Induced by Herpes Simplex Virus Infection in Mice

Herpes simplex virus (HSV) is the most probable cause of Bell's palsy. We succeded in producing a transient facial paralysis in the mouse due to herpes simplex viral neuritis simulating Bell's palsy. Type 1 HSV (strain KOS, 4.5×10^6 pfu/ml) was inoculated in the posterior aspect of the auricle. Fifty-six out of 104 mice (56.7%) developed facial paralysis on the inoculated side from 6 to 9 days after the inoculation. The facial paralysis continued for between and 7 days and healed spontaneously. In 36.8% of the animals with facial paralysis, HSV antigens were identified in the facial nerves of the involved side using immunohisto-chemical methods. No HSV antigen was proved in the facial nerve of the contralateral side and bilateral facial nerves of the animals without facial paralysis.

T. Sugita, S. Murakami, Y. Hirata, Y. Fujiwara, and N. Yanagihara
Department of Otolaryngology, Ehime University, Ehime, Japan

Eur Arch Otorhinolaryngology (1994) [Suppl]: S 504

M.R. Ghonim, A. El-Mongy, M.M. Moktar, S. Attia, and A. Tawfik

Ramsay Hunt Syndrome: Natural History

Thirty-nine patients with Ramsay Hunt syndrome (RHS) were seen over a 6-year period. There was a nonsignificant male preponderance and a nonsignificant peak between the ages of 40 and 60 years. There was a satisfactory recovery in 56.4% with a mean duration of 10.5 weeks, and 43.6% had an unsatisfactory recovery with various degrees of sequelae with a mean duration of 53.6 weeks. There was a strong correlation between severity of paralysis in the first 2 weeks and final facial recovery function ($p < 0.001$).

There was a remarkable tendency towards a satisfactory recovery within a few weeks of onset when the paralysis was incomplete or slowly progressed to a complete form during the first 2 weeks of onset. The chance of satisfactory recovery was very poor and the duration of recovery was longer when the paralysis was complete from onset. The correlation between other clinical findings and several tests in current use and the final facial function was studied.

M.R. Ghonim, A. El-Mongy, M.M. Moktar, S. Attia, and A. Tawfik
ORL, Neurology & Dermatology Departments, Faculty of Medicine, Mansoura University Mansoura, Egypt

Eur Arch Otorhinolaryngology (1994) [Suppl]:S 505

ABSTRACTS

N. Yanagihara, Y. Matsumoto, and T. Sugita

Evidence Suggesting the Viral Etiology of Bell's Palsy

Reactivation of the herpes simplex virus (HSV) type 1 virus has been regarded as a possible cause of Bell's palsy for the last 2 decades without verification. This paper presents the following three findings suggesting the viral etiology of Bell's palsy which were obtained in the recent research bone at the Dept. of Otolaryngology, Ehime University School of Medicine.

1. Experimental facial paralysis induced by viral neuritis: We succeeded in producing a transient facial paralysis in the mouse by inoculating herpes simplex type 1 virus into the auricle. The inflammatory changes took place in and around the geniculate ganglion, where the antigen of the HSV type 1 was proved to occur.
2. Lesion delineated by gadolinium-enhanced MRI: In the acute stage of Bell's palsy and Ramsay Hunt's syndrome the lesion was often clearly enhanced by gadolinium in MRI. In either disease marked enhancement was seen in the geniculate ganglion and its vicinity.
3. Surgical findings of the geniculate ganglion: Swelling and vascular congestion in the geniculate ganglion were a constant feature in severe Bell's palsy with preceding profound denervation. The findings resembled those of Hunt's syndrome.

The above findings are compatible with the reported histo-pathologic findings in the temporal bone obtained in the acute phase of Bell's palsy. Based on this evidence and the results of our clinical studies, the etiology and pathophysiologic aspects of Bell's palsy are discussed.

N. Yanagihara, Y. Matsumoto, and T. Sugita
Department of Otolaryngology, Ehime University School
of Medicine, Ehime, Japan

Bell's Palsy and Others

Eur Arch Otorhinolaryngology (1994) [Suppl]: S 509 – S 511

FREE PAPERS AND POSTERS

H. Tojima, M. Aoyagi, H. Inamura, H. Maeyama, H. Kohshu, Y. Tada, and Y. Koike

Management of Bell's Palsy Accompanied by Diabetes Mellitus

As is well known, it is not uncommon that Bell's palsy is accompanied by diabetes mellitus. On the other hand, it is obvious that administration of steroids is effective for treating patients with Bell's palsy. However, steroids should be given with much caution, because they cause the adverse effect of hyperglycemia. This report has two purposes. One is to clarify the methods for diagnosing diabetes mellitus in patients with Bell's palsy and for assessing diabetic control. The second is to describe a high-dose steroid therapy for diabetes in cases of Bell's palsy accompanied by diabetes.

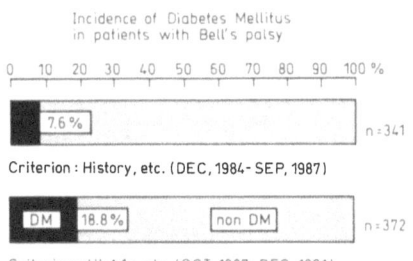

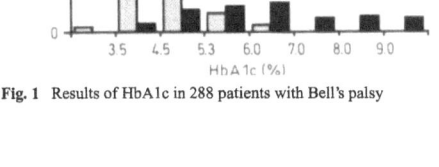

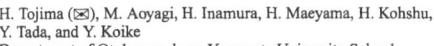

Fig. 2 Incidence of diabetes in patients with Bell's palsy, before, and after the introduction of HbA1c

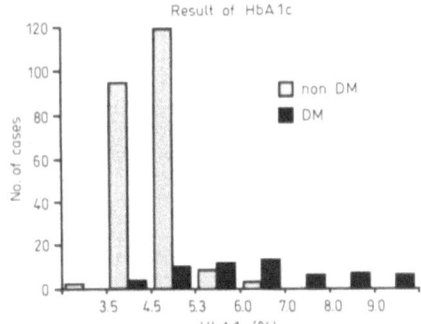

Fig. 1 Results of HbA1c in 288 patients with Bell's palsy

H. Tojima (✉), M. Aoyagi, H. Inamura, H. Maeyama, H. Kohshu, Y. Tada, and Y. Koike
Department of Otolaryngology, Yamagata University School of Medicine, Yamagata, Japan

Diagnosis of Diabetes and of Its Control

There are several methods of detecting diabetes mellitus. An important point in our screening test is the use of hemoglobin A1c (HbA1c). HbA1c is a product of hemoglobin and glucose through an irreversible nonenzymatic reaction. The value of HbA1c not only reveals how diabetes was controlled 1 or 2 months before the blood sample was taken, but is also useful for the screening of diabetes mellitus with a single blood test.

Figure 1 shows the results of HbA1c that were made to detect diabetes in 288 patients with Bell's palsy. It can be found that diabetics gave higher values of HbA1c than those without diabetics. Figure 2 shows the incidence of diabetes in patients with Bell's palsy, before and after the introduction of the HbA1c test. It is obious that the detection rate of diabetes has been recently increased to 18.8% after the introduction of the screening test of HbA1c. Figure 3 shows the results of the HbA1c levels in only diabetic patients with Bell's palsy. HbA1c is higher in fresh cases of diabetes. It is suggested that Hb1c is the useful test for detecting fresh diabetes. We have judged diabetic control

Diabetic Control in Diabetes-Accompanied Bell's Palsy

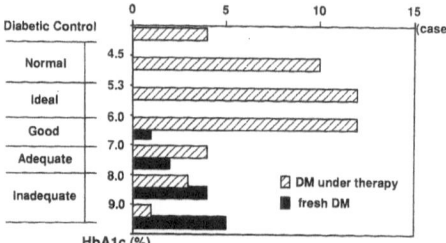

Fig. 3 HbA1c levels in only diabetic patients with Bell's palsy

using the levels of HbA1c of under 6%, ranging from 6% to 7%, from 7% to 8%, and over 8%, to be ideal, good, adequate, and inadequate control, respectively. The results emphasized that many diabetic patients under therapy showed ideal or good diabetic control. This indicated that Bell's palsy was not caused by worsening control of diabetes.

Effect of High-Dose Steroid Therapy

Table 1 is the protocol of the high-dose steroid therapy. This is our routine therapy for our patients with Bell's palsy. Prednisolone was given as described by Stennert, and hydroxyethyl starch was used in order to reduce blood viscosity and to improve microcirculation. In patients with diabetes, short-acting insulin was injected subcutaneously, using our sliding scale. Table 2 shows the responses of diabetes accompanied by Bell's palsy to therapies. In the case of complete palsy, the cure rate was 97.4% for the high-dose steroid therapy group and 58.3% for the no steroid group. Cure rate differed significantly between the two

Table 2 Responses of diabetes-accompanied Bell's palsy to therapie

	No. of cases	Cure cases	Cure rate (%)
Complete palsy			
High-dose steroid	36	35	97.4 ⎤ p < 0.01
No steroid	24	14	58.3 ⎦
Incomplete palsy			
No steroid	36	36	100

Table 3 Effects of high-dose steroid therapy

	No. of cases	Cure cases	Cure rate (%)
Bell's palsy			
With DM	36	35	97.5 ⎤*
Non DM	178	174	97.7 ⎦* ⎤
Hunt's syndrome	74	47	63.5 ⎦

*$p < 0.01$.

groups. Incomplete facial palsy could be completely cured without any drug administration. Table 3 shows the results of high-dose steroid therapy for complete facial palsy. The patients with Bell's palsy could be treated with high cure rates, whether diabetes was concomitant or not. On the other hand, the cure rate for Hunt's syndrome was significantly low, 63.5%. When response and effect of this therapy is considered, the pathophysiology of the facial palsy accompanied by diabetes was different from that of Hunt's syndrome.

Conclusions

1. HbA1c was useful for diagnosing diabetes mellitus and finding out how it was controlled.
2. Many patients with Bell's palsy accompanied by diabetes kept their diabetes under ideal or good control.

Table 1 High-dose steroid therapy

Days of treatment	Intravenous infusion		20% Mannitol (ml/day)	Prednisolone (oral) (mg/day)	Pentoxifylline (mg/day)
	Hydroxyethyl starch (ml/day)				
Inpatient					
1	1000	+	100/16 h	200	300
2	1000	+	100/16 h	200	300
3	1000	+	100/16 h	150	300
4	500	+	50/8 h	150	300
5	500	+	50/8 h	100	300
6	500	+	50/8 h	100	300
7	500	+	50/8 h	75	300
8	500	+	50/8 h	50	300
9	500	+	50/8 h	40	300
10	500	+	50/8 h	20	300

3. High-dose steroid therapy was highly effective in treating Bell's palsy accompanied by diabetes.

References

1. Koike Y (1990) Effect of early administration of high-dose steroids on Bell's palsy. The facial nerve. Kugler, Amstelveen, pp 395–400
2. Stennert E (1982) new concepts in the treatment of Bell's palsy. Disorders of the facial nerve. Raven, New York, pp 313–317

Eur Arch Otorhinolaryngology (1994) [Suppl]: S 512 – S 513

FREE PAPERS AND POSTERS

M. Mañós-Pujol, J. Nogues, A. Ros, J. Montero, J.M. Martinez-Matos, and M. Dicenta

Long-Term Results of Severe Facial Paralysis

Introduction

When axonal degeneration is present, prognosis of facial paralysis is bad. This finding may be obtained by electroneurography. Axonotmesis [1] is considered when the amplitude reduction of the evoked motor potential is bigger than 70% compared to the uninvolved side. As we are performing in our Department a prospective study to establish the influence of therapeutic attitude in the clinical evolution of Bell's palsy, the aim of the present study is to evalute the long-term functional status of patients who presented severe axonal degeneration.

Material and Methods

A series of 517 patients with peripheral facial paralysis of different etiologies treated at our hospital between 1984 and 1989 were studied retrospectively. In 63 of them (12.2%), the electroneuronographic study (ENoG) suggested axonotmesis and a severe initial clinical affectation. Of these 63 patients, 18 were lost, 10 died, 8 had operations on the facial nerve, and 2 received biofeedback rehabilitation. Therefore, only 25 patients, ranging in age from 12 to 73 years, underwent a prospective clinical evaluation. The etiologies of these 25 cases were: 11 Bell's palsy, 6 recurrent Bell's palsy, 2 Ramsay-Hunt syndrome, 2 delayed posttraumatic peripheral facial paralysis, 2 facial paralysis

post-acoustic-neuroma surgery, and 1 malignant otitis externa.

Clinical evaluation was performed according to the House grading system [2]. Electroneuronograhic studies were performed with a Medelec MS92 computer. Axonotmesis was considered when the average amplitude response was less than 30% of the results obtained from the contralateral side [3].

The data evaluated from all the cases were: (1) age at facial paralysis onset, (2) initial clinical examination according to the House grading [2] system (House 1), (3) EnoG results, (4) etiology of facial paralysis, (5) discharge from clinical examination [2], (6) 1992 clinical examination [2] (House 2), and (7) time period (months) between onset and 1992 evaluation.

Results

A clinical improvement was observed in all patients. Table 1 summarizes the results from Bell's palsy patients. The younger patients presented a near complete recovery of facial nerve function, while the older patients presented

M. Mañós-Pujol, J. Nogues, A. Ros, and M. Dicenta
Department of Otorhinolaryngology, Hospital P. Espanya,
C.S. Bellvitge, University of Barcelona, Spain

J. Montero and J.M. Martinez-Matos
Department of Otorhinolaryngology, Hospital P. Espanya,
C.S. Bellvitge, University of Barcelona, Spain

Table 1 Bell's Pallsy findings

N	Age	EnoG	House 1	House 2	Time (months)
1	69	25%	III	II	30
2	13	21%	IV	I	30
3	72	17%	VI	III	25
4	29	27%	VI	I	80
5	17	14%	VI	I	47
6	25	13%	VI	I	67
7	45	25%	VI	II	81
8	12	17%	V	II	82
9	73	15%	VI	IV	68
10	24	8%	VI	I	71
11	60	10%	VI	IV	96

Table 2 Recurrent Bell's palsy findings

N	Age	EnoG	House 1	House 2	Time (months)
1	11	8%	VI	II	73
2	27	24%	VI	III	92
3	18	6%	VI	II	58
4	48	25%	IV	II	86
5	29	16%	VI	III	72
6	66	22%	VI	III	46

Table 3 Ramsay-Hunt syndrome findings

N	Age	EnoG	House 1	House 2	Time (months)
1	54	20%	VI	III	33
2	68	10%	VI	III	59

Table 4 Postacoustic neuroma surgery facial paralysis findings

N	Age	EnoG	House 1	House 2	Time (months)
1	57	60%	VI	III	83
2	60	17%	VI	II	71

Table 5 Delayed Posttraumatic facial paralysis findings

N	Age	EnoG	House 1	House 2	Time (months)
1	48	10%	VI	V	25
2	18	20%	VI	I	67
3	18	11%	VI	III	75

Table 6 Otitis externa maligna facial paralysis findings

N	Age	EnoG	House 1	House 2	Time (months)
1	57	29%	VI	III	46

some residual sequelae. Table 2 shows the findings from the recurrent Bell's palsy group. In all cases a clinical improvement was observed but persistence of some sequelae was also noted. These findings were similar to those observed in Ramsay-Hunt syndrome cases (Table 3), postacoustic neuroma surgery patients (Table 4), delayed posttraumatic paralysis cases (Table 5), and otitis externa maligna patients (Table 6).

Discussion

An improvement of the facial nerve function was observed in all patients. However, there was an evident relationship between the degree of improvement and the age of the patient as reported elswhere [4]. The group of Bell's palsy patients also presented better results than the other groups. The long-term results of these groups of patients are important because they enable us to:

- Achieve better control of the patients.
- Make an accurate prognosis.
- Obtain better knowledge of the success of the treatments performed.
- Compare these results with other treatment and rehabilitation techniques and also with groups of patients, with no treatment.

References

1. Kimura J (1989) Stimulation of the facial nerve. In: Kimura J (ed) Electrodiagnosis in diseases of nerve and muscle. Davis, Philadelphia, pp 309–310
2. House JW (1983) Facial nerve grading system. Laryngoscope 93 : 1056–1069
3. Brown FW (1984) Electromyography and the cranial nerves. In: Brown FW (ed) The physiological and technical basis of electromyography. Butterworths, Boston, pp 429–458
4. Peitersen E (1982) Natural history of Bell's palsy. In: Graham MD, House WF (eds) Disorders of the facial nerve. Raven, New York, pp 307–312

Eur Arch Otorhinolaryngology (1994) [Suppl]: S514–S516

M. Aoyagi, O. Saito, H. Tojima, H. Maeyama, and Y. Koike

Distribution of Facial Nerve Conduction Velocities in Patients with Bell's Palsy

Introduction

The etiology of Bell's palsy remains unclear. Generally speaking, the thicker the myelinated nerve fibers, the faster the conduction velocity. Thick fibers with fast conduction velocity are considered susceptible to damage due to compression. Compression of the nerve in the fallopian canal may possible be the cause of Bell's palsy. To determine the distribution of facial nerve diameter in normal subjects, and to investigate the electrophysiological pathology of Bell's palsy, we developed a method for determining the distribution of nerve conduction velocities (DNCV) in facial nerve using the collision method of Hopf [1].

Method

Subjects

Distribution of nerve conduction velocities was measured by the collision method in 14 normal adults (19 sides) and 14 patients with Bell's palsy (14 sides), within 7–14 days following the onset of palsy.

Collision Method

Figure 1 shows the principle of the collision method. When electrical stimulation is applied to portion A on the peripheral side, compound muscle action potential [CMAP(A)] is obtained. When stimulation is given to

M. Aoyagi (✉), O. Saito, H. Tojima, H. Maeyama, and Y. Koike
Department of Otorhinolaryngology, Yamagata University School of Medicine, Iida-Nishi 2-2-2, Yamagata, 990-23, Japan

point B on the central side, CMAP(B) is obtained with slightly prolonged latency. When points A and B are stimulated simultaneously, the retrograde impulse induced by the stimulation of point A and antegrade impulse by the stimulation of point B collide with each other in the nerve, and disappear. Accordingly, the antegrade impulse induced by point A stimulation alone reaches the muscle and CMAP(A+B) is completely the same as CMAP(A).

In trace 4, point B is stimulated slightly after point A. Impulses from the two points collide only in nerve fibers with small diameter, because of the slow conduction velocity. In thick fibers with fast conduction velocity, the retrograde impulse induced by point A stimulation has already passed point B, and the antegrade impulse from point B is thus conducted to the muscle without collision. The waveform [CMAP(A+B)] thus includes CMAPs elicited with impulses from point A through thin and thick fibers and from point B through thick nerve fibers. CMAP induced by the antegrade impulse of point B stimulation can be obtained by subtracting CMAP(A) from CMAP(A+B).

When point B is stimulated after retrograde impulse from point A has passed point B in thin fibers with slow conduction velocity, impulses from point B can be conducted to the muscle without collision through all nerve fibers. The waveform of CMAP(A+B) thus includes CMAPs elicited with impulses from points A and B through thin and thick nerve fiberrs, and the second wave elicited with point B stimulation becomes prominent (Trace 5). A nerve consists of many fibers differing in diameter, and thus CMAP of nerve fibers with different conduction velocities can be recorded by changing the interstimulus interval (ISI) between the two points.

The amplitude of subtracted CMAP increases as a function of ISI, because CMAPs elicited with the stimulation conducted through the fibers with slow conduction velocity are added one after another. DNCV was determined from the rate of increase in amplitude, since this rate indicates the relative number of nerve fibers at each conduction velocity. When the amplitude increase of CMAP between an ISI of 2.0 and 2.25 ms is 20% of the full CMAP

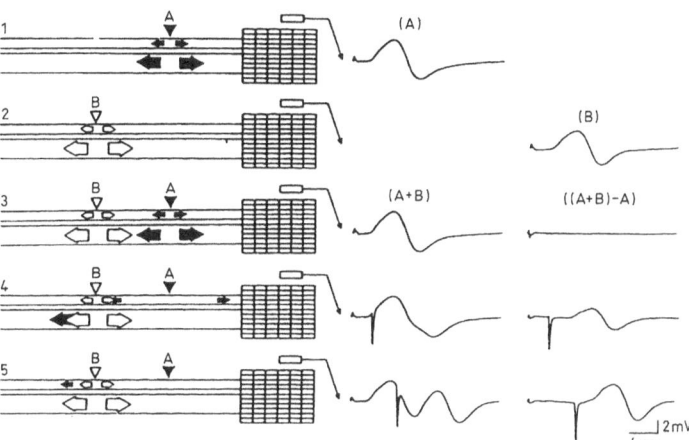

Fig. 1 Principle of the collision method. Traces 1 and 2, CMAPs elicited by stimulation at A and B are recorded from electrodes on the mentalis muscle [CMAP(A) and CMAP(B)]. Trace 3, When A and B are stimulated simultaneously, all impulses collide with each other. Trace 4, When stimulation B is slightly after stimulation A, only impulses of fiber with slow conduction velocity collide. Trace 5, When B is stimulated after all retrograde impulses from A had passed, all impulses from B reach the muscle. CMAP(A+B) is the actual recording with double stimulations and CMAP(A + B)-A) is the subtracted waveform

amplitude, the percentage of fibers with a conduction velocity of 20 – 22 m/s is 20% in the nerve.

Measurements

Stimulating electrodes were fixed at two points on the marginal mandibular branch of the facial nerve at an interval of 50 mm [2]. Electrical stimulation was a rectangular wave of 0.2 ms. The recording electrodes were placed bilaterally on the mentalis muscle. One on the opposite side served as a reference.

Results

Normal Subjects

Figure 2 shows the average and standard deviation of DNCV in 14 normal subjects. The abscissa shows conduction velocity and the ordinate the relative number of nerve fibers. DNCV showed unimodal distribution with a peak at 20 – 22 m/s. Minimum conduction velocity was 10 m/s and maximum 32 m/s.

Patients with Bell's Palsy

Figure 3 shows DNCVs in representative cases of Bell's palsy, compared with normal data. Electroneuronography (ENoG), the most reliable examination for determining the degree of wallerian degeneration in facial palsy, was conducted every 2 or 3 days at an early stage of palsy, and minimum ENoG was used as the index for evaluating

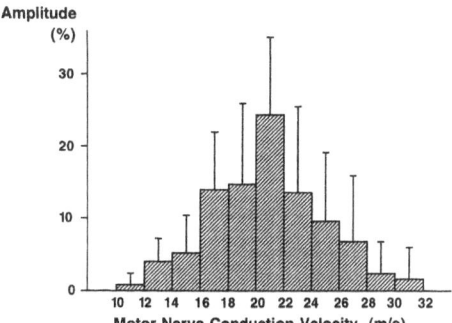

Fig. 2 Averages and standard deviations of DNCV in facial nerve in normal adults

degeneration. When expressing the DNCV in patients with Bell's palsy, the percentage in each conduction velocity was reduced by multiplying the value of ENoG.

We compared the distribution of NCV with the results of ENoG. For an ENoG of 30% – 50%, nerve fibers with a conduction velocity exceeding 20 m/s markedly decreased, and above 24 m/s, disappeared completely. This was observed in 12 of 14 cases. In patients with advanced wallerian degeneration, nerve fibers with slow conduction velocity decreased as did also those with fast conduction velocity.

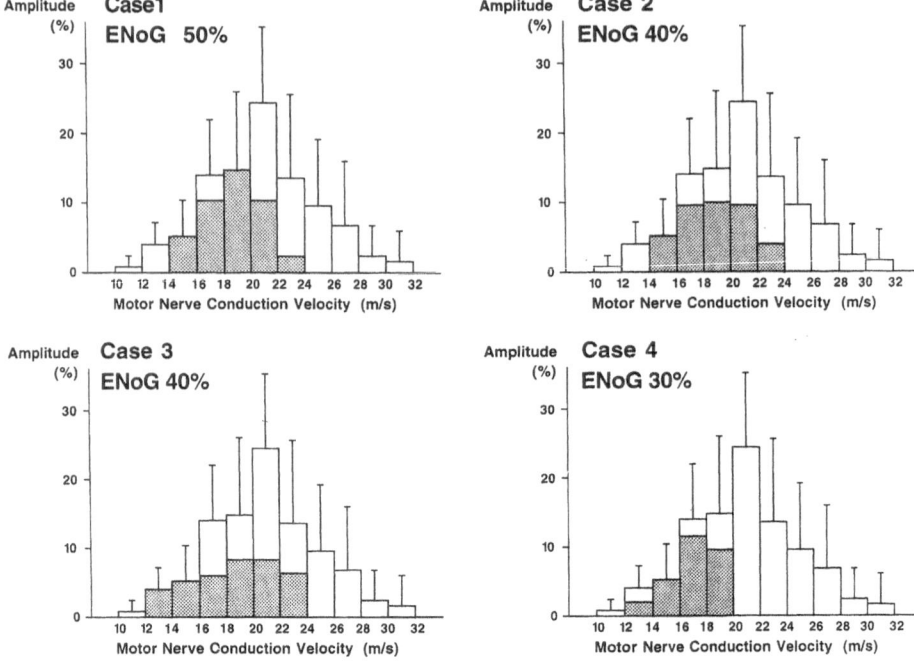

Fig. 3 DNCV in a patient with Bell's palsy (*shaded columns*) compared with a normal control (*open columns*)

Discussion

The average DNCV of facial nerve, as determined by the collision method of Hopf [1] using marginal mandibular branch and mentalis muscle, showed a unimodal distribution with a peak at 20–22 m/s in normal subjects. Minimal and maximal NCV were 10 and 32 m/s, respectively.

The results in the patients suggest that the number of thick fibers with fast conduction velocity decreases at first in Bell's palsy. In a previous study, the distribution of diameter of facial nerve fibers was histologically determined in normal guinea pigs and those with palsy induced by compression at the stylomastoid foramen. At 1 week after compression, thick fibers 4 µm or more in diameter had

markedly decreased and were considered more susceptible to damage induced by compression. Thin nerve fibers were considered less likely to be injured. Electrophysiological findings in the present study showed close agreement with the above histological findings. In the present study it was demonstrated that Bell's palsy is a compression neuropathy.

References

1. Hopf HC (1963) Electromyographic study on so-called mononeuritis. Arch Neurol 9:307–312
2. Tojima H (1988) Measurement of facial nerve conduction velocity and its application to patients with Bell's palsy. Acta Otolaryngol Suppl 446:36–41

Eur Arch Otorhinolaryngology (1994) [Suppl]:S517

M. Mañós-Pujol, R. Jimenez, E. Gil, J.P. Menen, A. Vidaller, and M. Dicenta

Tertiary Syphilis with Facial Paralysis

A 41-year-old man patient had peripheral facial paralysis, and osteolytic and osteoblastic lesions in the pelvis, skull, sternum, dorsal vertebrae, and left tibia. The cause of the disease was tertiary syphilis. Clinical and radiologic features are presented. This rare illness is discussed. Only nine cases of luetic facial paralysis have been reported in the literature since 1945, all of them of secondary syphilis. The prognosis for facial nerve functions is good with early correct antibiotic therapy.

M. Mañós-Pujol, R. Jimenez, E. Gil, J.P. Menen, and M. Dicenta
Department of Otorhinolaryngology, Ciutat Sanitaria de Bellvitge,
University de Barcelona, Spain

A. Vidaller
Department of Internal Medicine, Ciutat Sanitaria de Bellvitge,
University de Barcelona, Spain

Eur Arch Otorhinolaryngology (1994) [Suppl]: S518–S520

D. F. Hoffmann

Recurrent Facial Paralysis Associated with HIV Infection

Numerous head and neck manifestations of human immunodeficiency virus (HIV) and acquired immunodeficiency
disease (AIDS) have been reported [1–3]. These include
salivary gland lymphadenopathy and lymphoproliferative
disease [4–6]. Neurologic manifestations of AIDS, including cranial nerve neuropathies, have also been
described [7, 8]. We report the association of recurrent
facial paralysis and lymphoproliferative disease in two
patients with HIV.

Case Reports

Case 1 A 25-year-old homosexual male presented with a
1-day history of a left facial paresis. Two years previously
he had a left facial paralysis diagnosed elsewhere as Bell's
palsy. Complete recovery had occurred over several
months. On examination there was an incomplete left
facial palsy without synkinesis. An ill-defined fullness was
present at the angle of the mandible. Evoked electromyography showed an increased nerve conduction latency and
greater than 95% degeneration of the left facial compoud
action potential compared to the right. The audiogram was
normal except for loss of the left stapes reflex. An MRI
scan showed a well-circumscribed mass thought to be a
deep lobe parotid tumor. The mass could not be well visualized on CT scan. At 4 days after onset a complete facial
paralysis was present and evoked EMG was 0%. A needle
EMG showed evidence of a chronic left facial neuropathy
with evidence of degeneration and regeneration. Fine
needle aspiration biopsy showed salivary gland fragments

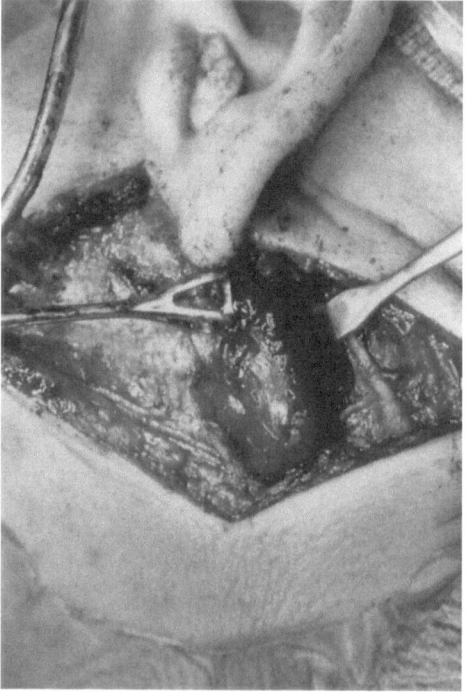

Fig. 1 Lymph node exposed deep to parotid gland

D. F. Hoffmann
Oregon Health Sciences University Portland, Oregon 97202, USA

and chronic inflammatory cells. HIV serology was obtained because of risk factors and proved to be positive.

The mass was approached as a probable malignant tumor. As the tail of the parotid gland was separated from the sternocleidomastoid muscle and the digastric muscle was exposed, a large lymph node became visible in the parapharyngeal space (Fig. 1). This was easily dissected out without performing a parotidectomy. The frozen section was suspicious for lymphoma and the procedure was terminated. CT scans of the abdomen and chest were normal, as was bone marrow aspiration. The final pathology was reported as chronic lymphadenitis with reactive hyperplasia. The final diagnosis was AIDS-related complex (ARC) with peripheral lymphadenopathy. Facial recovery was noted within 1 week postoperatively and by 4 months had progressed to grade II House-Brackmann recovery with mild synkinesis. At 6 months no further manifestations of AIDS had occurred.

Case 2 A 45-year-old white male presented with a history of recurrent facial paralysis. The onset of paralysis had been spontaneous and symptoms had occurred up to three times per week, lasting several hours each time for nearly 2 months. Then, 2 weeks prior to presentation, a complete paralysis developed without recovery. On examination there was a complete right facial paralysis with loss of tone. No masses were palpable. Stapes reflex was absent and evoked EMG was 0%. An MRI scan of the parotid and skull base was suspicious for an enhancing mass in the parotid gland. Past medical history was remarkable for HIV infection, which the patient stated was a result of a blood transfusion.

The mass was approached via a parotid incision for biopsy. The facial nerve was identified; however, it appeared to be about five times its normal diameter (Fig. 2). The surrounding parotid tissue appeared normal with the abnormality confined to the nerve itself. Analysis of the biopsy specimen from the nerve showed lymphoma, but the type could not be determined because the specimen was so small. Further testing to evaluate for lymphoma revealed disease in the liver. The association of lymphoma and HIV led to the diagnosis of AIDS. The patient was treated with several cycles of chemotherapy and azothioprim (AZT) over the subsequent 6 months. Nine months postbiopsy there was no evidence of lymphoma and the patient had grade III House-Brackmann recovery of facial function.

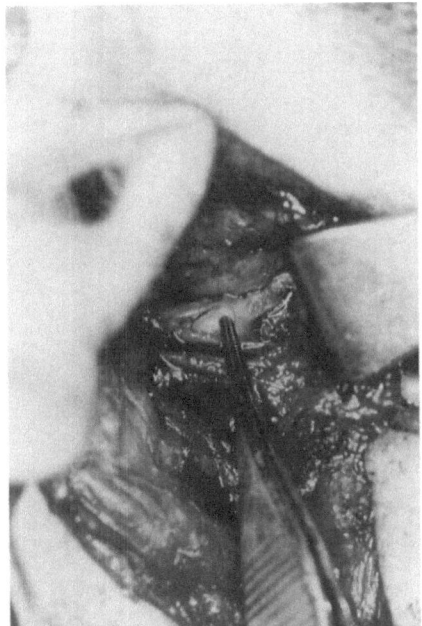

Fig. 2 Massive infiltration of main trunk of facial nerve with lymphoma

Discussion

Generalized lymphadenopathy is a well-known manifestation of HIV infection and AIDS. A number of reports have also documented the association of salivary gland lymphadenopathy and benign lymphoepithelial cysts in patients with HIV infection. Frequently these masses have been approached as salivary gland neoplasms and been found to be hyperplastic reactive lymph nodes. Recently the CT scan appearance of lymphoepithelial cysts in patients with HIV has been recognized as pathognomic and biopsy may not be necessary. Solitary masses in the parotid in patients with HIV must still be viewed with suspicion, however. Malignant lymphoma has a higher incidence in HIV-positive patients, and lymphomas involving the parotid gland in HIV-positive patients have been reported. The association of HIV and lymphoma leads to the diagnosis of AIDS. Certainly patients with risk factors for HIV who present with a parotid mass should be tested for HIV serology.

Case 1 illustrates a patient whose mass could have easily been missed on examination and who presented with sudden onset facial paralysis for a second time. The frequent recurrent paralysis in case 2 would have been less likely confused with Bell's palsy although no mass was palpable on examination. Without imaging studies and subsequent exploraton, neither diagnosis would have been apparent.

Conclusions

1. Patients with facial paralysis, particularly recurrent paralysis, should be queried as to HIV risk factors.
2. Despite the well-known association of HIV infection and benign parotid cysts, a parotid mass in an HIV-positive patient should be viewed with suspicion for a malignant lymphoproliferative disorder, particularly if associated with facial paralysis.

References

1. Marcusen DC, Sooy CD (1985) Otolaryngologic and head and neck manifestations of acquired immunodeficiency syndrome (AIDS). Laryngoscope 95 : 401 – 405
2. Rosenberg RA, Schneider KL, Cohen NL (1985) Head and neck presentations of acquired immunodeficiency syndrome. Otolaryngol Head Neck Surg 93 : 700 – 705
3. Wenig BM, Kuruvilla A, Goldrich MS, Heffner DK, Turr S (1990) Pathologic manifestations of acquired immunodeficiency syndrome in the head and neck. Ent J 69 : 406 – 415
4. Ryan RR, Ioachim HL, Marmer J, Loubeau JM (1985) Acquired immune deficiency syndrome – related lymphadenopathies presenting in the salivary gland lymph nodes. Arch Otolaryngol 111 : 554 – 556
5. DeVries EJ, Kapadia SB, Johnson JT, Bontempo FA (1988) Salivary gland lymphoproliferative disease in acquired immune disease. Otolaryngol Head Neck Surg 99 : 59 – 62
6. Shaha A, Thelmo W, Jaffe BM (1988) Is parotid lymphadenopathy a new disease or part of AIDS? Am J Surg 156 : 292 – 300
7. Gabuzda DH, Hirsch MS (1982) Neurologic manifestations of infection with human immunodeficiency virus. Ann Intern Med 107 : 383 – 391
8. Brown MM, Thompson A, Goh BJ, Forster GE, Swash M (1988) Bell's palsy and HIV infection. J Neurol Neurosurg Psychiatry 51 : 425 – 426
9. Holliday RA, Cohen WA, Schinella RA, Rothstein SG, Parsky MS, Jacobs JM, Som PM (1988) Benign lymphoepithelial parotid cysts and hyperplastic cervical adenopathy in AIDS-risk patients: a new CT appearance. Radiology 168: 439 – 441

Eur Arch Otorhinolaryngology (1994) [Suppl]: S 521 – S 524

A. Morelló, A. Olmo, A. López Soto, O. Biurrun, J. Pérez Villa, F. Sabater, J. Traserra Jr., and J. Traserra

Bilateral Facial Palsy in Wegener's Granulomatosis

Introduction

Peripheral facial paralysis has often been described in systemic diseases such as diabetes mellitus, hypothyroidism, periarteritis nodosa, Sarcoidosis, Takayasu's arteritis, and Wegener's granulomatosis (wa) [1]. However, this cranial nerve palsy occurs generally in patients with advanced disease and rarely marks the beginning of the clinical course [2]. We describe a patient who had WG with unilateral facial nerve palsy as the initial symptom. His audiogram demonstrated bilateral both air and bone conduction deficits. The evolution also involved the other side with bilateral facial palsy and he became profoundly deaf. Wegener's granulomatosis usually presents to the otolaryngologist with nasal manifestations, but peripheral nervous system symptoms can occur by chance in the clinical onset. This disease without treatment will proceed to death, while early recognition and proper treatment can induce long-lasting remissions. Thus, it becomes necessary for head and neck clinicians to become familiar with symptoms of the initial stage of the disease since they must help secure a proper diagnosis, particularly through biopsies when indicated [3].

Case Report

A previously fit 62-year-old man experienced a right-sided facial weakness of abrupt onset with tinnitus and occipital headache irradiated to both ears. Neurological examination showed a right-sided peripheral facial palsy. The patient was systemically treated with steroids for 2 weeks causing the facial palsy to disappear. Three months later, the patient experienced severe right hearing loss and a new episode of right-sided peripheral facial palsy that returned to normal with similar treatment within 1 week. His audiogram demonstrated a right mixed hearing loss. Three weeks later he developed the third episode of right facial palsy and his audiogram demonstrated bilateral mixed

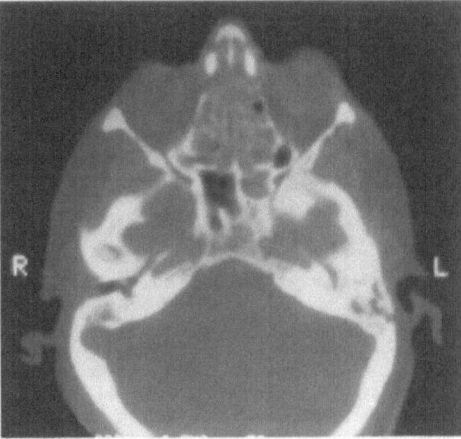

Fig. 1 Bilateral occupation of the middle ear, mastoid cavities, and ethmoidal, maxillary, and sphenoidal sinuses predominantly on the right side

A. Morelló (✉), A. Olmo, O. Biurrun, J. Pérez Villa, F. Sabater, J. Traserra Jr., and J. Traserra
Department of Otorhinolaryngology, Hospital Clinic,
Facultad de Medicina de Barcelona, C/Villarroell, 170,
08036 Barcelona, Spain

A. López Soto
Department of Internal Medicine, Hospital Clinic,
Facultad de Medicina de Barcelona, C/Villarroell, 170,
08036 Barcelona, Spain

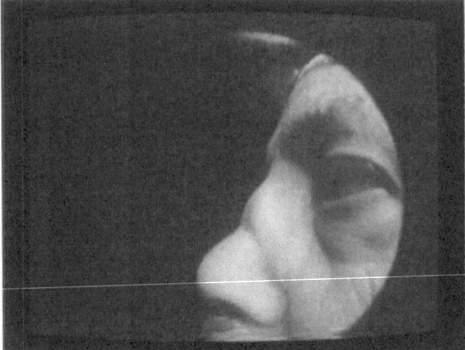
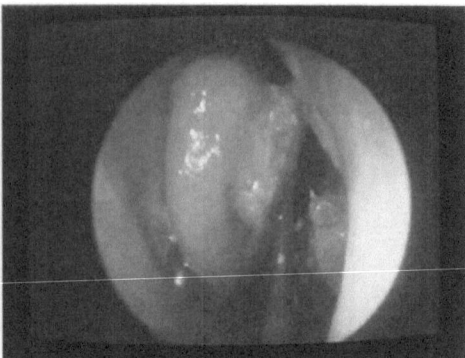

Fig. 2 Nasal deformity

Fig. 3 Mucopurulent rhinitis associated with mucosal crusting and necrosis of the septal cartilage

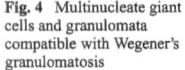

Fig. 4 Multinucleate giant cells and granulomata compatible with Wegener's granulomatosis

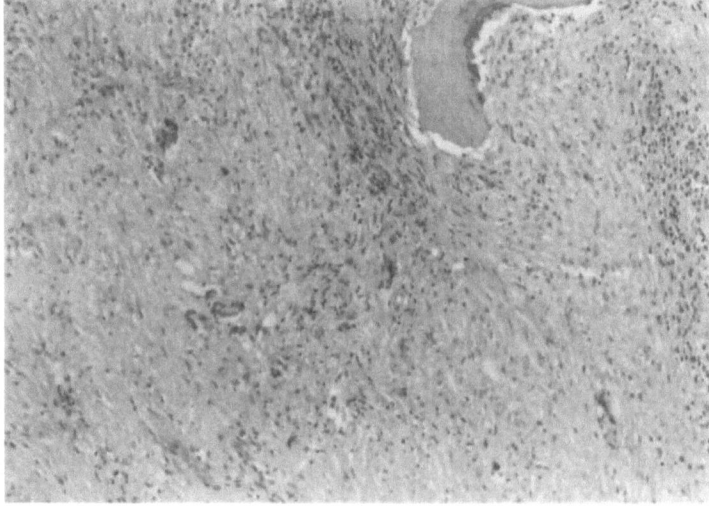

hearing loss. Furthermore he complained of nasal discharge. Examination by otoscopy showed a bilateral red and ballooned tympanic membrane. The nasal examination revealed an inflamed nasal mucosa. Ear-sinus radiographs and the CT scan demonstrated bilateral occupation of the middle ear, mastoid cavities, and ethmoidal, maxillary, and sphenoidal sinuses predominantly on the right side (Fig. 1). The surgical exploration of the right middle ear allowed facial decompression and granulation tissue biopsy. This and nasal mucosal biopsies showed a nonspecific inflam-matory infiltrate. On this occasion the treatment with steroids partially improved the facial palsy. The hearing loss continued to become progressively deeper. Six weeks later, during the fourth episode he became profoundly deaf and developed bilateral peripheral facial palsy. On examination he proved to have profound bilateral sensorineural deafness. Investigations at the time showed normal hemo-globin, white cell count, and platelets. His erythrocyte sedimentation rate was elevated to 70 mm/h. The auto-immune profile demonstrated a positive antineutrophil cytoplasmic antibody (ANCA) at 1 in 40. Rheumatoid factor and antinuclear antibody were negative. Repeat nasal biopsy showed nonspecific inflammatory tissue. He began taking cyclophosphamide (100 mg/day) and prednisolone (50 mg/day). Three months later he showed a slight improvement of hearing loss but continued to suffer from the bilateral facial palsy and complained of nasal and paranasal symptomatology such as rhinorrhea, diffuse nasal crusting, sinus pain, and nasal deformity (Fig. 2). The nasal endoscopy showed a mucopurulent rhinitis associated with mucosal crusting and necrosis of the septal cartilage (Fig. 3). This biopsy of the septum showed multinucleate giant cells and granulomata compatible with Wegener's granulomatosis (Fig. 4). He continued taking cyclophosphamide (100 mg/day) and prednisolone (30 mg/day) with almost total reversibility of his hearing loss and facial palsy within 4 months. He showed a residual slight sensorineural hearing loss with structurally normal brainstem auditory evoked potentials, and a weakness of both lower facial nerve branches. His disease has now stabilized, 25 mg/day cyclophosphamide and 10 mg/day prednisolone.

Discussion

Wegener's granulomatosis (WG) is a necrotizing vasculitis that is recognized for its distinctive clinicopathologic manifestations. The characteristic features of WG, which differentiate it from other vasculites, include necrotizing granulomatous vasculitis of the upper and lower respiratory tract, disseminated small vessel vasculitis, and focal necrotizing glomerulonephritis [4]. The etiology of WG is not known, although a cellular and humoral hypersensivity reaction to an unidentified antigen is suspected. In WG there is a slightly greater predilection for males and it may affect any age group, although it is rarely seen in the 1st decade of life. The incidence peaks during the 4th and 5th decades.

As in our case, for example, the otorhinolaryngologist may be the first physician called to examine these patients because WG often seems to have manifestations in the ear-nose-throat region, especially in the beginning. It is unusual to find advanced renal disease on initial presentation. Nose and paranasal sinuses are involved in more than 90 % of patients. The usual presentation is a mucopurulent rhinitis associated with mucosal crusting: on occasion necrosis of the septal cartilage occurs. Bacterial superinfections are a frequent complication in patients with severe sinusitis. Otological involvement occurs in 20 % – 40 % of cases [5]. Otitis media (OM) is common and occurs in 25 % of patients. The pathophysiology of OM relates to eustachian tube dysfunction and blockage resulting from inflammation caused by chronic rhinitis. Serous OM is the most common form of ear disease in WG. In addition to complications from eustachian tube

dysfunction, such as in our case, the ear may be a primary site for granuloma formation. Our patient had bilateral sensorineural deafness at the onset of the disease. This is rare in Wegener's granulomatosis [6]. McCaffrey et al., in a review of 112 patients with WG, showed that 9 also had sensorineural hearing loss; this was improved in 5 of the 9 patients after control of the disease with prednisone and cyclophosphamide. Schrader and Clements [7, 8] reported on a primary manifestation of WG of the ear with reversible sensorineural hearing loss. The mechanism may be vasculitis of the vasa nervorum, or inflammatory edema around the auditory nerve, but there are almost no pathological studies to demonstrate this. Two postmortem studies have been reported shortly after the onset of WG. They describe either granulomatosis tissue extending from the middle ear into the inner ear, or extensive hemorrhage in the inner ear. Yoon et al. [9] observed thick granulomatous changes in the middle ear, especially in the eustachian tube and the protympanum. However, characteristic necrotizing granulation tissue with multinucleated giant cells was not observed. In our case, the tympanotomy demonstrated inflammatory tissue in the middle ear, but the biopsies were not diagnostic. In the case described by Blatt and Lawrance, direct spread of granulomatous tissue through the round window resulted in destruction of the membranous labyrinth. However, the reversible condition of sensorineural hearing loss, such as in our case, pointed to multiple factors. Thus cochlear vessel involvement, granulomata compression of the acoustic nerve, and immune complex deposition in the cochlea have all been implicated in this process. In our case the brainstem auditory evoked potentials seemed to support the cochlear source of this sensorineural hearing loss.

In our case report the initial symptom was peripheral facial nerve palsy and the otolaryngologist was the first physician called upon to examine the patient. Palsy of the facial nerve has commonly been observed in WG [10], but only a few reports have mentioned facial nerve palsy as an initial symptom of WG [2]. Pathogenesis of the facial nerve palsy was related to vascular disturbances secondary to vasculitis of the vasa nervorum or perhaps related to granulomatous involvement of the facial nerve in WG [11]. A nude second portion of facial nerve, as in our case, is liable to show granulomata compression in the middle ear. However, the relapse of the palsy and the bilateral affection seem to show other possible mechanisms. An experimental study has demonstrated immunologic concepts in the pathogenesis of Bell's palsy [12]. Yoon et al. [9] observed histopathologic chances near the facial nerve, including inflammatory cell infiltrate and thickened blood vessels in the facial canal, in a patient with systemic vasculitis. So a potential mechanism in the VIIth alterations can be a lymphocytic infiltrate in areas of the facial and internal auditory canal, particularly distributed intraneuronally and perivascularly, leading either to reversible neuropraxia or to neural degeneration caused by vascular occlusion with subsequent ischemia of distal functional

S524

elements. It is interesting that similar fibrotic changes and formation of new bone in the inner ear have been observed in animal experiments after venous and arterial obstruction of the labyrinth and in humans who have systemic vasculitis, including WG and PAN [13]. Further studies in temporal bones are needed to understand the pathogenesis of this disease process.

Laboratory tests are not helpful in making a diagnosis of WG except for the anticytoplasmatic autoantibody (ANCA) blood test [14], which has been shown to be highly specific for WG. We have used the ANCA for corroboration of WG in our patient for whom at first tissue biopsies were not diagnostic. Also important is the knowledge that ANCA can be absent in the limited forms of WG.

In our case the CT scan demonstrated bilateral occupation of the middle ear and mastoid cavities, and ethmoidal and sphenoidal sinuses. Multiple biopsies of all these locations were not suggestive of WG, except for septal cartilage. Tissue biopsies may be nondiagnostic even in the presence of active disease. Repeated tissue samples from the upper respiratory tract are often required in order to establish the correct diagnosis since as many as 50% of the biopsies exhibit nonspecific acute and chronic inflammation with necrosis [15].

Although the disease was rapidly fatal as recently as 1970, treatment with cyclophosphamide and steroids has produced response rates of 93% [16].

Conclusions

- The potential otologic and facial involvement underscores the role of the otolaryngologist in the early diagnosis and treatment of WG [17].
- The prognosis of facial palsy and sensorineural hearing loss in WG can be improved with suppression of the vasculitis process by early treatment with combined cytotoxic-immunosuppressive therapy.
- Diagnosis, treatment, and follow-up of patients with WG is described as an example for the collaboration between the specialist for otorhinolaryngology and internal medicine. A long-term follow-up of patients with WG by specialists for ORL and IM seems to be absolutely necessary.
- The course of inner ear function, serum findings, and the success of immunosuppressive therapy in WG are comparable with immunologically mediated vasculitis in the inner ear [18]. The possibility of an underlying systemic autoimmunity should be considered in patients who have unexplained peripheral facial palsy and/or sensorineural hearing loss. Our patient's facial palsy and bone conduction loss is good evidence of peripheral facial and inner ear pathology. The almost total reversibility of these disturbances on treatment

makes it most important to consider the diagnosis of Wegener's granulomatosis in any case of unexplained facial palsy or sensorineural hearing loss.
- The otorhinolaryngologist must be aware of the varied manifestations of Wegener's granulomatosis and the availability of the anticytoplasmic autoatibody blood test as an aid in confirming the diagnosis [19].
- Repeated tissue biopsied from the upper respiratory tract are often required in order to establish the correct diagnosis.

References

1. Power WH (1974) Peripheral facial paralysis and systemic disease. Otolaryngol Clin North Am 7(2):397–405
2. Calonius IJ, Christensen CK (1980) Hearing impairment and facial palsy as initial sign of Wegener's granulomatosis. J Laryngol Otol 94:649–657
3. Dwyer J, Janzen VD (1981) Wegener's granulomatosis with otological and nervous system involvement. J Otolaryngol 10(6):476–480
4. Fauci AS, Haynes BF, Katz P: The spectrum of vasculitis: clinical, pathologica, immunologic and therapeutic considerations. Ann Intern Med 89:660–676
5. Kornblut AD, Wolff SM, DeFries HO, Fauci AS: Wegener's granulomatosis. Laryngoscope 90:1453–1465
6. Luqmani RA, Jubb R, Emery P, Reid A (1991) Adu dwomoa. Inner ear deafness in Wegener's granulomatosis. J Rheumatol 18(5):766–768
7. Schrader B (1986) Primary manifestation of Wegener's granulomatosis of the ear with reversible sensorineural hearing loss. Laryngol Rhinol Otol 65(1):29–31
8. Clements MR, Mistry CD, Keith AO, Ramsden RT (1989) Recovery from sensorineural deafness in Wegener's granulomatosis, J Laryngol Otol 103:515–518
9. Yoon MD, Paparella MD (1989) Schacherns Systemic vasculitis: a temporal bone histopathologic study. Laryngoscope 99:600–609
10. Campbell SM, Montanaro A, Bardana EJ (1983) Head and neck manifestations of autoimmune disease. Am J Otol 4:187–216
11. Steenerson RL (1986) Bilateral facial paralysis. Am J Otol 7(2):99–103
12. McGovern FH, Konigsmark BW, Sydnor JB (1972) An immunological concept for Bell's palsy. Experimental study. Laryngoscope 82:1594–1601
13. Kimura R, Perlman HB (1956) Extensive venous obstruction of the labyrinth. Cochlear changes. Ann Otol Rhinol Laryngol 65:332–351
14. Rasmussen N, Wiik A, Hoier-Madsen H, Borregaard N, van der Woude FJ (1988) Antineutrophil cytoplasm antibodies, 1988. Lancet 1:706–707
15. Fauci AS, Haynes BF, Katz P, Wolff SM (1983) Wegener's granulomatosis: prospective clinical and therapeutic experience with 85 patients for 21 years. Ann Intern Med 98:76–85
16. Govett GS, Amedee RG (1990) Wegener's granulomatosis of the head and neck. J La State Med Soc 142(5):13–16
17. Guyot JP, Baud C, Montandon P (1990) Wegener's granulomatosis with otological disorders as primary symptoms. ORL J Otorhinolaryngol Relat Spec 52(5):327–334
18. Kempf HG (1989) Ear involvement in Wegener's granulomatosis. Clin Otolaryngol 14(5):451–456
19. Colaço B, Statters D (1991) Deafness and vasculitis. Lancet 337:1602–1603

Eur Arch Otorhinolaryngology (1994) [Suppl]: S 525 – S 526

J. Pietruski

Facial Palsy in Equatorial Africa

The present paper is a short report on my observations of facial palsy during my stay in Africa. I have to stress the fact that an assessment and comparison of any epidemiologic factor in an underdeveloped country is verry difficult or almost impossible.

Zaire is an enormous country, 84 times larger than Belgium, and has no railways, roads, or telephone connections. The very poor medical service is interested mostly in tropical diseases and, recently, in acquired immunodeficiency syndrome (AIDS).

I have worked in Equatorial Africa in the south-east part of the former Belgian Congo (now Zaire) in Shaba (formerly known as Katanga) in the region called the Copperbelt. I was the only ENT specialist in this large region of about 500 000 km².

To date, there has been no work done on the problems in this part of Africa. I thought it would be interesting to present a short report.

Patients with facial palsy came to the Department of Otolaryngology mostly for other reasons. I collected 29 cases in Kipushi, Lubumbashi, Likasi, and Kolwezi between 1984 and 1988 with different etiologies (Table 1).

Table 1 Incidence of facial palsy (1984 – 1988)

Etiology	Women	Men	Total
Post-traumatic	–	2	2
External otitis	1	1	2
Chronic otitis media	2	3	5
Parotid and others tumors	4	5	9
Iatrogenic	1	3	4
Bell's palsy	4	2	6
Other	–	1	1
Total	12	17	29

J. Pietruski, UL. Etiudy Rew, 40/1, 02-643 Warsaw, Poland

In Table 1 there are only two cases of post-traumatic palsy; both were caused by falling from a truck. I would like to turn your attention to the two cases of external otitis, which I never seen before. Of long duration and scarring alternatively with no treatment, the circular scar closed the external auditory canal (EAC). As a consequence, the structures of the middle ear were destroyed and the facial nerve damaged. In three further cases, which are not included here, a fistula between the bone and the cartilage EAC saved the middle ear.

The other patients with chronic otitis media had discharge from the ear for many years. Of course they should have been operated on long ago, but they had never been to an ENT doctor. In two cases the tympanal part of the facial nerve was almost completely destroyed by cholesteatoma. I tried to restore the facial nerve continuity with a graft taken from the auricularis magnus nerve. Three other cases presented with the anatomy of the middle ear distorted by granulation, scar tissue, and hypertrophic mucous membrane. The lack of landmarks and bleeding makes dissection and looking for the nerve impossible.

There is a high percentage of parotid and other tumors. All these patients came to see me too late to be operated on.

I would like to mention the fact that before my arrival the method of parotidectomy with dissection and conservation of the facial nerve was unknown. During my first operation of the parotid mixed tumor according to the Göttinger tunnel method, the surgeons watching the operation were fascinated, because they did not even know that the facial nerve could be protected and saved.

There were four cases of iatrogenic palsy. I classify these cases separately in spite of the traumatic origin (two of them were the sequelae of a vertical incision of parotid gland abscess, and the two other were due to mastoidectomy performed many years ago).

Four patients with Bell's palsy had long-standig paralysis. The two remaining patients had been medically treated. The final patient in the series ("other") had long-standing paralysis after pregnancy.

Table 2 Age and sex of patients

Age group (years)	Men	Women	Total
12–20	4	5	9
21–30	6	4	10
31–40	5	2	7
41–52	2	1	3
Total	17	12	29

Table 3 First ENT Contact, $n = 29$

Below	3 m	Above
3	M	14
2	F	10
Total 5		24

The age and sex of patients is shown in Table 2. Facial palsy affects both sexes with a marked preference for men and for three early age groups: 12–20, 21–30, and 31–40 years. There are no patients over 52 years of age, because life survival time in Africa is short. 50 years is already old age, corresponding to about 70 years of age in Europe.

As for as the first visit to the ENT Department is concerned there, are two groups: before 3 months after onset (three men and two women) and after 3 months (14 men and ten women). The hghest incidence occurs in the second group, i.e., 24 cases. Only five patients in the first group were treated: three with Bell's palsy, one with chronic otitis media, and one with obliterative external otitis.

Conclusions

At the end of this short report, I would like to stress the following points: the postoperative period was mostly un-eventful, but I had no contact with my patients after they were discharged from the hospital. This is typical of African people in this region: they never return for check-ups or follow-up examinations.

I found no marked variations according to the season. The tropical climate exists all the year round and the daily fluctuations of temperature are between 10–15 °C, because the altitude above sea level is 1200–1500 m in this region.

I realize that this small number of cases is insufficient for any conclusions to be drawn. Because of the lack of any adequate record keeping for this type of disease, my aim was to obtain data which would serve as a starting point and be helpful in future research.

Eur Arch Otorhinolaryngology (1994) [Suppl]: S527

POSTERS

V. Azarova

Regeneration of Irradiated Rat Skeletal Muscle After Damage Under Different Experimental Conditions

It is known that ionizing radiation in high doses disturbs the posttraumatic regeneration of skeletal muscle. However, by means of experimental surgical methods the irradiated traumatized muscle recovers to a large extent. One method is autografting minced nonirradiated muscle tissue into the defect of the irradiated transected muscle. The aim of the present study was to use the preliminary denervated muscle for the above-mentioned autografting and to compare it with intact muscle. For histological and morphometric analyses the regenerates of rat m. gastrocnemius were examined for 2 months. The results showed that the skeletal muscle irradiated with 30 Gy after deep trauma was subject to atrophy or necrosis (control series). In most cases (72% of animals) indolent ulcers appeared on skin and shin muscle. The intact minced muscle tissue autografted in the area of injury onto irradiated transected muscle (first experimental series) promoted the recovery of neuromuscular junctions in the proximal and distal stumps of the muscle organ. The myogenesis of muscle fragments resulted in the development of myotubes and myofibers supplied with newly formed motor endings. The regenerates obtained contained much muscle tissue 2 months after irradiation and operation. By autografting fragments of preliminary denervated muscle tissue in the wound onto irradiated muscle (second experimental series) the processes of regeneration developed similarly, but more favorable morphometric indicators (relative muscle tissue content in regenerates depending on the area occupied by the tissue on the sections of irradiated operated m. gastrocnemius) were obtained. Thus, the denervated muscle, probably because of its metabolic characteristics, contributed to considerable restoration of tissue properties in skeletal muscle after irradiation and mechanical damage.

V. Azarove
Institute of Evolutionary Animal Morphology and Ecology, Moscow, Russia

Eur Arch Otorhinolaryngology (1994) [Suppl]: S 528

POSTERS

N. Bulyakova

Age Characteristics of Reinnervation of Skeletal Muscle Grafts

The recovery of innervation is one of the important conditions for successful skeletal muscle regeneration. The present communication deals with the age characteristics of motor and sensitive reinnervation in the rat gastrocnemius muscle 60 days after mincing or free grafting. The muscle grafts were examined in young rats (from newborn to 1 month old) and in rats aged 24–30 months.

The contractive function was not recovered in some young rat grafts. No infections were observed in those grafts. After mincing the noncontractile grafts were formed in all young rats. The number of such grafts was highest in newborn rats. After free grafting the noncontractile grafts were found only in newborns and in rats aged 1 week. In old rats all grafts contracted when the tibial nerve was stimulated. A large number of nervous fibers grew into grafts of young and old rats. However, re-establishment of nerve-muscle contacts was often impeded in rats operated upon in the early ontogenic stages; in grafts with unrepaired function few motor plates were found. In the contractile grafts of both young and old rats the numbers of motor endings were greater. They had more nuclei and a more diverse terminal arrangement. The sensory innervation comprised free terminal plexuses of sensory nerve fibers and modified sensory bulbs. More complex mechanoreceptors such as muscle spindles and Golgi tendon organs were not observed.

Thus, the results obtained demonstrated that grafted gastrocnemius muscle in rats within the first days after birth was reinnervated poorly compared not only with young rats aged 1 month, but also with old rats aged 24–30 months.

N. Bulyakova
Institute of Evolutionary Animal Morphology and Ecology, Moscow, Russia

Eur Arch Otorhinolaryngology (1994) [Suppl]: S529

FREE PAPERS AND POSTERS

P. Quesada, J.M. Fernández, M.L. Navarrete, and F. Crespo

Prediction of Surgical Criteria for Bell's Palsy on the Fifth Day of Evolution

One of the questions always posed with Bell's palsy patients needing surgical decompression is when to they have to be operated on. The final neurobiological purpose in achieving the absence of sequelae is to operate before endoneural degeneration. Supported by electroneuronographic follow-up studies, we have observed that on the 5th day of evolution we can evaluate which patients should undergo surgery.

P. Quesada, J.M. Fernández, M.L. Navarrete, and F. Crespo
Hospital Valle de Hebrón, Universidad Autonoma, Barcelona, Spain

Eur Arch Otorhinolaryngology (1994) [Suppl]: S530–S531

POSTERS

M. Kinishi, H. Hosomi, and M. Amatsu

Therapeutic Policy for Bell's Palsy and Hunt Syndrome

Introduction

To obtain satisfactory recovery in Bell's palsy and in Hunt syndrome, it is mandatory to commence the initial treatment within 1 week after onset. In 1979, Stennert proposed an excellent treatment modality with a high dose of cortisone and dextran and reported a high recovery rate [6]. Based on our experience [7, 2] with the modified modality (SD therapy) of the said protocol, however, this treatment was not always necessary for all patients with the disease. The present study was designed to evaluate the true benefit of SD therapy in treating Bell's palsy and Hunt syndrome.

Subjects and Methods

This study consisted of 295 patients with Bell's palsy and 93 patients with Hunt syndrome who were treated between July 1984 and December 1991. The patients studied were evaluated within 7 days of onset of the disease and were followed clinically until recovery occurred or for at least 6 months in cases of incomplete recovery. Of the 388 patients, 31 had chemical evidence of diabetes mellitus.

Evaluation of Facial Movement

The most reliable factor was the grade of palsy, i.e., incomplete or complete palsy, in prognostication of a palsy [1].

M. Kinishi, H. Hosomi, and M. Amatsu
Department of Otolaryngology, Kobe University School of Medicine, Kusunoki-cho, 7-5-1, Chuo-ku Kobe 650, Japan

For this reason, the evaluation of facial movement was done based on our scoring method modified from that of May [4, 5]. The patients underwent a ten-point examination; tone, wrinkling of the forehead, light and forced closing of the eyelids, blinking, wrinkling of the nose, grinning, whistling, puffing out of cheeks, and pouting of the lower lip. A score of 10 was given for each normal part, 5 if function was present but was weak, and 0 if movement was absent. The palsy was designated complete if the score of facial movement was less than 15 and incomplete if the score exceeded 20. Each patients with complete palsy was examined with a nerve excitability (NE) test at the first visit and again 1 week later. The extent of nerve function present was classified in one of the following three groups: good (with a difference of 3.5 mA or less between the minimal excitability thresholds on both sides); poor (with a difference of more than 3.5 mA between both sides and/or diminished response to a maximal stimulation); and absent (with no response to maximal stimulation).

The final recoveries were also categorized into two groups: complete and incomplete. Recovery was defined as complete if the score of facial movements exceeded 90 without sequelae and incomplete if the score was less than 85 and/or with sequelae.

Therapeutic Management

The therapeutic protocol of SD therapy is described elsewhere [7, 2]. For the first 7 days 500 ml dextran 40-lactated Ringer's solution was given daily within 3 h. Hydrocortisone was added directly to the dextran solution at a dose of 500 mg on the first day, 300 mg on the second day, 200 mg on the third and fourth days, and finally 100 mg on the next 3 days. Adenosine triphosphate (ATP) and vitamins B_6 and B_{12} were also added to the solution. Finally, pentoxifylline (300 mg/day) was administered orally during and after SD therapy. Oral vitamin B_{12} and ATP were also given each day.

Results

Bell's Palsy

Of the 295 patients treated with the SD therapy, 184 had complete palsy and 111 incomplete palsy. All patients with incomplete palsy recovered completely. Out of 184 patients with complete palsy, 162 (88%) had complete recovery and 22 partial recovery.

Of the 184 patients with complete palsy, 135 showed good NE, 37 poor NE, and 12 absent NE. All patients with good NE recovered completely. For the 37 patients with poor NE, recovery was complete in 27 cases (73%) and incomplete in ten cases. All patients with absent NE recovered partial facial movements.

Hunt Syndrome

Of the 93 patients treated with the SD therapy, 68 had complete palsy and 25 incomplete palsy. All patients with icomplete palsy had complete recovery. Of the 68 patients with complete palsy, 39 (57%) recovered completely and 29 incompletely.

Thirty-three patients showed good NE, 13 poor NE, and 22 absent NE. The good NE group showed complete recovery, except for one case. For 13 patients with poor NE, recovery was complete in seven cases (54%) and incomplete in six cases. The absent NE group showed partial recovery without exception.

Discussion

Although the etiology of Bell's palsy is still unknown, it is generally accepted that the major pathogenic factors are edema and primary or secondary ischemia of the facial nerve, leading to nerve compression and hypoxia. Stennert [6] proposed high dosages of cortisone for a strong anti-inflammatory and antiedematous effect and, additionally, low-molecular dextran in combination with pentoxifylline to increase peripheral nerve perfusion, with a high recovery rate. For the past 7 years we have been treating Bell's palsy [2] and Hunt syndrome [3] with a high dose of steroids and dextran (SD therapy) modified from Stennert's original protocol. In contrast to his patients, however, ours were treated as outpatients, given half the dose of hydrocortisone and a shorter duration of infusion during an overall shorter treatment span.

Out of 295 patients with Bell's palsy, 273 (93%) had complete recovery and 22 partial recovery. In contrast, 64 (69%) of 93 patients with Hunt syndrome recovered completely and 29 partially. This difference was statistically significant.

Complete palsy is a distressing condition, since recovery may be only partial in certain cases. As described previously [2, 3]. SD therapy is more effective than oral steroid therapy in Bell's palsy as well as in Hunt syndrome. This was confirmed by our experience. On the basis of these studies, it was concluded that SD therapy should be started immediately in cases of complete palsy.

As far as incomplete palsy is concerned, all patients recovered completely, regardless of the mode of treatment. Therefore, SD therapy was not always necessary for patients with incomplete palsy. Based on our experience with patients of initially incomplete palsy evaluated within 7 days after onset, however, the half of patients who were examined within 3 days of onset and whose score of facial movements ranged from 20 to 40 deteriorated into complete paralysis. For these cases, a daily check-up and SD therapy is advisable.

References

1. Hosomi H, Minatogawa T, Kokan T, Taniguchi (1975) Course of peripheral facial palsy and conservative treatment. Pract Otol Kyoto 68 : 655 – 662
2. Kinishi M, Amatsu M, Hosomi H (1991) Conservative treatment of Bell's palsy with steroids and dextran-pentoxiphylline combined therapy. Eur Arch Otolaryngol 248 : 147 – 149
3. Kinishi M, Hosomi H, Amatsu M, Tani M, Koike K (1992) Conservative treatment of Hunt syndrome. J Otolaryngol Jpn 95 : 65 – 70
4. Kinishi M, Matsui T, Hakozaki S, Nishiwaki I, Hosomi H (1983) Evaluating method for the degrees of facial palsy. Facial N Res Jpn 3 : 1 – 3
5. May M (1970) Facial paralysis, peripheral type: a proposed method of reporting. Laryngoscope 80 : 331 – 390
6. Stennert E (1979) Bell's palsy – a new concept of treatment. Arch Otolaryngol 225 : 265 – 268
7. Tani M, Kinishi M, Takahara T, Hosomi H, Amatsu M (1988) Medical treatment of Bell's palsy. Arch Otolaryngol (Stockh) [Suppl] 446 : 114 – 118

Eur Arch Otorhinolaryngology (1994) [Suppl]: S 532 – S 534

POSTERS

K. Murakawa, E. Ishimoto, K. Noma, K. Ishida, M. Nishijima, R. Izumi, H. Ishida, T. Minatogawa, F. Satomi, and T. Kumoi

Stellate Ganglion Block for Facial Palsy

Introduction

Although the cause of Bell's palsy has still not been clarified, its main pathophysiology is thought to be due to ischemic conditions of the facial nerves in the temporal bone. Since there is an extremely strong relationship between the pathophysiology of Bell's palsy and circulatory disorders of the nutrient blood vessels in the facial nerves, the main emphasis of the conservative treatment of this disorder by chemotherapy is aimed at circulatory improvement. On the other hand, at the pain clinic, improved blood flow to the facial nerve by stellate ganglion block (SGB) therapy is employed in treating patients with Bell's palsy. Its efficacy has already been adequately confirmed. The improved blood circulation during treatment of Bell's palsy by SGB is thought to be brought about by a vasculatory dilatation action due to the blocking effects on the sympathetic nerve. However, the detailed mechanism has not been adequately studied. Therefore, we report the effects of SGB on the common carotid artery blood flow volume and tissue blood flow volume in facial nerve tissue in patients at the acute stage of Bell's palsy and in experimental animals.

Materials and Methods

Clinical Study

Among patients at the acute stage of Bell's palsy, the onset of which occurred 1 week or less before, we selected 15 patients as our subjects. The main purpose and nature of the study were explained and all the patients gave willing consent for participation. The age of the patients (seven men and eight women) ranged from 15 to 69 years, with a mean value of 47.1 ± 4.6 years. The affected side was the left side in seven cases and the right side in eight cases. SGB was performed by the paratracheal approach, using 8 ml 1% mepivacaine. The success of SGB was confirmed by Horner's sign, hyperemia of the ocular conjunctiva, sensation of warmth in the face and upper limbs, and the stopping of sweating. The blood flow volume in the common carotid artery was measured (Fig. 1a) using an ultrasonic blood flow meter (Nikon Koden, FM1100) before performing SGB and 90 min after performing SGB.

Animal Study

Intravenous anesthesia with 10 mg pentobarbital and 4 mg pancuronium was administered to 18 mongrel dogs with a mean weight of 11.5 ± 1.7 kg. Tracheal intubation was performed, and artifical respiration with room air was conducted. Skin incisions were made on the anterior cervical region and the common carotid artery was exposed and attached to an electromagnetic flowmeter Nihon Koden, MFV 3200). Skin incisions were also made on the lateral cervical region and at the ectopic region from the stylomastoid foramen; the facial nerves were exposed, and the tissue blood flow volume in the facial nerves was continuously measured using a laser Doppler tissue blood flowmeter (Advance, ALF 2100). The cervicothoracic ganglion corresponding to the stellate ganglion in humans

K. Murakawa (✉), E. Ishimoto, K. Noma, K. Ishida, M. Nishijima, R. Izumi, and H. Ishida
Department of Anesthesiology, Hyogo College of Medicine, 1-1 Mukogawa-cho, Nishinomiya, Hyogo, 663, Japan

T. Minatogawa, F. Satomi, and T. Kumoi
Department of Otolaryngology, Hyogo College of Medicine, 1-1 Mukogawa-cho, Nishinomiya, Hyogo, 663, Japan

was punctured, 1 ml 1% mepivacaine was infusec, thus making experimental SGB, and the effects on the blood flow in the common carotid artery and the facial nerve tissue were studied (Fig. 1b, c).

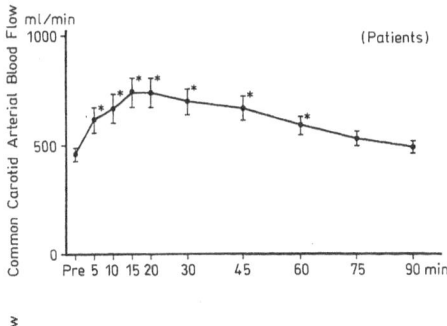

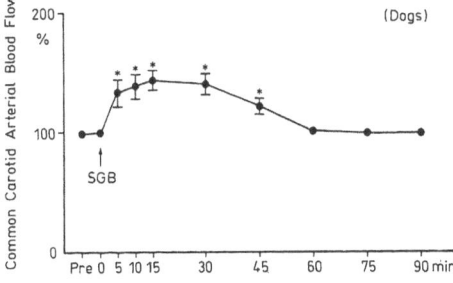

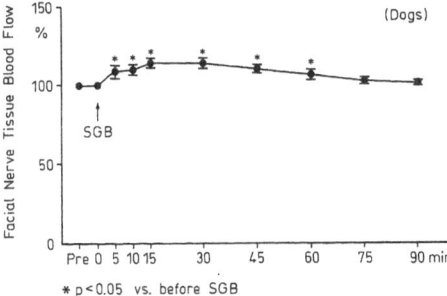

* p<0.05 vs. before SGB

Fig. 1a–c Blood flow in the common carotid artery in patients (**a**) and dogs (**b**) and in the facial nerve tissue in dogs (**c**)

Results

Clinical Study

Prior to performing SGB, the blood flow volume in the common carotid artery was 482.3 ± 41.0 ml/min, but from 5 min after performing SGB it increased markedly, and at 20 min it was 787.6 ± 92.5 ml/min (163.3%). Thereafter, a gradual decline, but with still significant increases compared to the pre-SGB level, continued up to 75 min after. Blood pressure and heart rate showed no significant changes even after SGB.

Animal Study

At the time of performing SGB, arterial pressure rose transiently, but thereafter displayed no marked changes. The blood flow volume in the common carotid artery increased markedly immediately after SGB, and after reaching a peak of $143.3 \pm 7.7\%$ at 15 min, it gradually declined, but the significant increases continued until 45 min after. Also, the tissue blood flow of the facial nerves almost paralleled that in the common carotid artery. From 5 min after performing SGB it increased significantly and reached peak values of $114.0 \pm 2.7\%$ and $114.0 \pm 2.6\%$ at 15 and 30 min, respectively. Thereafter, a gradual decline, but still significant increases compared to the pre-SGB level, continued up to 60 min after.

Discussion

The main pathological conditions of Bell's palsy are thought to be due to ischemic conditions of the facial nerves inside the temporal bone, and the mechanism for the developmet of paralysis is thought to be due to edema and compression caused by ischemic changes in the nerve. The main center of nutrient blood vessels to the facial nerves inside the temporal bone is anatomically the external carotid artery system, and a close relationship between the onset of Bell's palsy and circulatory disorders in the common carotid artery system has been reviewed. Limited reports have implicated circulatory disorders of the external carotid system in the possible mechanism for the onset of Bell's palsy. In our previous study in patients at the acute stage of Bell's palsy, SGB markedly increased the blood flow through the external carotid artery and the common carotid artery at 30 min after performing SGB due to dilatation of the peripheral blood vessels in the external carotid arery and the nutrient blood vessels to the facial nerve. It became clear that blood flow almost doubled, and it was evident that SGB in Bell's palsy patients markedly increased the blood flow to the nutrient blood vessels of the facial nerve [1]. In this study, along with studying the effects on blood flow through the common carotid artery due to SGB, we studied changes in blood flow in the facial nerve in experimental animals using a laser Doppler tissue blood flowmeter. By this technique, in which the laser light is dispersed by the erythrocytes inside the tissue, it is possible to continuously measure microcirculation by analyzing cyclic count changes [2]. Our results indicate that parallel to the increase in blood flow through the common carotid artery due to SGB, the tissue blood flow in the facial nerve also clearly increased, confirming that SGB markedly increases blood flow in the nutrient blood vessels of the facial nerve. Thus, due to its sympathetic nerve-blocking action, since SGB dilates blood vessels both on the arterial side and venous side, SGB is thought to be effective in treating not only neural damage of blood flow stoppage due to vascular constriction, but also in the regeneration of nerve fibers that have already undergone Wallerian degeneration and secondary disorders due to entrapment as well. Since in this study it was confirmed that a marked increase was observed in the common carotid artery blood flow and the facial nerve tissue blood flow and that the circulatory improvement effects of SGB extend as far as the facial nerve itself, SGB is considered to be an extremely effective treatment for Bell's palsy.

References

1. Murakawa K et al. (1990) Effects of stellate ganglion block on the blood flow through the external carotid artery in idiopathic facial palsy. Facial N Res Jpn 10 : 195–198
2. Nilsson GE et al. (1980) Evaluation of a laser Doppler flowmeter for measurement of tissue blood flow. IEEE Trans Biomed Eng 27 : 597–604

Eur Arch Otorhinolaryngology (1994) [Suppl]: S 535 – S 536

POSTERS

R. Ferreira Bento, P. Bogar, and M. C. Lorenzi

Treatment Comparison Between Dexamethasone and Placebo for Idiopathic Facial Palsy

Introduction

Idiopathic facial palsy (Bell's palsy) was first described by Charles Bell in 1883 [1]. Since then, the treatments employed have been empirical in some way, as no etiological cause has been well established. Some theories are widely accepted such as viral, ischemic, and autoimmune origin [2–4]. All of them are based on vascular changes causing edema with neural compression and then neuropraxia. The drug most commonly used is cortisone, with the finality of aging on the edema. In the literature we have found no citations about the use of dexamethasone, although it is known to have an excellent effect in acute processes of the central nervous system because of its fast efficacy and aggregation on neuronal membrane. We observed that many patients treated with different drugs had a good evolution too. The aim of this study is to find out the real advantage of treating patients with dexamethasone by analyzing the final evolution of the paralysis and the recuperation time.

Method

A double-blind study was performed in 79 sequential patients with diagnosis of Bell's palsy, seen in the ENT Department of the Hospital das Clinicas da Universidade de Sao Paulo from 1989 to 1990. In the study, the following patients were excluded: (a) those with any previous drug treatment; (b) diabetic or hypertensive patients; and (c) patients with acute or chronic otitis media.

We performed clinical and subsidiary examinations. All patients underwent a subjective clinical examination in order to classify the intensity of the palsy [5]. For the purpose of confirming the Bell's palsy diagnosis, additional factors were taken into account: patients' history, clinical examination, audiometry, impedance, immune blood serum exams for syphilis, fasting blood sugar, and tomography with special focus on the fallopian canal. The patients were randomly selected; one group of patients received dexamethasone (0.13 mg/kg per day) and the others placebo. The patients were evaluated weekly until their final recovery. The patients were divided into two groups of 20, and 39 patients were excluded because they did not come for the follow-up. The results were evaluated by the Kruskall-Wallis method, and the rate adopted was 0.05%.

Results

The two groups were similar in age, sex, start of treatment, and initial clinical grade (Table 1).

The average time until recovery was 61.45 days for the group treated with dexamethasone (ranging from 7 to 240 days) and 40.95 days for the group treated with placebo (ranging from 8 to 70 days). Figure 1 shows the comparison between dexamethasone and placebo regarding recuperation time. Figure 2 shows the results of the patients in whom medication was initiated less than 4 days after onset of palsy, and Fig. 3 the patients in whom it was initiated after 5 days or more. By the statistical method adopted there were no differences between the two groups ($p < 0.05$).

Discussion

The literature review showed similar studies with cortisone [6]. Adour made a double-blind study with prednisone and

R. Ferreira Bento, P. Bogar, and M. C. Lorenzi
Department of ENT, Faculdade de Medicina da Universidade de São Paulo, Av., Dr. Eneas de Carvalho Aguiar, 255 – 6º andar, sala 602, CEP 05403, Brazil

Table 1 Patients' details

Treatment group	Age (years)		Treatment start after onset (days)		Initial grade		Sex (n)	
	Median	Range	Median	Range	Median	Range	m	f
Dexamethasone	30.95	5–53	3.8	0–15	6.4	3–14	12	8
Placebo	27.1	10–55	2.75	0–9	7.45	3–16	6	14

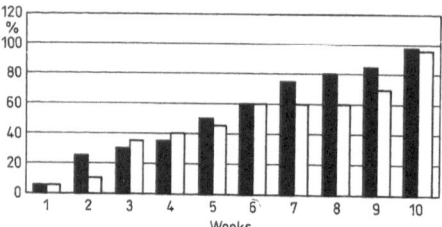

Fig. 1 Comparison between the dexamethasone (*shaded bars*) and placebo (*black bars*) groups regarding recuperation time in terms of percentage recovery

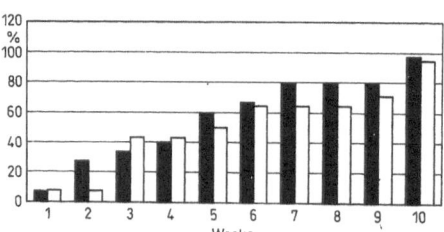

Fig. 2 Comparison between patients in the dexamethasone group in whom medication was initiated less than 4 days after onset of palsy (*shaded bars*) and the placebo group (*black bars*) in terms of percentage recovery

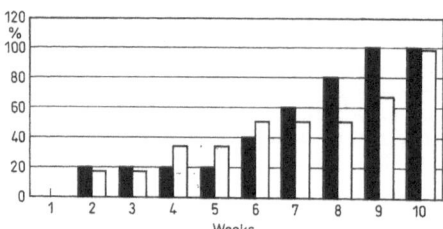

Fig. 3 Comparison between patients in the dexamethasone group in whom medication was initiated 5 days or more after onset of palsy (*shaded bars*) and the placebo group (*black bars*) in terms of percentage recovery

placebo [7], and Taverner and Leeds used cortisone acetate and placebo [8]. These authors showed better results with cortisone concerning the recuperation time, which was not observed in our investigation. There is no doubt that in those cases with pain the dexamethasone acted better. The exclusion of the patients who already had more than 15 days of pathology was based on the fact that it takes 15 days for the Wallerian degeneration to develop. The exclusion of diabetic and hypertensive patients was due to the possibility of another cause of paralysis (such as diabetic neuritis or vessel pathologies) as well as related contraindications of the drug. At a first glance the number of 40 patients that finished the study seems too small to draw statistical conclusions, but this was due to the strict criteria drawn up for patient inclusion. A total of 39 patients out of 79 that had startd the protocol were excluded during the study, mainly because they did not come for the follow-up. This fact led us to believe that their recovery was so satisfactory that they saw no necessity to come back.

Conslusions

We conclude that there were no significant differences between the two groups based on final appearance or the recuperation time.

References

1. Bell C (1883) The nervous system of the human body. Green, Washington, pp 46–51
2. Mcgovern FH (1968) A review of the experimental aspects of Bell's palsy. Laryngoscope 78 : 324–333
3. Hilger JA (1949) The nature of Bell's palsy. Laryngoscope 59 : 228–235
4. Blunt MJ (1956) The possible Role of vascular changes in the etiology of Bell's palsy. J Laryngol Otol 70 : 701–713
5. Bento RF (1990) Anastomose do nervo facial (intratemporal) com adesivo tecidual fibrínico. Estudo em doentes portadores de paralisia facial traumatica. Thesis, Faculty of Medicine, University of Sal Paulo
6. Taverner D et al. (1971) Comparison of corticotrophin and prednisone in treatment of idiopathic facial paralisis (Bell's palsy). BMJ 2 : 20–22
7. Adour KK et al. (1972) Prednisone treatment for idiopathic facial paralysis (Bell's palsy). N Engl J Med 287 : 1268–1272
8. Taverner D, Leeds MRCP (1954) Cortisone treatment of Bell's palsy. Lancet 20 : 1052–1054

Eur Arch Otorhinolaryngology (1994) [Suppl]: S 537 – S 539

POSTERS

P. G. Heymans

Emotions in the First 99 Days After the Onset of Facial Paralysis: A Single Case Study

Research Questions

How does a young, pretty woman cope emotionally with a peripheral facial paralysis? Surgical removal of an acoustic neurinoma robbed our 25-year-old female patient of one of her most important tools for dealing with social situations: her attractive face.

She was intensively followed from 2 weeks preoperation until 99 days after the medically successful operation. Among other data, daily measurements were collected concerning 117 emotions she had experienced during the day.

Emotions are important because they serve as clues toward the more basic concerns which are touched in the aftermath of the facial damage. From a strictly biological point of view, the patient was cured after the successful removal of the tumor, but from her perspective things have only just started, as she becomes aware of the need to socially adjust to the new situation.

Specific questions are: (a) what preoperation fears did the patient have?; (b) what do the trajectories of the 117 emotions over 99 days look like? (c) what is the course of her emotional involvement? (d) what is the course of the emotional quality or tone of each day in this period?; and (e) what are her basic, underlying concerns and what do their arousal trajectories look like over these 99 days?

Method

At the end of each day, the patient completed a checklist regarding 117 emotions, indicating with a number from 1 (not present) to 9 (very intensely) how she had experienced each emotion that day. Moreover, at selected intervals she

P. G. Heymans
Department of Developmental Psychology, Rijks Universiteit
Utrecht, The Netherlands

indicated on a separate checklist what the pattern of emotions would look like for an "ideal day." These patterns turned out to be very stable. Two weeks before the operation, an extensive biographical interview was held. The patient was asked at regular intervals to give informed consent for continuing with the investigation. Data analyses were performed with the SPSS-pc statistical package.

Results

The following list shows the anxieties the patient expressed 2 weeks before the operation:

1. I don't know how strong I am.
2. I don't know whether I am strong enough to carry the consequences of the operation.
3. How awkward is it not hearing with one ear?
4. How much mental/physical misery do I have to endure after the operation?
5. How much forced gratitude toward others do I have to show?
6. Will it still be possible to interact as an equal with people, especially the ones who have helped me?
7. How dependent will I be on others?
8. Will I not doubt the integrity of the people around me?
9. Will my vanity not be hurt by the consequences of the operation?
10. Will I continue trying to become happy?
11. Will I not relapse into bulimic eating episodes?
12. Will my life continue in the same chaos as before?
13. Will others recognize me as a complete person?
14. Will I not feel stared at by others/strangers?
15. Will my life after the operation not be of a lesser/inferior quality, and will I be able to adjust to such a life?

Interestingly, when asked about any preoperation anxieties on day 27 *after* the operation, she could not remember any of them. When confronted with the list, she only recognized anxiety item 6.

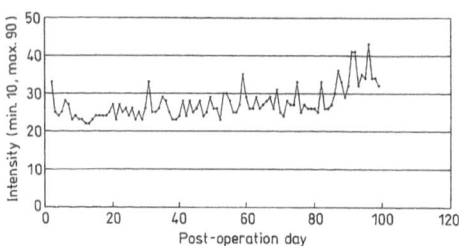

Fig. 1 Emotional involvement averaged over 117 emotions in the postoperative period

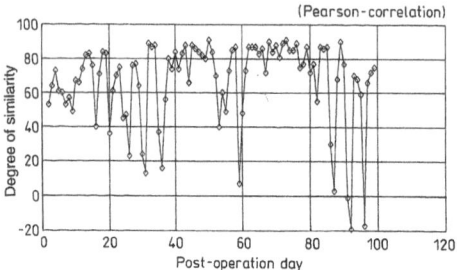

Fig. 2 Emotional tone of postoperative days, i.e., compared with "ideal" day

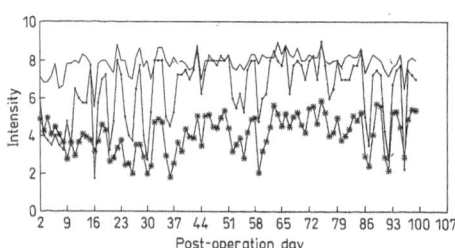

Fig. 3 Related basic emotions: —, feeling safe; -■-, happiness; -*-, being in control of your life

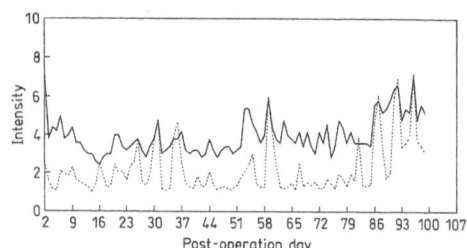

Fig. 4 Related basic emotions: -, vulnerability; —, worries about moral failure

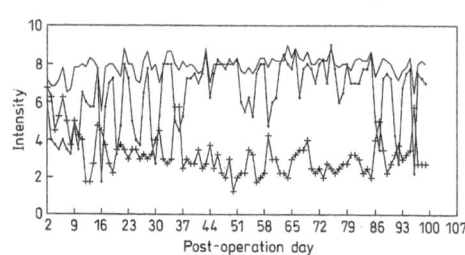

Fig. 5 Related basic emotions: —, feeling safe; -■-, happiness; -+-, dependency

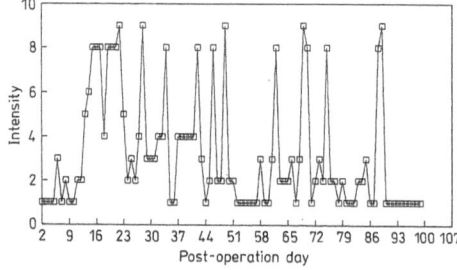

Fig. 6 Intensity of desire for sex in the postoperative period

Figure 1 shows the total involvement in emotions, averaged over the 117 emotions. An upward trend is present.

The emotional tone of a day is the similarity between the reported emotion pattern for a day and the pattern for an "ideal" day. The course of the emotional tone is shown in Fig. 2. The first 10 days (during which the patient was in the hospital recovering) with their rather constant positive emotional tone are noteworthy. After being released from hospital, a strong cyclicity is present in the data: 3 "good" days followed by 2 or 3 "bad" days. The patient suffers from bulimia. She was able to stop this habit immediately before the operation and during 4 weeks after the operation. On day 31, her first bulimic relapse occurs. All dips in the curve for emotional tone below 0.40 are associated with bulimic tendencies. The return of bulimic eating signals the intrusion of "normal life" in the life of this patient.

The trajectories for the 117 emotions cannot be shown here. They were subjected to cluster analyses to detect groups of emotions with a similar trajectory. These clusters were inspected for theoretical coherence. Nine clusters were found, of which one is an artifact as it consists of 36 emotions which were all nearly absent over the 99-day period.

The remaining eight clusters or basic emotions were interpreted as: (1) a concern for feeling safe, (2) vulnerability, (3) volatile moods, (4) desire for sex, (5) fear and sorrow over personal failures, (6) happiness, (7) dependency, and (8) being in control of your own life. The trajectories for these basic emotions are shown in Fig. 3–6. As can be seen, these eight basic emotions are interrelated. "Feeling safe" and "happiness" (r, 0.74) form the concern "security" and are in opposition to "dependency" (r, 0.51, 0.62) (see Fig. 5). Moreover, "being in control of your own life" covaries with security, as shown in Fig. 3. Together, these four basic emotional concerns seem to correspond to the attachment/exploration system, one control system for human behavior. The patient in this study seems to alternate between bouts of active exploration in which she feels in control and experiences pleasure and bouts of dependency on others.

"Desire for sex" shows a pattern which is completely independent of all other basic emotion clusters. In the 2 weeks after the operation this index of vitality achieves its first peak (see Fig. 6). "Being vulnerable" and "worring over one's moral failures" (indicated by emotions such as shame, guilt, frustration, fear, feeling damaged) are also related (r, 0.69), as shown in Fig. 4. These two basic emotions are, as a group, also independent of the other ones. Other data from this patient indicate that the peaks in both curves are related to her thinking over the medical procedures she is going through, more especially prospects for rehabilitation derived/constructed by her on the basis of the information provided. Continued research will have to clarify this hypothesis.

Concluding Remarks

With the daily administration of a simple emotion checklist, insights can be obtained into the degree to which basic emotions or concerns are touched upon in the aftermath of a surgical removal of a tumor, resulting in facial paralysis. The registration of patients' emotions does not only serve as a means for research, but is also experienced by the patients as a rehabilitation service. Perhaps in the future, graphs like the ones shown here will be used for improving the communication between patients and their medical doctor in the rehabilitation period.

Eur Arch Otorhinolaryngology (1994) [Suppl]: S 540

POSTERS

G. Morello-Castro, M. Junyent, J. Bel, and A. Morrello

Facial Paralysis in Children

Facial paralysis (FP) in children is most often idiopathic; however, many diverse and identifiable etiologies exist. We present four cases of facial paralysis in children and newborns seen in a 12-month period during 1991. Causes of FP in this series included: Bell's palsy, Melkersson-Rosenthal syndrome, and forceps trauma. Curre approaches to diagnosis (facial nerve latency test, scanning the facial nerve) and treatment, including pharmacological treatment with sterids and surgical treatment, are described. Two of them recovered good facial activity and no secondary effects were found during treatment.

G. Morello-Castro
Department of ENT, Medecin University, Sant Llorens, 21,
43201 Reus Tarragona, Spain

Eur Arch Otorhinolaryngology (1994) [Suppl]:S 541 – S 544

K. Yuen, S. Kawakami, T. Ogawara, I. Inokuchi, M. Maeta, and Y. Masuda

Evaluation of Facial Palsy by Moiré Topography

Introduction

To evelute facial nerve function, several visual assessment methods have proposed by May, Yanagihara, Stennert, House, Brackman, among others, and the score method is widely accepted as a simple and useful method for examination to evaluate roughly the degree of facial palsy. However, it is difficult to capture fine changes with the score method when precise evaluation is required, and it is limited as a form of objective and reporducible assessment. Therefore, it is not a very suitable method to follow up the process of the recovery in facial nerve palsy.

We were able to solve these problems with moiré topography. Moiré topography is based on light itnerference theory and allows visualization in three dimensions of an object's surface contours, like a geograhic map, with high precision. Because it measures without direct contact, it is particularly useful for measuring any object, such as flesh, which is readily deformed by little force. This method has been used since 1970 to measure rough-surfaced materials in three dimensions. We have applied this method to assess facial palsy for two reasons:

1. As an addition of a objective form of evaluation to subjective macroscopic evaluation.
2. For quantitative evaluation and detailed analysis of the degree of improvement because of very wide range of partial paralysis.

Method

Using the lattice irradiation type moiré camera FM3013 connected to a CCD camera and a monitoring device, the face was measured and a photographic record was made by thermal video printer FTI-200 after confirmation of moiré strips. The interval between moiré strips was set to show 2.0 mm in depth and the face was fixed so as to make the oculoauricular surface horizontal. Photographs were then taken as front pictures. To observe the function of each branch of the facial nerve, we took five moiré photographs each while the patient performed one of the following actions: wrinkling the forehead, closing eyes lightly, blowing out the cheeks, grinning, and at reat (Figs. 1 – 5). In the case of infants and young children, who cannot willfully change their expression, two moiré photographs were obtained: one while crying and one at rest (Fig. 6a, b).

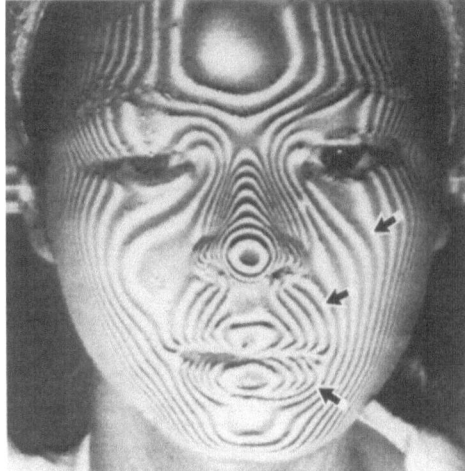

Fig. 1 At rest. Moiré strip, running through cheek and mental point becomes flat. Winding pattern of moiré strips around mouth angle does not appear on palsy side. Interval of moiré strip between subnasal point and lower lip becomes wide

K. Yuen, S. Kawakami, T. Ogawara, I. Inokuchi, M. Maeta, and Y. Masuda
Department of Otolaryngology, Okayama University Medical School, 2-5-1 Shikata-cho, Okayama-shi, Okayama, 700 Japan

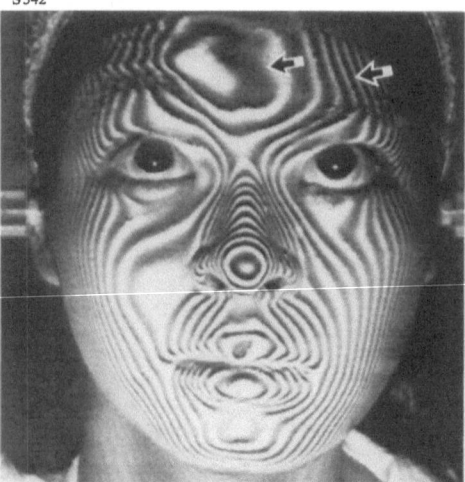

Fig. 2 Wrinkling the forehead. Remarkable asymmetry of stripy on forehead. No winding pattern of moiré strips is formed by wrinkling forehead on palsy side

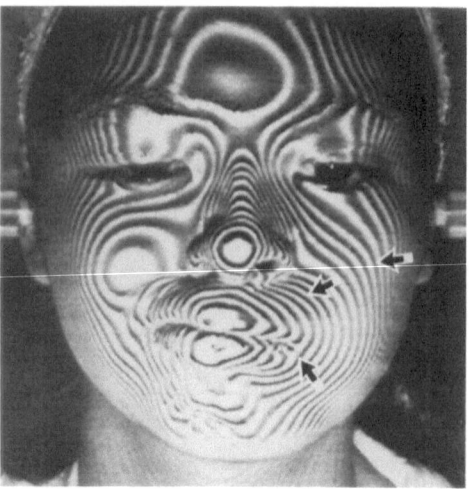

Fig. 4 Blowing out the cheeks. Moiré strip running through cheek and mental point becomes flat. Winding pattern of moiré strips around mouth angle does not appear on palsy side. Interval of moiré strip between subnasal point and lower lip becomes wide

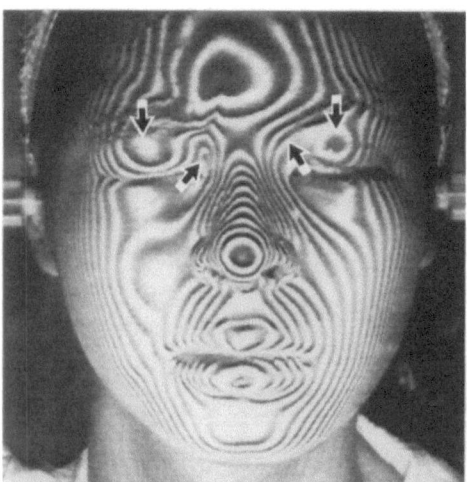

Fig. 3 Closing eyes lightly. Moiré strip on superior eyelid has different heights. Winding pattern of moiré strips, running from canthus to superior eyelid, is less on palsy side

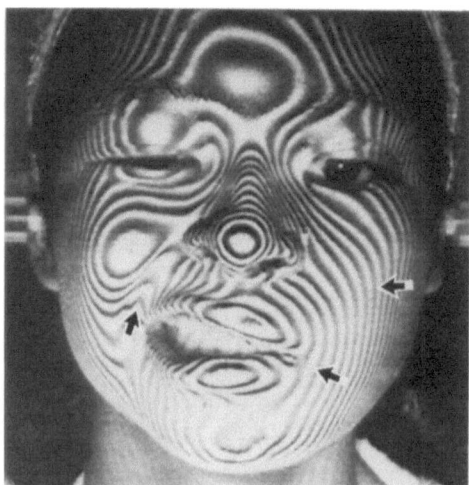

Fig. 5 Grinning. Moiré strip running through cheek and mental point becomes flat. Winding pattern of moiré strips by nasolabial groove is less on palsy side. Winding pattern of moiré strips around mouth angle does not appear on palsy side

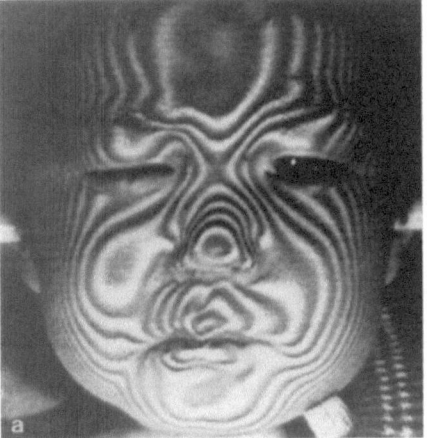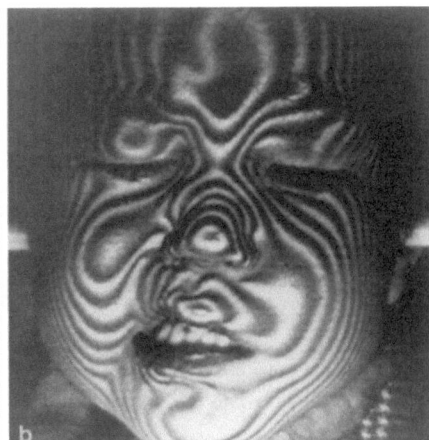

Fig. 6 a, b Infant at rest (**a**) and crying (**b**)

We calculted the asymmetry index (AI) as follows: on these photographs, we considered the line down through the center of the bilateral canthus (medial angles of eye) and the subnasal point as the median line. We then established seven reference lines, each perpendicular to the median line, through through measuring points; glabellar superior, infraorbital, nasal tip, subnasal, superior labial, inferior labial, and mental point. Bilateral symmetry indices were compared and measured as grades of facial palsy at these measurig points. The AI were expressed as the average percentage of the value; it was calculated by dividing the smaller difference in distance up to the two right and left cross-points, i.e. reference line and moiré strip of same level, by the bigger one. Total AI were expressed as the average AI of these items. To measure and calculate the AI, we used a personal computer PC9801 and digitizer KD4300.

Result

The following characteristic patterns of moiré strips are observed:

1. Remarkable asymmetry of strips on forehead were noted.
2. No winding pattern of moiré strips was formed by wrinkling the forehead on the palsy side.
3. Moiré strips overlying the superior eyelid were at different heights.
4. Moiré strips running through the cheek and mental point became flat.

5. The interval between moiré strips between the subnasal point and lower lip became wide.
6. The winding pattern at the nasolabial groove was less pronounced on the palsy side.
7. The winding pattern around the mouth angle was not present on the palsy side.

The patterns noted above disappeared gradually as the paralysis recovered. Comparing the score method to the AI method, cases of severe paralysis judged by a three-stage grading system such as May's or Yanagihara's method had a 20%–25% AI, cases of partial paralysis had 12%–19%, nearly normal cases had 5%–10% and normal cases had an AI of less than 5%. Patients who had the same score differed in the AI.

Discussion

Because the site and grade of palsy was obviously expressed from patterns of moiré strips as a visual image and the AI as a value, objective and well-reproducible assessment of the recovery process could be made without a practiced doctor; it was also very useful in explaining the palsy to patients. Using five moiré photographs obtained while wrinkling the forehead, closing eyes lightly, blowing out the cheeks, grinning, and at rest, we can readily visualize the extent of paralysis and notice any change in characteristic moiré strip patterns. The difference between right and left AI was more marked for severe paralysis and partial paralysis. Of course, cases with improved points in other visual assessment showed obvious changes in moiré patterns and marked improvement in the AI. In cases with an unchanged score in which the patient and the doctor nevertheless felt that a improved ment had taken place, information from the moiré method expressed a change for better.

In this study, we determined the characteristic moiré strip patterns and measured the difference between the right and left sides at seven points to provide a simple approach.

Conclusions

The score method is widely accepted as a simple and useful examination for roughly evaluating the degree of facial palsy; however, it is limited in its objectivity and reproducibility.

The moiré method is much better than other visual methods in providing a quantitative and objective evaluation of facial palsy.

References

1. Takasaki H (1970) Moiré topography. Appl Optics 9 : 1467 – 1472
2. Inokuchi I, Kawakami S, Maeta M, Masuda Y (1991) Evaluation of facial palsy by moiré topography. Proc Holography Interferometry Optical Pattern Recognition Biomed SPIE 1429 : 39 – 45
3. Maeta M, Inokuchi I, Kawakami S, Kinosita S, Masuda Y (1991) Evaluation of facial palsy by pattern of moiré strips. Facial nerve Res Jpn 11 : 199 – 202
4. Inokuchi I, Kawakami S, Maeta M, Yorizane S, Masuda Y (1991) Evaluation of facial palsy in infants by moiré topography. Facial Nerve Res Jpn 11 : 203 – 206
5. Inokuchi I (1992) Quantitative assessment of facial palsy by moiré topography. J Otolaryngol Jpn 95 : 715 – 725

Eur Arch Otorhinolaryngology (1994) [Suppl]: S 545

E. Berrut-Marechaud, M. R. Magistris, and R. Häusler

Bell's Palsy: Steroid Therapy in Chosen Cases?

The usefulness of steroids in the treatment of Bell's palsy remains controversial. We evaluated retrospectively 112 patients who presented with Bell's palsy, 64 treated with prednisone (800 mg in 20 dayd) and 48 with vitamins. The two groups were homogeneous accordign to age, sex, degree of palsy, and type of nerve lesion as assessed by electroneuromyography. Of the 112 patients, 15% had mostly neurapraxia, 30% mostly axonotmesis, and 55% had both. Altogether, recovery was good in 68%, fair in 24%, and poor in 8%. In the case of neurapraxia and patients with both types of lesions, steroids did not appear to improve recovery (good in 80% with prednisone, 76% with vitamins), while in axonotmesis they do seem to influence the outcome (good in 68% with prednisone, 29% with vitamins).

We conclude that steroids may be useful in Bell's palsy with marked axonotmesis. As electroneuromyography allows such patients to be identified around 7 days after onset of symptoms, we suggest that in each case steroids should be started, with the possibility of stopping them if neurapraxia appears to dominate.

E. Berrut-Marechaud and M. R. Magistris
Division of Clinical Neurophysiology, University Hospital, Geneva, Switzerland

R. Häusler
University Clinic of ENT, Head and Neck Surgery, Bern, Switzerland

Eur Arch Otorhinolaryngology (1994) [Suppl]:S546

ABSTRACTS

S. Hashimoto, M. Toshima, S. Koike, M. Ishigaki, and T. Takasaka

Result of High-Dose Steroid Therapy (Stennert) in Facial Palsy

Since 1988, more than 100 patients have been treated in our clinic by high dose steroid therapy, which was first introduced by Stennert in 1979. We have slightly modified the method from the original. The initial dose of prednisolone is 200 mg/day in adults and 2 mg/kg per day in children. Hydroxyethyl starch instead of dextran 40 is used in order to reduce liver dysfunction. In patients with Ramsay-Hunt syndrome, acyclovir is used for 5 days. The cure rate is 94% and most patients showed complete recovery within 8 weeks. Ten patients showed denervation in NET before or during the treatment bur five patients among them recovered completely. All children recovered completely and more quickly than adults. No severe side effects were observed during the treatment. Liver dysfunction was often observed but recovered quickly after the treatment.

S. Hashimoto, M. Toshima, S. Koike, M. Ishigaki, and T. Takasaka
Department of Otolaryngology, Tohoku University School
of Medicine, Sendai 980, Japan

Eur Arch Otorhinolaryngology (1994) [Suppl]: S 547

ABSTRACTS

E. Peitersen

Natural History of Bell's Palsy

The aim of this Copenhagen facial nerve study is to explain the spontaneous course of the idiopathic facial nerve palsy without any kind of treatment. Today Bell's palsy is the accepted term for specifying an acute monosymptomatic peripheral facial palsy of unknown etiology. Acute unilateral, and idiopathic without involvement of other peripheral nerves are specific requirements for the diagnosis.

The material included 1701 patients seen during a 25-year period. At the first consultation a standard ENT examination was performed including a thorough description of the grade and localization of the pareses. Furthermore taste, stapes reflex, and lacrimation tests together with acoustic-vestibular examinations were made. After 1 year the checks were discontinued. If the slightest suspicion of any systemic disease occurred relevant investigations were made to verify these conditions.

The first examination revealed 30% with incomplete pareses while the remaining 70% were complete. The initial examination of taste, stapes reflex, and lacrimation showed reduced or abolished function in 83%, 72%, and 11%, respectively. The spontaneous course showed that all patients' muscular function recovered and I cannot stress too strongly that none of the 1701 patients without treatment remained totally paretic; 85% got the function back within 3 weeks. The remaining 15% obtained function between 3 and 5 months after the onset of the palsy. Seventy percent recovered normal mimimal function of the face, and 12% had insignificant sequelae. The last 18% had permanently more or less diminished function with contracture and associated movements. Normal function for taste, stapes reflex, and lacrimation was obtained in 80%, 86%, and 97%, respectively.

E. Peitersen
Department of ENT, University of Copenhagen,
Hvidovre Hospital 2650 Hvidovre, Denmark

The Facial Nerve Nucleus

Eur Arch Otorhinolaryngology (1994) [Suppl]: S551 – S554

G. Lamas, S. Poignonec, I. Fligny, J. Soudant, and J.C. Willer

Central and Peripheral Rearrangements Following Hypoglossal-Facial Crossover: An Electrophysiological Study

Introduction

Hypoglossal facial crossover is the most common procedure performed to rehabilitate a paralysed face, when the trunk of the facial nerve is not available for end-to-end anastomosis. This technique always gives at least a symmetrical face at rest. Independent movements allowing smiling and closing of the eye could be the best end result. This present work was performed to study the central and peripheral arrangements, following a hypoglossal-facial crossover. The peripheral changes were studied with classical electromyography. The central changes were studied with the Blink reflex. In this way we demonstrated the presence of central connections between the trigeminal and hypoglossal nuclei.

Patients and Methods

Patients

Eight patients with hypoglossal-facial crossover were included in this series. The facial palsy was secondary to surgery (acoustic neuroma, seven cases; cholesteatoma of the petrous bone, one case). In seven cases, the facial nerve was sacrificed during surgery. Surgical repair was performed as soon as possible according to the postoperative status (from day 7 to day 90; mean, 27.6 days). In one case, the facial nerve was anatomically intact but was still not functional after 15 months. In all cases, a XII – VII crossover was proposed to the patient [5]. Except in two cases with a poor result, though symmetry was good at rest, the

Table 1 Main clinical findings

No. patients	Sex	Age (years)	Delay of crossover (days)	Delay of study (months)	Synkinesis	Facial spasm
1	F	47	7	14	0	+/–
2	F	44	18	21	+	+/–
3	F	57	20	52	+	+/–
4	M	53	21	55	–	+/–
5	M	50	90	15	+	+
6	F	60	10	24	+	+
7	M	69	27	12	0	+
8	M	58	455	45	+	+

G. Lamas, S. Poignonec, I. Fligny, and J. Soudant
Department of ENT, Hopital de la Pitié Salpétrière, Paris, France

J.C. Willer
Department of Neurophysiology, Hopital de la Pitié Salpétrière, Paris, France

postoperative results showed a good functional improvement. The main clinical findings concerning the patients are shown in Table 1. The first signs of regeneration appeared at 4 months, with good improvement of the facial tone giving facial symmetry. Follow-up was always longer than 12 months. The following points were noted: a symmetrical face at rest with marked contraction in two cases (Nos. 5 and 7), reasonable eye closure except in two cases (Nos. 5 and 7), and synkinesia except in one case (No. 1), especially while swallowing and moving the tongue.

Methods

We studied all our cases in two ways: first, a classical electrophysiological investigation was done and the blink reflex test was performed. During the first session, classical routine electrophysiological investigations were done to assess the peripheral function of the XII–VII crossover (on the operated side) were stimulated in the pretragal region with two surface electrodes, the cathode being distal. The electrical stimulus was a 0.2-ms rectangular shock delivered at a rate of 0.5 Hz by a constant current stimulator. The direct motor responses were recorded with the surface bipolar electrodes successively applied on the orbicularis oculi, orbicularis ori, and mentalis muscles on normal and operated sides. For the motor response of each muscle previously mentioned were studied: the threshold (mA), maximum amplitude from spike to spike (mV), and latency (ms) measured from the stimulus to the first deflection of the baseline. The blink or trigeminal-facial reflex was recorded during the second session. The method used has been well described elsewhere [1, 8]. The supraorbital nerve was stimulated through the skin with two needle electrodes. As previously describe, the stimulus was a 0.2-ms rectangular shock delivered at a rate of 0.15 Hz by constant current stimulation. The reflex responses were recorded with surface electrodes on a cleaned skin overlying the orbicularis oculi muscle. In this way the dif-

ferent characteristics (threshold, latency, amplitude) were studied for the reflex responses on the right and the left side, following stimulation of the right and left supraorbital nerve.

Results

Results of the Peripheral Investigation

We studied and compared the electrophysiological characteristics (latency, threshold, amplitude) of the direct motor responses of the facial muscles during stimulation of the normal facial nerve on the normal side and the XII–VII nerve anastomosis on the operated side. The results are summarized in Table 2. On the normal side the latencies and amplitudes were identical for the three muscles (orbicularis oculi, orbicularis ori, and mentalis), but on the operated side the three parameters were slightly different according to the muscle explored. In the orbicularis oculi, the latency was shorter than in the other muscles but its threshold was higher and its amplitude lower. On the other hand, in the mentalis the latency was longer but the threshold lower and the amplitude uppermost. The values recorded for the orbicularis ori were mid way. These electrophysiological results show that the mentalis seems to be the first muscle to recover its physiological function. This was confirmed by unitary investigations of facial muscles by means of a needle electrode successively inserted into the three muscular groups. Therefore reinnervation seems to occur according to a decreasing gradient from the mentalis to the orbicularis oculi.

Results of the Central Study

As for the direct motor response, the elementary electrophysiological characteristics (latency, threshold, and amplitude) were studied for each component of the blink reflex. Electrical stimulation of the supraorbital nerve on the normal side was consistent with a classical reflex re-

Table 2 Summary of results

	Normal side			Operated side		
	Latency (ms)	Threshold (mA)	Amplitude (mV)	Latency (ms)	Threshold (mA)	Amplitude (mV)
Orbicularis oculi	3.29 +/- 0.38	1.8 +/- 0.19	4.19 0.88	4.50 +/- 0.83	4.9 +/- 0.56	0.59 +/- 0.47
Orbicularis ori	3.71 +/- 0.28	1.73 +/- 0.25	4.25 +/- 0.9	5.18 +/- 1.4	4.66 +/- 0.9	0.93 +/- 1.26
Orbicularis mentalis	3.71 +/- 0.36	1.75 +/- 0.21	4.63 +/- 0.87	6.33 +/- 1.24	3.65 +/- 0.61	2.66 +/- 1.96

Table 3 Parameter individual and mean values

Patients	Normal side			Operated side		
	Latency (ms)	Threshold (mA)	Amplitude (mV)	Latency (ms)	Threshold (mA)	Amplitude (mV)
1	10.70	2.00	1.25	14.50	5.50	0.15
2	11.20	1.80	2.80	13.90	5.90	0.20
3	10.70	2.10	1.60	12.30	6.00	0.15
4	11.00	2.00	1.80	13.00	5.30	0.16
5	10.40	2.10	1.00	No reflex response		
6	10.10	1.60	1.30	10.10	5.50	0.50
7	11.60	1.50	0.90	No reflex response		
8	10.60	1.60	1.10	11.30	6.70	0.15
Mean ± SEM	10.79 ± 0.16	1.84 ± 0.08	1.46 ± 0.20	12.52 ± 0.61	5.82 ± 0.19	0.22 ± 0.05

sponse with two components R1 and R2 in the ispilateral orbicularis oculi. It is important to note that stimulation of the supraorbital nerve on the normal side produced no reflex response in the orbicularis oculi on the opposite side (operated side). Electrical stimulation of the supraorbital nerve on the operated side produced an R1-type response in six out of eight cases. In comparison to the homologous response with the normal side, this R1 response had a significantly lower latency, a much higher threshold, and a lower amplitude. The individual and mean values for these parameters are shown in Table 3. In only one patient (case No. 1) was an R2-type response (latency = 65 ms, threshold, 6 mA, amplitude = 0.4. mV) observed during stimulation of the supraorbital nerve on the operated side. On the other hand, such a stimulation also produced a contralateral R2 response on the healthy side in all patients. The electrophysiological characteristics of this cross R2 response were identical to the R2 response.

Discussion

This electrophysiological study shows that two important groups of results are noted following a XII–VII nerve anastomosis.

Peripheral Nervous Changes Produced by the XII–VII Nerve Anastomosis

We showed that stimulation of the tragal region gives different motor responses according to the recorded muscle. In the orbicularis oculi the response latency was shorter but the threshold higher and the amplitude lower. In the mentalis, the threshold was lower, the amplitude the highest, and the latency the longest. We recorded intermeditae values in the orbicularis ori. High-amplitude and low-threshold responses corresponded to a good motor recovery. Axonal regeneration and muscular reinnervation proceeded differently, better in the lower facial area, less

marked in the upper area. With regard to the axonal regeneration the mulitplication of Schwann cells and the grwth of Bungner bands occurred preferentially in the inferior fibers going to the inferior facial territory. Certain trophic factors (NGF or BDNF) might be preferentially produced in the inferior territory.

Central Nervous Changes Produced by the XII–VII Nerve Anastomosis

In normal subjects and on the normal side in our eight patients, electrical stimulation of the supraorbital nerve caused a reflex response with two components, R1 early (around 11 ms) ipsilateral to the stimulus and R2 late (around 34 ms) bilateral related eye closure [4]. On the operated side in six out of the eight patients, an R1 response was recorded in the orbicularis oculi when the ipsilateral supraorbital nerve was stimulated. This is surprising because there is no anatomical connection between the trigeminal cutaneous afferents and the motoneurons of the hypoglossal nerve. Therefore a synaptic rearrangement would take place. It is tempting to suggest that the CII nerve motoneurons were sending messages upward to the trigeminal afferents following their peripheral information about their new end course. This would produce a heterotopic reafference with a subsequent functional recovery in the reflex pathway. This observation is most interesting because this rearrangement is secondary to a lesion on the efferent fibers [6, 7].

References

1. Boulou PH, Willer JC, Cambier J (1981) Analyse electrophysiologique du réflexe de clignement chez l'homme. Rev Neurol (Paris) 137 (8/9): 523–533
2. Carpenter MB, Sutin J (1983) Human neuroanatomy. Williams and Wilkins, Baltimore
3. Kimura J (1973) The blink reflex as a test for brain stem and higher central nervous function. In: Desmedt JE (ed) New devel-

opments in electromyography and clinical neurophysiology, vol 3. Karger, Basel, pp 682–691

4. Kugelberg E (1952) Facial reflexes. Brain 75:385–396
5. May M (1986) The facial nerve. Thieme, New York
6. Polistina DC, Murray M, Goldberger ME (1990) Plasticity of the dorsal root and descending serotoninergic projections after partial deafferentation of the adult rat spinal cord. J Comp Neurol 299:349–363

7. Raisman G (1985) Synapse formation in the septal nuclei of adult rats. In: Cotman CE (ed) Synaptic plasticity. Guilford, New York, pp 13–38
8. Willer JC, Lamour Y (1977) Electrophysiological evidence for a facio-facial reflex in the facial muscles in man. Brain Res 119:459–464

Eur Arch Otorhinolaryngology (1994) [Suppl]: S 555 – S 556

G. Lamas, S. Poignonec, I. Fligny, J. Soudant, and J.-C. Willer

Recovery of Normal Excitability of the Facial Motor Nucleus Following Facial Nerve Decompression in Hemifacial Spasm

In a previous study it was shown that a central and widespread hyperexcitability of the facial motor nucleus was a common feature of the affected side of patients with hemifacial spasm (HFS). It was thus concluded that the patients' abnormal reactions would depend on the existence or not of a background activity in the facial motoneurons. This background activity would be increased in HFS by a permanent neuronal antidromic excitation originating from the ectopic focus and ephaptic transmission on the facial nerve itself. These data raise the following question: what happens to the facial motoneuron hyperexcitability when the ectopic ephaptic excitation of the facial nerve has been removed?

Thus, the aim of the present work was to test the functional relieving effect of facial nerve decompression on the central hyperexcitability of facial motoneurons demonstrated in a patient (the first of this series) affected with left HFS. The patient was a 65-year-old man, treated and stabilized by regular insulin injections with no neurological or traumatic past history. In February 1991, when emerging from a hypoglycemic coma due to an intercurrent infection, the patient developed left HFS within 2 – 3 h for no apprent and obvious reason. Clinical examinations showed typical left HFS with a major hypertonia affecting all left facial muscles associated with watering of the left eye while the right side was clinically completely normal. Scan and MRI gadolinium explorations revealed no abnormality.

G. Lamas, S. Poignonec, I. Fligny, and J. Soudant
Department of ENT, Groupe Hospitalier Pitié-Salpêtrière, 75013 Paris, France

J.C. Willer
Lab. Neurophysiology, Groupe Hospitalier Pitié-Salpêtrière, 75013 Paris, France

In a first set of preoperative experiments, we studied the trigeminofacial reflexes elicited by electrical stimulation of supraorbital nerves on both the right and left side according to a procedure described previously [2, 4]. The study of the blinking reflex in orbicularis oculi muscles showed abnormal crossed R1 components on both right (normal) and left (HFS) sides elicited by contralateral supraorbital nerve stimulation, respectively. Furthermore, on the left side, supraorbital nerve stimulation elicited blink-type R1-R2 reflex responses in the orbicularis oris and mentalis muscles but not on the normal (right) side. We therefore analyzed the facial motoneuronal excitability of the R1 response. For this purpose, as in the companion paper [3], we used a classical double-shock technique fully described elsewhere [5]. Results were unambiguous and showed that in all the facial muscles where an R1 reflex was recorded (left and right orbicularis oculi, left orbicularis oris, and left mentalis muscles) the conditioning stimulus induced an abnormally high facilitatory effect on this R1 component. For example, in the orbicularis oculi muscles, the facilitation was much higher (+150%) than that usually observed in normals. It occurred for a shorter interstimulus interval ($\Delta t = 0$ ms) and remained for a longer delay period ($\Delta t = 100$ ms) than that currently observed in normals ($\Delta t = 30$ ms and 20 ms, respectively).

In March 1991, the patient underwent decompressive surgery of the facial nerve via the left middle fossa approach. At the level of the geniculi ganglion, the nerve was found to be compressed by an inflammatory process of the nerve sheath. This latter was opened along the first and second portion of the nerve as well as at the level of the geniculi ganglion. The day following surgery, clinical investigations revealed that all clinical signs of HFS had totally disappeared and no facial palsy was detected. One month postoperatively, since the patient was still in relief, electrophysiological investigations showed a complete normalization not only on the peripheral aspect of the facial nerve (normal distal latencies and potentials, and amplitudes), but also on facial reflexes. The crossed R1 blink responses were not detectable in orbicularis oculi muscles, along with the abnormal extopic reflex responses in orbicularis oris and mental muscles. The excitability curves of the R1 component of the blink reflex were similar on the left and right side and were comparable to those from normal subjects showing a recovery of normal excitability in the facial motor nucleus. It is concluded that these electrophysiological investigations provide useful sensitive and quantitative tools for careful exploration of patients with HFS.

Acknowledgements This work was supported by INSERM (CRE), AP-HP(CRC 92–93), and by la Fondation pour Recherche Médicale.

References

1. Holstege G, (1990) Neuronal organization of the blink reflex. In: Paxinos G (ed) The human nervous system. Academic, New York, pp 287–296
2. Kugelberg E (1952) Facial reflexes. Brain 75:385–396
3. Poignonec S, Vidailhet M, Lamas G, Fligny I, Soudant J, Jedynak P, Willer JC (1992) Electrophysiological evidence for central hyperexcitability of facial motoneurons in hemifacial spasm. Eur Arch Otol Rhinol Laryngol (submitted)
4. Willer JC, Lamour Y (1977) Electrophysiological evidence for a facio-facial reflex in the facial muscles in man. Brain Res 119:459–464
5. Willer JC, Roby A, Boulu P, Bourau F (1982) Comparative effects of electroacupuncture and transcutaneous nerve stimulation on the human blink reflex. Pain 14:267–278

Eur Arch Otorhinolaryngology (1994) [Suppl]: S 557

POSTERS

O. Guntinas-Lichius, A. Gunkel, E. Stennert, and W. F. Neiss

Astroglial Response in Facial and Hypoglossal Nucleus After Hypoglossal-Facial Anastomosis in the Rat

Introduction

Following axotomy of a peripheral motor nerve, within 24 h glial fibrillary acidic protein (GFAP) immunoreactive astrocytes are activated in the nucleus of origin. Astrocytic processes are interposed between the axotomized neurons and presynaptic terminals. This reaction is thought to protect the neurons during repair. We investigated the astroglial response in the facial and hypoglossal nucleus after hypoglossal-facial anastomosis (HFA) in comparison to facial-facial and hypoglossal-hypoglossal anastomosis and resection of the nerves.

Material and Methods

In 213 rats either a HFA was performed microsurgically (regeneration of the hypoglossal nucleus with change of function and degeneration of the facial nucleus) or a facial-facial or hypoglossal-hypoglossal anastomosis (regeneration of the respective nucleus) or both nerves were transected and 10 mm of the distal portion removed (degeneration of both nuclei). Four to 112 days after the operation (dpo) all rats wre fixed by perfusion and the GFAP reactivity was evaluated in 6-μm paraffin sections using a polyclonal antibody against GFAP.

Results

Four days after HFA some GFAP-positive astrocytes were seen in the hypoglossal nucleus. The GFAP immunoreactivity had slightly increased at 7 dpo, reached its maximum at 14 dpo, decreased at 28 and 42 dpo, and had disappeared at 56 dpo.

The GFAP reactivity was stronger in the facial nucleus after HFA as well as after resection of the peripheral nerves than in the hypoglossal nucleus: many GFAP-positive astrocytes were already observed at 7 dpo, the reaction intensity had further increased at 14 dpo and reached its maximum at 28 dpo. Up to 56 dpo a distinct GFAP reactivity was seen; at 112 dpo the reaction had disappeared.

Following facial-facial or hypoglossal-hypoglossal anastomosis, GFAP was less expressed in the regenerating nucleus than in the hypoglossal nucleus after HFA: after these single anastomoses GFAP was notably increased at 4 dpo, reached its maximum at 7 dpo, and had almost disappeared at 42 dpo.

Conclusion

The astrocytic reaction increased *and* decreased faster during regeneraton than during degeneration. The reaction appeared less intense in the regenerating nucleus after hypoglossal-facial anastomosis than after facial-facial or hypoglossal-hypoglossal anastomosis. The highest GFAP reactivity occured during degeneration after resection of the peripheral nerves.

Acknowledgement This work was supported by the Deutsche Forschungsgemeinschaft (Ne 412/1-1).

O. Guntinas-Lichius, A. Gunkel, E. Stennert, and W. F. Neiss
Department I for Anatomy and Department of Otolaryngology, University of Cologne, Joseph-Stelzmann-Str. 9, 50924 Cologne, Germany

Eur Arch Otorhinolaryngology (1994) [Suppl]:S 558

POSTERS

O. Guntinas-Lichius, A. Gunkel, E. Stennert, and W.F. Neiss

Synaptic Stripping in Facial and Hypoglossal Nucleus after Hypoglossal-Facial Anastomosis in the Rat

Introduction

Axonal transection causes a separation (stripping) of intact synaptic terminals from the perikarya of axotomized neurons in the facial and hypoglossal nucleus by activated microglia. During regeneration, this displacement of boutons is reversed. We investigated synaptic stripping in the facial and hypoglossal nucleus after hypoglossal-facial anastomosis (HFA) in comparison to facial-facial and hypoglossal-hypoglossal anastomosis and the resection of both nerves.

Material and Methods

In 213 rats either a HFA was performed microsurgically (regeneration of the hypoglossal nucleus with change of function and degeneration of the facial nucleus) or facial-facial or hypoglossal-hypoglossal anastomosis (regeneration of respective nucleus) or both nervs were transected and 10 mm of the distal portion removed (degeneration of both nuclei). Four to 112 days after the operation (dpo) all rats were fixed by perfusion and the presynaptic boutons were stained in 6-μm paraffin sections by a monoclonal antibody against synaptophysin (an integral membrane protein of synaptic vesicles).

Results

After HFA and to a greater extent after hypoglossal-hypoglossal anastomosis, synaptic stripping occurred in the hypoglossal nucleus within 7 dpo and remained constant up to 14 dpo. Rebuilding started at 28 dpo and finished at 56 dpo. At no time wre motoneurons with complete loss of axosomatic terminals observed.

In the facial nucleus, HFA or resection of the peripheral nerves caused nearly complete synaptic stripping within 7 dpo and almost no axosomatic treminals were present from 14 to 42 dpo. Rebuilding started at 56 dpo and was still incomplete at 112 dpo.

From 7 to 28 days after facial-facial anastomosis, facial motoneurons were observed that completely lacked axosomatic synapses.

Conclusion

Synaptic stripping was more intense during degeneration after resection than during regeneration after nerve anastomosis, but it was reversible in both conditions. Hypoglossal-facial anastomosis caused less stripping and faster restoration of axosomatic synapses in the hypoglossal nucleus than hypoglossal-hypoglossal anastomosis. Facial-facial anastomosis caused the facial nucleus to react in a slightly different way.

Acknowledgement This work was supported by the Deutsche Forschungsgemeinschaft (Ne 412/1-1).

O. Guntinas-Lichius, A. Gunkel, E. Stennert, and W.F. Neiss
Department I for Anatomy and Department of Otolaryngology,
University of Cologne, Joseph-Stelzmann-Str. 9,
50924 Cologne, Germany

Eur Arch Otorhinolaryngology (1994) [Suppl]: S 559

POSTERS

W. F. Neiss, E. Schulte, O. Guntinas-Lichius, A. Gunkel, and E. Stennert

Response of Nissl Substance in the Facial and Hypoglossal Nucleus After Hypoglossal-Facial Anastomosis in the Rat*

After axotomy of a peripheral motor nerve, structural alterations of Nissl's substance in the neuron are observed. This reaction – classically termed chromatolysis – is considered as a response to the changed metabolism of the injured neuron; its regeneration seems to cause restoration of Nissl's substance. We performed a quantitative investigation of Nissl's substance in the facial and hypoglossal nucleus after hypoglossal-facial anastomosis (HFA) in comparison to facial-facial (FFA), hypoglossal-hypoglossal (HHA) anastomosis, and resection of the nerves.

Material and Methods

In 213 rats either an HFA was performed microsurgically (regeneration of the hypoglossal nucleus with change of function and degeneration of the facial nucleus) or a facial-facial or hypoglossal-hypoglossal anastomosis (regeneration of the respective nucleus) or both nerves were transected and 10 mm of the distal portion removed (degeneration of both nuclei). Four to 112 days postoperation (dpo) all rats were fixed by perfusion and the entropy (E) of Nissl's substance was evaluated in 6-μm paraffin sections using a VIDAS image analyzer (Kontron, FRG).

Results

Transection of the nerve leads to an increase of E in the corresponding nucleus and – to a smaller degree – in the contralateral nucleus; whereby maximum entropy is reached 56 dpo. The second pair of nuclei remains unaffected. Restoration of Nissl's substance with decrease of entropy is observed after HHA and HFA, the latter yielding in slower restoration. In both cases contralateral hypoglossal nuclei show an increase and decrease of E, thus paralleling the reaction in the operated nucleus. Increase of E is less pronounced in the contralateral nucleus. For both sides E is not restored to normal values after 112 dpo.

Conclusions

The alteration of Nissl's substance indicates neuronal damage and neuronal repair after transection and anastomosis of motor nerves. The corresponding contralateral nuclei show a coreaction. The entropy of Nissl's substance is a highly sensitive structural parameter with great discriminative power for differentiation between neurons by means of high-resolution image analysis.

W. F. Neiss and O. Guntinas-Lichius
Department I for Anatomy, University of Cologne,
Cologne, Germany

A. Gunkel and E. Stennert
Department of Otolaryngology, University of Cologne,
Cologne, Germany

E. Schulte
Anatomische Anstalt der Universität München, Munich, Germany

* Supported by the Deutsche Forschungsgemeinschaft (Ne 412/1-1) and by Kontron Elektronik GmbH, Eching, Germany.

Eur Arch Otorhinolaryngology (1994) [Suppl]: S 560

D. Lopez Aguado, B. Perez, J. Rivero, M.-E. Campos, R. Gutierrez, and L. Diaz-Flores

New "Perineurial Cells" in the Compartmentation
of the Regenerated Nerves

After transection of the nerve trunk resulting in scarring, numerous axonal sprouts arise from both the tips of the axon and the proximal nodes of Ranvier. A compartmentation of groups of the sprouting axons occurs with formation of many miniature fascicles. The origin of the new cells which surround the groups of the axons is not clear. Among the possible cellular sources are the endoneurial fibroblasts, Schwann cells, and perineurial cells. In the present work, a segment of the epineurium and underlying perineurium of the rat facial nerve was removed (n, 20). The histologic characteristics of the newly formed cover and the subjacent tissue were studied 3, 5, 7, and 15 days after surgery and proliferation of the remaining perineurial cells was observed. The present study suggests that performed perineurial cells, together with Schwann cells and endoneurial cells, grow during nerve regeneration. The former contribute to the origin of the new cover of the groups of axon. By means of this procedure, numerous miniature fascicles are created and the normal endoneurial environment is restored.

D. Lopez Aguado, B. Perez, J. Rivero, M.-E. Campos, R. Gutierrez, and L. Diaz-Flores
Catedra de ORL, Facultad de Medicina, Ofra, La Laguna, Tenerife, Spain

Eur Arch Otorhinolaryngology (1994) [Suppl]: S 561

ABSTRACTS

R. Pallini, E. Fernandez, L. Lauretti, and E. Marchese

Somatotopic Changes of the Stylohyoid Muscle Subnucleus After Section and Repair of the Facial Nerve

Peripheral nerve injury induces a series of changes along the circuit levels of the involved nerve, from the cortex to the periphery. Functional regeneration should be influenced by these changes. In the present work, the rat facial nerve was sectioned and repaired at the stylomastoid foramen. From 3 to 21 monts after surgery, the somatotopic rearrangement of the motor facial nucleus was studied. Horseradish peroxidase (HRP) was injected in the isolated stylohyoid muscle to retrogradely label the parent motoneuron pool in the brain stem. The most important findings can be summarized as follows: (1) the volume of the subnucleus was markedly increased after regeneration because of the more dispersed motoneuron pattern as compared to the intact controls; (2) more than 80% of the HRP-labeled motoneurons were located outside the borders of the control stylohyoid subnucleus overlying the other subnucleus either in the main nucleus of the facial nerve and dorsally to the main nucleus or outside the borders of the accessory nucleus of the facial nerve; (3) the stylohyoid muscle subnucleus showed a bilateral somatotopic representation in 50% of the operated animals because of HRP-labeled motoneurons in the contralateral facial nerve nucleus; (4) the number of HRP-labeled motoneurons was increased twofold with respect to the intact controls; (5) the mean soma diameter of motoneurons was similar in both the operated and intact control rats. This study provides original information on the plastic changes which occur in the stylohyoid muscle subuclecus following regeneration of the facial nerve. These data provide the basis for comparative anatomofunctional studies.

R. Pallini, E. Fernandez, L. Lauretti, and E. Marchese
Department of Neurosurgery, Catholic University, Rome, Italy

Eur Arch Otorhinolaryngology (1994) [Suppl]: S 562

ABSTRACTS

R. Laskawi and J.R. Wolff

Axotomy of the Facial Nerve Not Only Induces Changes in the Facial Nucleus But Also in Remotely Related Brain Regions

It is well established that following lesion of the rats facial nerve, changes are found in its nuclear region involving motoneurons, their afferent synapses, microglia, and astroglia. Functional changes in remote brain regions such as the motor cortex have been reported shortly after lesion of a peripheral motor nerve (Sanes et al. 1988). Mechanisms involved are not yet well known. Such possible mechanisms might be important for comprehension of facial dyskinesias (hemifacial spasm, blepharospasm, synkinesis). In the present study we transected the right facial nerve in adult rats. To demonstrate reactions of glial and neuronal structures, we studied immunohistochemical changes in S100-protein glial fibrillary acidic protein (GFAP), and phosphorylated and nonphosphorylated neurofilaments in various brain regions and after various survival times. Following facial nerve lesion we not only found changes in the facial nucleus but also in remotely related brain regions, especially in the neocortex. These include quickly appearing side differences in the accumulation of glial markers (S100, GFAP). Preliminary results also show that cortical reactions of facial nerve lesions can be modified by previous lesion of the trigeminal nerve, and that it is possible that side differences also occur after blocking the neuromuscular junction by botulinum toxin.

R. Laskawi and J.R. Wolff
Department of ENT, Department of Anatomy,
Universität of Göttingen, 37075 Göttingen, Germany

Eur Arch Otorhinolaryngology (1994) [Suppl]:S563

POSTERS

R. S. van Gelder, B. G. E. S. Bernard, P. G. Heymans, and M. Wiggers

Peripheral Facial Paralysis:
Evaluation of Effects in a Case-study

In our laboratory we had the, unique, opportunity to study a 40-year old male patient who, on his own initiative, made contact with the laboratory prior to being operated upon for a tumour in the ear. This operation unfortunately led to partial damage to the right facial nerve, resulting in paralytic phenomena on the right side of the face. A facial paralysis is characterised by clear asymmetry between the two sides of the face, both during rest and during movement. A facial paralysis can also give rise to psychological and social problems.

Method

The patient was followed for a period of approximately two years during which the process of spontaneous remission of facial function as well as myofeedback facial muscle training took place.

Video-recordings and EMG-registrations of the process of spontaneous remission were made as discussed in Wiggers et al. (1987) [3]. Wiggers et al. used the Facial Action Coding System (Ekman and Friesen 1978), an observational method, and an Electromyography based approach. Both methods can be used to describe changes over time. However, Electromyography appears to be more useful to detect low levels of asymmetry which are not yet visible and therefore not measurable with the Facial Action Coding System. On the other hand, in some cases the latter

R. S. van Gelder (✉)
Schoolstraat 41, 1111 BP Diemen, The Netherlands

B. G. E. S. Bernard
Bergkristal 14, 6922 NP Duiven, The Netherlands

P. G. Heymans
Department of Developmental Psychology, Rijksuniversiteit Utrecht, Heidelberglaan 2, De Uithof, 3584 CS Utrecht, The Netherlands

M. Wiggers
Hazenkampseweg 135, 6531 NE Nijmegen, The Netherlands

system appeared to offer a more reliable criterion than Electromyography for the assessment of visible asymmetry.

To be discussed here are the photographs and psychological assessments made at the following points in time:

1. Before operation
(Operation)
2. After operation – 2 months
3. After operation – 4 months
4. After operation – 10 months
5. After operation – 14 months
6. After operation – 20 months
7. After operation – 21 months
(Start of Myofeedback)
8. After 1 week
9. After 2 weeks
(End of Myofeedback)
10. After treatment – 1 month

Evaluation-methods

A. Measurements were made directly from the photographs of the asymmetries in facial expression, as outlined in: van Gelder et al. (1990) [1].

B. A questionnaire evaluating subjectively experienced feelings of "well-being", derived from Luteijn's (1974) NPV, measured:

– level of self-confidence;
– satisfaction in social interaction.

Details are described in van Gelder et al. (1984) [2].

Results

A. Measurements of asymmetries were shown to be reliably executed. The results will be presented for three facial expressions:

1. measurement of eye-brow asymmetry during raising of the eyebrows,
2. measurement of eye-lid asymmetry and mouth-corner asymmetry during closing of the eye-lids, and
3. measurement of mouth-corner asymmetry and eye-lid asymmetry during "smiling".

General comments on resulting asymmetries in *intended* movements on the following moments:

After operation: strong increase of asymmetry due to paralysis.
Before treatment: at first decrease, later increase presumably partly due to reinnervation, partly to forming of connective tissue on the damaged side (i.e. contracture).
After treatment: no systematic effects.

General comments on resulting asymmetries in *unintended* movements on the following (same) moments:

After operation: no systematic effects.
Before treatment: at first decrease, later increase of asymmetry; for mouthcorner asymmetry during eyeclosure this increase may be due to prolonged reinnervation on the damaged side causing pathological synkinesis; for eyelid asymmetry during smiling this increase may be due to a stronger action of the eyelids on the healthy side (normal synkinesis).
After treatment: no systematic effects.

B: The (reliable) questionnaire consisted of two scales: the IN-adequacy scale, measuring level of self-confidence and the S(ocial) I(nadequacy) scale measuring satisfaction in social interaction.

General comments:
The patient did not appear to lack in self-confidence or to feel inadequate in social interaction situations. Quite the contrary, he felt even better on both scales than the average healthy subject.

Conclusions

By means of photography in a single case-study it was possible to detect fair instabilities in asymmetry during facial movements two years after incidence of a peripheral facial paralysis, even after intervention with myofeedback. Causes for these instabilities are not yet clear and need to be researched.

Psycho-social problems, often seen with peripheral facial paralysis, could not be demonstrated in this patient. This may be due to the fact that this subject was not, as indicated by his strong motivation to collaborate in this project, a typical example of the patient-population.

References

1. Van Gelder RS, Philippart SMM, Bernard BGES, Devriese PP, Whiting HTA, van Wieringen PCW (1990) Effects of myofeedback and mimetherapy on peripheral facial paralysis. International Journal of Psychology 25:191–211
2. Van Gelder RS, Zegers JG, van Wieringen PCW, Devriese PP, Whiting HTA, Bronk J, Kobus MH (1984) Psycho-social effects of mimetherapy in the rehabilitation of patients with a peripheral facial paralysis. Paper presented at the 6th International Congress of Psychomotricity, June 1984, The Hague
3. Wiggers M, van Gelder RS, Heymans PG (1987) The evaluation of facial paralysis: a case study using the Facial Action Coding System and Electromyography. Journal of Clinical and Experimental Neuropsychology 9:278–279

Subject Index

Authors Index